VOLUME TWO

Stereoscopic Atlas of

MACULAR DISEASES

diagnosis and treatment

VOLUME TWO

Stereoscopic Atlas of
MACULAR
DISEASES
diagnosis and treatment

J. DONALD M. GASS, M.D.
Professor of Ophthalmology
Department of Ophthalmology and Visual Sciences
Vanderbilt University
School of Medicine
Nashville, Tennessee

Professor Emeritus
Bascom Palmer Eye Institute
University of Miami
School of Medicine
Miami, Florida

FOURTH EDITION

*with 2866 illustrations
and 124 stereoscopic pairs in full color*

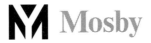

St. Louis Baltimore Boston Carlsbad Chicago Naples New York Philadelphia Portland
London Madrid Mexico City Singapore Sydney Tokyo Toronto Wiesbaden

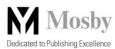
Mosby

Dedicated to Publishing Excellence

A Times Mirror
Company

Publisher: Anne S. Patterson
Senior Editor: Laurel Craven
Developmental Editor: Kimberley Cox
Project Manager: Patricia Tannian
Project Specialist: Ann E. Rogers
Layout Artist: Jeanne Genz
Book Design Manager: Gail Morey Hudson
Manufacturing Supervisor: Karen Lewis

FOURTH EDITION

Copyright © 1997 by Mosby–Year Book, Inc.

Printed in the United States of America
Composition by Graphic World, Inc.
Color separation by Jefferson/Keeler Printing Company
Printing/binding by Maple-Vail Book Mfg Group

Mosby–Year Book, Inc.
11830 Westline Industrial Drive
St. Louis, Missouri 63146

International Standard Book Number 0-8151-3416-9

Gass, J. Donald M. (John Donald M.), 1928-
    Stereoscopic atlas of macular diseases: diagnosis and treatment/
  J. Donald M. Gass. — 4th ed.
      p.   cm.
    Includes bibliographical references and index.
    ISBN 0-8151-3416-9 (set)
      1. Macula lutea — Diseases — Atlases.   I. Title.
    [DNLM: 1. Macula Lutea — pathology — atlases.   WW 17 G251s 1997]
  RE661.M3G37   1997
  617.7′3 — dc20
  DNLM/DLC
  for Library of Congress   96-29166
                                                                       CIP

96 97 98 99 00 / 9 8 7 6 5 4 3 2 1

To
Margy Ann
my high school sweetheart, dear wife,
and best friend.

And to my
colleagues
whose sharing of their patients and
knowledge has made this book possible.

Preface to the Fourth Edition

The enormous expansion of the literature concerning diseases of the ocular fundus has made each revision of this book more difficult. Although the updated text includes more than 6500 citations, I am certain that I have overlooked many important contributions. The organization of this edition is the same as that of previous ones. For the first time printed stereoscopic color photographs rather than reels of stereoscopic color transparencies are used to illustrate disorders of the fundus. A few stereoscopic black and white fluorescein angiograms are illustrated throughout the book. Stereographs may be viewed with the viewer provided or with stereoscopic spectacles or other viewing devices.

New to this edition are discussions and illustrations concerning the following concepts and disorders.

- ▶ The clinical and histopathological features of two distinct types of choroidal neovascularization: type I subretinal pigment epithelial neovascularization and type II subsensory retinal neovascularization, and the importance of recognition of these types in regard to the feasibility of their surgical excision.

- ▶ Update of the pathogenesis and surgical treatment of age-related macular hole.

- ▶ Demonstration of the potential for systemic corticosteroid treatment to cause severe exudative detachment of the retina and pigment epithelium in otherwise healthy patients with idiopathic central serous chorioretinopathy as well as in patients being treated for systemic disease.

- ▶ Clinical and histopathological evidence that retinal arteries, ordinarily not affected in patients with systemic atherosclerosis, may develop focal yellowish atheromata at sites of focal damage to their endothelium, associated with a variety of ocular disorders, including toxoplasmosis retinitis, acute retinal necrosis caused by herpes zoster virus, acquired retinal artery macroaneurysms, idiopathic bilateral acquired recurrent branch retinal artery occlusions, large-cell non-Hodgkin's lymphoma, as well as at sites of impacted arterial emboli.

- ▶ Peculiar fundus changes associated with dominantly inherited Müller cell internal limiting membranous dystrophy, ring 17 chromosome, and benign fleck retina syndromes.

- ▶ Toxic chorioretinopathy associated with use of clofazimine, bleomycin, cisplatinum, and orally ingested silver salts.

- ▶ Intraocular infection with gnathostoma and trematodes, further evidence to implicate cat-scratch bacillus as a cause of focal retinitis and neuroretinitis, and *Ancylostoma caninum* as a cause of diffuse unilateral subacute neuroretinitis. In AIDS patients choroiditis caused by *Pneumocystis,* multifocal retinitis and choroiditis caused by histoplasmosis and tuberculosis, and progressive outer retinal necrosis caused by herpes zoster virus.

- ▶ Acute zonal occult outer retinopathy and its relationship to the multiple evanescent white dot syndrome, punctate inner choroiditis, and acute macular neuroretinopathy.

- ▶ Preliminary evidence of the effectiveness of treatment of patients with serpiginous choroiditis treated with acyclovir and of those with diffuse unilateral subacute neuroretinitis, minimal vitritis, and no detectable nematode treated with a scatter pattern of laser photocoagulation placed in the zone of outer retinal lesions to decrease the blood–inner retinal barrier before the administration of antihelminthic agents.

The author wishes to thank Mrs. Reva Hurtes, who prepared and verified the references; Mrs. Ditte Hess, Mrs. Kazuka Forman, Mr. Rick Stratton, and the other members of the photography department of Bascom Palmer Eye Institute; and Dr. Debra Husain, Dr. Wanda Pak, and the other members of the resident house staff of the Department of Ophthalmology, Vanderbilt Medical School, for their assistance in preparation of the manuscript.

J Donald M Gass

August 1996

Preface to the First Edition

The accessibility of the tissues of the inner eye to close scrutiny by the physician is unequaled by any other organ of the body. Having acquired a knowledge of ocular pathology and the skills of ophthalmoscopy and biomicroscopy, the physician is able to record his in vivo observations of the ocular fundus in gross pathologic terms with reasonable accuracy. This becomes of particular importance in evaluating the patient with loss of central vision resulting from alterations in the structure of the macula. The physician should attempt to determine as far as possible the anatomic changes present, such as choroidal atrophy, choroidal thickening, choroidal wrinkling, change in color of the pigment epithelium, serous detachment of the pigment epithelium, serous detachment of the retina, hemorrhagic detachment of the pigment epithelium and retina, cystoid retinal edema, intraretinal hemorrhage, loss of retinal transparency, retinal wrinkling, and preretinal membrane. He should also attempt to determine the locus of the primary disease process—choroid, retinal pigment epithelium, retinal, or vitreous. Only after making these determinations can the physician evaluate the significance of the patient's ocular, medical, and family history in arriving at a diagnosis, prognosis, and course of therapy.

A variety of ancillary studies may be helpful in certain instances. The use of intravenous fluorescein is of particular value in detecting and defining certain physiologic as well as anatomic changes in the ocular fundus.

The purpose of this atlas is to utilize black and white fundus photographs, stereo color fundus photographs, fluorescein angiographs, and photomicrographs to illustrate some of the anatomic and physiologic alterations produced by a variety of intraocular disease processes affecting the macular region.

After a discussion of the normal macular region (Chapter 1), the diseases affecting this region will be considered in the following order according to the primary tissue involved: diseases of the choroid (Chapters 2 to 4), pigment epithelium (Chapter 5), retina (Chapters 6 to 10), vitreous (Chapter 11), and congenital pit of the optic nerve head (Chapter 12). This subdivision is somewhat arbitrary in that it is not possible in some instances to know which of the ocular tissues is primarily involved by a particular disease process. Stereophotographs of some of the fundus photographs are included in fifteen reels, each containing seven views, attached to the back cover of the book. The appropriate reel number (Roman numeral) and view number (Arabic numeral) are indicated in the lower right-hand corner of the black and white photographs.

All fundus photographs were made with the Zeiss fundus camera. Fluorescein angiography was done utilizing modifications[1,2] of the technique described by Novotny and Alvis.[3] Kodak Kodachrome II and Kodak Tri-X film was used.

With a single exception, the fundus photographs used in this atlas were obtained from the photographic files of the Bascom Palmer Eye Institute of the University of Miami. Most of the patients were examined by me.

I wish to thank Dr. Edward W.D. Norton, Chairman of the Department of Ophthalmology, the members of the full-time and resident staff, and the many other physicians whose patients are

---

[1]Gass, J.D.M., Sever, R.J., Sparks, D., and Goren, J.: A combined technique of fluorescein funduscopy and angiography of the eye, Arch. Ophthalmol. **78**:455-461, 1967.

[2]Haining, W.M., and Lancaster, R.C.: Advanced technique for fluorescein angiography, Arch. Ophthalmol. **79**:10-15, 1968.

[3]Novotny H.R., and Alvis, D.L.: A method of photographing fluorescence in circulating blood in the human retina, Circulation **24**:82-86, 1961.

illustrated in this book. I am particularly indebted to Mr. Johnny Justice, Jr. and his assistants, Mr. Kenneth Peterson, Mrs. Dixie Sparks Gilbert, and Mr. Earl Choromokos for their skill in fundus photography, and to Mr. Joseph Goren and Miss Barbara French for preparation of the illustrations.

Finally, I wish to thank Mrs. Margaret Bertolami, Dr. Alexander R. Irvine, Mrs. Reva Hurtes, and Miss Beth Railinshafer for their help in preparing and editing the manuscript.

J. Donald M. Gass

Contents

7

Inflammatory Diseases of the Retina and Choroid

Infectious agents may be carried from elsewhere in the body and cause one or more foci of infection in the retina and less often in the choroid in one or both eyes. In the case of bacteria and fungi, the nature of the agent can often be established by blood cultures. If treated early with specific antibiotics, the ocular damage may be minimized (Fig. 7-1). Untreated, endophthalmitis may develop rapidly. In some instances when bacteria and fungi gain entrance into the vitreous, either endogenously or exogenously, vitritis with or without periphlebitis may be the earliest sign of an endophthalmitis.[9]

Infectious and noninfectious inflammatory diseases involving primarily the choroid, for example, histoplasmosis, tuberculosis, toxocariasis, cysticercosis, serpiginous choroiditis, Harada's disease, and sympathetic uveitis, often cause visual loss associated with exudative detachment of the posterior retina. See Chapter 3 for a discussion of these choroidal inflammatory disorders.

▼ PYOGENIC CHORIORETINITIS

Septic emboli containing bacteria derived from focal areas of infection such as diseased heart valves, or focal abscesses involving the teeth, skin, or other organs, may lodge in the retina and produce focal white areas of retinitis and overlying vitritis (Fig. 7-1). These may be accompanied by white-centered hemorrhages (Fig. 7-1, *B*). Less frequently the septic emboli lodge in the choroid and may produce a subretinal abscess. (See Fig. 3-47, *A* to *C*.) Most patients with bacterial retinitis will have signs and symptoms of systemic illness, including fever, chills, elevated white blood cell counts, petechiae, splinter hemorrhages of the nail bed, and physical findings pointing to the primary site of the infection. Roth described white retinal lesions and separate hemorrhages in patients with sepsis.[1,4-11] Litten described white-centered hemorrhages in patients with endocarditis and called them "Roth's spots."[6] The white center may contain organisms, although most are sterile and are composed of white blood cells. In many instances the white center is composed of fibrin occurring at the site of extravasation of blood from the retinal blood vessels.[3,10] Roth's spots occur most frequently in patients with severe anemia from any cause, including leukemia and subacute bacterial endocarditis. If bacterial sepsis is suspected, prompt medical evaluation, including blood cultures, a search for the primary site of the infection, and institution of antibiotic therapy, may

FIG. 7-1   Bacterial Septic Embolization of the Retina and Optic Nerve Head.

A to **F**, This 12-year-old girl noted blurred vision during an acute febrile illness. Visual acuity was 15/400. There was massive intraretinal and subretinal exudation in the macular and juxtapapillary regions (**A**). There were peripheral patches of retinitis surrounded by multiple Roth's spots (**B** and **C**). Angiography revealed leakage of dye from the lesion at the temporal margin of the optic disc (**D**). Coagulase-positive staphylococci were cultured from the blood and a dental root abscess. She received intravenous antibiotic therapy. One year later (**E** and **F**), visual acuity had improved to 20/25. *Arrow* indicates a vitreous veil on the optic nerve head secondary to posterior separation of the vitreous. Focal chorioretinal scars remained at the site of some of the areas of retinitis (compare **C** and **F**).

G to **L**, Metastatic bacterial retinitis, macular star, and papillitis (**G** and **H**) occurring in a 32-year-old man who was receiving AZT and Zovirax because of HIV positivity for 10 years. He complained of decreasing vision in his right eye of 2 months' duration. Medical workup, including blood cultures, was negative. Visual acuity was 20/400 in the right eye. There were minimal vitreous cells. Six weeks after treatment with doxycycline the lesions showed evidence of early resolution. Note the angiomatous appearance of the optic disc lesion (**I** and **K**). Three months later the lesions had resolved (**L**). His visual acuity, however, had improved only slightly to 20/80.

succeed in preservation of useful vision in some patients (Fig. 7-1).

▼ FOCAL INDOLENT METASTATIC BACTERIAL RETINITIS IN ACQUIRED IMMUNE DEFICIENCY SYNDROME (AIDS)

Patients with AIDS may develop multifocal, discrete, yellow-white patches of bacterial retinitis that enlarge slowly over weeks and accumulate large amounts of subretinal fluid and fibrinous exudate with minimal inflammatory cell reaction in the overlying vitreous (Fig. 7-1, *G* to *L*).[2] This form of indolent bacterial retinitis is caused by relatively nonpathogenic bacteria, such as *Rhinococcus equi* and *Bartonella* (see discussion of cat-scratch disease in the next section), that usually respond to oral doxycycline. In immunosuppressed patients the retinal lesions may be mistaken for the more frequently encountered retinal infections caused by Herpes viruses, *Candida, Cryptococcus,* and *Toxoplasma* organisms.

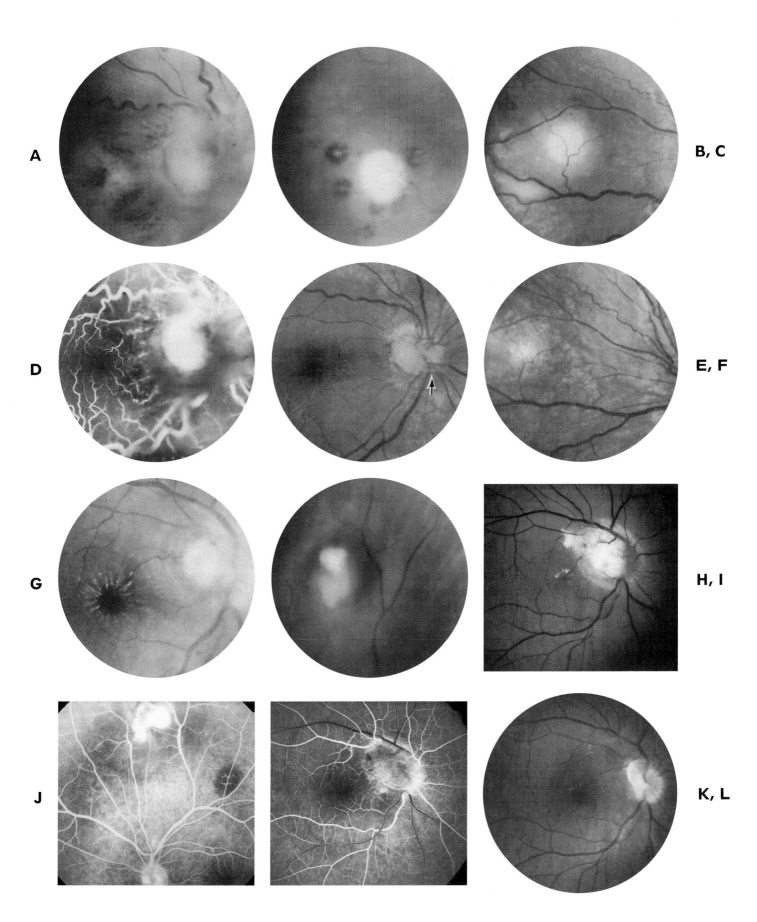

A

B, C

D

E, F

G

H, I

J

K, L

603

▼ CAT-SCRATCH DISEASE (CSD)

Cat-scratch disease (CSD) classically is described as tender regional lymphadenopathy developing in association with a primary skin lesion received as the result of contact with cats. This may be accompanied by generalized aching, malaise, anorexia, and occasionally fever. Whereas a scratch is the common mode of transmission of CSD it may be transmitted by cat bites, licking, or handling of objects associated with cats, particularly kittens. CSD is caused by a pleomorphic gram-negative bacillus, referred to previously as the English-Wear bacillus, the *Rochalimaea* bacillus, and recently *Bartonella*.[15a,25] *Bartonella henselae* and *B. quintana* belong to the order Rickettsiales and are thought to be responsible for trench fever and bacillary angiomatosis, as well as CSD.[15a] In 1977 and 1987 the author noted the association of CSD in patients with Leber's stellate neuroretinitis and multifocal retinitis, and this relationship has been documented by others more recently.[13-15,17-19,24,26] CSD is probably an important, but not the only, cause of the clinical syndrome of self-limited acute idiopathic multifocal retinitis and neuroretinitis (Fig. 7-2) (see p. 700 and Leber's idiopathic stellate neuroretinitis, Chapter 13, p. 996). The focal white retinal lesions may occur anywhere in the fundus but have some predilection for occurring adjacent to and obstructing major retinal arteries and less often veins (Fig. 7-2, *A* to *H*). These retinal lesions, as well as similar lesions involving the optic nerve head, may be associated with an angiomatous-like proliferation of capillaries (Fig. 7-2, *I* to *L*).[16,22] The white lesions typically involve the inner half of the retina and may or may not be associated with overlying vitreous cells. They may simulate cotton-wool ischemic spots, but their distribution in the fundus is not necessarily associated with the distribution of a first-order arteriole as is the case with cotton-wool spots. The focal white retinal and optic disc lesions, swelling of the optic disc, and macular star figure typically clear spontaneously within several weeks or months and the visual acuity usually returns to normal or nearly normal. Most of the retinal lesions resolve without causing RPE damage.

The CSD bacillus may also cause acute encephalopathy and other neurologic and systemic manifestations in otherwise healthy patients and in patients with AIDS.[13,14,22] Ocular and CNS involvement typically occurs in children or young adults. Patients with CNS involvement may manifest convulsions and fever in approximately 50% of cases and neuroretinitis in 10% to 15% of cases.[14] Spontaneous recovery of vision and neurologic deficits occurs in nearly all cases, usually within 3 months. Biopsy of enlarged lymph nodes may reveal evidence of the infection. The bacillus may be demonstrated by the Warthin-Starry stain or culture from skin or lymph node specimens. Detection of antibodies to the cat-scratch bacillus is helpful in the diagnosis.[13,14] The indirect fluorescent antibody assay for *Bartonella henselae* and *B.*

FIG. 7-2 Benign Multifocal Retinitis and Papillitis Caused by Cat-Scratch Bacillus and Other Bacteria or Viruses of Low Pathogenicity.

A to **D,** This 32-year-old woman noted floaters and a paracentral scotoma in the right eye soon after two episodes of chills and fever. Her visual acuity was 20/20, right eye, and 20/25, left eye. In both eyes she had multiple focal areas of inner retinal whitening. One of these (*arrows,* **A**) was associated with obstruction of an inferior temporal branch retinal artery. A focal lesion was present nasally on the left optic disc (*arrow,* **B**). All of the lesions stained (*arrows,* **C** and **D**). Medical evaluation was unremarkable except for some elevation of cardiolipin antibody. One year later she was well and had 20/20 visual acuity bilaterally.

E, This 21-year-old woman in the second trimester of pregnancy noted floaters and visual loss in the left eye 2 weeks following an episode of fever of unknown origin. She owned seven cats but could recall no history of being scratched. Visual acuity in the left eye was counting fingers only. One to 2 + vitreous cells were present in the left eye. Multifocal white lesions interpreted as inner retinitis were present in both eyes (*arrows*). One of these was associated with obstruction of the supertemporal branch retinal artery in the left eye. Medical evaluation, including blood cultures, was negative.

F to **H,** This 28-year-old man with AIDS noted blurred vision in the left eye associated with multiple foci of retinitis and papillitis (*arrows,* **F** to **H**). One lesion (*lower arrow,* **F**) caused obstruction of the inferior branch retinal artery.

I to **L,** This healthy 22-year-old male had a 3-week history of blurred vision right eye. He owned many household cats, was frequently scratched, but denied recent illness. Visual acuity was 20/200, right eye, and 20/20, left eye. Note the hemimacular star, exudative retinal detachment, and focal retinitis (*arrow,* **I**) enveloping but not obstructing the inferior branch retinal artery. A similar but smaller focal area of retinitis was present in the left eye (*arrow,* **J**). Note the pseudoangiomatous appearance of the active lesion angiographically (*arrow,* **K**). Both lesions stained (**L**). Within several weeks he recovered normal vision without treatment.

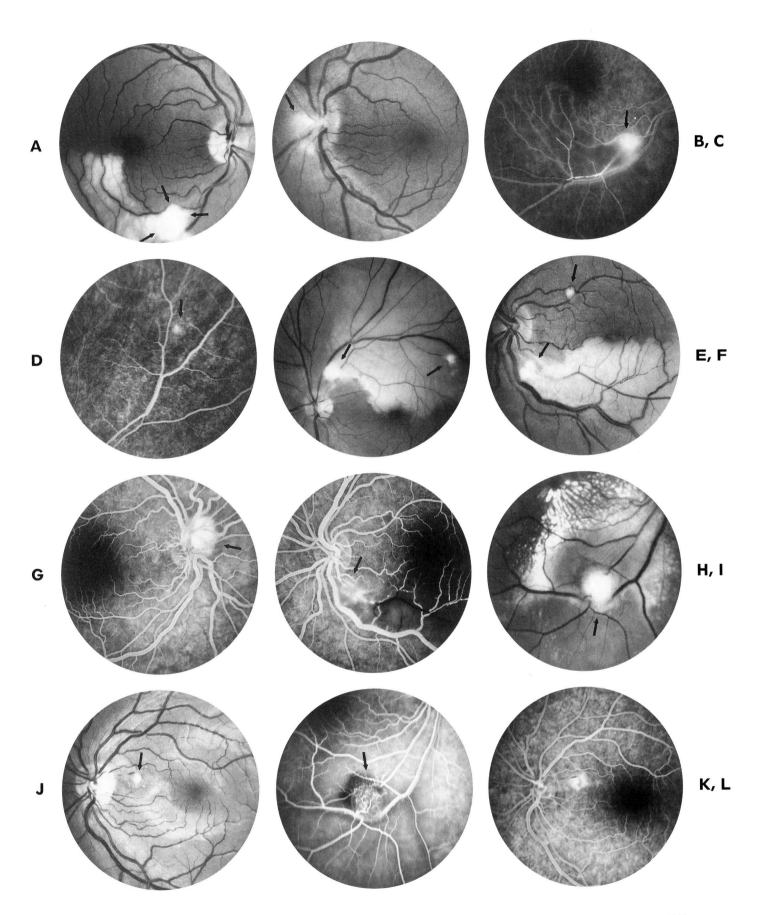

A

B, C

D

E, F

G

H, I

J

K, L

605

quintana, available through the Centers for Disease Control and Prevention in Atlanta, is sensitive for the diagnosis of CSD.[15a] The favorable prognosis without treatment makes evaluation of treatment with doxycycline, ciprofloxacin, and prednisone difficult.

The tendency for some of the retinal and optic nerve inflammatory lesions to appear very vascular biomicroscopically and angiographically may be an important feature of cat-scratch infection (Fig. 7-2, *J* to *L*). Angiomatous-like masses referred to as epithelioid angiomatosis and caused by cat-scratch bacillus have occurred on the skin and mucous membranes of patients with AIDS.[12,20-23] In these patients the lesions may appear similar clinically to Kaposi's sarcoma. In the eye the lesions may simulate capillary angiomas or astrocytic hamartomas of the retina (Fig. 7-2, *I* to *L*).

▼ RETINOCHOROIDITIS CAUSED BY *MYCOBACTERIUM TUBERCULOSIS* IN IMMUNOSUPPRESSED PATIENTS

The eye in the immune competent individual with pulmonary tuberculosis is infrequently affected. Patients with miliary tuberculosis may develop multifocal choroidal granulomas and, less often, endophthalmitis. Patients with AIDS and tuberculosis, however, may develop severe multifocal retinochoroiditis, caused by *M. tuberculosis* (Fig. 7-3, *A* and *B*), as well as by the ordinarily less pathogenic *M. avium.*[1]

▼ LYME BORRELIOSIS

Lyme borreliosis is a tick-transmitted disorder caused by the spirochete *Borrelia burgdorferi.* This disorder usually begins with a characteristic ex-

FIG. 7-3 *Mycobacterium tuberculosis* **Retinochoroiditis.**

A and B, This patient, who had AIDS, died soon after these photographs because of disseminated infection with tuberculosis. Note multifocal choroidal and retinal lesions that were present in both eyes.

Lyme Disease

C to H, Iritis, vitritis, snow-bank exudates on the pars plana, cystoid macular edema, and retinitis proliferans bilaterally in a 25-year-old man with serologic evidence of Lyme disease.

(**A** and **B** from Blodi et al.[1]; **F, G,** and **H** from Smith et al.[66])

panding red maculopapular annular skin lesion. After several weeks the organism may spread systemically and be associated with secondary annular skin lesions, meningitis, cranial or peripheral neuritis, migratory musculoskeletal pain, and carditis. The patient often does not recall a tick bite. Months to years later intermittent or chronic arthritis, or chronic neurologic or skin abnormalities may develop.

A miscellaneous group of fundus pictures, including pars planitis, retinal vasculitis, bilateral diffuse choroiditis, acute posterior multifocal placoid pigment epitheliopathy, macular edema, papilledema, and Leber's stellate neuropathy, have been reported in patients with systemic illness and serologic evidence of previous exposure to *Borrelia burgdorferi.*[57-67] Only pars planitis associated with snow-bank exudates, and anterior uveitis, however, have occurred with sufficient frequency to suggest a significant relationship to Lyme disease (Fig. 7-3, *C* to *H*).[60,66,68]

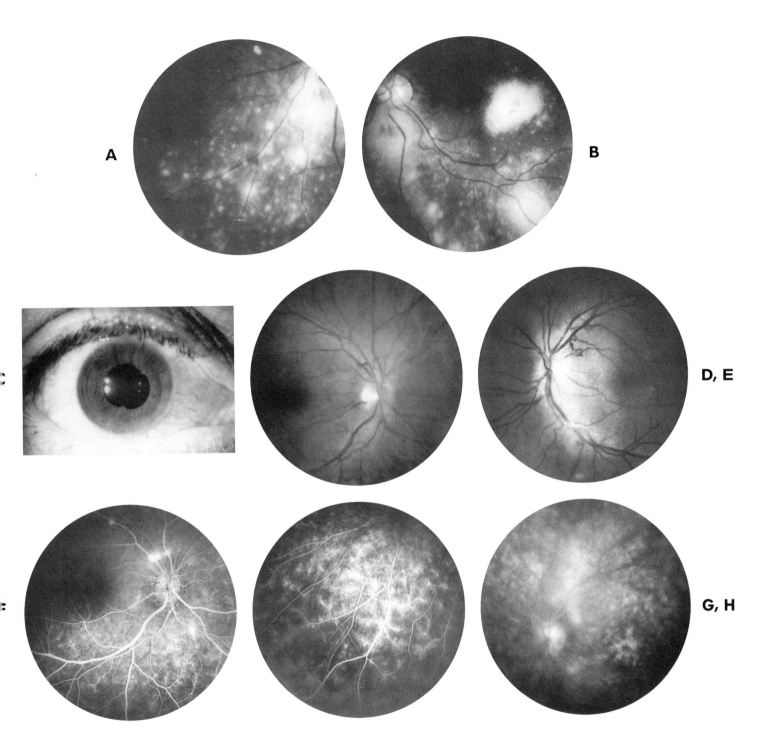

A

B

C

D, E

G, H

607

▼ LUETIC CHORIORETINITIS

Many different fundus lesions have been described in congenital and acquired syphilis (Figs. 7-4 and 7-5). Salt-and-pepper changes affecting primarily the peripheral retina are the most frequent alterations described with congenital syphilis. Severe involvement of the ocular fundus, however, may occur and produce a picture simulating retinitis pigmentosa (Fig. 7-5, *E* and *F*). In acquired syphilis, particularly in patients with secondary syphilis, several acute funduscopic pictures should suggest the possibility of syphilis. Secondary syphilis occurs 6 weeks to 6 months after the primary inoculation, which particularly in homosexuals may be overlooked. During the secondary stage of syphilis there is widespread dissemination of the spirochetes and the patient often experiences malaise, fever, hair loss, papular macular rash, condyloma lata, mucous patches, and generalized lymphadenopathy (Fig. 7-4, *J* to *L*). Approximately 5% of patients with secondary syphilis will show evidence of panuveitis.[40,45] Probably the most common fundus change is that of vitreous cellular infiltration and either single or multiple, nonelevated, geographic, yellow-white, ill-defined, chorioretinal lesions that often are confluent in the posterior pole and midperiphery of the fundus (Fig. 7-4, *B* and *G*).* Both eyes are affected in half of all cases. In some patients the chorioretinal lesions may be largely confined to the area around the optic disc. They may be associated with superficial, flame-shaped hemorrhages. The fundus picture may simulate the early stages of the acute retinal necrosis syndrome.[44] Secondary retinal detachment and choroidal detachment develop in some patients.[31] The active yellow-gray placoid outer retinal and choroidal lesions fade centrally and often there is clumping of the RPE in a leopard-spot configuration (Fig. 7-4, *D, H,* and *I*).[37] These pigment clumps may become less apparent over a period of months. The clinical course is variable. In some cases the chorioretinitis resolves spontaneously and the appearance of the fundus and retinal function may return to near normal. In others widespread areas of chorioretinal atrophy and loss of retinal function occur (Fig. 7-5, *A* to *C*). Migration of RPE into the overlying retina in a bone-spicule pattern may occur many months later. Choroidal neovascularization developing at the edge of a chorioretinal scar may be a late complication (Fig. 7-5, *D*).[39]

---

*References 27, 32, 33, 36, 37, 46, 52, 53, 55, 56.

FIG. 7-4   Luetic Chorioretinitis.

A to F, Acute posterior placoid chorioretinitis in both eyes of this 42-year-old homosexual man with a 2-week history of blurred vision and floaters in both eyes. Approximately 6 weeks previously he had noted a skin eruption on the sole of his left foot and perirectal pruritus. Visual acuity was 20/20 in the right eye and 20/30 in the left eye. There was evidence of bilateral anterior and posterior uveitis with many vitreous cells and opacities in the left eye (**A**). Because of the presence of irregular retinal whitening in the periphery of the left eye, a diagnosis of possible acute retinal necrosis was made. Four weeks later he noted marked visual loss in the right eye. Visual acuity was 8/200. There were several large zones of gray-white change at the level of the RPE and outer retina in the macula (**B**) and periphery (**C**) of the right eye. Angiography (**D** and **E**) revealed these lesions to be hypofluorescent early and to stain later. A leopard-spot pattern of background hypofluorescence was apparent in the macular area (**D**). The blood and cerebrospinal fluid serology were positive for syphilis. Following intravenous penicillin, the fundus changes and uveitis cleared promptly, leaving a coarsely mottled pattern of pigmentation in the macular area. He experienced a rapid recovery of vision. Four months later his visual acuity was 20/15 in the right eye and 20/20 in the left eye. There was mild pigment mottling in both macular areas.

G to I, Acute posterior placoid chorioretinitis, vitritis, and maculopapular dermatitis caused by secondary syphilis in a 48-year-old man whose visual acuity was 6/200. Fluorescein angiography revealed a leopard-spot pattern of nonfluorescence in the area of partial fading of the gray-white lesion, that was nonfluorescent early and stained late (**H** and **I**). His left eye became involved several days later. The lesions resolved promptly after treatment with penicillin and his acuity returned to 20/30 right eye and 20/20 left eye within 4 weeks.

J to L, Alopecia (**J**), and maculopapular dermatitis (**K** and **L**) in patients with acute visual loss associated with acute posterior placoid chorioretinitis caused by secondary syphilis.

(G to K from Gass et al.: Ophthalmology 97:1288-1297, 1990[37]; L from Passo and Rosenbaum: Am J Ophthalmol 106:1-6, 1980.[47])

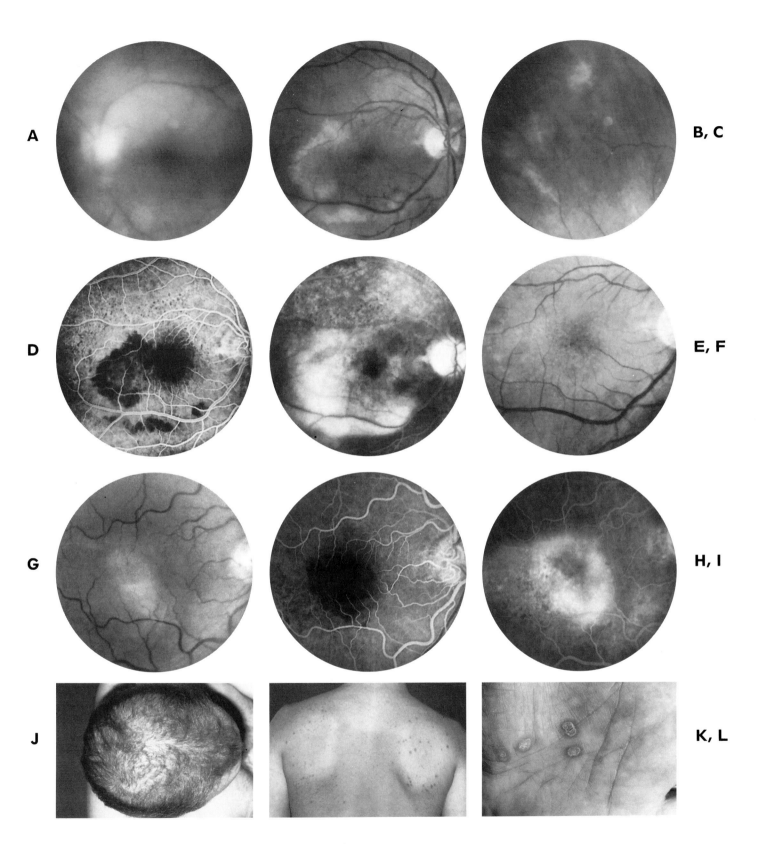

Fluorescein angiography in the region of the active yellow-white chorioretinal lesions show initially evidence of hypofluorescence followed by late staining at the level of the RPE (Fig. 7-4, *D, E, H,* and *I*). Fluorescein staining of the optic disc and major retinal veins is frequent. During the early stages of resolution of the active chorioretinal lesions, the leopard-spot change in the RPE may be more apparent angiographically than ophthalmoscopically.

The acute placoid chorioretinal retinal lesions of secondary syphilis may be mistaken for those of acute placoid multifocal pigment epitheliopathy and serpiginous choroiditis.[37] Eliciting a history of and/or the detection of any of the nonocular manifestations of secondary syphilis, and institution of prompt treatment with penicillin, is important in making the correct diagnosis and in preventing permanent visual loss. Return of visual function may be dramatic. The patient should be evaluated for evidence of AIDS, which often accompanies secondary lues.[37,41,43,47,54] Syphilis may be accelerated and neurosyphilis encountered earlier in patients with AIDS.[41]

In some patients with acquired syphilis the fundus picture is primarily that of retinal vasculitis with retinal hemorrhages,* occlusive arterial disease, and retinitis proliferans (Fig. 7-5, *G* and *H*).[28,46] Many different funduscopic changes have been attributed to syphilis, including neuroretinitis,[35] disciform scar,[49] acute retinal necrosis,[44] pseudo–retinitis pigmentosa, and optic atrophy.[50] Syphilis has been called the "great imitator."[55] Since it is a common infection, however, care must be used in assigning it as the cause of an ocular disease solely on the basis of positive serologic tests for syphilis. These include the nonspecific reagin tests, such as VDRL, or more specific tests, including FTA-ABS and MHA-TP. There is some controversy concerning the criteria for diagnosis of neurosyphilis and for the dosage and route of

FIG. 7-5   Luetic Chorioretinitis.

A to **C,** Bilateral chorioretinal scars caused by secondary luetic chorioretinitis.

D, Subretinal neovascularization *(arrow)* in the macula of a patient with chorioretinal scars following chorioretinitis caused by secondary syphilis.

E and **F,** Congenital luetic chorioretinopathy in a 41-year-old woman with poor vision all of her life, interstitial keratitis, +FTA, and 20/80 visual acuity. Note the narrowing of the retinal vessels, optic disc pallor, and pseudo–retinitis pigmentosa change peripherally.

G and **H,** Presumed luetic retinal vasculitis in this 30-year-old homosexual man with a 10-day history of blurred vision in his right eye. The left eye was amblyopic since birth. Five years previously he had primary syphilis. Sixteen months previously he developed a skin rash on the feet and hands. This was diagnosed as syphilis 3 months before the onset of visual symptoms and he received intramuscular penicillin. His visual acuity was 20/50 in his right eye and hand motions only in the left eye. He had widely scattered retinal hemorrhages, perivascular exudation (**G**), and angiographic evidence of multiple sites of retinal vascular obstruction, predominantly affecting the veins (**H**). There was perivascular staining in the late photographs.

administration of penicillin in these patients.[29] Because of the high incidence of positive reaction of the spinal fluid to the serologic tests for syphilis during the secondary stages of the disease, spinal fluid examination is usually not recommended for patients presenting with the ocular manifestations of secondary syphilis. Recommended treatment for patients with active chorioretinal disease caused by syphilis is intensive high-dose intravenous aqueous penicillin G, 2.4 million units every 4 hours for at least 6 days, followed by intramuscular injection of benzathine penicillin every week for 3 weeks.[35,46,48]

*References 28, 30, 34, 38, 40, 42, 46, 51.

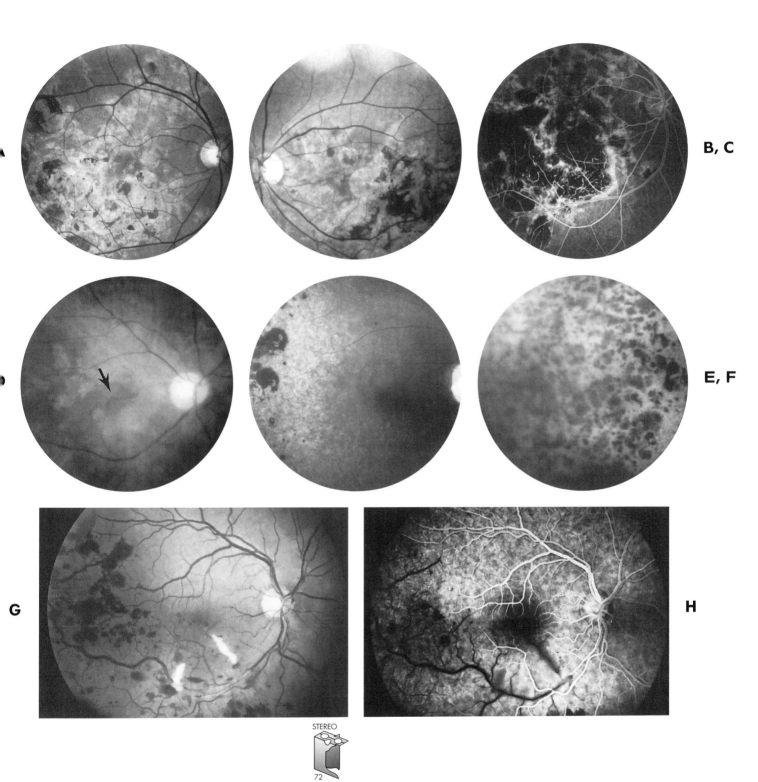

A

B, C

E, F

G

H

STEREO
72

611

▼ FUNGAL RETINOCHOROIDITIS

Certain fungi either involve primarily the retina or extend rapidly from the choroid into the retina where they produce white intraretinal fungal abscesses (*Aspergillus fumigatus, Candida albicans, Trichosporon beigelii,* and *Sporothrix schenckii*). Others produce primarily yellow-white multifocal choroidal infiltrates that may cause serous and hemorrhagic retinal detachment (*Histoplasma capsulatum, Blastomyces dermatitidis, Coccidioides immitis,* and *Cryptococcus neoformans.*) These latter diseases, which may be associated with disciform retinal detachment, are discussed in Chapter 3.

Candida retinochoroiditis

Hospitalized patients, particularly those with postoperative complications of abdominal surgery receiving prolonged intensive antibiotic treatment by an intravenous catheter, are prone to develop candidemia and focal white retinal abscesses (Fig. 7-6, *A* to *F*).* The focal white retinal lesions are typically superficially located in the retina and are frequently associated with small cottony balls in the vitreous overlying the primary lesion (Fig. 7-6, *D*). Other predisposing factors for development of retinal candidiasis include intravenous drug abuse, chemotherapy, corticosteroid administration, malignancy, bone marrow transplantation, diabetes, severe burns, endocrine hypofunction, other debilitating diseases, contaminated intravenously administered medications, and maternal birth canal infection.† The appearance of the fundus lesion is strongly suggestive of the diagnosis. The diagnosis may be confirmed by cultures of the site of the intravenous administration, blood cultures, or vitreous aspiration. Multiple white-centered superficial retinal hemorrhages may also occur.[73] The white centers may be caused by microabscesses containing the fungi,[95] or by sterile fibrin–platelet aggregates (see previous discussion of pyogenic bacterial infection). The disease may respond to systemically administered amphotericin B or 5-fluorocytosine or both.[70,81,92-94] Intravitreal injection of amphotericin B has been used successfully as a primary form of treatment[71,72,81,94] and as an adjunct to systemic treatment (Fig. 7-6, *C* to *F*).[92] Spontaneous resolution of *Candida* retinal abscesses may occur.[76] For this reason patients with mild retinal involvement and no evidence of other organ involvement may be followed for evidence of

*References 69, 73, 76, 77, 79, 80, 82-85, 90-95.
†References 69, 70, 73-76, 79, 80, 88, 89.

FIG. 7-6 *Candida* **Septic Chorioretinitis.**

A, Focal *Candida* retinal abscess *(arrows)* with "cotton ball" vitreous opacities.

B, Histopathology of focal *Candida* chorioretinitis. Note the predominantly granulomatous inflammation of the choroid, retina, and vitreoretinal juncture. The RPE is destroyed. The overlying vitreous contains predominantly histiocytes. Special stains revealed evidence of *Monilia.*

C to **F,** *Candida* endophthalmitis in a 50-year-old man with chronic alcoholism who noted pain and redness in his right eye. Visual acuity was 20/50. Note the string of white vitreous opacities (**C** and **D**). *Candida albicans* was cultured from the vitreous and from an ulcer on the bottom of his foot (**E**). At the time of vitrectomy intravitreal amphotericin B was given and systemic administration of ketoconazole was begun. Six weeks later, visual acuity was 20/25 and the fundus was normal (**F**).

Aspergillus Chorioretinitis

G to **H,** This 33-year-old man with a history of "bruised ribs and chills," intravenous drug abuse, and a 1-day history of eye pain and visual loss in the right eye, had a visual acuity of 2/200, right eye, and 20/20, left eye, mild iritis, vitritis, and a subhyaloid *(top arrow,* **G**) and subretinal hypopyon *(bottom arrow,* **G**) associated with a subretinal hemorrhagic inflammatory mass in the right macula. Cultures of the aqueous humor and blood, echocardiography and HIV serology were negative. An intravitreal injection of amphotericin B, 5 µg, was done. Vitreous culture was positive for *Aspergillus flavus.* He received intravenous amphotericin B for 3 weeks. Eleven months later his visual acuity was 20/400 and there was a flat scar in the right macula (**H**).

Histoplasmosis Retinochoroiditis.

I to **K,** This 29-year-old-man with AIDS died because of complications associated with cytomegalovirus pneumonitis and systemic histoplasmosis. He complained of a hazy spot in his left eye. He had multiple white foci of retinitis in both eyes (**I**). Microscopic examination of his eyes revealed multifocal areas of necrotizing perivascular retinitis (**J**) and choroiditis associated with *H. capsulatum* organisms *(arrow,* **K**).

(**A** and **B** from Griffin et al.[84]; **G** and **H** from Weishaar et al.[101a]; **I** to **K** from Specht et al.: Ophthalmology 98:1356-1359, 1991.[107])

progression.[77] The development of retinal striae around a focal retinal monilial abscess is a sign suggesting early resolution of the lesion.[78] If the retinal lesion(s) progress or if evidence of more advanced disease is present, the administration of 5-fluorouracil, which is relatively nontoxic, may be effective. Development of resistance to 5-fluorouracil, however, is frequent. To avoid renal

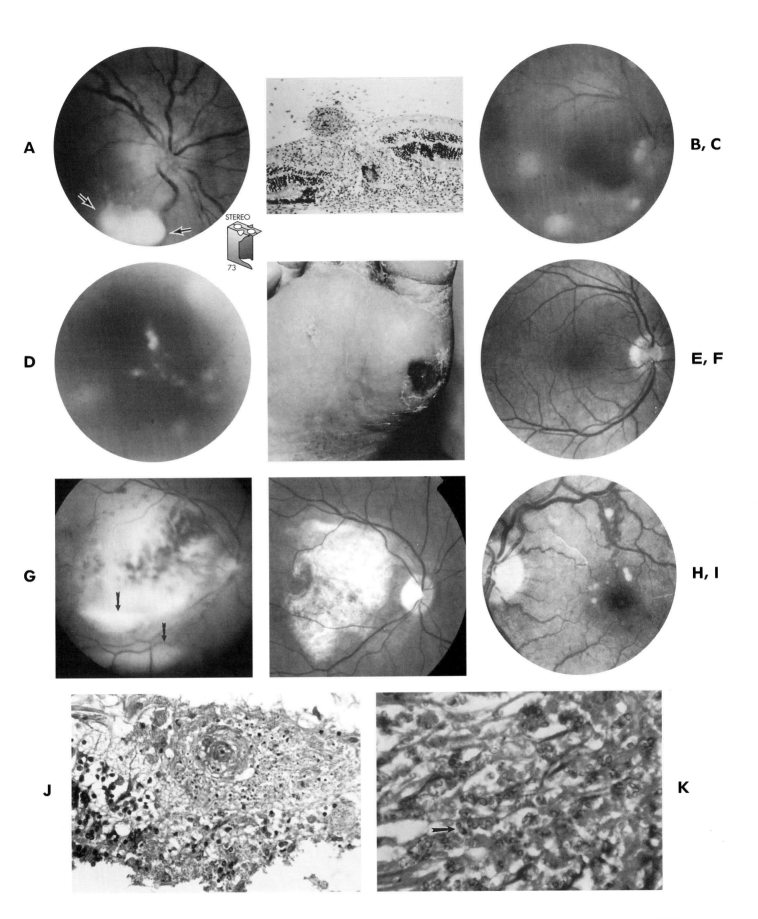

toxicity associated with treatment with systemic amphotericin B, some patients with ocular involvement in the absence of evidence of other organ involvement with monilial infection, may be successfully managed with pars plana vitrectomy and intravitreal injection of amphotericin B.[70,72,86,92,94]

The development of epiretinal membranes may be the cause of visual loss in some patients otherwise successfully treated for chorioretinal monilial infection. Surgical removal of these membranes may result in partial restoration of visual function.[87]

Aspergillosis

Intravenous drug abuse is the primary cause of intraocular infection with *Aspergillus.* In these patients it ranks only behind *Candida* as the cause of endogenous fungus endophthalmitis. Ocular involvement is typically the first manifestation of the infection except when it occurs in immune incompetent individuals.[96-101] The patients present with subacute visual loss, mild pain, and redness of the eye that may be associated with a varying degree of anterior chamber reaction. Chorioretinitis and endophthalmitis caused by *Aspergillus* have characteristic clinical features. Preretinal or subretinal exudation may be accompanied by a hypopyon as a result of layering of inflammatory cells (Fig. 7-6, *G* and *H*).[101a] A hemorrhagic retinal vasculitis may be present.[98,99] Isolated retinal hemorrhages and preretinal fluffy vitreous opacities may obscure fundus details. In some cases only a mild vitritis may be present initially. A variety of species of *Aspergillus* may be responsible for human infection. Pars plana vitrectomy and intravitreal injection of amphotericin B are the first choice in treatment of *Aspergillus* infection of the inner eye. The use of amphotericin B intravenously, in the absence of any other evidence of systemic infection, is controversial.[98-100]

Retinochoroiditis caused by other fungi

Other fungus diseases, such as trichosporonosis[103] and sporotricosis,[102] may cause chorioretinal lesions and endophthalmitis similar to that produced by *Candida.*

Histoplasmosis retinochoroiditis in immune incompetent patients

Histoplasma capsulatum may cause multifocal, active, white, retinal, subretinal, and choroidal lesions in one or both eyes of patients with AIDS (Fig. 7-6, *I* to *K*) or other immune incompetent

FIG. 7-7 Congenital Toxoplasmosis Retinitis.

A to **D,** Heterotopia of the macula and dragging of the retinal vessels of the right eye (**A** and **B**) caused by congenital toxoplasmosis retinitis in a 29-year-old woman with intracranial calcification and focal chorioretinal scars (**B** and **C**). Note angiographic evidence of retinochoroidal anastomosis at the site of the scar in the left eye (*arrow,* **D**).

E to **F,** Macular scars in an HIV-positive infant presumed to be caused by congenital toxoplasmosis. Visual acuity was 20/20, right eye, and 20/40, left eye.

G to **I,** Presumed congenital toxoplasmosis in a 32-year-old woman with poor vision since birth. Note the deep excavation of the scar in the right macula (*Stereo* **G** and **H**).

J and **K,** Multiple chorioretinal scars of uncertain cause in both eyes of this 9-year-old child who had good vision until recently when she developed evidence of subretinal neovascularization in the left macula. She was the product of an 8-month pregnancy that was terminated because of retarded intrauterine growth.

states (see Fig. 3-43, *A* to *C*).[104-107] In immune competent individuals histoplasmosis may cause focal choroiditis that typically results in multiple focal atrophic chorioretinal scars without producing ocular symptoms. These scars later in life may be the site of development of subretinal neovascularization and visual loss. (See presumed ocular histoplasmosis syndrome in Chapter 3.)

Phycomycosis (mucormycosis)

See Chapter 6, p. 464.

▼ TOXOPLASMOSIS RETINITIS

Toxoplasmosis is the most frequent cause of focal necrotizing retinitis in otherwise healthy human individuals (Figs. 7-7 to 7-10).* The protozoan *Toxoplasma gondii* is either transmitted to the fetus in utero when the mother acquires the infection during pregnancy or, less commonly, it infects the retina following ingestion of the organism. There is a predilection for infection of the central nervous system and the retina. In congenital toxoplasmosis the retinal lesion may occur as part of a generalized severe infection (encephalomyelitis, convulsions, fever, jaundice, cerebral calcification, hydrocephalus, and paralyses of various types) or more frequently as part of a mild subclinical infection. Large, atrophic, often excavated, chorioretinal

*References 108, 110, 111, 114, 119, 121, 123, 125, 127-132, 136, 141-145, 148, 150, 151, 153, 158, 162, 164-166, 169, 170, 174, 176, 179.

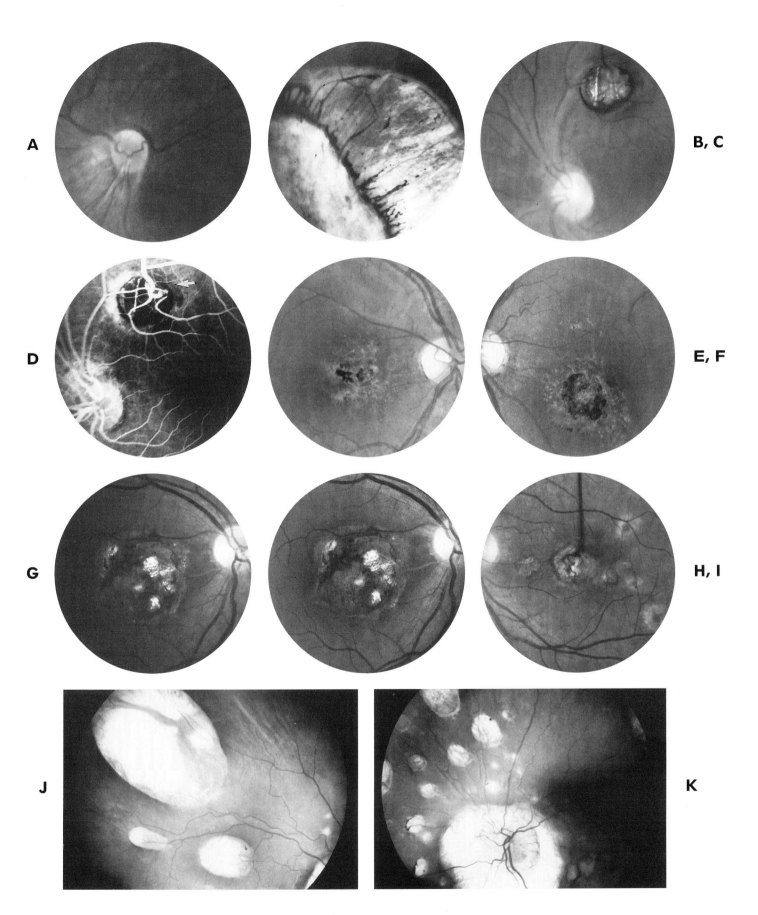

A

B, C

D

E, F

G

H, I

J

K

scars centered in or near the macular area or elsewhere in the fundus in children and adults are probably caused in many cases by congenital toxoplasmosis (Fig. 7-7, *B, C, H, J,* and *K*). When they are symmetric, however, these macular lesions must be differentiated from similar appearing inherited dystrophic lesions (see Fig. 3-38). Whether acquired in utero or postnatally, the *Toxoplasma* organisms may lie dormant in the encysted form in the apparently normal retina either adjacent to or remote from chorioretinal scars. When the organisms become unencysted one or more acute, white, necrotizing lesions may occur in a previously normal-looking retina or at the margin of an old chorioretinal scar (Fig. 7-8). The lesions usually involve the full thickness of the retina but in some cases may be confined to either the inner or, less frequently, the outer half of the retina. In the former they are associated with overlying vitreous inflammatory cell infiltration. When the retinitis involves primarily the outer retina, serous detachment of the underlying retina is frequently present (Fig. 7-8, *A* to *I*). When the acute lesion includes a major retinal vessel, it may cause either a branch retinal arterial occlusion (Fig. 7-9, *A* to *C*)[114,127,130] or a venous occlusion (Fig. 7-9, *D* and *E*).[130] Most patients with acute retinitis are seen initially because of a history of floaters and less often because of loss of central vision caused by foveal involvement by focal retinitis (Fig. 7-8), cystoid macular edema, or detachment associated with paracentral focal retinitis. Focal periarterial exudates and arterial atheromatous plaques (Kyrieleis' arteriolitis) simulating arterial emboli may occur either in the immediate vicinity of the acute retinitis or remote from it (Fig. 7-9, *F* to *I*).[127-129,142,153,175] Fluorescein angiography shows no permeability alterations or evidence of artery obstruction in the area of the arterial plaques but demonstrates marked fluorescein staining in the area of the retinitis (Figs. 7-8, *B, C, E, H,* and *I,* and 7-9, *C*). The periarterial plaques may fade or may persist following resolution of the retinitis. Occasionally acute multifocal arterial wall opacification is widespread throughout the fundus and may be accompanied by similar multifocal gelatinous-appearing opacities scattered along the major retinal veins. Ophthalmoscopic and angiographic evidence of diffuse perivenous exudation may occasionally occur in areas remote from the acute retinitis. The presence in these patients with retinal vasculitis of reduced levels of antibody affinity to retinal S-antigen with normal levels of circulating immune complexes suggests

FIG. 7-8 Serous Macular Detachment Caused by Active Outer Retinal Toxoplasmosis and by Subretinal Neovascularization Arising at Toxoplasmosis Chorioretinal Scar.

A to **E,** This 18-year-old woman developed floaters associated with a focal area of acute retinitis (*arrow,* **A**) and widespread periphlebitis in the right eye. Angiography showed intense staining in the area of the retinitis and leakage of dye from the major retinal veins and optic disc (**B** and **C**). Several years later, she developed visual loss caused by serous retinal detachment in the macula associated with multiple foci of outer retinitis near the edge of the old scar and in the papillomacular bundle area (*arrows,* **D**). Angiography (**E**) revealed early staining of the foci of retinitis and late diffuse staining of the subretinal fluid.

F to **I,** Serous macular detachment caused by recurrence of retinitis (*arrows,* **F** and **G**) near a scar. Note late staining of the subretinal fluid.

J to **K,** Serous macular detachment caused by recurrence of retinitis (*arrow,* **J**) in a patient with bilateral macular scars.

L, Serosanguinous retinal detachment caused by subretinal neovascularization arising at the inferior edge of a toxoplasmosis scar.

a defective regulation of antiretinal autoimmunity.[140] Swelling of the optic disc and angiographic evidence of staining of the disc may accompany focal areas of retinitis or, in some cases, may be the presenting manifestation of toxoplasmosis (Fig. 7-9, *J* to *L*). Multiple, small, gray deposits (presumably inflammatory cells) may develop along the inner retinal surface in the vicinity of the acute retinitis, and it may be difficult to distinguish these from small foci of active retinitis. If the vitreous separates from the retina near the acute lesion, these gray deposits usually remain attached to the posterior surface of the vitreous.

The active focus of retinitis usually enlarges for a period of 1 to 2 weeks before gradually fading over a period of several months, usually leaving in its wake a pigmented atrophic chorioretinal scar. Segmental optic disc pallor may develop in the zone of nerve fiber atrophy caused by the retinitis.

In some patients the onset of the disease is characterized by the development of multifocal small foci of retinitis, largely confined to the outer retinal layers (Fig. 7-10, *A*).[121,146] After resolution, some of these small lesions may leave no chorioretinal scarring. There may be a series of remissions and exacerbations before development of the larger, more typical, full-thickness focus of acute retinitis (Fig. 7-10, *A* to *D*). Another atypical presentation is that of an acute papillitis before the

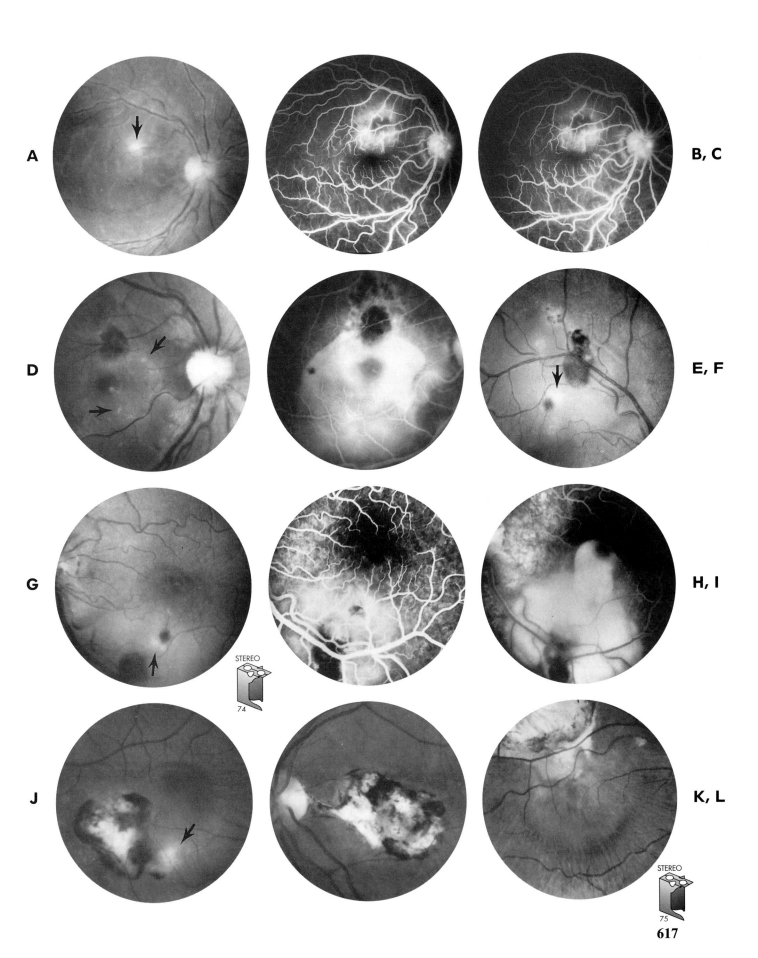

development of a focal area of retinitis (Fig. 7-9, *J* to *L*).[124,125,145,179] Findings that should suggest that disc swelling may be caused by toxoplasmosis are severe vitreous inflammation, fluffy white peripapillary lesions, nerve fiber bundle defect, and often good visual acuity.[124,125]

The clinical diagnosis of ocular toxoplasmosis is always a presumptive one. Most patients will demonstrate skin test and serologic evidence of previous contact with the organism.[161] The diagnosis of acute toxoplasmosis is very likely in otherwise healthy patients with a focus of acute retinitis in an eye with one or more chorioretinal scars. Even in the absence of another scar, a solitary focus of acute retinitis in a healthy patient occurs most often in patients with serologic evidence of the infection; a few do not, and the titers may be low in many patients. In addition to the ELISA, the immunofluorescent antibody test, and the Sabin-Feldman dye test (rarely done anymore), detection of evidence of toxoplasmosis in the aqueous humor may be accomplished using the polymerase chain reaction.[109,115,178] Cytologic diagnosis of toxoplasmosis may occasionally be made from vitreous biopsy.[134]

Most chorioretinal scars caused by toxoplasmosis are atrophic, partly pigmented, and associated with postinflammatory changes in the overlying vitreous and a nerve fiber bundle visual field defect. Hypertrophic disciform scars, however, develop in some patients (Fig. 7-10, *E* and *F*). In rare cases reactive proliferation of the RPE in these scars may be mistaken for a melanoma.[139] Remodeling of the retinal circulation caused by previous occlusion of vessels passing through the area of retinitis is often present (Fig. 7-9, *D* and *E*). Evidence of retinochoroidal anastomosis may develop (Fig. 7-9, *D*).[141,153,163] Development of subretinal neovascularization, usually type 2, at the edge of an inactive scar may cause loss of central vision (Fig. 7-8, *L*).[118,128] The large macular chorioretinal scars seen in children and attributed to congenital toxoplasmosis usually do not show evidence of postinflammatory changes in the vitreous. Unusual and unexplained associations with toxoplasmosis retinitis are the development of Fuchs' heterochromic cyclitis and either unilateral or bilateral zones of retinitis pigmentosa–like fundus changes.[120,143,168,172]

Familial involvement with ocular toxoplasmosis is rare. In southern Brazil (Alto Uraguai region), however, familial ocular toxoplasmosis is endemic.[133,171] The prevalence of ocular toxoplasmosis there is 30 times higher than elsewhere.[133] The

FIG. 7-9 Toxoplasmosis Retinitis.

A to **C**, Branch retinal arterial occlusion caused by acute retinitis, presumed to be toxoplasmosis (**A**). Angiography showed evidence of branch artery obstruction (*arrow,* **B**) and late staining in the area of retinitis (**C**).

D and **E**, Retinochoroidal anastomosis (*arrows*) in two patients following venous obstruction caused by toxoplasmosis retinitis.

F to **I**, Chorioretinal scars (**H**) and marked periarterial plaque deposition persisting for years following multiple areas of acute retinitis presumed to be caused by toxoplasmosis in a 30-year-old man whose visual acuity was 20/20 in both eyes. Angiography showed evidence of the periarterial plaques and minimal evidence of obstruction to blood flow (**I**).

J to **L**, Presumed toxoplasmosis papillitis in a 7-year-old boy with acute loss of vision in the right eye (**J**). Angiography revealed staining of the optic disc (**K**). Within several months the disc swelling resolved and optic atrophy was evident. Twenty-one months later he had further loss of vision in the right eye caused by acute retinitis in the macula (**L**).

frequent ingestion of raw or undercooked pork has been suggested as a possible explanation for this.

Histopathologic examination of an acute toxoplasmosis lesion in eyes of immune competent patients reveals a focal necrotizing retinitis associated with an underlying acute and chronic granulomatous choroiditis and scleritis (Fig. 7-10, *G* and *H*).[137] The inflammatory reaction surrounding the necrotizing retinitis is markedly reduced in immunosuppressed patients (Fig. 7-10, *I* and *J*). In spite of the presence of scleritis that may be evident ultrasonographically beneath the focal retinitis in immune competent patients, only occasionally do they complain of pain.[167] The encysted and free forms of *Toxoplasma* organisms are found in the relatively normal retina surrounding the necrotic retina (Fig. 7-10, *J* and *K*).[150,157] They are occasionally found in the choroid in immunosuppressed patients.

The value of pyrimethamine (Daraprim), sulfadiazine, clindamycin, minocycline, trimethoprim-sulfamethoxazole, and corticosteroids in the treatment of active lesions in immune competent humans is uncertain.* Treatment probably has no value in preventing recurrences.[160] These drugs have been demonstrated to be effective in experimental infections with *Toxoplasma* in animals. There is only minimal evidence, however, that they are of value in the treatment of toxoplasmosis in

---

*References 108, 117, 122, 152, 156, 159, 160.

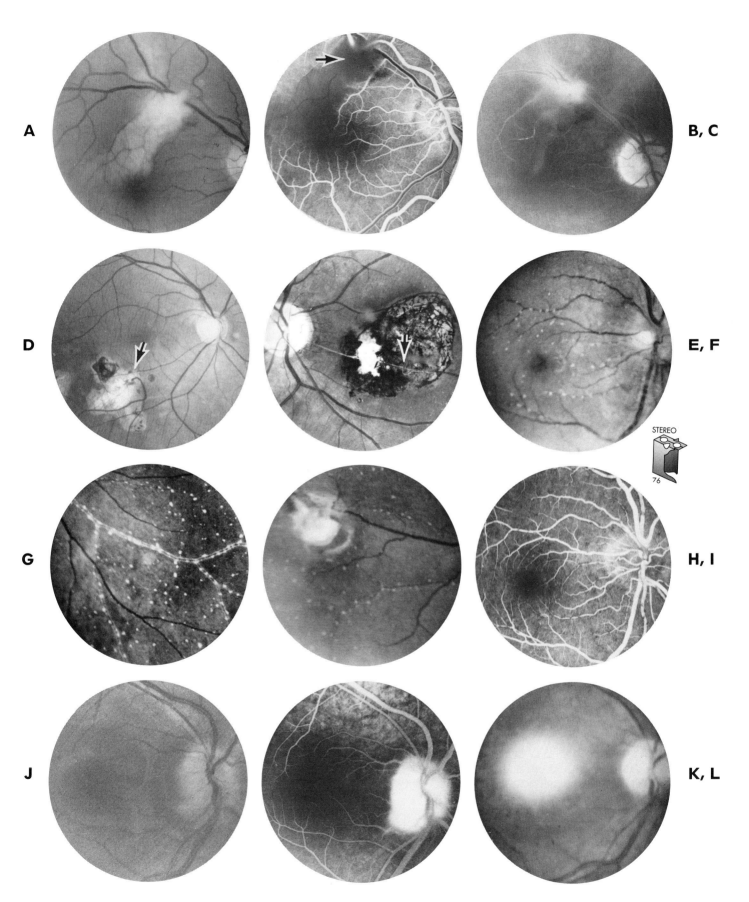

A

B, C

D

E, F

G

H, I

J

K, L

STEREO
76

619

immune competent humans.[119] Most authors agree that treatment is unnecessary and inadvisable in lesions outside the macular area. In cases where the center of the macula is threatened, use of one or more of the antibiotics in combination with systemic corticosteroids is probably advisable. Topical corticosteroids and mydriatics are indicated in the presence of accompanying iridocyclitis.

In patients with AIDS or who are immune compromised for other reasons, toxoplasmosis may cause a fulminant and widespread necrotizing retinitis as well as encephalitis.* Features of toxoplasmosis retinitis in patients with AIDS that differ from those in immune competent patients are multiple active lesions, infrequency of acute lesions arising adjacent to inactive scars, frequent involvement of both eyes, and frequent evidence of central nervous system involvement. Some of these patients present with multifocal, small, widely scattered lesions that may rapidly become confluent and produce a clinical picture identical to acute retinal necrosis.[154] Vitritis is usually present but may be less than that seen in immune competent patients with similar size retinal lesions. Clinically the retinal lesions may simulate those caused by cytomegalic inclusion disease,[135] although typically retinal hemorrhages are less prominent and vitritis more evident in lesions caused by toxoplasmosis. Toxoplasmosis encephalitis is a leading cause of death in patients with AIDS. Approximately 10% to 20% of patients with intracranial toxoplasmosis develop retinal lesions.[138] Involvement of the brain often occurs in the absence of ocular involvement. Toxoplasmosis may cause either a diffuse necrotizing encephalitis or discrete space-occupying intracranial lesions. In the former, computerized tomography may be normal; in the latter, it may show focal lesions with ring-shaped enhancement after contrast infusion.[138] Coinfections of the retina and choroid may occur.[135,138] The retinal and the brain lesions caused by *Toxoplasma* respond favorably to pyrimethamine and sulfadiazine, but recurrence of the infection is common after cessation of treatment.[135,138] Corticosteroid treatment may be necessary to reduce cerebral edema but probably is unnecessary in treatment of the retinitis since the intensity of the inflammation is less than in normal patients.[138] The results of serologic tests in patients with AIDS are unreliable. The presence of elevated IgM in as many as

---

*References 112, 113, 116, 126, 135, 138, 147, 149, 151, 154, 155, 173, 177, 180.

FIG. 7-10   Toxoplasmosis Retinitis.

A to **D,** Multifocal subacute recrudescent retinitis presumed to be caused by toxoplasmosis in a 17-year-old girl who was seen initially with a 1-month history of blurred vision in the right eye (**A**). Visual acuity was 20/100 in the right eye and 20/20 in the left eye. There were no vitreous cells. Note the multiple, small, gray lesions in the foveolar area *(arrows)*. Angiography at that time showed no evidence of fluorescein staining. Photographs taken at 2- to 3-month intervals over the subsequent several years showed a frequent change in the position of the gray lesions and no evidence initially of residual RPE changes (**B**). The visual acuity remained unchanged. Seven years after her initial examination, she returned with acute loss of vision in the right eye. There was a large area of acute retinitis in the right macula (**C**). Over the subsequent 9 years, she had other acute attacks. When the patient was last seen, visual acuity was 20/200 and a large atrophic macular scar was present (**D**).

E and **F,** Active toxoplasmosis retinitis (**E**) resolved and produced an elevated hypertrophic scar with retinochoroidal anastomosis (**F**).

G, Acute toxoplasmosis retinochoroiditis in an immune competent patient. Note the necrotic retina separated by Bruch's membrane *(arrow)* from a focal area of thickening of the choroid by granulomatous inflammation.

H, Focal area of granulomatous choroiditis and scleritis underlying toxoplasmosis retinitis in an immune competent adult.

I and **J,** Photomicrographs of acute focal necrotizing toxoplasmosis retinitis in the macular area of an immunosuppressed patient. Note the disturbance of the underlying RPE and the minimal nongranulomatous inflammatory reaction in the underlying choroid (**I**). A high-power view of the lesion in **J** shows encysted organisms *(left arrow,* **J**) and free organisms *(right arrow,* **J**) at the junction between viable and necrotic retina.

K, Electron micrograph showing encysted toxoplasma organisms.

G, courtesy Dr. Andrew P. Ferry, presented at Verhoeff Society, 1987; **H** from Hogan and Zimmerman[137]; **I** and **J** from Nicholson and Wolchok[150]; **L,** courtesy Dr. W. Richard Green.

12% of these patients suggests a high incidence of acquired infection.[148]

Solitary active toxoplasmosis retinitis may be simulated by other infections (*Candida,* pyogenic bacteria, bacteria of low pathogenicity in patients with AIDS, cat-scratch disease bacillus), ischemic retinopathy, and neoplasia (large-cell lymphoma, metastatic carcinoma to the retina). Retinal artery occlusion caused by a focal area of toxoplasmosis may appear similar to that occurring in patients with acute multifocal retinitis associated with cat-scratch disease or of unknown cause (Fig. 7-2), and patients with bilateral idiopathic recurrent

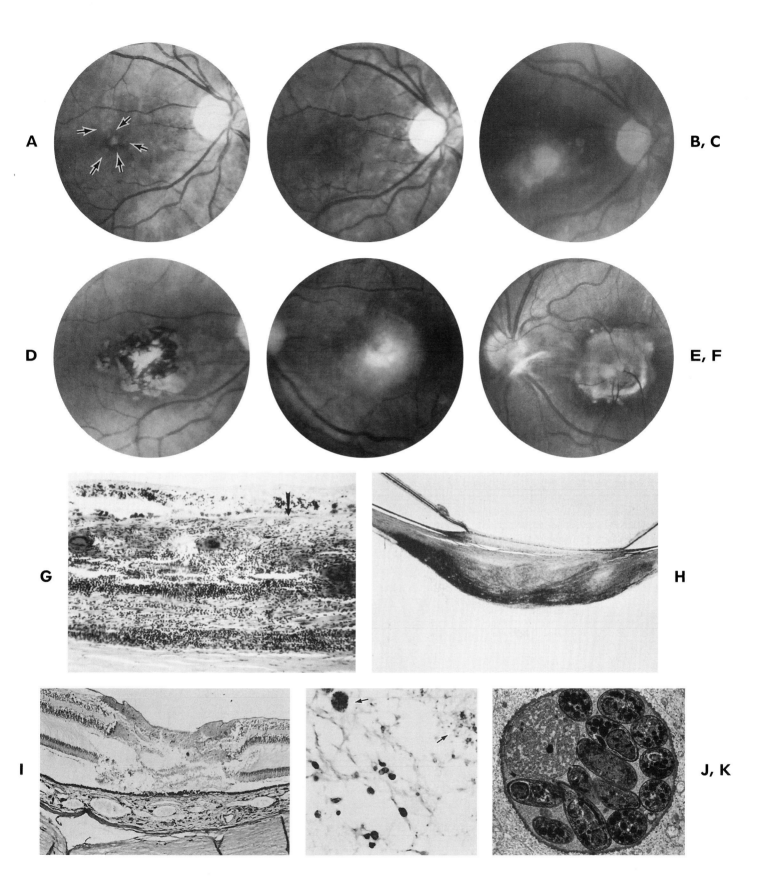

branch retinal artery occlusion (see Figs. 6-10 and 6-11). Multifocal outer toxoplasmosis may simulate punctate inner choroiditis (pseudo–presumed ocular histoplasmosis) (see Fig. 7-41), and diffuse unilateral subacute neuroretinitis (Figs. 7-11 and 7-12).

▼ MALARIA

Cerebral involvement with *Plasmodium falciparum* malaria major is an important cause of mortality, particularly in children in tropical regions.[181] Those manifesting papilledema and outer retinal edema outside the major retinal vascular arcades are more likely to die or survive with neurologic sequelae. Other fundus findings include retinal hemorrhages, cotton-wool spots, intraretinal edema, narrowed and obstructed arteries and small capillaries in the macula, and venous distension and tortuosity.

▼ TOXOCARIASIS CHORIORETINITIS

See Chapter 3.

▼ DIFFUSE UNILATERAL SUBACUTE NEURORETINITIS

Diffuse unilateral subacute neuroretinitis (DUSN) is a clinical syndrome characterized early by visual loss, vitritis, papillitis, retinal vasculitis, and recurrent crops of evanescent gray-white outer retinal lesions and later by progressive visual loss, optic atrophy, retinal vessel narrowing, and diffuse RPE degeneration occurring in one eye of otherwise healthy patients (Figs. 7-11 to 7-13).[186,188,189] DUSN is caused by at least two as yet unidentified species of nematodes that may wander in the subretinal space for 4 years or longer and cause progressive ocular damage.[186,188,204-207]

FIG. 7-11   Diffuse Unilateral Subacute Neuroretinitis (DUSN).

A to **C,** Note the subretinal motile nematode *(arrows)* and the subretinal gray-white inflammatory lesions in the inferior portion of the macula of a 14-year-old boy with acute visual loss in his right eye. Visual acuity was 20/200.

D to **G,** This young girl experienced rapid loss of vision in the right eye and was misdiagnosed as having acute posterior multifocal placoid pigment epitheliopathy. Note the coiled subretinal nematode *(arrow,* **D**). Angiography showed the subretinal lesions to be nonfluorescent early (**E**) and to stain later (**F**). Note also evidence of the retinal perivasculitis. The presence of the worm was unrecognized at the time of initial examination. Twenty-eight months later the patient's visual acuity was counting fingers only. Note the optic atrophy, narrowing of the retinal vessels, and diffuse degenerative changes in the RPE (**G**).

H and **I,** Late stages of DUSN in a 15-year-old Black boy whose visual acuity was 20/400. Note the optic atrophy, severe narrowing and sheathing of the retinal arteries (**H**), and widespread mottled depigmentation of the RPE with relative sparing of the macula angiographically (**I**).

J to **L,** Perivasculitis in a 27-year-old man with mild loss of vision in the right eye. The left eye was normal. The candle wax–dripping exudates suggested sarcoidosis (**J**). Medical evaluation was negative. Angiography revealed extensive staining (**K**). Four months later, the exudates had cleared (**L**). There was a vitreous tag *(arrow),* pallor of the optic disc, and multiple focal as well as diffuse changes in the peripheral RPE. A 700 μm motile subretinal nematode was found at the equator and was killed with argon laser. Six weeks later the visual acuity was 20/25 and there was no evidence of active retinitis.

(**D** to **G** from Gass J.D.M. et al.: Diffuse unilateral subacute neuroretinitis, Ophthalmology 85:521, 1978.[188])

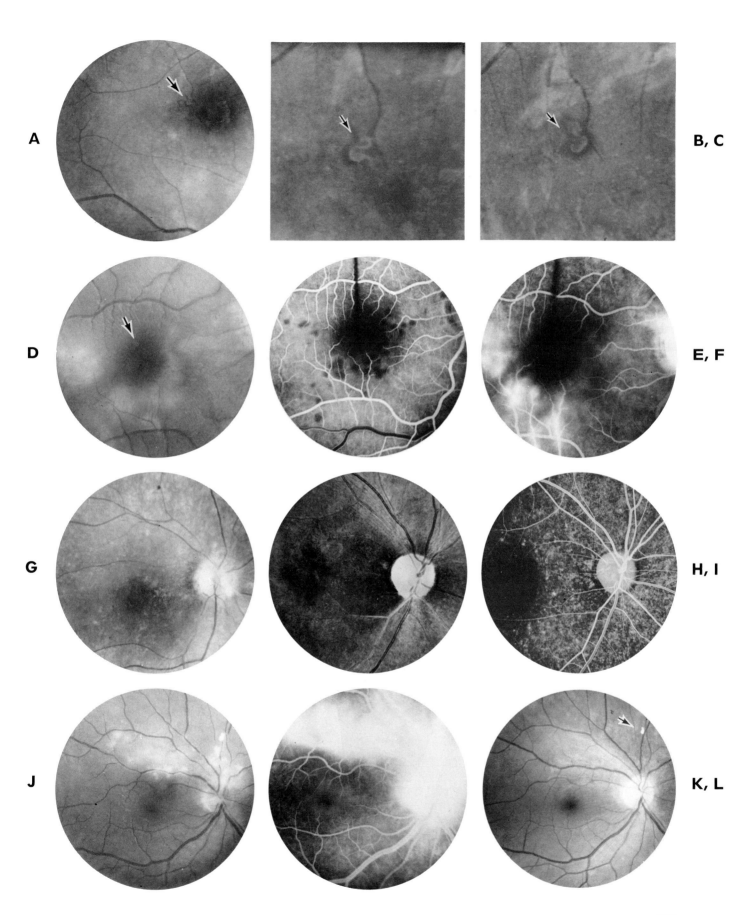

A

B, C

D

E, F

G

H, I

J

K, L

623

Patients may be seen initially during the early or subacute stage of the disease because of acute visual loss in one eye. Vitreous cells are invariably present but in some patients may be few in number. There may be mild to moderate swelling of the optic disc in the affected eye. There may or may not be any other visible changes in the fundus at that time. Visual acuity may be mildly or severely affected. A Marcus Gunn pupil reaction is usually present. A few patients may demonstrate a mild ciliary flush, anterior chamber cells, flare, and keratic precipitates. An occasional patient may have a hypopyon. Usually within several days or weeks, careful observation of these patients will disclose focal, gray-white or yellow-white lesions with fuzzy borders that involve the external layers of the retina and RPE (Figs. 7-11, *A* and *D;* 7-12, *A, B, D, F, G,* and *J;* and 7-13, *A* to *C*). The lesions are typically confined to a single zone frequently in the macular or juxtamacular areas. They typically fade from view, usually within several days, leaving minimal ophthalmoscopic evidence of change in the underlying RPE. Successive crops of these lesions may occur from week to week in the same or adjacent areas of the fundus (Fig. 7-12) and in some cases these may completely resolve only to recur again. Focal retinal hemorrhages, perivenous exudation similar to that seen in sarcoidosis (Fig. 7-11, *J*), and occasionally localized serous detachment of the retina may occur. In some patients during the early course of the disease the visual acuity may be normal or minimally affected. Over a period of weeks or months, diffuse as well as focal depigmentation of the RPE occurs (Fig. 7-11, *G* to *I*). These changes are usually least prominent in the central macular area. The multifocal areas of depigmentation, which are most numerous in the midperipheral fundus, may simulate those seen in the presumed ocular histoplasmosis syndrome. Accompanying these progressive changes in the RPE is a gradual narrowing of the retinal arterioles and increasing pallor of the optic disc (Fig. 7-11, *D* to *I*). Pigment migration into the overlying retina is uncommon. In many cases, particularly in young children, the disease is not detected until the defective vision is found on a school vision examination. Choroidal neovascularization and disciform lesions may occur in some patients. In general the degree of optic disc pallor and retinal vessel narrowing parallels that of central visual loss, but striking exceptions occur.

The disease is caused by a motile, white, often glistening nematode that is gently tapered at both ends and varies in length from 400 to 2000 μm, with

FIG. 7-12   Diffuse Unilateral Subacute Neuroretinitis.

A to **C,** This 14-year-old boy was hospitalized because of suspected ocular histoplasmosis or toxoplasmosis. He had noted rapid loss of vision in the left eye. Over a 5-week period, crops of evanescent gray-white subretinal lesions appeared and disappeared (**A**) before a motile subretinal nematode (*arrows,* **B** and **C**) was noted. The nematode disappeared, and 3 years later the patient's visual acuity was counting fingers only. He had optic atrophy, some narrowing of the retinal vessels, and diffuse changes in the RPE.

D to **I,** This young man developed acute visual loss in the right eye associated with a few vitreous cells and multiple outer retinal lesions confined to the macula of the right eye. These lesions obstructed choroidal fluorescence early and stained late (**E**). The diagnosis was acute posterior placoid multifocal pigment epitheliopathy. Over the next 11 days the crops of white lesions moved inferotemporally. The subretinal worm (*arrow,* **D,** and *inset,* **E** and **F**) was found in retrospective review of photographs and photocoagulation (**H**) resulted in a focal scar (**I**) and resolution of the disorder.

J to **L,** This 16-year-old girl presented with a 3-month history of visual loss in the right eye. Visual acuity was 20/40 and there was a 2+ afferent pupillary defect. Vitreous inflammation and multifocal outer retinal lesions were present in the right macula. A subretinal worm was suspected (*arrow,* **J**) but did not show movement. One week after 2 g of thiabendazole daily for 2 days, all of the subretinal lesions had disappeared except for the area of intense retinitis and vitreous reaction (**K**), presumably caused by death of the worm. Five months later her acuity was 20/25. Note the scar at the site of the focal retinitis (*arrow,* **L**).

(A to C from Gass J.D.M. et al.[188]; J to L from Gass et al.[187])

its largest diameter being approximately ¹⁄₂₀ of its length (Figs. 7-11, *A* to *D;* 7-12, *B, C, F,* and *G;* 7-13, *A* to *D* and *G* to *L*).[186,188,204-208] It propels itself by a series of slow coiling and uncoiling movements and less often by slithering snakelike movements in the subretinal space. It may be found during any stage of the disease and should be looked for even in patients with advanced optic atrophy, narrowing of the retinal vessels, and degenerative changes in the RPE.[188] The second eye is rarely affected. There are at least two endemic areas in the United States for this disease. In the southeastern United States, the Caribbean islands, and Latin America the nematode varies in length from approximately 400 to 700 μm.[183,186] In the other endemic area, the north midwestern United States, it measures approximately 1500 to 2000 μm in length (Fig. 7-13, *A* to *F*). Individual cases have been reported from Germany and Ghana.[182,199,203] A careful search

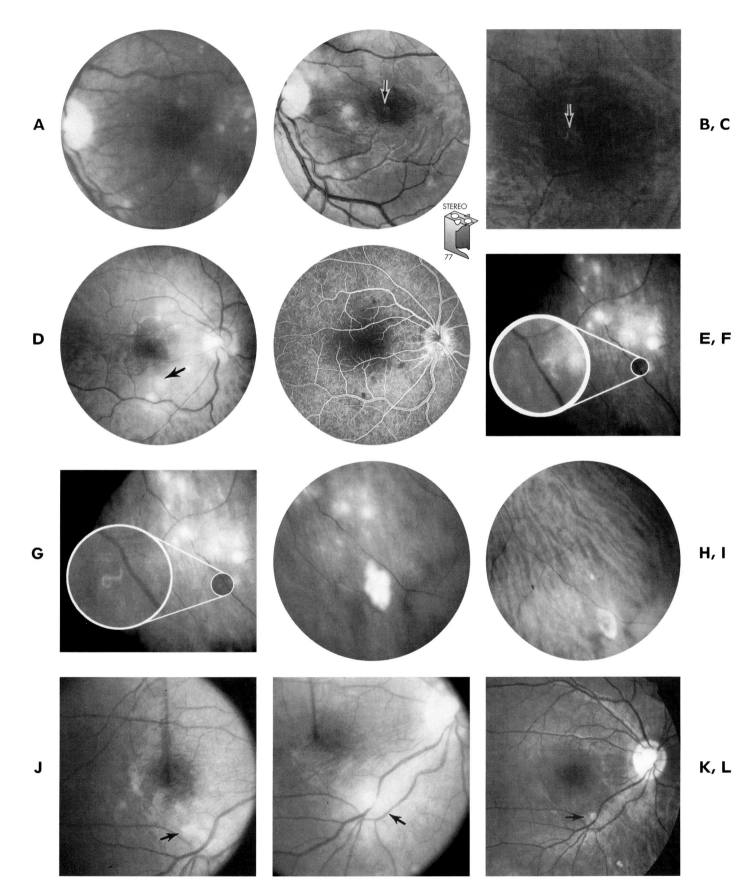

A

B, C

D

E, F

STEREO
77

G

H, I

J

K, L

with a fundus contact lens is required to locate the smaller worm, which is only barely visible with indirect ophthalmoscopy using a 15-diopter lens. The larger worm is relatively easy to detect using indirect ophthalmoscopy. The worm is most likely to be found somewhere in the vicinity of active deep retinal white exudative lesions that probably are caused by a toxic inflammatory reaction to material left in the wake of the wandering nematode. These lesions and the worm are more frequently located in the extramacular areas. The magnification and wide field of view provided by a fundus contact lens and the fundus camera are ideal for locating these worms.

Fluorescein angiography in the early stages of the disease usually demonstrates leakage of dye from the capillaries on the optic nerve head. The gray-white areas of active retinitis are nonfluorescent early but stain during the later phases of angiography (Figs. 7-11, *E* and *F,* and 7-12, *E*). Prominent perivenous leakage of dye may occur in some patients in the earliest stage of the disease (Fig. 7-11, *K*), and there may be minimal or no angiographic evidence of damage to the RPE. As the disease progresses, greater evidence of loss of pigment from the RPE is manifested angiographically as an irregular increase in the background choroidal fluorescence (Fig. 7-11, *I*).

The electroretinogram in the affected eye is usually reduced in all stages of the disease and often is moderately or severely reduced, with the b-wave being affected more than the a-wave in the later stages of the disease.[188,189,198] Rarely the ERG may be extinguished.

The identification of the worm is unknown. Serologic tests for *Toxocara canis* are typically negative.[186] The stools are free of ova and parasites. Eosinophilia is infrequently detected. These patients do not manifest evidence of systemic disease. A small nematode was excised by means of eye-wall biopsy in one patient (Fig. 7-13, *G* to *I*). Although there were some features that suggested the possibility of *Ancylostoma caninum,* its precise identification could not be made.[185] Cunha de Souza recently extracted the subretinal nematode through a retinotomy after pars plana vitrectomy (Fig. 7-13, *L*).[183a] Unfortunately, because of poor fixation, definite identification of the worm was not possible. Grossly it showed similar features to the worm removed in Miami,[185] and to a 380-μm-long subretinal worm successfully aspirated from the eye of a patient by professor Kuhnt in 1886 (Fig. 7-13, *K*).[200] Dr. Dwight D. Bowman recently reviewed the pictures of the worm removed by Cunha

FIG. 7-13 Diffuse Unilateral Subacute Neuroretinitis (DUSN).

A to F, These figures illustrate large subretinal nematodes associated with DUSN in patients, all of whom were from the midwestern United States. **A** shows the nematode *(arrow)* in a 65-year-old woman who experienced rapid loss of vision in her right eye. **B** and **C** illustrate movement of a similar-sized subretinal worm *(arrows)* in a 13-year-old boy with rapid loss of vision in the right eye. Note the blurred optic disc margin and coarse mottling of the RPE. **D** to **F** illustrate argon laser photocoagulation of a large worm *(upper arrow,* **D**) in a 23-year-old man. Note that the S-shaped RPE imprint of the worm *(lower arrow,* **D**, and *arrow,* **E**) in the central macular area, where it apparently had lain for some time before moving superiorly, has disappeared in **F**.

G to J, Small subretinal nematode *(arrow),* that initially was located in the macula of a 18-year-old Puerto Rican boy (**G**). Several months later the patient's visual acuity was counting fingers and the nematode had migrated to the midperiphery of the fundus. Reversed C-shaped applications of argon laser photocoagulation (**H**) were used to chase the worm anterior to the equator. An eye-wall resection was done. Note the worm lying in the subretinal space *(arrows,* **I** and **J**).

K, In January 1886 Professor H. Kuhnt in Jena aspirated a nematode from the posterior vitreous eye of a 31-year-old man (his drawing, **K**). He interpreted the worm, which was 0.38 mm in length, as either a filarial worm or adolescent form of *Strongylus.* In 1986 Dr. P.C. Beaver's interpretation of Kuhnt's drawing was probable *Toxocara canis* (personal communication).

L, This worm (600 μm long and 30 μm wide) was extracted from the subretinal space via pars plana vitrectomy in a patient with the typical findings of DUSN. On gross examination it was initially interpreted as a probable third stage of *Toxocara canis* but more recently has been interpreted as *Ancylostoma caninum.* Unfortunately the worm decomposed before microscopic examination could be done. The patient had no serologic evidence of having toxocariasis.

(**A to C** and **G** from Gass J.D.M. and Braunstein R.A.: Arch. Ophthalmol. 101:1689, 1983; copyright 1983, American Medical Association[186]; **D** to **F** from Raymond et al.[206]; **K** from Kuhnt[200]; **L** from Cunha de Souza et al.[183a]; Bowman.[181a])

de Souza (Fig. 7-13, *L*) and concluded that it is most likely *Ancylostoma caninum.*[181a] It is of interest that three of the last 10 patients with a subretinal worm identified at the Bascom Palmer Eye Institute had cutaneous larval migrans months or several years before the onset of ocular symptoms. *Ancylostoma caninum,* a hookworm of dogs, is a common cause of cutaneous larval migrans in the southeastern United States. The infective third-stage larva of *A. caninum* is approximately

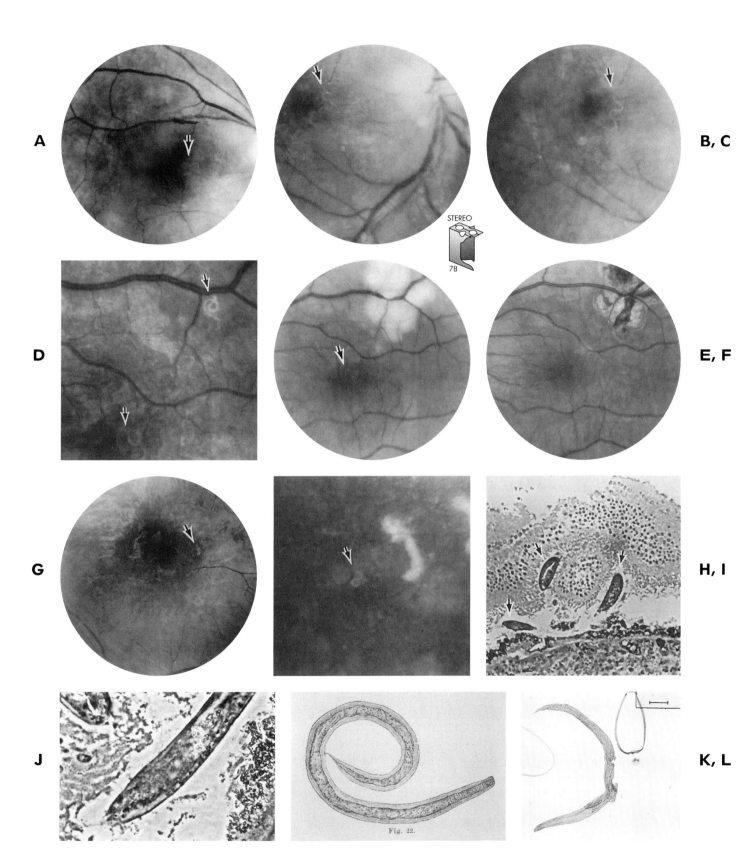

STEREO
78

Fig. 22.

650 μm in length and is capable of surviving in host tissue, including that of humans, many months and probably years without changing size or shape.[202] The second-stage larvae of *Baylisascaris procyonis,* a nematode found in the intestinal tract of raccoons, has been suggested as a possible cause for DUSN.[184,190,191,193-197] Although this nematode, whose larval stage measures 1000 to 1500 μm in length, is a common cause for meningoencephalitis in other animals, it has been rarely incriminated in similar disease in humans.[184,191] The infrequent history of exposure to raccoons and the absence of central nervous system involvement in over 100 patients with DUSN seen at Bascom Palmer Eye Institute make *Baylisascaris* highly unlikely as a cause for DUSN in the southeastern United States, the Caribbean, and Latin America.[201] In DUSN the size of the nematodes, the geographic distribution of reported cases, the clinical picture, and the infrequency of serologic evidence of infection with *Toxocara canis* make it unlikely that *T. canis* is the cause of DUSN.

The pathogenesis of DUSN appears to involve a local toxic tissue effect on the outer retina caused by worm byproducts left in its wake as well as a more diffuse toxic reaction affecting both the inner and outer retinal tissues.[186,188,189,192] This latter reaction is manifest initially by rapid loss of visual function and alteration of the electroretinogram and later by evidence of loss of the ganglion cells (optic atrophy) and narrowing of the retinal vessels. The variability of the inflammatory signs and tissue damage seen in these patients suggests great differences in host immune response to the organism.

Only one eye believed to be affected by DUSN has been studied histopathologically.[189] The eye was enucleated 15 months after the onset of the disease, which was clinically suggestive of the early acute and subacute phases of DUSN. This occurred at a time before recognition of the cause of this syndrome, and it is probable that the subretinal worm was lost during sectioning of the eye during gross examination. Histopathologically the eye showed evidence of a nongranulomatous vitritis, retinitis, and retinal and optic nerve perivasculitis with extensive degeneration of the peripheral retina, mild degeneration of the posterior retina, mild optic atrophy, mild degenerative changes in the RPE, and a low-grade, patchy, nongranulomatous choroiditis. No evidence of eosinophilia or a worm was present. Failure to find sufficient structural retinal and optic nerve damage to account for the patient's light perception–only vision at the time of enucleation suggested that the loss of visual function was partly explained on a pathophysiologic rather than an anatomic basis.

Photocoagulation, the treatment of choice, is effective in destroying the worm without causing significant intraocular inflammation (Figs. 7-12, *H,* and 7-13, *E*). Locating the worm, which is always found in the vicinity of the white outer retinal lesions when they are present, may require prolonged and repeated examinations. When migrating in the subretinal space, the worm is relatively isolated from the effect of orally administered thiabendazole or diethylcarbamazine, except in those patients with moderate to severe vitreous inflammation.[186] In these latter patients, thiabendazole has been successful in causing death of the worm (Fig. 7-12, *J* to *L*).[187] The presence of a focal area of intense retinitis and fading of the other white lesions 7 to 10 days after oral administration of thiabendazole is evidence of success of the treatment and is followed by rapid and permanent resolution of the disease. Another strategy for treatment that has proved successful in one patient, after numerous unsuccessful attempts to locate the worm in an eye with minimal inflammation, was the application of scatter laser applications surrounding and within the zone of outer retinal white lesions, to disrupt the blood–retinal barrier before administration of thiabendazole.

Diffuse unilateral subacute neuroretinitis is a great imitator. In the acute and subacute stages, it may simulate diseases associated with unilateral papillitis, papilledema, retrobulbar neuritis, and vitritis. When associated with perivasculitis, it may simulate retinal sarcoidosis (Fig. 7-11, *J* to *L*). When associated with active outer retinal white lesions, it may mimic acute multifocal posterior placoid pigment epitheliopathy (Fig. 7-11, *D*), serpiginous choroiditis, evanescent white dot syndrome, Behçet's disease, multifocal outer toxoplasmosis, and the pseudo–presumed ocular histoplasmosis syndrome (Fig. 7-12, *A* and *B*). In the later stages it may be misdiagnosed as unilateral optic atrophy caused by retrobulbar or intracranial lesions, the presumed ocular histoplasmosis syndrome, unilateral retinitis pigmentosa, posttraumatic chorioretinopathy, and chorioretinal atrophy after ophthalmic artery occlusion (Fig. 7-11, *H* and *I*). It is important to consider the diagnosis in patients with the early findings of the disease because photocoagulation of the worm will prevent further loss of visual function and occasionally will be followed by visual improvement.

▼ ONCHOCERCIASIS

Epidemiologic studies have suggested that onchocerciasis may be responsible for an ocular syndrome that occurs frequently in patients living in endemic areas, particularly in western equatorial Africa.[209-211,214-217,220] Symptomatically and ophthalmoscopically this syndrome closely simulates some of the tapetoretinal dystrophies. The patient's primary complaints are loss of peripheral vision and night blindness. The primary funduscopic findings consist of varying degrees of atrophy of the RPE, choroid, and retina, with the most prominent involvement being initially in the posterior fundus, particularly in the juxtapapillary area and often in rather discretely outlined zones temporal to the macular area (Fig. 7-14). These changes are usually associated with progressive pallor of the optic disc and occasional optic disc swelling and focal areas of slight swelling of the choroid. Longitudinal studies of lesions of the posterior segment in patients with untreated onchocerciasis have demonstrated progressive changes that include live microfilaria, intraretinal hemorrhages, cotton-wool patches, intraretinal pigment, white and shiny intraretinal deposits, RPE window defects, and progressive depigmentation at the edge of chorioretinal scarring at rates up to 200 μm/year.[218] Ivermectin and mebendazole therapy did not appear to alter the progression of depigmentation of the scars. These observations suggest that onchocercal chorioretinitis is associated with early changes in the retina and RPE, and that the retinal disease may progress rapidly. Angiographically, both the optic disc and the area of choroidal swelling show evidence of fluorescein staining. Varying degrees of RPE hyperplasia and subretinal fibrosis occur. Disciform detachment of the macula is not part of the picture. Peripheral visual field loss is often out of proportion to the atrophy of the choroid and retina, and much of the visual loss is believed to be caused by optic nerve damage. Microfilaria 100 to 200 μm in length have been observed biomicroscopically within or beneath the retina in patients with normal fundi and visual function.[214] The fact that organisms occur in the choroid of these patients who have filaria throughout the body

does not necessarily prove that they are the cause of the fundus changes. The observations, however, of acute transient multifocal areas of staining at the level of the RPE and progressive changes in the optic nerve in these patients following treatment with diethylcarbamazine citrate lend some support to the concept that *Onchocerca volvulus* is responsible for the fundus changes occurring chronically in these patients.[211,220] There is some evidence to suggest that these fundus changes may be more prominent in patients who have received treatment over a prolonged period of time, compared to those who have not. Thus, it appears that onchocerciasis, either alone or in concert with some other organisms or genetic factors, is responsible for a night-blinding disease and, in at least some endemic areas, is responsible for severe disabling posterior ocular disease. The pathogenesis of this disease may prove to share some features with that of the pseudo–retinitis pigmentosa sine pigmenti that occurs in patients with diffuse unilateral subacute neuroretinitis (see p. 622). It is uncertain whether autoimmune mechanisms play a role in the pathogenesis of onchocercal chorioretinitis.[212,222]

Unlike diethylcarbamazine, which quickly eliminates microfilaria from the eye and is associated with reactive and occasionally functional ocular changes, ivermectin eliminates microfilaria slowly from the anterior chamber of the eye over a period of 6 months and causes minimal ocular inflammatory reaction or functional deficit. This slow action of ivermectin may be attributed in part to its inability to cross the blood–aqueous barrier,[213] and or the mode of action of ivermectin, which may inactivate (paralyze) rather than kill the microfilaria.[221] A single dose of ivermectin, 150 μg/kg, repeated once a year leads to marked reduction in skin microfilaria counts and ocular involvement. It has no long-term effect on adult worms. There is no significant exacerbation of either anterior or posterior segment eye disease. Treatment leads to a marked and prolonged improvement in the ocular status. Safety and effectiveness permit its use on a massive scale and it promises to revolutionize treatment of this disease.[219,223]

▼ DIROFILARIASIS

There are many species of *Dirofilaria* in wild and domestic animals worldwide. All species found in the subcutaneous tissues of humans are accidental zoonotic infections. *Dirofilaria repens* and *D. immitis* have been removed from the vitreous of the human eye.[224-228] The adult *D. immitis* varies in length from a few centimeters to 35 cm. It is possible that the large intraocular nematode illustrated in Fig. 7-15, *J* to *L,* may have been a dirofiliarial worm.

FIG. 7-14   Chorioretinal Degenerative Changes Seen in Patients with Onchocerciasis.

A to **E,** Chorioretinal degeneration presumed to be caused by onchocerciasis in an African. Note in the composite (**A**) and macular area (**B**) of the left fundus, the narrowing of the retinal vessels, pallor of the optic disc, and the large geographic areas of atrophy and hyperplasia of the RPE. Similar changes were present in the right eye (**C**). Angiography reveals some loss of the choriocapillaris in the areas of geographic RPE atrophy (**D** and **E**).

F to **H,** Similar but less severe changes with relative sparing of the central macular area in another patient with onchocerciasis.

(Courtesy Dr. Hugh R. Taylor.)

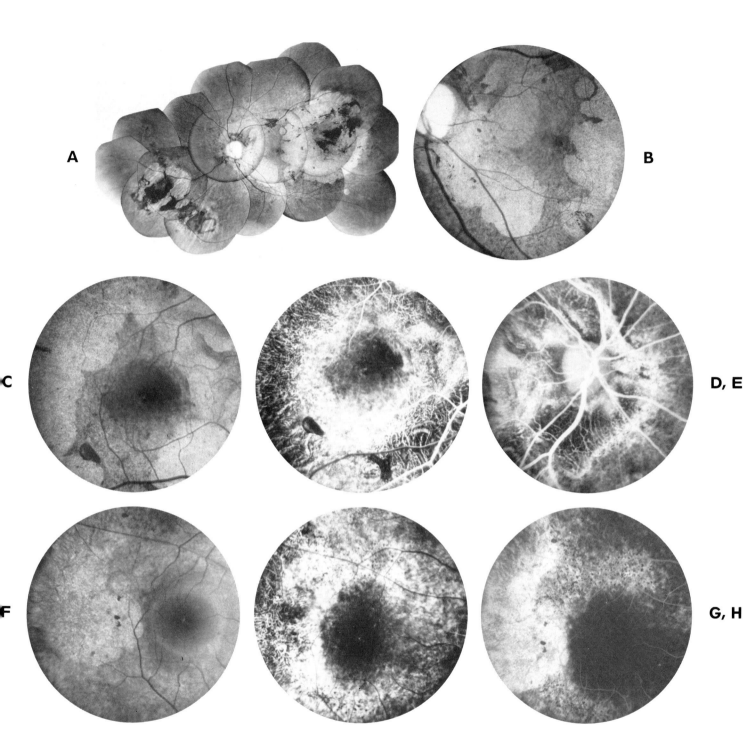

▼ GNATHOSTOMIASIS

Gnathostoma spinigerum is the most common species known to cause human gnathostomiasis. The worm is primarily found in Asia. The definitive hosts are cats and dogs. It has been reported in mammals in North America. Its life cycle involves three larval stages that develop in fresh water. In the first stage, as a free-living form, it is ingested by copepods and matures to the second larval stage. The copepods are ingested by fish, snakes, and other animals that drink contaminated water. The worm completes its third larval stage in them. At this stage humans may become facultative hosts by eating the raw infected intermediate host. It is at the third stage that the larvae may migrate for many years in humans, causing inflammation in multiple organ systems, including the skin, lungs, central nervous system, and eye (Fig. 7-15, *A* to *E*).[229-232] The worm has involved the posterior ocular segment in at least two instances.[229,232] In two cases the worm was successfully removed by vitrectomy (Fig. 7-15, *A* to *E*).[229]

▼ OTHER NEMATODE INFECTIONS OF THE EYE

Goodhart and associates[233] have reported the successful removal of a 9-mm nematode, either *Porrocaceum* or *Hexametra,* from the subretinal space of a young man with uveitis and total retinal detachment (Fig. 7-15, *F* to *I*). The adult stages of these large ascarid larvae are found in the stomach and intestine of carnivorous reptiles, birds, or mammals. The larvae ordinarily develop within the tissues of small mammals before becoming infective for the final host. This patient probably ingested the eggs from soil or water contaminated with the feces of an owl, hawk, snake, or other carnivorous final host.

FIG. 7-15   Gnathostomiasis.

A to C, Faintly visible macular star (**A**) and intravitreal *Gnathostoma* (**B** and **C**) in a young Vietnamese girl complaining of blurred vision in the right eye. Her visual acuity was 20/60. *Arrows* indicate the mouth of this nematode, whose body is filled with red blood. Note the stomal end of the worm is attached to a vitreous strand. The worm was initially mistaken for a partly occluded retinal vascular anomaly. The worm was successfully removed via the pars plana.

D to **E**, Intravitreal gnathostoma with arrows indicating the stoma.

Subretinal *Porrocaceum* or *Hexametra*.

F to **I**, This large subretinal nematode was surgically removed via the pars plana in this 27-year-old man who presented with a 3-week history of blurred vision and floaters and a 3-day history of only light perception in his left eye. A 9000-μm-long nematode (**G**, *arrows*) was found in the subretinal space at the time of surgery. After a retinotomy the nematode was grasped with forceps (**H**) and was extracted from the eye. Ten months later the vitreous was clear (**I**) and his visual acuity was 20/80.

Large Subretinal Nematode of Uncertain Type.

J to **L**, A long, coiled, motile subretinal nematode, estimated to be approximately 25 mm long (*arrows,* **J**), was found in the eye of this Latin American air force pilot who noted recent loss of vision in his left eye. Note the unusual pattern of fluorescein staining of the subretinal exudate enveloping the nematode. Several weeks later examination in Miami revealed a pigment figure in the left macula, and a nonmotile, partly decomposed worm in the subretinal space (*arrows,* **K** and **L**) at the temporal edge of the left macula. Note the swollen end segment of the worm *(small arrows)* and the small-diameter, tightly coiled loops of the worm *(large arrow,* **L**). The type of nematode could not be identified.

(**A** to **C**, courtesy of Dr. Stephen R. Fransen; **D** to **E** from Bathrick et al.[229]; **F** to **I** from Goodhart et al.[233])

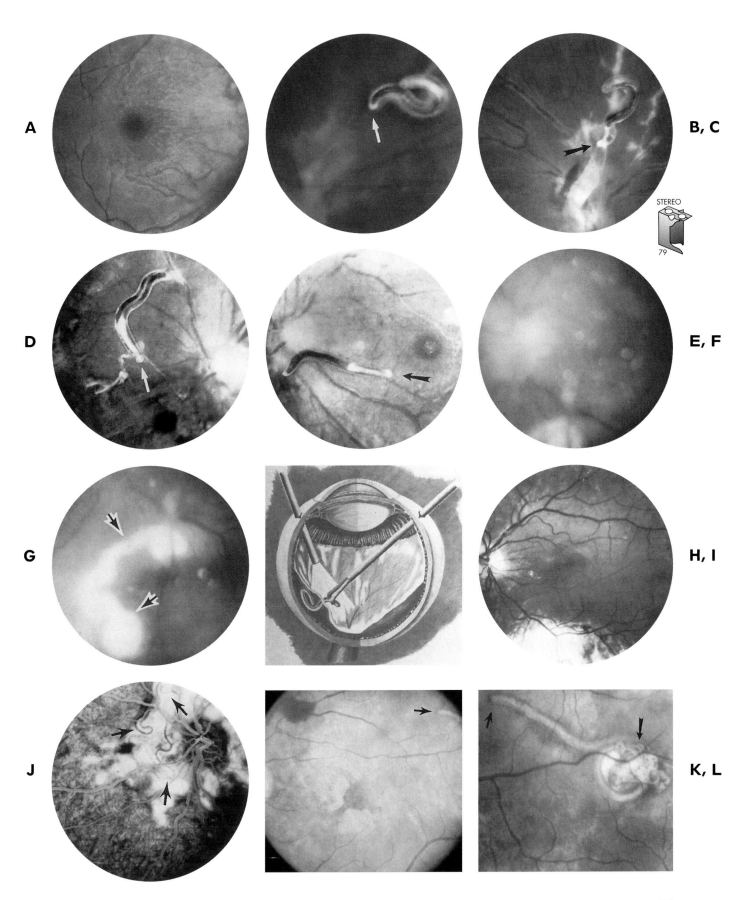

▼ OPHTHALMOMYIASIS

The term "myiasis" describes the invasion of the living vertebrate organism by the larval form (maggot) of certain flies in the order Diptera. The larvae responsible for intraocular invasion (ophthalmomyiasis interna) belong mostly to those genera that are obligatory tissue parasites, that is, those that exclusively require living host tissue for the completion of their larval development. These include the cattle, sheep, horse, deer, reindeer, rodent, squirrel, chipmunk, rabbit, and human botflies.[249] Flies identified as causes of ophthalmomyiasis interna include *Hypoderma bovis, Cuterebra* sp., *Gastrophilus intestinalis, H. lineatum, Oedemagena tarandi, Oestrus ovis, Cochliomyia hominivorax,* and *Rhinoestrus purpureus.*[237,239,241,249,252,259] The rodent botfly maggot *Cuterebra* (Fig. 7-16, *J* and *K*) and *Hypoderma* are probably responsible for most cases of ophthalmomyiasis interna in the United States of America.[234a,239,241,252,255] The eggs or larvae may be transported to the human corneal or conjunctival surface either by the adult fly, by a secondary vector such as a tick or a mosquito, or by the patient's hands. Most patients give no history of being struck in the eye by a fly. The maggots either may remain in the periocular tissues (ophthalmomyiasis externa)[235,250,256,263] or may bore their way through the ocular coats and come to lie in the anterior chamber, posterior chamber, or subretinal space (Figs. 7-16 and 7-17).* The reaction of the eye to the larval invasion varies. Signs of inflammation usually develop only after the death of the maggot. In some cases the maggot gains entrance into the subretinal space and over a period of months makes many excursions back and forth across the breadth of the fundus, creating an unusual pattern of cross-hatching or "railroad" tracks in the RPE (Figs. 7-16 and 7-17).[241,243,245] During its entrance through the sclera and choroid and its course beneath the retina it may cause one or more small subretinal hemorrhages (Fig. 7-16, *D* to *F*). In some cases it exits from the eye without causing any symptoms, despite widespread damage to the RPE in the macular area (Figs. 7-16, *A* to *C,* and 7-17, *A* and *B*).[245,245a] In one case a *Cuterebra* maggot was found in the conjunctiva of a boy who presented with a subconjunctival hemorrhage and subretinal hemorrhage and tracks.[245a] In some cases the maggot may die in the subretinal space

*References 234, 239-245, 247, 248, 251, 254, 257-262.

FIG. 7-16   Ophthalmomyiasis Interna.

A to C, This asymptomatic 16-year-old girl had a visual acuity of 20/10 bilaterally. Her left eye was normal. Note the crisscrossing tracks throughout the right eye. These tracks were demonstrated best with fluorescein angiography (**B** and **C**). The maggot had exited the eye.

D, Motile subretinal maggot associated with a small amount of subretinal blood.

E, Submacular hemorrhage caused by a maggot that has migrated into the vitreous cavity.

F, Maggot lying on the anterior surface of the retina. Note the surrounding subretinal tracks and the round retinal hemorrhages *(arrows)*.

G to I, Subretinal tracks in a Black woman with a history of loss of central vision for many months in the right eye. Visual acuity in the right eye was 20/200 and in the left eye was 20/20. Note the cross-hatched subretinal tracks and optic atrophy in the right eye (**G** and **H**) and the normal left fundus (**I**). No maggot was identified in the right eye.

J, Scanning electron micrograph of first instar larva of the rodent botfly, *Cuterebra.*

K, *Cuterebra jellisoni* botfly.

(**D** from Fitzgerald C.R., Rubin M.L.: Arch. Ophthalmol. 91:162 1974; copyright 1974 American Medical Association[243]; **E,** courtesy Dr. T. F. Schlaegel Jr; **F,** courtesy Dr. W. S. Grizzard; **G to I,** courtesy Dr. Ralph F. Hamilton Jr; **J** from Custis et al.[239]; **K** from Baird.[234a])

and cause a localized toxic reaction and a scar. In other cases it may enter the vitreous cavity, where usually it dies soon afterward, probably from lack of nutrition. The inflammatory reaction that follows varies from a minimal vitritis to an intense endophthalmitis. The caliber of the retinal vessels and the color of the optic nerve head are usually unaffected. Optic atrophy and visual loss in a few cases, however, may occur (Fig. 7-16, *G*).[240] Invasion of the cornea has occurred.[253] Only rarely are both eyes affected, and this occurred in a patient from Guam.[261] (See discussion of Lytico-Bodig after this section.)

Linear and arcuate tracks in the ocular fundus should always suggest the possibility of ophthalmomyiasis. The tracks are less numerous and more easily recognized in the peripheral fundus. In the posterior pole the tracks may be so numerous that their confluence may be mistaken for a variety of diffuse inflammatory, traumatic, or degenerative diseases affecting the RPE (Figs. 7-16, *A,* and 7-17, *A* and *B*). In such cases fluorescein angiography is especially valuable in silhouetting the tracks (Figs. 7-16, *B* and *C*). Although other organisms, such as *Toxocara canis,*

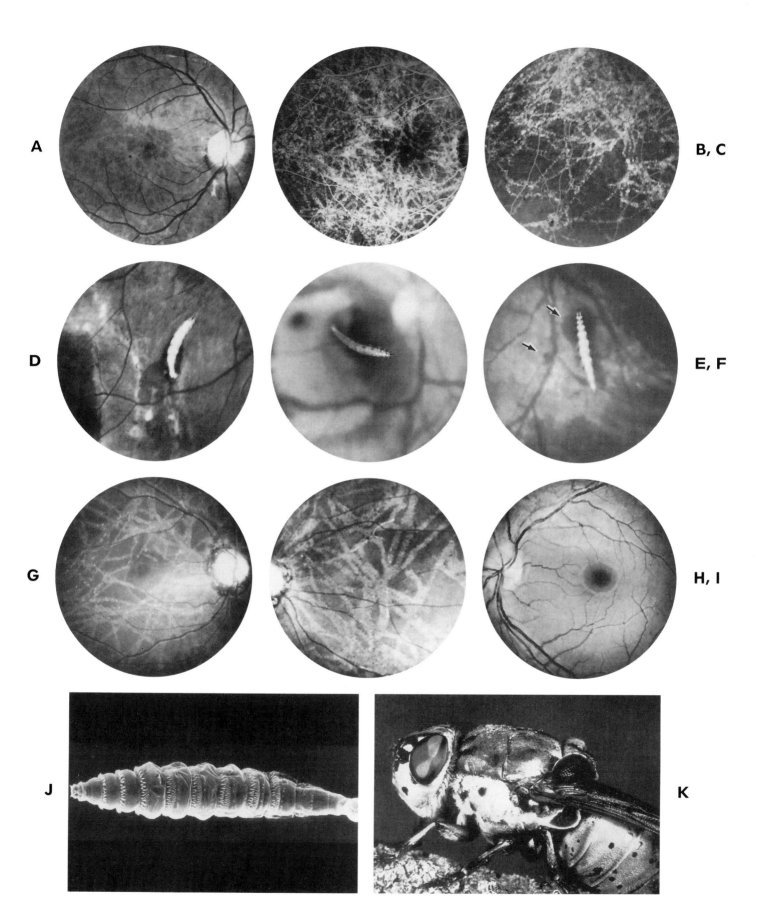

635

the nematodes responsible for diffuse unilateral subacute neuroretinitis, and trematodes, may migrate into the subretinal space, they do not produce the widespread pattern of broad RPE tracks that are believed to be pathognomonic for myiasis. The larger of the nematode larvae responsible for diffuse unilateral subacute neuroretinitis may produce a curvilinear arrangement of hypopigmented spots that simulates slightly that of subretinal tracks. The curvilinear depigmented bands or beadlike arrangement of atrophic chorioretinal scars that may occur, usually at the equator in the presumed ocular histoplasmosis syndrome (POHS) and pseudo-POHS may be mistaken for the tracks in myiasis (see Fig. 3-39, C).[251] I have seen two patients with an extensive network of subretinal fibrous strands and demarcation lines following spontaneous reattachment of a chronic rhegmatogenous retinal detachment incorrectly diagnosed as myiasis. A positive clinical diagnosis of ophthalmomyiasis can be made only with the visualization of the white or semitranslucent segmented maggot, tapered slightly at both ends (Figs. 7-16, D to F, and 7-14, A).

In the presence of significant intraocular inflammation, the initial treatment of intraocular myiasis should be directed toward the reduction of inflammation with the use of corticosteroids. If inflammation cannot be controlled, surgical removal of the maggot is indicated. If the maggot is alive and the eye is free of inflammation, the clinician may elect to observe the patient carefully for spontaneous exit of the maggot from the eye. If treatment of a subretinal maggot is elected, photocoagulation is probably preferable to removal of the organism by sclerotomy. The maggot should be watched until it moves beyond the macular and juxtapapillary area before photocoagulation treatment is begun. In two patients treated with photocoagulation, no unusual inflammatory reaction occurred.[243,244]

A pigmentary retinopathy simulating ophthalmomyiasis interna is endemic in the native Chamorro Indians (Fig 7-17, C and D).[236,238,246,261] This retinopathy is particularly prevalent in patients who also have Lytico-Bodig (also known as amyotrophic lateral sclerosis-Parkinsonism-dementia complex of Guam). No maggot has been

FIG. 7-17 Ophthalmomyiasis Interna.

Time-lapse composite photographs showing movement of a maggot (arrow) in the subretinal space. This worm was destroyed with photocoagulation without causing significant intraocular inflammation.

B, A composite photograph of an asymptomatic patient who was seen for glasses. His visual acuity was 20/20. Note the extensive pattern of subretinal tracks and the clumps of pigmentation temporal to the macula and surrounding the optic disc (arrows). No maggot was visible in the eye. The patient was seen again several years later, and the visual function and fundi were unchanged.

Subretinal Tracks in Lytico-Bodig.

C to D, Subretinal tracks (**C** and **D**) presumed to have been caused by a fly maggot in two Chomoro Indians from Guam. Note the "dead-end" track (arrow, **C**).

E, Histopathology of a track observed clinically in a Chomoro Indian shows hypopigmentation of the pigment epithelium (between the arrows), a few subretinal pigment-laden macrophages, and some thickening of Bruch's membrane.

(**A,** courtesy Dr. Constance R. Fitzgerald; **B** from Gass and Lewis[245]; **C** and **D,** courtesy Dr. S. D. Thomas Hanlon.)

observed in any of these patients. Histopathologic examination of eyes with the tracks has revealed focal attenuation of the RPE but no evidence of inflammation or a larva (Fig. 7-17, E).[236] Population surveys in Guam suggest that all of the patients with the subretinal tracklike lesions are 50 years of age or older.[246] Other than the frequent association of the retinopathy in patients with Lytico-Bodig, there is no other evidence that the retinal and central nervous system share a common etiology. The pathogenesis of both disorders is unknown. The remarkable similarity of the retinopathy to that in myiasis suggests that it may have been caused by a fly that was prevalent in Guam before the Japanese occupation in World War II. The decimation of livestock and other wildlife hosts, during the occupation, in addition to the widespread use of insecticides at the end of the war, may have eradicated all of the botflies, which are no longer found in Guam.[246]

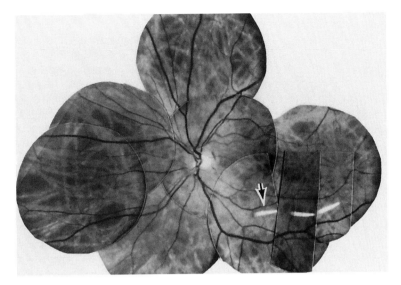

A

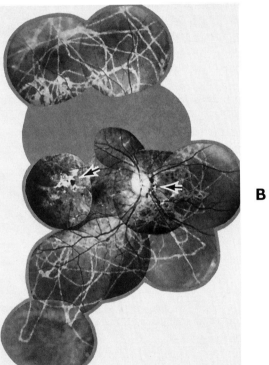

B

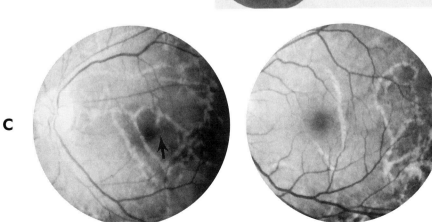

C

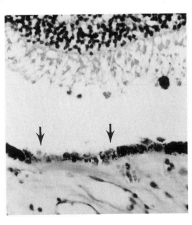

D, E

▼ CYSTICERCOSIS

See Chapter 3.

▼ ECHINOCOCCOSIS

Taenia echinococcus lives in the intestine of the dog, from which its eggs may be transmitted to the human stomach. From here the young embryos penetrate the intestinal tract and may be carried to various organs, rarely the eye. The hydatid cysts have been described beneath the retina and within the vitreous.[264,265]

▼ INTRAOCULAR TREMATODA

Trematode infection of the human eye is uncommon and most cases have involved lung flukes (*Paragonimus* species) and schistosomiasis.[266] There are several reports of human infection with the migratory larvae (mesocercariae) of *Alaria* in North America and the eye was involved in three patients.[267-269] Ocular manifestations include pigmentary retinal tracks, areas of active or healed retinitis, retinal hemorrhages, and signs of diffuse unilateral subacute neuroretinitis (Fig. 7-18). The trematodes may persist in the retina and vitreous for at least several years after onset of the ocular infection (Fig. 7-18).[268] *Alaria* species occur as adults in the intestine of carnivorous mammals. Their life cycle involves a succession of three hosts: the snail, the first intermediate host; a tadpole or frog, the second intermediate host; and a carnivore definitive host. The most common means of human infection is by eating inadequately cooked frogs' legs.

Schistosomiasis

Trematodes that inhabit the blood vessels of humans are referred to as schistosomes. Dickinson and coworkers reported an unique case of eccentric multifocal choroiditis that resembled acute posterior multifocal placoid pigment epitheliopathy and serpiginous choroiditis in a 17-year-old man with visual loss and an itchy rash on his forehead of 2 weeks' duration. He had recently returned from Tanzania.[266] Histologic examination of the skin lesions revealed ova of *Schistosoma mansoni*.

▼ RETINOPATHY ASSOCIATED WITH RICKETTSIAL DISEASES

Rocky Mountain spotted fever is an acute febrile eczematous disease caused by *Rickettsia rickettsiae* and transmitted by the wood and dog tick. It is not

FIG. 7-18   Intraocular Trematode.

A to E, Subretinal trematode causing gray subretinal exudation (*arrows,* **A** and **B**) in the right macula of a healthy 35-year-old Asian man. Note evidence of peripheral irregularly pigmented tracks caused by the trematode (**A**). Magnified views of the right macular area show movement of the subretinal trematode (*arrows,* **C** to **E**). The trematode was destroyed with laser photocoagulation.

F to I, Vitritis and periphlebitis (**F**) caused by a subretinal trematode in a healthy 38-year-old Asian man complaining of visual loss in the left eye. His visual acuity was 4/200. Following treatment with sub-Tenon's capsular corticosteroids his vision improved and irregular pigmentary tracks became evident (**G**). Twenty-one months after recurrent episodes of vitreous inflammation, a motile trematode (*arrow,* **H**) that was encysted was found in the vitreous (**H**) and was removed via pars plana vitrectomy. The trematode was identified as *Alaria mesocercaria* (**I**). Note the oral sucker *(left arrow),* ventral sucker *(right arrow),* and penetration glands *(P).* The patient's visual acuity returned to 20/50.

(**A** to **I** from McDonald et al.[268])

confined to the Rocky Mountain area, with nearly half of the cases occurring in the south Atlantic states.[273] Ocular findings that may accompany the acute illness include petechial lesions on the bulbar conjunctiva, conjunctivitis, anterior uveitis, papilledema, retinal venous engorgement, cytoid bodies, retinal hemorrhages, and retinal vascular occlusion.* Fluorescein angiography shows evidence of capillary nonperfusion in the region of the cottonwool patches, leakage of dye from the retinal vessels in the vicinity of the patches, and evidence of venous obstruction. In exanthematous cutaneous lesions, the organisms invade the nuclei of the capillary endothelial cells, proliferate, and destroy the capillary endothelial cells. Necrosis of the intima and media causes thrombosis and microinfarcts. It is probable that the pathogenesis of the retinal vascular changes is similar. The fundus findings usually resolve without causing visual loss following treatment of the disease with antibiotics, such as chloramphenicol and tetracycline.

Similar fundus findings have been reported in other rickettsial diseases, including endemic typhus.[270,274,275,278]

---

*References 271, 272, 276, 277, 279, 280.

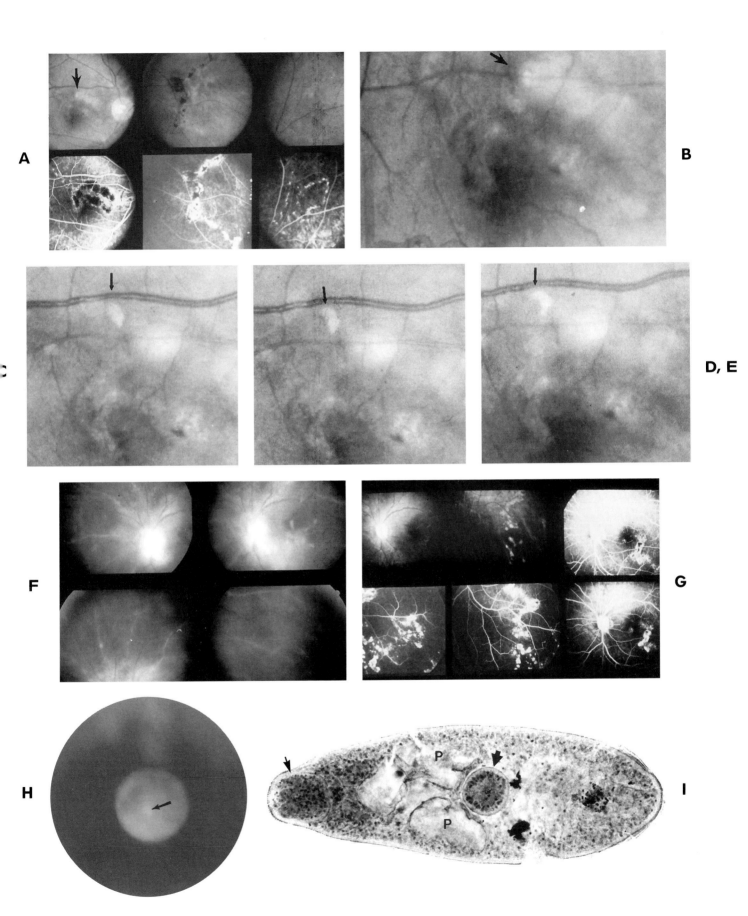

▼ VIRAL DISEASES

Herpes virus retinochoroiditis

The herpes family of viruses under a variety of circumstances causes a funduscopic picture of necrotizing retinochoroiditis that is sufficiently characteristic to suggest strongly the diagnosis. This family includes the herpesvirus simiae, which only rarely infects humans. These viruses also produce a similar histopathologic picture of necrotizing retinitis and underlying choroiditis. In areas adjacent to, as well as remote from, the areas of retinal necrosis, intranuclear inclusion bodies may be found by light microscopy, and viral particles by electron microscopy in the retina, RPE, and optic nerve cells. Specific identification of the particular herpesvirus depends on viral cultures, immunofluorescent histologic studies, and polymerase chain reaction for the detection of virus genome.[439] Vitreous or chorioretinal biopsy and culture may be indicated in patients with suspected herpes infection or other infection, macular threatening lesions, suspicion of malignancy, and when the results are expected to influence therapy or patient care. Ideally the specimen should be divided into three parts for light and EM study, immunohistochemistry, and microbiology and tissue culture. Biopsy should only be undertaken if there is support of an experienced immunopathologist and the availability of necessary laboratory capabilities, including immunohistochemistry, electron microscopy, and tissue culture.[286] The quality of the cytologic material obtained from vitreous biopsy is probably similar in specimens obtained by needle aspiration and vitreous suction cutter aspiration done without infusion solution.[289]

Herpes simplex retinochoroiditis

Herpes simplex retinochoroiditis occurs most often in neonates with herpes simplex encephalitis.[282,283,290,295] It is usually caused by herpes simplex type 2 and is acquired from the mother's genital tract at birth. The risk of a newborn acquiring infection from a mother with herpes infection is approximately 50%.[292] Ocular involvement occurs in approximately 20% of neonatal infants with herpes simplex virus (HSV). It varies widely in severity from conjunctivitis to necrotizing retinochoroiditis.[291] The retinitis begins as multicentric areas of retinal opacification that frequently become confluent (Fig. 7-19). It is associated with variable amounts of retinal hemorrhage. The disease in infants is usually fatal. In some patients chorioretinal scars may be evident at birth.[295] Hypopigmented skin lesions, brain lesions, and

FIG. 7-19   Herpes Simplex Retinochoroiditis and Encephalitis.

A to F, This 18-month-old boy had a 4-day history of lethargy and low-grade fever accompanied by seizures on the second day of his illness. He was comatose on admission to the hospital. A lumbar puncture revealed 219 white blood cells with 63% monocytes in the cerebrospinal fluid. The protein was 189 mg/dl. Computed tomography revealed a left temporal lobe lesion. Funduscopic examination revealed multifocal areas of retinitis, perivasculitis, and hemorrhage (**A** and **B**). The patient died on the fourteenth day of his illness. Gross examination of the eyes revealed hemorrhagic retinitis (**C**). A photomicrograph showed retinal necrosis, retinitis (**D**), perivasculitis, choroiditis, and viral intranuclear inclusions (*arrow,* **E**) that were most common in the inner nuclear layer. Electron microscopy revealed intranuclear viral particles typical of herpesvirus (*arrow,* **F**). Similar findings were present in the brain.

(**A** and **F** from Cibis et al.[282])

quiet retinal scars suggest that intrauterine infection probably occurred during the second trimester.[295] First trimester infection probably produces teratogenic defects. Third trimester infection produces active neonatal HSV infection. Late ophthalmologic manifestations of neonatal herpes simplex virus infection include optic atrophy, chorioretinal scars, corneal scars, and cataract.[284,295,296] Coarse hyperpigmented areas may occur preequatorially in clinically silent cases. There is a high incidence of ocular changes in those patient with neurologic disease resulting from neonatal herpes simplex. Visual impairment in patients who are severely neurologically handicapped as a result of HSV infection is caused mainly by cortical blindness.[284]

Herpes simplex retinochoroiditis may occur alone or in association with encephalitis in either healthy adults* or immunosuppressed patients.[293,298] Herpes simplex virus has been isolated from eyes with the acute retinal necrosis syndrome in otherwise healthy adult patients with primary HSV-1 or recurrent HSV-1.[294,297] Magnetic resonance imaging studies may show evidence of spread of the virus posteriorly to both optic tracts and lateral geniculate ganglia.[288] Thus, the clinical disease shares many features with the "von Szily" experimental model for HSV retinitis in the mouse.[299]

---

*References 281, 285, 287, 288, 293, 297, 322.

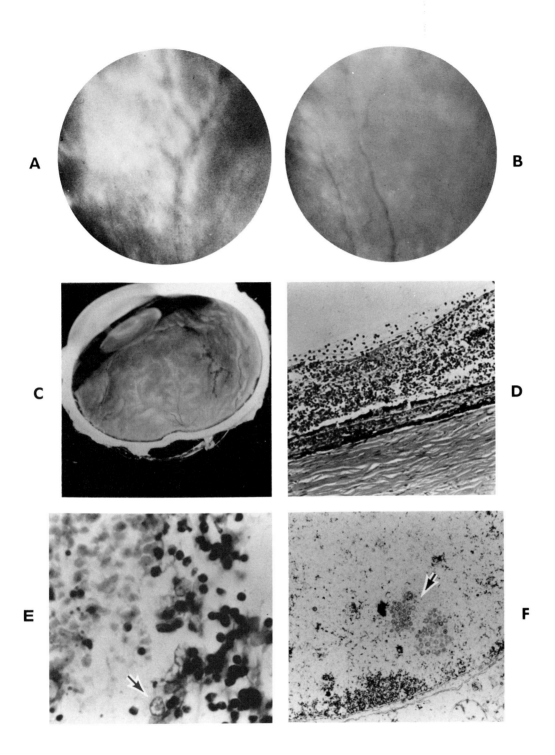

Herpesvirus B

Herpesvirus simiae (herpes B virus) is an alpha herpesvirus endemic in monkeys of the *Macaca* species, in which it causes stomatitis and conjunctivitis.[300-303] The virus is extremely virulent in humans, 75% of whom die of an ascending myelitis. It may cause multifocal necrotizing retinitis, optic neuritis, and panuveitis in one or both eyes of humans.[301,302]

Cytomegalovirus retinochoroiditis and optic neuritis

Although as many as 81% of adults have complement fixation antibodies indicating previous exposure to cytomegalovirus (CMV), manifest disease is rare in otherwise healthy individuals and occurs primarily in the unborn infant and the immunosuppressed patient.[315,358]

Congenital cytomegalic inclusion disease is characterized by a syndrome of prematurity, microcephaly, intracranial calcification, chorioretinitis, optic atrophy, hepatosplenomegaly, anemia, and thrombocytopenia.[365]

Postnatally acquired infections occur most commonly in immunosuppressed individuals with the acquired immune deficiency syndrome (AIDS; see p. 656), renal allografts, or systemic malignancies or while receiving high-dose corticosteroids.* Approximately 30% of patients with AIDS will develop CMV retinitis.[342] Cytomegalovirus retinitis is the first manifestation of AIDS in approximately 2% of patients and results in the initial diagnosis of AIDS in approximately 15% of patients.[362] Survival after the diagnosis of AIDS may be significantly shorter if CMV retinopathy is the initial manifestation of syndrome.[341] The ophthalmoscopic features of the acute stage of necrotizing retinitis include multiple granular yellow-white areas that become confluent and are associated with retinal hemorrhages, vascular sheathing, and sharp margins separating the active area of necrotizing retinitis from the surrounding retina (Fig. 7-20, *A, E,* and *F*). The funduscopic appearance has been likened to that of pizza. The segmental distribution of the hemorrhagic lesions along major retinal vessels may be mistaken for branch vein occlusion.[307] Cytomegalovirus retinitis infrequently begins in the central macular area.[335,370] The retinitis spreads much like a brush fire, leaving an atrophic retina and a mottled RPE along its trailing edges (Fig. 7-20, *D*). Vitreous cells may or may not

*References 304, 306, 307, 309-313, 316, 317, 320, 321, 327, 350, 351, 354, 356, 357, 371.

FIG. 7-20 Cytomegalovirus (CMV) Retinitis in Patients Receiving Corticosteroid and Antimetabolite Therapy Following Renal Transplantation.

A to D, This 35-year-old woman noted paracentral scotomata in both eyes. In the right eye she had an active wedge-shaped area of retinitis associated with hemorrhages and perivascular cuffing (**A**). In the left eye she had large geographic areas of chorioretinal scarring at sites of previous retinitis (**D**). Angiography of the area illustrated in **A** revealed widespread collapse of the retinal vascular bed in the area of acute retinitis and multiple focal areas of staining within the lesion (**B** and **C**). Eleven years later, visual acuity in the right eye was 20/200. She had extensive peripheral chorioretinal scarring, vitritis, and cystoid macular edema. The left eye had a dense cataract, and visual acuity was only light perception.

E and F, A wedge-shaped area of hemorrhagic necrotizing retinitis in the inferior macular region of the right eye of a 36-year-old woman. She died soon afterward, and histopathologic section of the eye depicted in **E** showed a sharp junction between the relatively normal retina and the thickened retina in which the normal retinal elements were replaced by extensive infiltration of large mononuclear cells containing prominent intranuclear inclusions (**F**). Note the discrete line of juncture between the involved and uninvolved RPE *(arrow)*.

Cytomegalovirus (CMV) Retinitis in Patients with AIDS.

G to I, Progressive CMV retinitis and optic neuritis occurring over a 2-month period. Note the extensive exudation into the macular area (**H**) 1 month after photograph in **G**, and evidence of early resolution of the retinitis after ganciclovir treatment in **I**.

J, Smoldering slowly progressive CMV retinitis. Note active gray border *(arrows)* surrounding the atrophic retina.

K to L, Frosted branch angiopathy accompanying CMV retinitis.

(**E** and **F** from DeVenecia et al.[321])

accompany the retinitis. Cytomegalovirus retinitis infrequently poses an immediate threat to loss of vision on presentation.[335] It is a slowly progressive, necrotizing retinitis that appears in either a fulminant hemorrhagic or granular pattern. As the infection progresses, the leading edge of the infection is followed by a healing process that results in a thin fibroglial scar. Small refractile deposits and larger yellow-white plaquelike deposits occur within areas of healed CMV retinitis. These large plaques do not appear calcified or refractile, yet histologically these fibroglial scars may be highly calcified.[324,326] It is important not to mistake these lesions clinically for active lesions of CMV. Early spontaneous resolution of CMV reti-

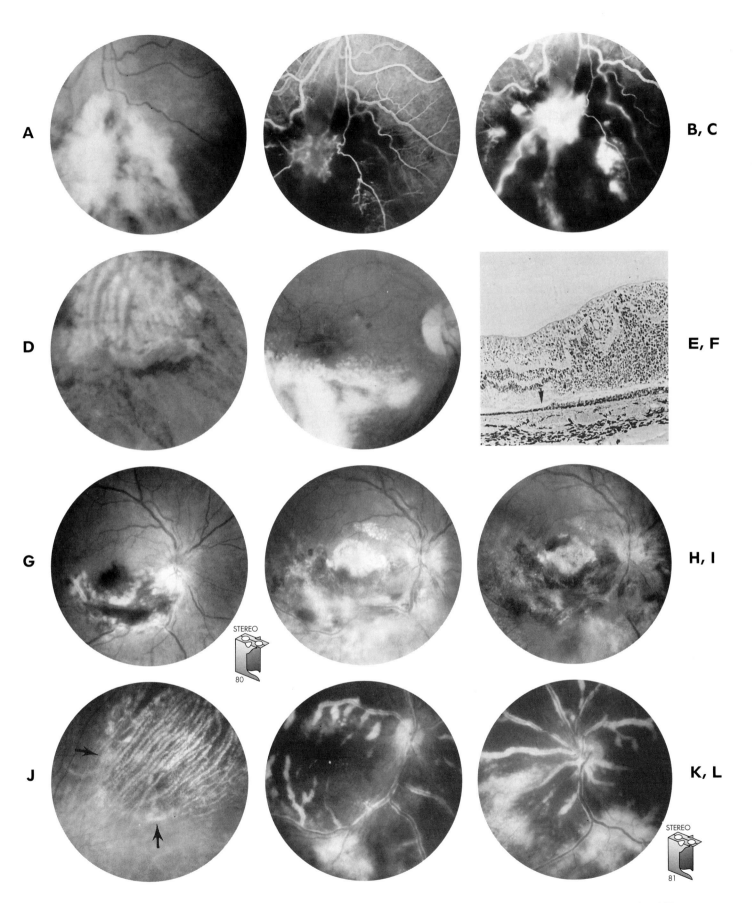

A

B, C

D

E, F

G

H, I

J

K, L

STEREO
80

STEREO
81

643

nitis may account for chorioretinal scars found on initial examination of patients with AIDS.[326]

Infection of the optic disc and juxtapapillary retina is often associated with severe visual loss (Fig. 7-20, *G*).[336] In some cases involvement of the optic disc and juxtapapillary retina causes visual loss as the result of intraretinal exudation and macular star formation and with exudative macular detachment (Fig. 7-20, *H*).[332] Patients with low CD4+ counts, usually less than 100, are at increased risk for developing CMV retinitis and HIV-related noninfectious retinal vasculopathy.[347] Fluorescein angiography demonstrates evidence of retinal vascular occlusion and permeability alterations in the areas of hemorrhagic and necrotizing retinitis (Fig. 7-20, *B* and *C*).

Severe sheathing of the retinal vessels appearing like frosted branches of a tree, simulating that occurring in idiopathic frosted retinal periphlebitis, may accompany CMV retinitis (Fig. 7-20, *K* and *L*).[333,334,341,360,367] This may be associated with signs of vitreous and anterior chamber inflammation. Fluorescein angiography shows no occlusion or stasis but does demonstrate late leakage from the sheathed vessels. This perivasculitis usually clears within several weeks after antiviral and corticosteroid treatment.[334,355] Corticosteroids may not be necessary.[355] The CMV retinitis, however, often continues to show evidence of graying along its margin (Fig. 7-20, *J*). This smoldering retinitis may extend slowly and is a sign of persistent activity. Cystoid macular edema occurs infrequently in patients with AIDS, particularly in those with less severe states of immunosuppression.

Disc neovascularization may develop in patients with CMV retinitis, and it may regress spontaneously.[348] Exudative and rhegmatogenous retinal detachment may complicate CMV retinitis.[323,330-332,339,343,361] Approximately 15% to 30% of patients with CMV retinitis develop a rhegmatogenous retinal detachment. The differential diagnosis may be difficult because small or ragged holes may be difficult to visualize.[312,350] Patients with chronic vitritis may lose central vision because of cystoid macular edema.

Histopathologically, the areas of active retinitis are sharply circumscribed from the normal-appearing retina (Fig. 7-20, *F*).[311,321,364] The retina is thickened, and its laminar architecture is markedly disrupted by the presence of many enlarged cells containing prominent Cowdry type A intranuclear eosinophilic inclusions with surrounding clear zones, giving the cells an owl's-eye appearance. The underlying RPE is typically disrupted and varying degrees of chronic inflammatory cells are present in the underlying choroid. Intranuclear inclusions may be identified in RPE, optic nerve, and vascular endothelial cells of the choroid. Electron microscopy demonstrates viral particles typical of the DNA viruses as well as prominent electron-dense cytoplasmic bodies.[309,321]

The clinical diagnosis is made by demonstrating virus in the patient's urine and by a rise in complement fixation and neutralization titers. The virus can be cultured from the anterior chamber in eyes with hypopyon,[313,317] saliva, buffy coat of the blood, tears,[320] vitreous, and the retina.[309,371]

Dual infection of retina with human immunodeficiency virus type 1 and cytomegalovirus occurs but its role in producing fundus changes or in the enhancement of other infections is uncertain.[325,363] Autopsy studies of patients with AIDS have shown evidence suggesting that bilateral CMV retinitis may be a marker for HIV encephalitis.[325] These studies have failed to demonstrate evidence that HIV is a cause for cotton-wool patches.

Ganciclovir is the treatment of choice in patients with CMV retinitis.* Eighty percent to 90% of patients with CMV retinitis will demonstrate evidence of prompt resolution of the retinitis following induction dosages of intravenously administered ganciclovir. Those with visual loss associated with exudative detachment often experience improvement in visual acuity.[332] Thirty percent to 50% will reactivate while on maintenance treatment.[338,340] Ganciclovir is a viral static drug that does not eliminate the virus or suppress expression of all virus genes.[353] It appears to function by limiting viral DNA synthesis and subsequent packaging of viral DNA into infectious units.[353] There is also evidence that decreasing the amount of corticosteroid therapy has a favorable effect on CMV retinitis in some cases. Approximately 33% of patients with AIDS receiving ganciclovir for CMV retinitis will demonstrate evidence of persistent smoldering retinitis, that is, graying along margins of the zones of retinitis. The smoldering retinitis may slowly extend without evidence of other activity seen in retina (Fig. 7-20, J). In some cases, however, this persistent gray border may not progress and biopsy of such lesions has shown no evidence of viral particles.[345] Fundus photographs and visual fields are helpful in detecting evidence of progression.[308,335,341]

Intravitreal administration of ganciclovir appears to be a safe and effective alternative in the management of CMV retinitis in patients with AIDS.[314,319,329,337] It is particularly useful in patients with severe neutropenia, and those wishing to remain on systemic ZDV.[318,319] The potential value of sustained-release intravitreal ganciclovir in the treatment of CMV retinitis has been demonstrated clinically, experimentally, and pathologically.[305,359,366] Combination treatment with foscarnate and ganciclovir may be helpful in the 10% to 20% of patients whose CMV retinitis is resistant to ganciclovir alone.[328,346,349] Side effects of ganciclovir treatment include frequent bone marrow toxicity, indefinite intravenous treatment required, and frequent relapses on maintenance treatment; the drug cannot be used with AZT because of bone marrow toxicity.[357,369] Foscarnate may be used with AZT, which may also have a favorable effect on CMV retinitis.[326,328] Ganciclovir and foscarnate appear to be equivalent in controlling CMV retinitis and preserving vision, however, patient survival is somewhat longer with foscarnate.[369]

The mean survival of patients with AIDS after development of CMV retinitis has increased since 1981.[341] Patients treated with ganciclovir live longer after diagnosis (median 7 months) than untreated patients (median 2 months). Location of retinal lesions appears to have no prognostic significance for survival. The interval from diagnosis of AIDS to diagnosis of CMV retinitis (median 9 months) has not increased.

Surgeons often use vitrectomy and silicone oil in the management of retinal detachment in patients with AIDS because this technique is effective in these complicated detachments and the operating time is reduced.* Disadvantages of this technique include hyperopic shift, reduction in accommodative amplitudes, and cataract. The visual results after surgery are generally poor and they continue to worsen after surgery. Indications for repair will change with advances in medical treatment of AIDS.[339] Ocular toxoplasmosis and herpes zoster virus (HZV) are other causes of detachment in AIDS. Retinal detachment occurs more frequently after HZV than after CMV retinitis. The mean survival after repair of retinal detachment caused by CMV retinitis in patients with AIDS varies from 4 to 37 months.[323,331]

Use of laser treatment to prevent the progression of CMV retinitis appears to be ineffective.[368]

Herpes zoster virus (HZV) retinochoroiditis and optic neuritis

Most patients with herpes zoster ophthalmicus and chicken pox demonstrate no involvement of the choroid, retina, and optic nerve. Nevertheless there are several clinical syndromes in which chorioretinal and optic nerve involvement by the HZV may cause severe visual loss.†

---

*References 323, 331, 339, 343, 350, 352, 361.
†References 376, 388, 394, 415, 421, 438, 450.

---

*References 314, 319, 335, 338, 340-342, 344, 348, 350.

645

Focal choroiditis

During the convalescent stage of chicken pox or herpes zoster ophthalmicus an occasional patient may develop one or more yellow-white placoid choroidal lesions throughout the posterior fundus (Fig. 7-21, *A* to *C*).[377] (See also Chapter 3.)

Congenital varicella syndrome

Infants of mothers who had varicella infection during the second trimester may demonstrate, at birth or soon afterward, systemic findings included bulbar palsy, mild hemiparesis, cicatricial skin lesions, developmental delay, and learning difficulties as well as ocular manifestations including chorioretinal atrophy, chorioretinal scars simulating toxoplasmosis, hypoplastic optic discs, attenuated electroretinographic and evoked occipital potential amplitudes, congenital cataract, and Horner's syndrome (Fig. 7-21, *C*).[426] The HZV titer to IgM is typically negative.

Focal retinitis, neuroretinopathy, ischemic optic neuropathy, and retinal vascular occlusion

In children and adults the external manifestation of herpes zoster ophthalmicus or chicken pox may be associated occasionally with optic disc swelling, macular star, branch or central retinal artery or vein occlusion, and multifocal retinitis (Fig. 7-21, *D* to *I*).[383,385,387,402,418] In children and adults HZV can cause a granulomatous arteritis and an ocular syndrome similar to that produced by cranial arteritis, including ophthalmoplegia, ischemic optic neuropathy, hypotony, phthisis bulbi, and contralateral hemiplegia (Fig. 7-21, *J* to *K*).[372,406,438,459]

Acute retinal necrosis (herpetic thrombotic retinochoroidal angiitis and necrotizing neuroretinitis)

Herpes zoster virus is probably the primary cause of acute retinal necrosis, a clinical syndrome that develops in one or both eyes of typical healthy individuals of all ages. Initially, it is characterized by the development of mild anterior uveitis, followed within a few days by vitreous inflammation, pain, occasionally glaucoma, and usually a rapid decline in visual function caused by a rapidly progressing occlusive retinal arteritis, necrotizing retinitis, and optic neuritis associated with progressive inflammatory infiltration of the vitreous (Figs. 7-22 to 7-24).* The retinal whitening often begins

---

*References 375, 376, 380, 382, 397, 401, 403, 404, 407, 412, 413, 417, 420, 425, 427, 432, 440, 444, 448-450, 454, 456-458, 461.

646

FIG. 7-21   Herpes Zoster–Varicella Virus Chorioretinitis.

A and **B,** This 37-year-old woman with chicken pox developed episcleritis, visual loss, exudative macular detachment and focal choroiditis in the left eye. She showed rapid improvement of all signs and symptoms following treatment with acyclovir.

C, This patient sustained marked visual loss following a severe episode of chicken pox when she was 4 years of age. Her visual acuity was 20/200 bilaterally.

Ischemic Optic Neuropathy in Association with Herpes Zoster Ophthalmicus.

D to **G,** Acute loss of vision in the right eye occurred 2 days after development of herpes zoster ophthalmicus in this 40-year-old HIV-positive man with evidence of ischemic optic neuropathy and mild central vein obstruction. His visual acuity was light perception and progressed to no light perception within several days. Doppler studies revealed evidence of stenosis of the ophthalmic artery. MRI scan of the brain was normal. Two months later he had some anterior chamber reaction in the right eye, which was still blind.

H and **I,** This 7-year-old boy with a 6-day history of herpes zoster ophthalmicus noted acute loss of vision caused by anterior ischemic optic neuropathy (**H**). His visual acuity was 20/100. He had a dense superior altitudinal scotoma and marked contraction of the inferior visual field. He was treated with oral prednisone, 50 mg/day. Four years later (**I**), note the optic atrophy. His acuity was 20/60.

J to **L,** Photomicrographs showing postischemic cavernous atrophy of the optic nerve (**J**) caused by granulomatous arteritis (**K** and **L**) in a blind, painful eye removed from a patient who had herpes zoster ophthalmicus.

---

in multifocal areas that become confluent in the peripheral fundus (Fig. 7-22, *A*). It is typically associated with perivascular infiltration, vascular occlusion, and hemorrhage (Figs. 7-22, *D* to *F*, and 7-23, *E* to *H*). The occlusive vasculitis may affect the major retinal and optic nerve head arteries posterior to the zones of full-thickness necrotizing retinitis (Fig. 7-23, *A* to *D*). Retinal opacification rapidly spreads posteriorly, frequently sparing the macula (Fig. 7-22, *F*). Multiple posterior white lesions occasionally occur early in the course of the disease. These may involve either or both the inner and outer retina. Marked yellow atheromatous cuffing, narrowing, and occlusion of the major branch retinal arteries may develop (Fig. 7-23, *A* to *D*). Widespread necrotizing retinitis is the predominant fundus finding in most patients; however, some show evidence of extensive retinal arteritis preceding development of large areas of retinal

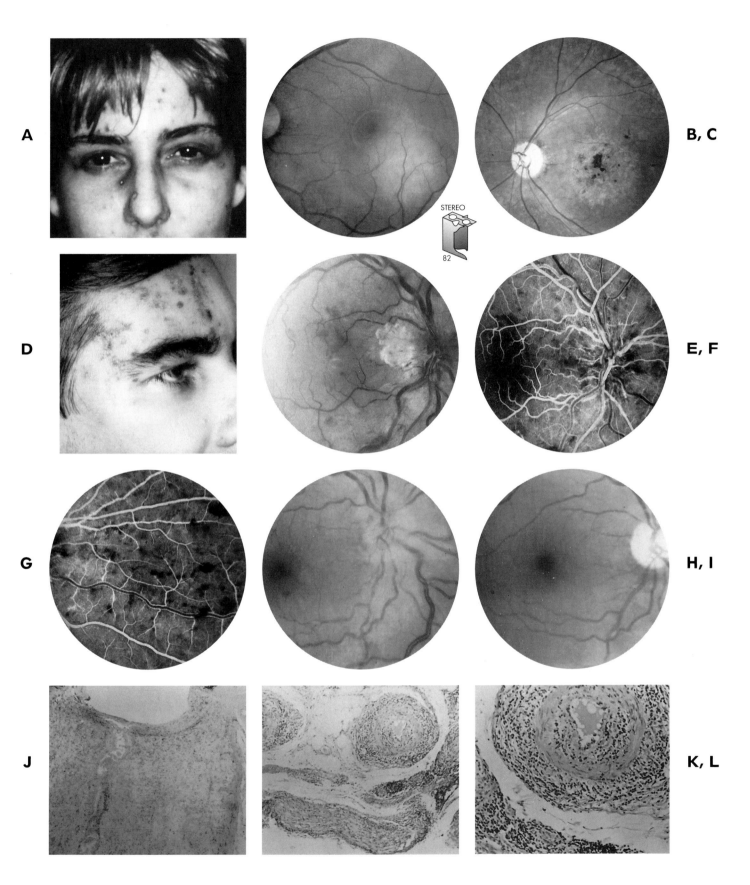

A

B, C

D

E, F

G

H, I

J

K, L

necrosis (Fig. 7-23, *A* to *D*). In some patients visual loss is caused primarily by branch or central retinal artery occlusion, and the presence of either an arcuate pattern or diffuse retinal whitening and cherry-red spot along with the atheromatous changes may be misinterpreted as embolic occlusion of the retinal arteries secondary to carotid artery disease (Fig. 7-23, *A* to *D* and *G* to *I*).[389,404,430,447] Some patients may demonstrate a milder progression and severity of the disease.[373,436]

Fluorescein angiography demonstrates reduced perfusion in the areas of retinal necrosis and retinal capillary permeability alteration as well as evidence of focal choroidal inflammatory cell infiltration and RPE damage in areas uninvolved by retinal necrosis (Fig. 7-23, *B* and *I*). After a few days the necrotic retina crumbles and sheds into the vitreous and a sharply outlined pattern of usually mild pigment mottling is left in the area of previous retinal necrosis (Fig. 7-22, *B* and *G*). Even as the areas of retinitis are clearing, the patient may experience further sudden and profound loss of vision caused by thrombotic arterial occlusion within or near the optic nerve head (Fig. 7-23, *A* to *D*). In approximately two-thirds of eyes, large irregular retinal holes develop in the necrotic retina and are followed by vitreous organization, traction, and extensive retinal detachment (Fig. 7-22, *C*). The detachment typically occurs 6 to 12 weeks after the onset of the disease. The overall prognosis for visual acuity is generally poor, with only 30% of affected eyes achieving an acuity of better than 20/200.

Risk factors for severity of the disorder early in the course of the disease are retinal arteritis, reduced electroretinographic amplitudes, and elevated circulating immune complexes.[435] Central vision, however, may be retained in those patients who do not develop retinal detachment because of the tendency for the retinitis and choroiditis to spare the posterior pole (Fig. 7-22, *F* and *G*).

Approximately two-thirds of patients with the acute retinal necrosis syndrome are males. The second eye becomes involved in approximately one-third of patients, usually within 6 weeks of onset in the first eye. Involvement of the second eye may be delayed for as long as 19 years.[445,449] In patients receiving early treatment with Acyclovir, the likelihood of involvement of the fellow eye is reduced.[441] Most patients have no antecedent systemic disease. Herpes zoster ophthalmicus, the Ramsay-Hunt syndrome, and chicken pox may occur in some patients shortly before the onset of

acute retinal necrosis.* Herpes simplex virus, aphthous ulcers, and intravenous cocaine have been implicated in the development of acute retinal necrosis in several patients.[395,397,433,458]

Histopathologic examination of the eyes of immune competent patients with the early stage of acute retinal necrosis caused by the HZV reveals two major components: (1) sharply defined zones of full-thickness necrotizing retinitis associated with replicating herpes virus (Fig. 7-24) and (2) occlusive vasculitis affecting the choroidal and retinal vessels unassociated with evidence of replicating virus within the blood vessels (Fig. 7-24).[389,390,404] The thickened necrotic retina involving all layers seen histopathologically corresponds with the zones of dense retinal whitening seen clinically (Fig. 7-23). In the areas adjacent to the necrotic retina where the retina is partly preserved, numerous intranuclear inclusion bodies typical of the herpesviruses are evident by light and electron microscopy in the retina and RPE (Fig. 7-24, *G* and *H*). Immunocytopathologic staining techniques, immunofluorescence, and polymerase chain reaction techniques have been used to identify the virus as herpes zoster.[390,439,442,448,452]

FIG. 7-22   Acute Retinal Necrosis Syndrome.

A to **C,** Fundus painting depicting the frequent peripheral distribution of the necrotizing retinitis early in the course of the disease (**A**), the RPE changes after its resolution (**B**), and retinal detachment with large, ragged, retinal holes that typically occurs 6 to 12 weeks after the onset of the disease (**C**).

D to **G,** Extensive peripheral necrotizing retinitis in a healthy 79-year-old woman. Note the confluent areas of retinitis in the periphery associated with perivascular hemorrhage (**D** and **E**) and the patchy involvement posteriorly with sparing of the center of the macula (**F**). There was marked narrowing of the retinal vasculature and pallor of the optic disc. The right fundus was normal. The retinitis resolved spontaneously. Seven weeks later, visual acuity was 20/50. There was complete closure of all of the nasal retinal vessels (**G**) and extensive closure of the peripheral vasculature temporally. She maintained this vision over the subsequent 3 years, when she was lost to followup.

H to **I,** This man was blinded in both eyes by the acute retinal necrosis syndrome several years previously. Note the optic atrophy and threadlike remnants of the retinal vessels (**H**) that barely perfuse with fluorescein (**I**).

(A to C from Young and Bird.[461])

---

*References 382, 390, 391, 401, 419, 420, 423, 434, 450, 458, 460.

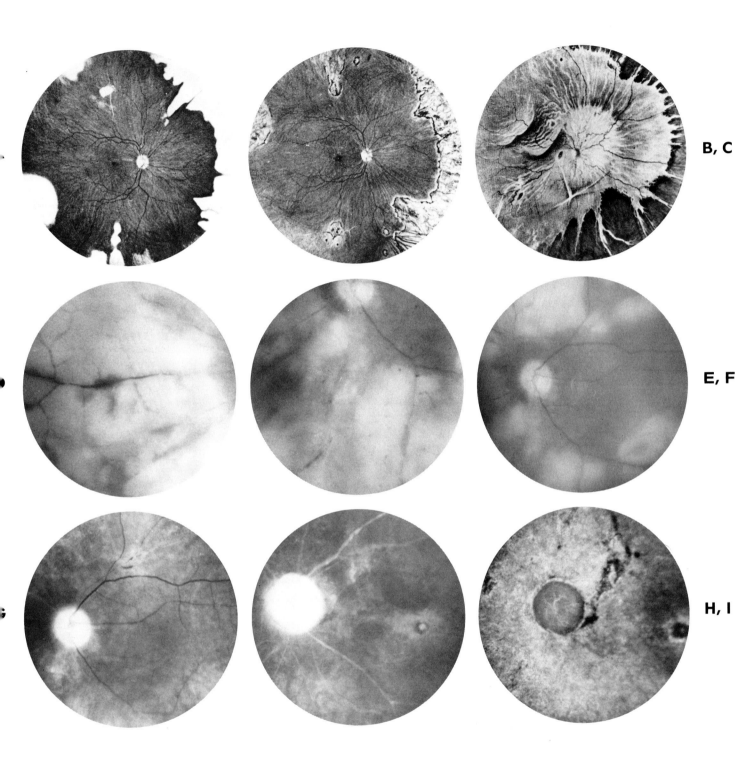

B, C

E, F

H, I

In areas where the white necrotizing retinitis has faded from view clinically, only skeletal remains of partly thrombosed major retinal vessels may be found (Fig. 7-24, C). The major retinal arteries may be occluded as a result of infiltration of the arterial walls by acute and chronic inflammatory cells as well as lipid-laden macrophages (Fig. 7-24, B). The choroid may be focally and diffusely thickened by acute and chronic inflammatory cells and occlusive vasculitis that involves both the choroidal arteries and the choriocapillaris (Fig. 7-24, C, D, and F). This vasculitis may be associated with necrosis of the overlying pigment epithelium and outer retina (Fig. 7-24, F). A necrotizing optic neuritis may be found (Fig. 7-24, *E*). No virus has been identified in the uveal tract or in the walls of the retinal vessels. It is probable that the HZV does not invade the retinal and choroidal blood vessels but instead induces an acute reactive inflammatory granulomatous response within the retinal arterial wall, as well as in the choroidal vasculature, that plays an important role in the ischemic damage to the inner and outer retina apart from the necrosis inflicted by direct intraretinal spread of the replicating virus. This reactive immune-induced vasculitis is probably largely responsible for the panuveitis and the necrotizing optic neuropathy accompanying this disorder (Fig. 7-24, *E*). The same explanation may be invoked for the giant cell arteritis associated with ischemic optic neuropathy (Fig. 7-21, *E* to *L*) and contralateral hemiplegia that occurs in some patients with herpes zoster ophthalmicus.[406,413,428] Clinically the marked choroidal involvement (Fig. 7-24, *A, C, D,* and *F*) in patients with acute retinal necrosis is largely occult because of the loss of transparency of the overlying ischemic retina. On histopathologic examination of two eyes enucleated many months after partial resolution of acute retinal necrosis caused by HZV, the author found a smoldering retinochoroiditis and a giant-cell reaction in the vicinity of Bruch's membrane and the internal limiting membrane of the retina.[405,448] This granulomatous response to these collagenous membranes is similar to that which may occur around Descemet's membrane in patients after HZV keratitis.[408,414]

Although most cases of acute retinal necrosis are probably caused by the HZV, the herpes simplex virus, cytomegalovirus, and *Toxoplasma* have been incriminated in a few cases.[395,433,446] Establishing the cause of acute retinal necrosis can be difficult. In addition to serial determination of serum and intraocular fluid HZV antibody levels and viral culture, the newly developed immunocytopathologic techniques have improved our ability to identify HZV infection in tissue sections.[390,439,442,452] Biopsy of the retina at the junction of the necrotic and unaffected retina during plana vitrectomy is occasionally used for diagnosis.[399,400,455] Our failure to recognize the acute retinal necrosis (ARN) syndrome before approximately 20 years ago suggests that a mutation in the HZV may have occurred. The phenotypes HLA-DQw7A and HLA-BW62,DR4 occur in 55% and 16%, respectively (controls 19% and 3%), of patients with ARN.[416]

Although the necrotizing retinitis typically appears initially in the peripheral fundus, it may begin

FIG. 7-23 Acute Retinal Necrosis.

A to **D,** Unilateral acute retinal necrosis in a 55-year-old man who was receiving antimetabolite therapy for lymphocytic lymphoma when he noted blurred vision in the left eye. When seen initially, he had extensive peripheral necrotizing retinitis, macular ischemia, vitritis, and iridocyclitis that were initially attributed to the ischemic ocular syndrome caused by carotid artery obstruction. There was extensive yellowish opacification of the retinal arterial walls posteriorly (**A**). The early phases of angiography revealed multiple filling defects in the choroid and evidence of extensive peripheral retinal occlusive disease (**B** and **C**). Carotid arteriography was within normal limits. Over the subsequent 5 days, the patient developed further evidence of central retinal arterial thrombosis and occlusion (**D**).

E and **F,** Bilateral acute retinal necrosis syndrome in a healthy 42-year-old man with a 3-week history of loss of vision in the right eye and a 1-day history of loss of vision in the left eye. His visual acuity in the right eye was no light perception and in the left eye was 20/70. In the right eye he had massive hemorrhagic necrotizing retinitis in the peripheral fundus associated with a pale optic disc and narrowing of the retinal vessels (**E**). In the left eye he had swelling of the optic nerve head, retinal hemorrhages, and scattered deep white retinal lesions (**F**). The right eye was enucleated for diagnostic purposes, and the pathologic findings were identical to those illustrated in Fig. 7-24. A convalescent titer for herpes zoster performed by the anticomplement immunofluorescence test was 1:256 for IgG and negative for IgM. The patient was treated with intravenous acyclovir, aspirin, and intravenous methylprednisolone. His vision decreased within 24 hours to bare light perception and then subsequently returned to 5/200. Ten weeks later he developed a rhegmatogenous retinal detachment that was successfully repaired. Electron microscopic and immunocytopathologic stains of the right eye revealed evidence of herpes zoster. Varicella zoster virus was cultured from the vitreous.

G to **I,** Acute retinal necrosis in a 67-year-old man whose findings were initially attributed to the ischemic ocular syndrome caused by carotid artery obstruction. Nine days after the onset of symptoms the vision in his left eye had decreased to no light perception. He had massive necrotizing retinitis with relative sparing of the macula (**G** and **H**). There was narrowing of the retinal arterioles and pallor and swelling of the optic disc. Early phases of fluorescein angiography revealed patchy areas of nonfilling of the choroid (**I**) and extensive occlusion of the peripheral retinal vasculature. Because of the development of a small area of retinitis in the right eye, the left eye was enucleated. Light and electron microscopic findings are illustrated in Fig. 7-24. Immunocytopathologic stains showed the virus to be herpes zoster.

(**E** and **F** from Culbrtson W.W. et al.: Varicella zoster virus as a cause of the acute retinal necrosis syndrome. Ophthalmology 93:559, 1986[390]; **G** from Culbertson W.W. et al.: The acute retinal necrosis syndrome. II, histopathology and etiology. Ophthalmology 89:1317, 1982.[389]; **H** and **I** from Gass.[404])

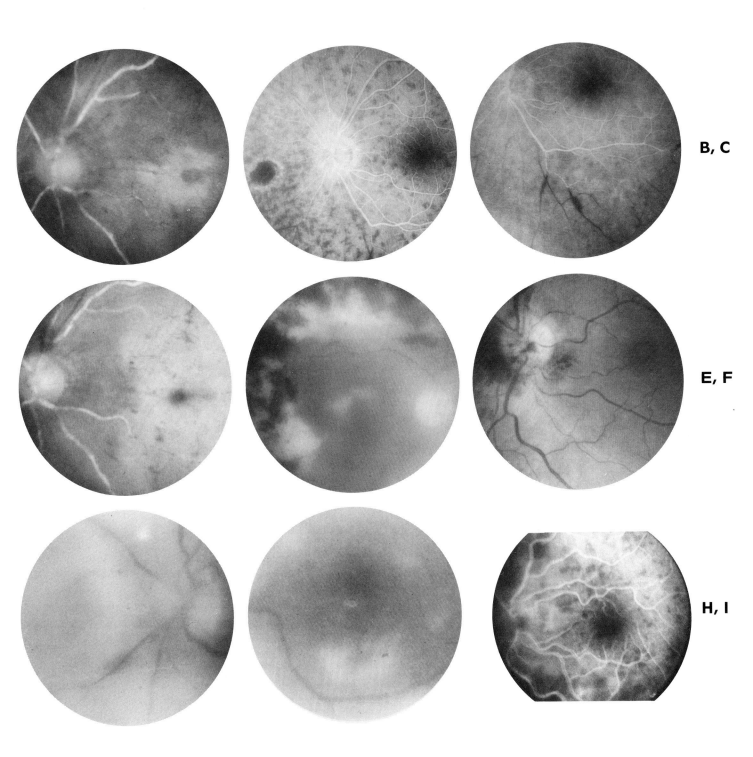

B, C

E, F

H, I

as multifocal lesions in the macula. Whereas progression of the disease is usually rapid, in some cases a slow progression may simulate that seen in other diseases such as toxoplasmosis or reticulum cell sarcoma. During the acute stages of the disease the differential diagnosis includes (1) cytomegalic inclusion disease, which almost always occurs in immunosuppressed individuals, is typically less widespread, progresses at a slower rate, and is usually associated with more retinal hemorrhage and less evidence of retinal arterial occlusion; (2) primary herpes simplex retinitis, usually seen in infants but occasionally in adults with encephalitis[294]; (3) bacterial or fungal retinitis; (4) large-cell non-Hodgkin's lymphoma (reticulum cell sarcoma), usually in elderly patients; (5) diffuse toxoplasmosis, usually in patients receiving long-term corticosteroid therapy or otherwise immunosuppressed; (6) Behçet's disease; (7) sarcoidosis; (8) retinoblastoma in infants; (9) pars planitis and nematode endophthalmitis in children and young adults; (10) traumatic retinopathy (commotio retinae); (11) central retinal artery occlusion in association with severe carotid artery disease (ischemic ocular syndrome); (12) retinal necrosis in X-linked lymphoproliferative disease[409]; and (13) acute multifocal hemorrhagic retinal vasculopathy.[381] Ophthalmoscopic pictures identical to acute retinal necrosis have been reported in immunosuppressed patients with Hodgkin's disease,[392] central nervous system toxoplasmosis,[446] cytomegalic inclusion disease,[454] Behçet's disease,[461] and giardiasis.[424] In some of these cases the acute retinal necrosis may in fact have been caused by herpes zoster.

During the healed stage of acute retinal necrosis, the pigmentary changes, chorioretinal atrophy, severe vascular narrowing and sheathing, and optic atrophy simulate those seen in ophthalmic artery occlusion, Behçet's disease, severe diffuse unilateral subacute neuroretinitis, severe atypical retinitis pigmentosa, and posttraumatic chorioretinal scarring.

The diagnosis of acute retinal necrosis is based primarily on the clinical picture and the exclusion of other causes of retinal whitening and retinal vascular occlusion. There are no consistent laboratory findings of diagnostic importance. Vitreous specimens are unlikely to show evidence of intranuclear inclusions, and viral cultures may be negative. Retinal biopsies in this disease have a significant chance of missing the limited areas where the diagnostic inclusions are present in viable but inflamed retinas. A biopsy specimen should include the edge of a recently developed white area of retinitis and its adjacent normal-appearing retina.

Acyclovir appears to be effective in the treatment of acute retinal necrosis, and it reduces the risk of fellow eye involvement.[380,390,441,443] The treatment regimen presently being used at the Bascom Palmer Eye Institute for the treatment of the acute stage of acute retinal necrosis includes intravenous acyclovir and, 2 to 3 days later, oral prednisone; these drugs are continued until all signs of the acute retinal necrosis have disap-

peared. Acetylsalicylic acid is given by mouth to reduce the hyperaggregation of platelets that has been demonstrated in these patients.[374] Resolution of the active retinitis typically begins 3 to 5 days after initiation of acyclovir. Treatment with acyclovir does not prevent retinal detachment. Prophylactic photocoagulation to delimit the zones of retinal necrosis may be effective in reducing the risk of retinal detachment.[411,453] Approximately two-thirds of the patients respond well to scleral-buckling procedures, which may be supplemented with vitrectomy in some cases.[378,379,384,386,437] Retinal and optic disc neovascularization may occasionally occur and may respond favorably to panphotocoagulation.[410] There seems to be little rationale for consideration of optic nerve sheath decompression in the treatment of ARN optic neuropathy.[451]

FIG. 7-24 Light and Electron Microscopic Findings in the Acute Retinal Necrosis Syndrome Caused by Herpes Zoster (Same Case Illustrated in Fig. 7-23, G to I).

A, Thrombotic occlusive retinal arteritis of the optic nerve head.

B, Note vacuolated cells, either lipid-laden endothelial cells or macrophages (arrow), in the wall of this occluded retinal artery.

C, Retina nasal to the optic disc showing thrombosed retinal artery and marked necrosis of the retina. (Compare with Fig. 7-23, **G.**)

D, Thrombotic occlusion of the choriocapillaris and large choroidal artery (arrow) underlying necrotic RPE.

E, Segmental infarction and inflammation of the nasal half of the retrolaminar optic nerve.

F, Temporal retina showing sharp junction of necrotizing retinitis and relatively normal retina. Note the extensive underlying choroiditis. The retina in the macular area (not shown) was well preserved, and the choroiditis was multifocal rather than diffuse.

G, Temporal retina showing eosinophilic intranuclear viral inclusions within retinal and RPE cells (arrows).

H, Electron micrograph showing intranuclear viral particles in retinal cells.

(**A** to **C** and **F** to **H** from Culbertson W.W. et al.: The acute retinal necrosis syndrome. II. Histopathology and etiology. Ophthalmology 89:1317, 1982[389]; **D** and **E** from Gass.[404])

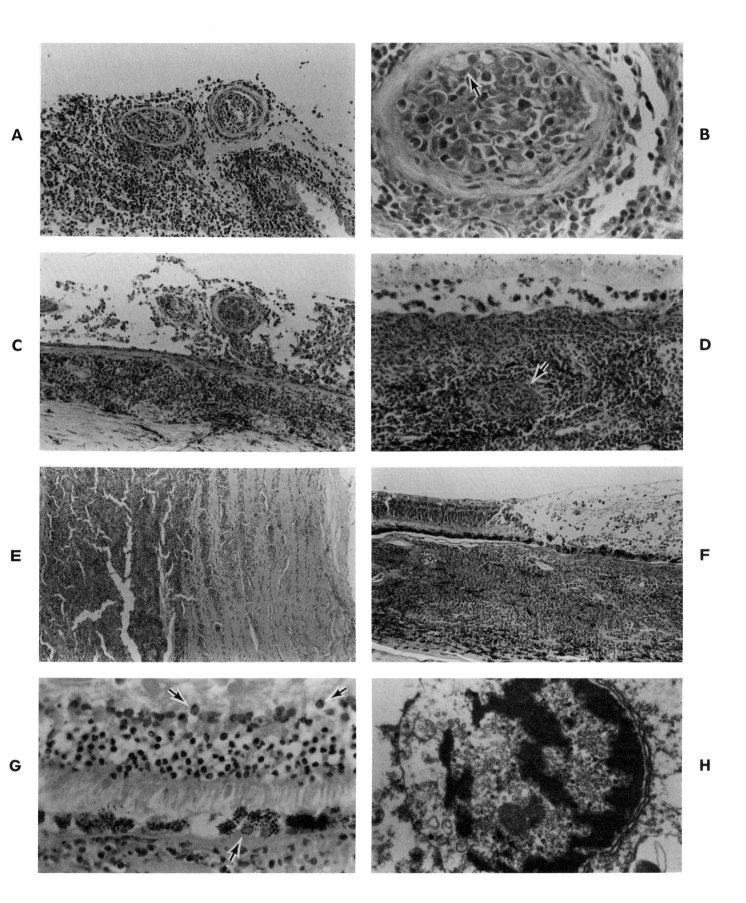

Acute retinal necrosis in immune incompetent patients

Immune incompetent patients, particularly those with AIDS, often develop an atypical clinical picture of acute retinal necrosis characterized by fewer inflammatory signs, frequent involvement of the macula, less involvement of the retinal and choroidal blood vessels, rapid progression of the necrotizing retinitis, poor response to antiviral agents, and severe bilateral visual loss (Fig. 7-25).[393,396,398,422,429] Whereas some have emphasized outer retinal involvement (posterior outer retinal necrosis or PORN syndrome), there is clinical and histopathologic evidence that the necrotizing viral retinitis involves the inner retina early in these patients (Fig. 7-25, *A* to *E* and *J* to *K*).[429] Because these patients are immunosuppressed, the acute reactive granulomatous retinal and choroidal arteritis typically seen in immune competent patients with HZV ARN is less severe, but the replicating virus causes severe rapidly progressing retinal necrosis involving all retinal layers.

▼ EPSTEIN-BARR VIRUS

Epstein-Barr virus (EBV) infects virtually everyone by adulthood, and a lifelong latency is maintained. It infects children silently, whereas the majority of adolescents develop infectious mononucleosis (IM). Thus the clinical outcome of EBV infection is age dependent. Children with primary immune insufficiency can have fatal or chronic IM, malignant B-cell lymphoma, virus-associated hemophagocytic syndrome, aplastic anemia, or acquired hypogammaglobulinemia. Part of the predilection for AIDS and other immunosuppressed patients to develop B-cell lymphomas may result from EBV infection. Acyclovir and immunoglobulin therapy can be of value in some patients with active EBV infection.[464] Ocular involvement seldom occurs in patients with other clinical manifestations of EBV. A variety of ocular disorders associated with EBV infection have been reported, including acute necrotizing retinitis,[463] outer punctate retinitis simulating toxoplasmosis,[464] multifocal choroiditis and panuveitis,[465] anterior uveitis, severe panuveitis with optic disc swelling, and macular edema.[466] There is conflicting information concerning the incidence of serologic evidence of recent EBV infection in patients with multifocal choroiditis and panuveitis. (See multifocal choroiditis and panuveitis, p. 688.)

FIG. 7-25 Atypical Acute Retinal Necrosis Caused by Herpes Zoster Virus in AIDS (Progressive Outer Retinal Necrosis, PORN Syndrome).

A to **G,** Acute visual loss occurred in this 49-year-old man who was HIV positive. Note the multifocal lesions surrounding paracentral zones of retinal whitening that involved the inner as well as the outer retina (**A** and **B**). Angiography showed evidence of perifoveolar retinal vascular occlusion and incomplete staining of the white paracentral lesions (**C** to **E**). Two weeks later he had severe visual loss and progression of the retinitis (**F**) and 5 weeks after the onset of symptoms he was virtually blind. Note the severe retinal vascular narrowing, optic disc pallor, and relative sparing of the choroid (**F**). The left eye was enucleated and HZV was cultured and identified with immunofluorescent staining with a monoclonal antibody to varicella–zoster virus.

H to **K,** Visual loss occurred in this 39-year-old man with AIDS and a history of two episodes of herpes zoster dermatitis. Note the multifocal white retinal lesions (**H** and **I**). There was minimal vitreous inflammation. One week later his visual acuity was 20/300 in the right eye and hand movements only in the left eye. Vision progressed rapidly to no light perception in the right eye, which was enucleated for diagnostic purposes. Histopathologic examination (**J** and **K**) revealed extensive necrosis of the retina that in many areas was more marked in the inner than outer retina. Note the absence of the retinal and choroidal vascular inflammatory response and compare it with the severe inflammatory response that occurs in the immune competent patient with ARN caused by HZV (Fig. 7-24).

(**A** and **E** from Margolis et al.[431]; **G** to **J** from Dr. Curtis E. Margo.[429])

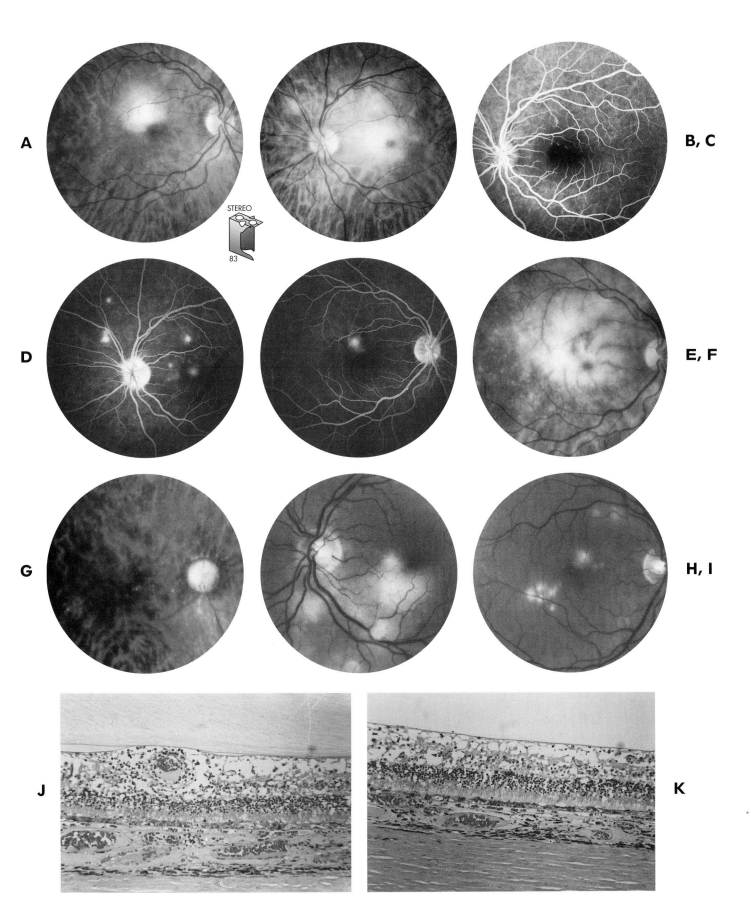

A

B, C

D

E, F

G

H, I

J

K

STEREO
83

▼ HUMAN IMMUNODEFICIENCY VIRUS (HIV) AND ACQUIRED IMMUNE DEFICIENCY SYNDROME

Acquired immune deficiency syndrome (AIDS) first became apparent in 1975 but has rapidly become a global pandemic. It is transmitted primarily by sexual contact that can be homosexual, bisexual, or heterosexual; by parenteral transmission, by transfusion of infected blood products or injection using blood-contaminated needles or syringes; and perinatally before, during, or after delivery.* The definition of AIDS that was formally based primarily on the acquisition of one or more "indicator diseases" associated with HIV infections such as infection by opportunistic organisms, lymphomas, and encephalopathy now includes asymptomatic patients with CD4+ T-lymphocyte counts of less than 200 cells/μl.[473a]

AIDS is caused by infection with the retrovirus Human immunodeficiency virus (HIV), which causes a profound immunodeficiency resulting primarily from a progressive quantitative and qualitative deficiency of the CD4+ subset of T-lymphocytes referred to as the helper or inducer T-cells. There is an associated elevation of circulating immune complexes and elevated serum IgA and IgG levels. The median time from HIV exposure to the development of AIDS is approximately 11 years.[496a] Patients often are seen initially because of fever, generalized lymphadenopathy, a wide variety of severe opportunistic infections, and, in approximately 30% of patients, the development of a progressive form of Kaposi's sarcoma. Ocular findings occur in 50% to 70% of patients. The most common ocular finding is one or more cotton-wool patches (approximately 50% to 70% of cases) (Fig. 7-26, A), retinal hemorrhages and Roth's spots (approximately 40%), microaneurysms (approximately 20%), and cytomegalic retinitis (approximately 25%) (Fig. 7-26).[490,494,505] The cotton-wool patches are similar to those occurring in other retinal vascular diseases except that they are generally smaller in size.[498] They regress in 4 to 6 weeks. They may appear early in the course of the disease, and their appearance is unrelated to specific infections or the general status of the patient. When these patches are viewed by fluorescein angiography, they are identical with cotton-wool patches seen from other causes.[500] Histopathologically, they are cytoid bodies associated

FIG. 7-26   Acquired Immune Deficiency Syndrome.

A, Cotton-wool spots.

B and **C,** Photomicrographs of cotton-wool patch. Note cytoid body, which is partly calcified (*arrows,* **B;** hematoxylin and eosin). Some of the calcified tissue (pale area) was dislodged during sectioning. The whole cytoid body stained positively for calcium (**C,** von Kossa stain).

D and **E,** Cytomegalic inclusion disease retinitis.

F, Cytomegalic inclusion papillitis.

G, Photomicrograph of eye illustrated in **F** showing necrosis of the juxtapapillary retina and nasal half of the optic nerve, which contained many cytomegalic cells.

H, Kaposi's sarcoma of the lower eyelid.

I and **J,** Clinical photograph (**I**) and photomicrograph (**J**) of Kaposi's sarcoma of the inferior conjunctival *cul-de-sac.*

K and **L,** Kaposi's sarcoma of the conjunctiva in a patient with AIDS before (**K**) and several weeks after subconjunctival injection of 0.5 ml of 3 million IU interferon alfa-2a.

(**B** and **C** from Tannenbaum et al.[511]; **K** and **L** from Hummer et al.[491])

with arteriolar obstruction, basal laminar thickening, endothelial cell swelling, and degeneration of the pericytes.[500] We have observed calcification histopathologically within cytoid bodies in two patients with AIDS (Fig. 7-21, *B* and *C*).[511] Although structures resembling *Pneumocystis carinii* were identified in a cotton-wool patch in one case,[496] there is minimal evidence to support an infectious cause for the arteriolar obstruction. Vascular damage from a circulating immune complex deposition has been suggested as the cause.[500] The HIV-1 virus has been demonstrated in the retina, conjunctiva, tears, iris, and cornea of patients with AIDS.[404,471,506] The role of this virus in causing cotton-wool patches, microaneurysm and hemorrhages,* nonstaining CME, macular star, optic neuropathy, or otherwise unexplained visual loss in some patients with AIDS,† and in potentiating the effects of opportunistic infections is uncertain.[501]

Most opportunistic infections occur in patients with a CD4+ T-lymphocyte count of less than 200 cells/μl. For opportunistic infections associated with AIDS see the following: bacteria, see p. 602; cytomegalovirus, p. 642; herpes zoster virus and acute retinal necrosis, p. 654; mycobacterium, p. 606; cat-scratch disease, p. 604; cryptococcosis, p. 148; histoplasmosis, p. 614; pneumocystis, p. 152.

Cytomegalic retinitis and optic neuritis are the most serious ocular complications of AIDS from

---

*References 467-475, 477-479, 483, 485, 486, 489-500, 503, 505, 506, 508-510, 513.

*References 480, 482, 501, 502, 505, 512.
†References 469, 481, 488, 502, 507, 515.

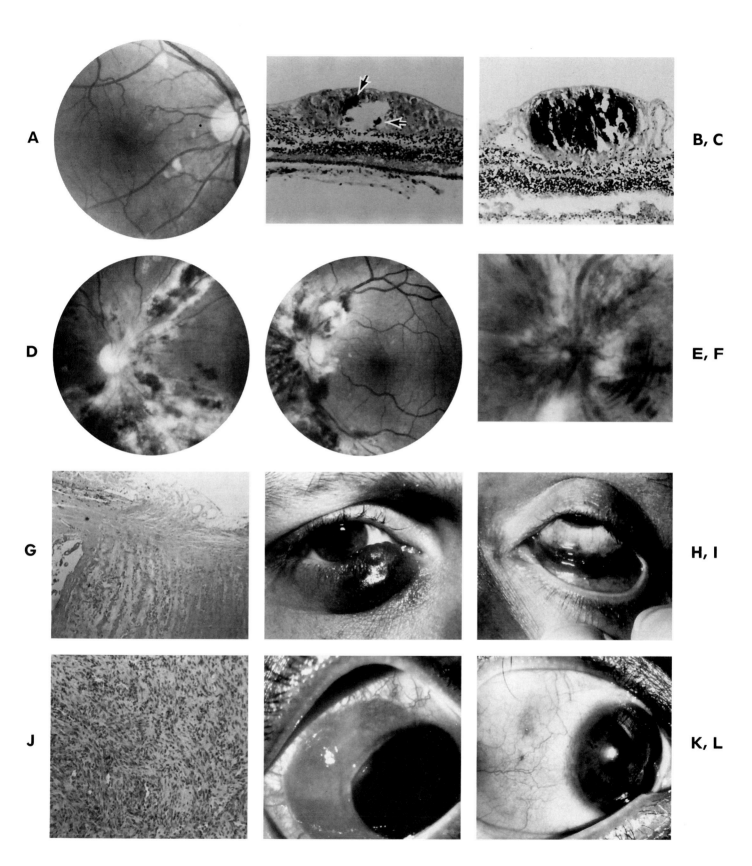

the visual as well as the overall prognostic standpoint (Fig. 7-20, *G* to *L*). Cytomegalic retinitis develops late in the course of the disease, is progressive, and, before the use of antiviral agents, was usually followed several weeks after its discovery by death caused by systemic infection with *Cytomegalovirus* or one or more of the following: *Pneumocystis carinii* pneumonia, *Cryptococcus neoformans* meningitis, *Toxoplasma gondii* encephalitis, and disseminated *Mycobacterium avium, Mycobacterium intracellularis,* and *Candida albicans.**

Kaposi's sarcoma appears as one or more erythematous violaceous masses that may involve the conjunctiva, skin of the lids, and occasionally the orbits (Fig. 7-26, *H* to *L*).[472,483,491] Progressive involvement of the skin, mucous membranes, internal organs, and lymph nodes may be the major cause of death in approximately 9% of patients. Burkitt's lymphoma of the orbit and a variety of neuroophthalmologic complications usually caused by intracranial infections may occur.[470]

Therapy in patients with AIDS is directed toward inhibition of replication of HIV and control of opportunistic infections (see pp. 152, 642, 654). Chemotherapy, cryotherapy, local excision, and tumor injection with alpha-interferon are used to control Kaposi's sarcoma (Fig. 7-26, *K* and *L*).[491]

▼ HUMAN T-LYMPHOTROPIC VIRUS TYPE 1

The human T-lymphotropic virus type 1 (HLTV-1) is a human retrovirus that causes adult T-cell leukemia and lymphoma and HTLV-1-associated myelopathy (HAM). Both are endemic and are prevalent in the Caribbean, Italy, sub-Saharan Africa, and Kyushu and Okinawa islands.[516] These patients may develop uveitis and retinal vasculitis,[517-520] and occasionally multiple white retinal lesions.[516]

▼ RUBELLA RETINITIS

Children born of mothers who contracted rubella during the first trimester of pregnancy may show a variety of anomalies of development of the eyes and other organs (Fig. 7-27).[521-535] In these children there is a high incidence of what has been described as salt-and-pepper mottling of the RPE (Fig. 7-22, *D* to *L*).[524,530] This is often most prominent in the posterior fundus. Both eyes are affected in 80% of cases.[530] Early progression of

*References 476, 490, 497, 504, 505, 510.

FIG. 7-27 Congenital Rubella.

A, This child had microphthalmos and cataract in the left eye, rubella retinopathy in the right eye, hearing loss, dental hypoplasia, and congenital heart disease.

B to **E,** Dental hypoplasia (**B**), iris stromal and RPE atrophy (**C**), and rubella retinopathy (**D**) in a 4-year-old boy whose mother had rubella in the first trimester of pregnancy. Note the extensive derangement of the RPE (**D**). His visual acuity was normal. At age 11 years, the RPE changes were less apparent (**E**).

F to **I,** Rubella retinopathy (**F** and **G**) in a 9-year-old boy who developed loss of vision in the right eye secondary to subfoveal choroidal neovascularization (*arrow,* **F**). His mother received gammaglobulin injections during the first trimester of pregnancy because of exposure to an epidemic of rubella. His visual acuity in the left eye was 20/15. His electrooculographic and electroretinographic findings were normal. Angiography in the right eye showed evidence of choroidal neovascularization (**H**) and widespread alterations of the RPE in both eyes (**H** and **I**).

J to **K,** Compare the prominent RPE mottling associated with rubella in an 11 year old (**J**) with that of the more subtle mottling in a 37-year-old man (**K**). Angiography in the man shows evidence of marked hypopigmentation of the RPE. Visual acuity was normal in both patients.

the pigment mottling in childhood may be caused by persistence of the rubella virus within the RPE. Pigment mottling, however, becomes less prominent in adulthood. This pigmentary change of the fundus may be accompanied evidence of pigment loss from the pigment epithelium of the irides, which in some cases will transilluminate in an irregular fashion (Fig. 7-27, *C*). These alterations of the RPE may occur alone or may be associated with other ocular abnormalities, such as cataracts and microphthalmos, and systemic abnormalities, including deafness and congenital heart disease (Fig. 7-27, *A* and *B*). In patients with evidence of RPE involvement only, the visual acuity is usually normal. Choroidal neovascularization and disciform macular detachment may be a late complication of rubella retinopathy (Fig. 7-27, *F* to *I*).[523,524,527,534] The electroretinographic and electrooculographic findings, color vision, and visual fields in most patients are normal. Fluorescein angiography shows mottled hyperfluorescence caused by extensive and irregular loss of pigment from the RPE (Fig. 7-27, *H* and *I*) and may be helpful in detecting early choroidal neovascularization (Fig. 7-27, *H*). Pathologically, the salt-and-pepper changes in the fundus are caused by altered pigmentation and some atrophy of the RPE.[522] The retina and choroid are unaffected. Rubella retinopathy may be mimicked by inherited dystrophies

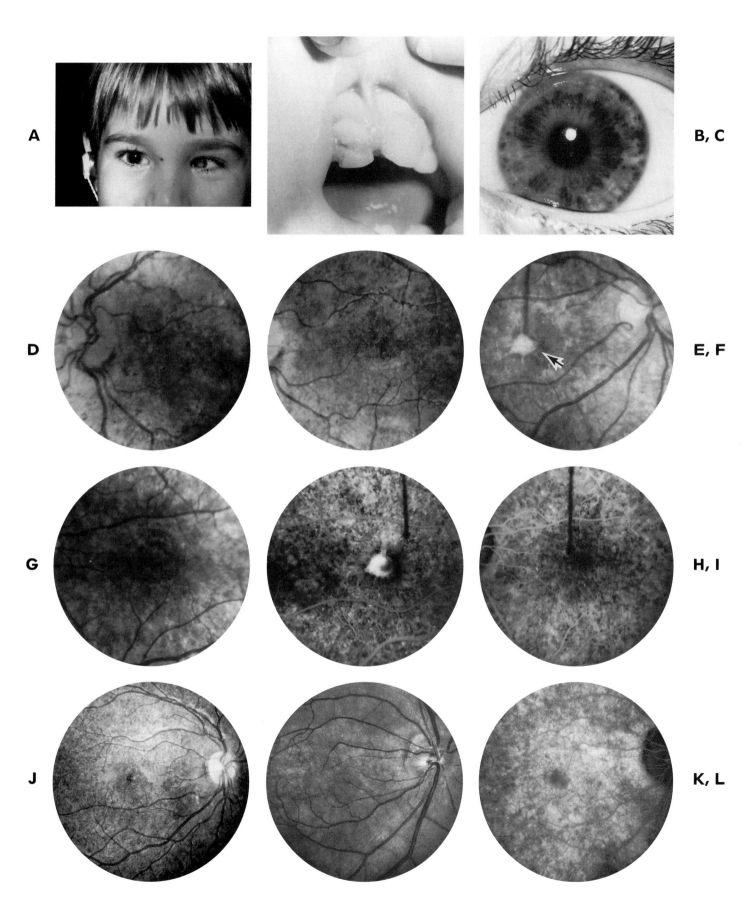

A

B, C

D

E, F

G

H, I

J

K, L

of the RPE (see Fig. 4-5), the carrier state of X-linked ocular albinism (see Fig. 5-37, *J*), X-linked choroideremia (see Fig. 5-28, *E* and *F*), and toxic diseases of the RPE (see Fig. 9-2).[525]

▼ SUBACUTE SCLEROSING PANENCEPHALITIS

Subacute sclerosing panencephalitis (Dawson's encephalitis) is a progressive neurologic disease that typically occurs in children and young adults with a mean age of 7 years. Males are affected three times as often as females. Personality and behavioral changes are usually followed by dementia, seizures, myoclonus, and death. It occasionally occurs in young adults, who may recover with only minimal neurologic deficit (Fig. 7-28, *C* to *I*). Fifty percent of patients will have involvement of the visual system. Visual complaints often antedate the onset of neurologic symptoms by several weeks.[536,537,548] Neurologic symptoms may be delayed as long as 22 months.[536,539] Most patients have a history of preceding measles (rubeola infection) usually before 2 years of age. The patients may be seen initially because of loss of central vision caused by one or more small, flat, focal, white retinal lesions or larger more ragged gray-white areas (Fig. 7-28, *A* to *D*).[540,541,547] Either one or both eyes may be affected. When the retinitis involves the center of the macula, a cherry-red spot may be present.[544,545] The white retinal lesions resolve rapidly and are replaced by irregular areas of RPE atrophy, gliotic scarring of the retina, radiating retinal folds, and occasionally retinal hole formation (Fig. 7-28, *B* and *G* to *J*). The pigmentary changes may be misinterpreted as heredomacular dystrophy. The pigmentary changes are not always confined to the macula.[546] There is minimal evidence of choroidal involvement. The vitreous is relatively free of inflammation. The optic disc may be swollen or atrophic.[540] Angiography is helpful in detecting subtle changes in the RPE.[542,543]

FIG. 7-28   Retinitis Caused by Subacute Sclerosing Panencephalitis.

A and **B,** This 12-year-old boy had several patches of acute retinitis in the right macula (**A**). He had similar lesions in his left eye. His visual acuity was 20/400 in the right eye and finger counting at 4 feet in the left eye. Note the cherry-red spot. Ten days later there was partial clearing of the central lesion and evidence of a larger lesion temporally (**B**). At that time he had no neurologic symptoms and the neurologic evaluation was normal. During the next month, however, he became lethargic, mute, and blind. He died 2 months later of cardiopulmonary arrest. He had been exposed to measles at age 5 and had received attenuated measles virus vaccine 5 months before the onset of visual symptoms.

C to **I,** A healthy 21-year-old man had a 1-week history of blurred vision in his left eye. At that time there was evidence of retinal whitening associated with some hemorrhage (**C**). The right fundus was within normal limits except for the presence of a small hemorrhage in the macula. A medical evaluation that included spinal fluid examination revealed a rubeola IgG titer in the cerebrospinal fluid of 1:64, which was thought to be diagnostic of subacute sclerosing panencephalitis. The patient's past medical history was negative for measles or immunization against rubeola. Three years previously he had been hospitalized for brain fever of uncertain etiology. Two weeks after visual loss in the left eye he noted loss of vision in the right eye. Examination revealed an irregular area of necrotizing retinitis (**D**). A fluorescein angiogram revealed evidence of perivascular leakage of dye and some staining of the lesions (**E** and **F**). The retinal lesions in his left eye had partly faded (**G**). An electroencephalogram revealed findings compatible with subacute sclerosing panencephalitis. Six months later there was irregular scarring and thinning of the retina in the macular area of both eyes (**H** and **I**). Visual acuity was counting fingers at 3 feet.

J and **K,** Irregular pigmentary disturbances of the macula and mild papilledema caused by subacute sclerosing panencephalitis (**J**) in an 8-year-old boy who 4 weeks previously became lethargic, incontinent, and finally comatose. He died 3 weeks later, and histopathologic examination of the macular region revealed an atrophic thinned retina containing large masses of multinucleated syncytial giant cells containing numerous intranuclear eosinophilic inclusions (**K**).

(**A** and **B** from Landers and Klintworth[544]; **C** to **I,** courtesy of Dr. W. Sanderson Grizzard and Dr. Andrew K. Vine; **J** and **K** from Font et al.[538])

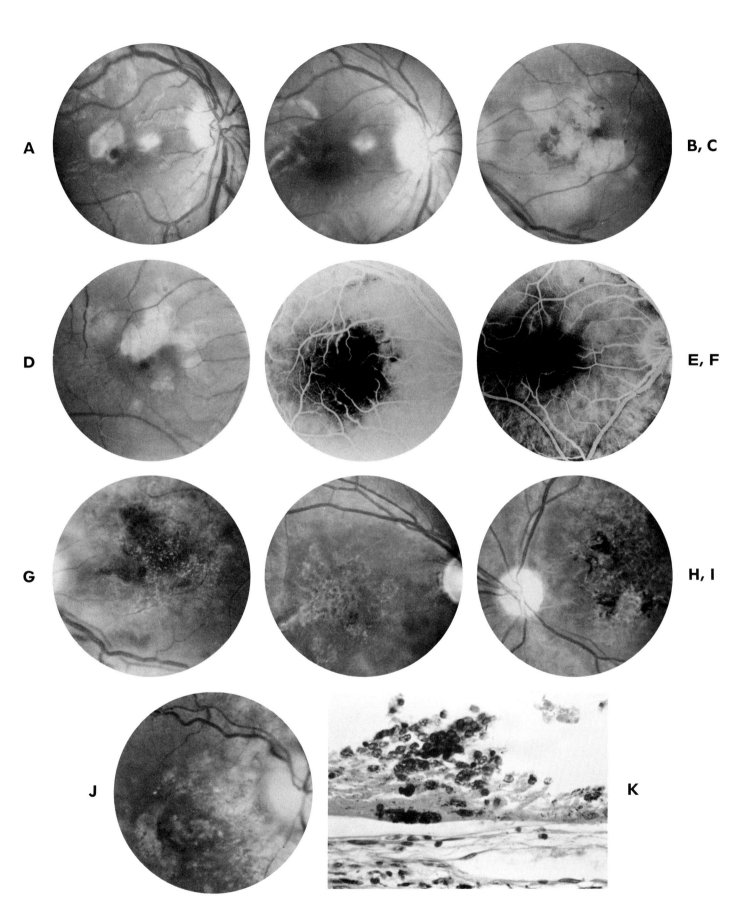

Histopathologically, the acute stage of subacute sclerosing panencephalitis is characterized by patchy focal areas of retinal necrosis, pigment-laden macrophages, minimal evidence of inflammation in the retina, loss of pigment from the RPE, and minimal inflammation in the choroid.[538,544] Later the retina may show focal areas of atrophy of the inner, outer, or both layers with disruption and hyperplasia of the RPE and the presence of Cowdry type A and Cowdry type B intranuclear inclusions as well as some intracytoplasmic inclusions (Fig. 7-28, K).[538,541,544] Viral particles typical for measles virus have been identified in both the retina and the brain of these patients.[541,544] Evidence of measles virus has been demonstrated in the retina utilizing immunofluorescent techniques.[538,544] The demonstration of high levels of measles antibody in the serum and cerebrospinal fluid is helpful in establishing the diagnosis. The electroencephalogram shows bursts of high-amplitude, sharply contoured, slow-wave complexes. There is much evidence that subacute sclerosing panencephalitis is caused by an altered form of the measles virus. There is no treatment. The acute stage is most likely to be confused with toxoplasmosis, cytomegalovirus infection, Rift Valley fever retinitis, acute posterior multifocal placoid pigment epitheliopathy, or one of the sphingolipidoses. The later pigmented stage of the disease is most likely to be confused with Vogt-Spielmeyer disease (neuronal ceroid lipofuscinoses; see p. 412) or Stargardt's disease.

Subacute sclerosing panencephalitis may be precipitated during cytotoxic and immunosuppressive treatment or in immunodeficiency states, which lower the resistance of the host to the measles virus.[541]

▼ MUMPS NEURORETINITIS

Papillitis and neuroretinitis usually associated with clinical evidence of meningoencephalitis occasionally develop in patients with mumps.[549,550] One or more foci of retinitis may also be present. Most patients recover normal visual function.

▼ RIFT VALLEY FEVER RETINITIS

Rift Valley fever is an acute disease primarily affecting cattle and sheep caused by a specific arthropod-borne virus that is endemic in the western one-third of Africa. Epidemics involving humans have occurred, the most severe of which caused the death of over 600 people in Egypt during 1977 and 1978. In humans this is typically an acute febrile illness with biphasic temperature elevations mimicking dengue fever. It is associated with muscle and joint pains, headaches, and occasionally nausea and vomiting. Conjunctivitis and photophobia are common during the early phases of the disease. Visual loss occurs often days or weeks after subsidence of the fever and is associated with multiple areas of what appear to be acute necrotizing and hemorrhagic retinitis in the macular and paramacular areas, similar to that seen in subacute sclerosing panencephalitis and the herpes viruses.[551-555] Vitritis and occlusion of the major retinal arteries are common. This latter change is presumed to be related to proliferation of the retinal vascular endothelium. Vitreous hemorrhage and retinal detachment may occur in some patients. The natural course of the disease is variable. The patients may recover normal acuity or may have severe permanent visual loss, depending on the location and severity of the retinal involvement. The most severe systemic complications are encephalitis and hemorrhagic hepatitis.

The virus is an RNA type and is believed to be transmitted by an insect, possibly the mosquito. Human infection can also occur by handling diseased or dead animals or contaminated specimens. The diagnosis is based on a demonstrated rise in the hemagglutination antibodies of the Rift Valley fever virus and the complement fixation test.

▼ RETINAL VASCULITIS AND PERIVASCULITIS

The terms "retinal vasculitis" and "retinal perivasculitis" are used interchangeably as clinical names to describe the funduscopic picture of exudative gray-white sheathing of the major retinal blood vessels. The retinal veins or arteries or both may be primarily affected. Fluorescein angiography shows evidence of perivenous or periarterial staining and may show evidence of vascular obstruction. In using these terms, we recognize that the primary cause of the fundus and angiographic findings may be immune-induced damage rather than inflammatory cell damage to the permeability and patency of the retinal blood vessels. Retinal vasculitis and perivasculitis may occur as part of well-defined ocular diseases of known cause (toxoplasmosis, pp. 614-622; diffuse subacute neuroretinitis, pp. 622-628; cytomegalovirus retinitis, pp. 642-645; syphilis, pp. 608-611) or well-defined syndromes of unknown cause (sarcoidosis, pp. 698-700; Behçet's disease, pp. 702-704; acute posterior multifocal placoid pigment epitheliopathy, pp. 668-675; acute zonal occult outer retinopathy, pp. 682-683; pars planitis, pp. 705-707; multiple sclerosis,[563,565] p. 706; idiopathic recurrent branch retinal artery occlusion, pp. 458-462; and Eales' disease, pp. 534-538). Other more recently described or less well-defined clinical syndromes associated with retinal vasculitis and perivasculitis are retinal phlebitis and panuveitis associated with viral-like upper respiratory disease,[558] frosted branch retinal angiitis and acute multifocal hemorrhagic retinal vasculitis.[381,556,559,562,566-568]

Acute retinal periphlebitis and panuveitis associated with viral-like upper respiratory disease

Acute bilateral visual blurring associated with inflammatory cellular infiltration of the anterior and posterior ocular chambers and fluorescein angiographic evidence of periphlebitis may occur in some patients during or immediately following an upper respiratory or flulike illness (Fig. 7-29, A to D).[557,558,560,561,564] Visual blurring usually disappears in 1 to 2 weeks in association with return of the fundus and angiographic findings to normal. An adenovirus was cultured from the stool of one such patient (Fig. 7-29, A to D).

Frosted branch angiitis

Patients with frosted branch angiitis present with visual symptoms associated with a striking ophthalmoscopic picture in one or both eyes of widespread prominent perivascular infiltration that in most patients is confined to the major retinal veins (Fig. 7-29, E to L).[556,559,562,566-568] This may or may not be associated with retinal hemorrhages, serous macular detachment, and optic disc swelling. Most previously reported patients have received systemic corticosteroid treatment, but some patients may recover without treatment.[567] Although the visual prognosis is generally good, some patients may develop severe perivascular hemorrhage, extensive retinal vascular closure, retinitis proliferans, vitreous hemorrhage, and rubeosis of the iris (Fig. 7-29, G to L).[562] These latter patients become indistinguishable from patients with acute multifocal hemorrhagic retinal vasculitis (see following discussion).

Acute multifocal hemorrhagic retinal vasculitis

Otherwise healthy patients with acute multifocal hemorrhagic retinal vasculitis develop loss of vision associated with mild anterior uveitis, multifocal areas of retinal vasculitis (predominantly venular) with marked intraretinal hemorrhage, retinal capillary nonperfusion, retinal neovascularization, optic disc swelling, and vitritis.[381] Retinal necrosis is not a prominent part of this syndrome. Oral prednisone appears to be of some benefit in treatment of this disorder, which is unresponsive to treatment with acyclovir. Photocoagulation of the neovascular complications may be necessary. The etiology of this disorder, which shares some features with Behçet's disease, Eales' disease, and acute retinal necrosis, is unknown.

FIG. 7-29 **Acute Retinal Periphlebitis and Panuveitis.**

A to D, This 9-year-old boy complained of blurred vision while recovering from an acute respiratory infection. Visual acuity was 20/25. There were cells in the anterior chamber and vitreous. Note the retinal striae in the macular region (**A**). The left eye showed identical changes. Adenovirus was cultured from his throat, and spinal fluid examination revealed pleocytosis. Angiography revealed leakage of dye from the optic disc and the major retinal veins (**B**). Six weeks later visual acuity, the fundi, and fluorescein angiography were normal (**D**).

E to L, Frosted branch angiitis occurred in this 25-year-old woman who noted blurred vision as she was recovering from an upper respiratory infection. Her visual acuity was 20/40 right eye and 20/25 left eye. She had vitreous cells, sheathing of the retinal veins, and mild optic disc edema bilaterally (**E and F**). She was treated with 80 mg daily of prednisone orally. Two weeks later her visual acuity was finger counting at 1 foot, right eye, and at 5 feet, left eye. She had severe hemorrhagic retinopathy that was more marked in the right eye (**G to I**). Angiography (**J to L**) showed marked closure of the peripheral retinal vasculature. She subsequently developed severe proliferative retinopathy that required panretinal photocoagulation and vitrectomy.

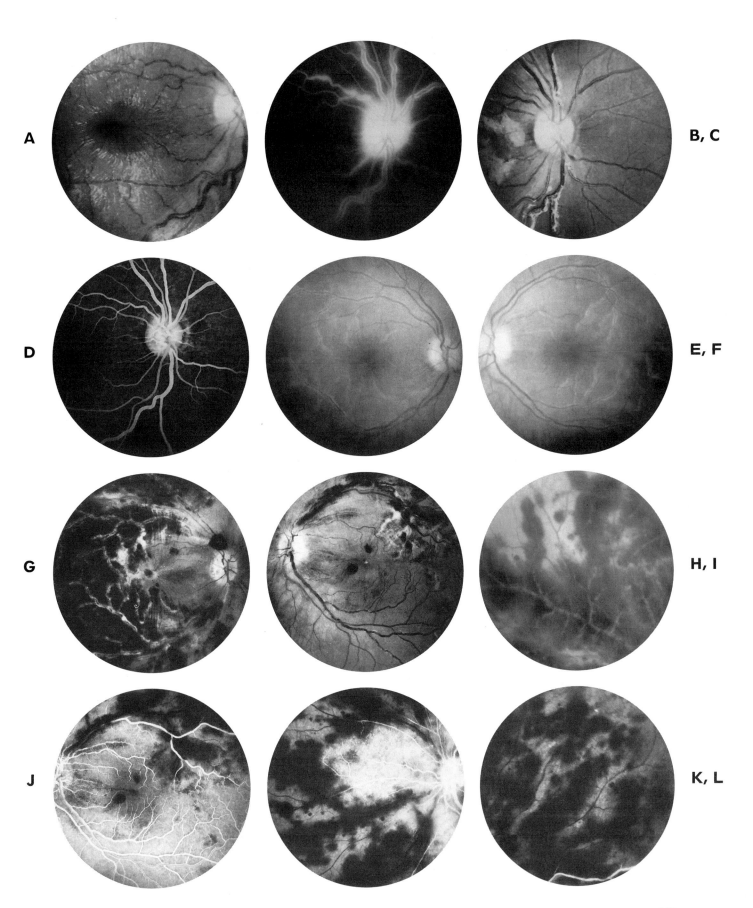

▼ RETINOCHOROIDAL DEGENERATION ASSOCIATED WITH PROGRESSIVE IRIS NECROSIS

Margo et al. described progressive pigment epithelial and retinal atrophy that began in the macula and juxtapapillary retina (Fig. 7-30, *A* to *D*), mild iritis, elevated intraocular pressure (IOP), severe pain, progressive iris atrophy (Fig. 7-30, *E*), progressive decrease in ERG amplitudes, and complete blindness within 3 years in a healthy 34-year-old man whose extensive medical workup was negative.[569] Histopathology revealed pigment granules and pigment-laden macrophages in the AC, severe ischemic necrosis of the iris *(F)* chronic inflammatory cells in the uveal tract, and marked chorioretinal atrophy, with only a thin strand of glial tissue resting on an atrophic choroid. There were patchy areas of preservation of the inner retina posteriorly (Fig. 7-30, *G*) and some preservation of the retina and choroid peripherally, where thrombi were found in some of the choroidal blood vessels. Electron microscopy revealed no viral particles or evidence of a storage disease. The authors found no clues as to the pathogenesis of the disorder.

FIG. 7-30 Retinochoroidal Degeneration Associated with Progressive Iris Necrosis.

A to **G,** This healthy 34-year-old man became bilaterally blind within 3 years after the onset of an unusual retinochoroidal degenerative disease. Within five months of the onset of symptoms his visual acuity declined to 20/300. There was severe mottling of the RPE in the macula bilaterally (**A** and **B**). Dark adaptation studies, VEP, and ERG were normal. Eighteen months later there was extensive degeneration of the retina, counting fingers visual acuity, and severe ocular pain bilaterally (**C** and **D**). The third year of his illness was characterized by severe retinal vascular narrowing, mild iritis, progressive iris atrophy (**E**), modest elevation of the intraocular pressure, and blindness. Both eyes were enucleated because of severe pain. Histopathologic examination revealed severe ischemic necrosis of the iris (**F**), mild nongranulomatous uveitis, and marked chorioretinal atrophy and degeneration postequatorially. There were a few areas of preservation of the inner retina posteriorly (**G**). Electron microscopy revealed no viral particles.

(From Margo et al.[569])

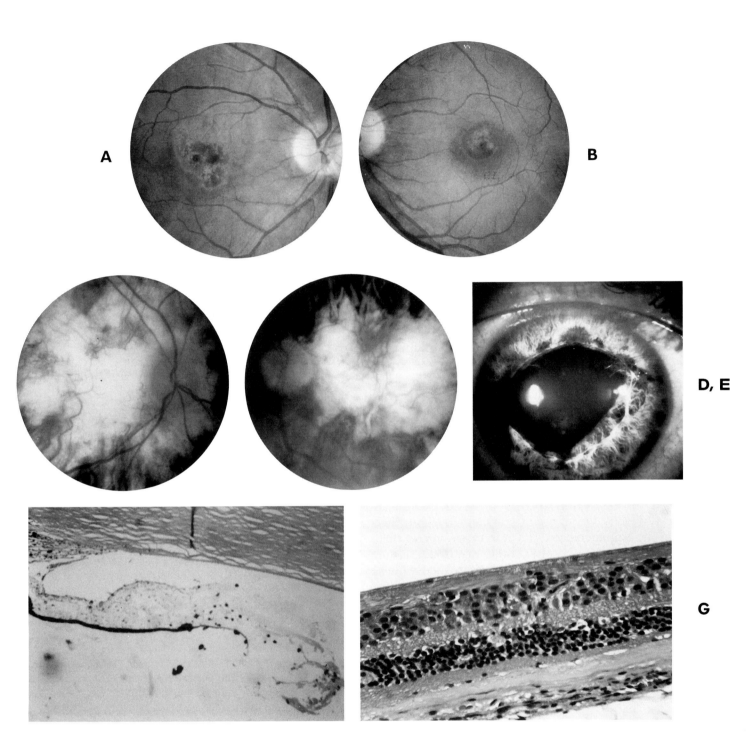

▼ ACUTE POSTERIOR MULTIFOCAL PLACOID PIGMENT EPITHELIOPATHY

Acute posterior multifocal placoid pigment epitheliopathy (APMPPE) typically affects young healthy male or female patients (average age approximately 25 years), who develop rapid loss of vision in one or both eyes secondary to multiple postequatorial, circumscribed, flat, gray-white, subretinal lesions involving the RPE (Figs. 7-31 to 7-33).* These lesions are rarely associated with retinal detachment or with retinal hemorrhage (Fig. 7-32, B and C).[591,595] The overlying retina usually appears normal. Inflammatory cells in the vitreous may be present in 50% of the patients. Approximately one-third of the patients give a history of a flulike syndrome antedating the onset of visual symptoms.† In one case it followed a mild hypersensitivity reaction to swine flu vaccine.[594] APMPPE has occurred in patients with thyroiditis,[596] cerebrovasculitis,‡ adenovirus type 5 infection,[572] lymphadenopathy,[591] hepatomegaly (Fig. 7-31, K and L),[591] erythema nodosum,[583,591,615] regional enteritis,[591] sarcoidosis,[575,585] acute nephritis,[602] lupus erythematosus,[598] serologic evidence of Lyme disease,[576,621] and spinal fluid pleocytosis and elevated protein.[577,588,589,595,610] Two patients with evidence of CNS vasculitis died within several weeks after onset of APMPPE as systemic corticosteroids were being tapered.[593,618] Autopsy in one case revealed evidence of granulomatous arteritis in the leptomeninges.[618] These cases suggest that APMPPE may be the initial manifestation of primary CNS angiitis, which is associated with a high mortality rate of approximately 95% if untreated, 46% if treated with corticosteroids, and 8% if treated with corticosteroids and cytotoxic agents.[578]

---

*References 571-573, 577, 581-583, 588-592, 594-597, 600, 601, 603-610, 615, 617, 624.
†References 572, 589, 591, 595, 608, 619.
‡References 570, 587, 595, 599, 610-614, 616, 618.

FIG. 7-31   Acute Posterior Multifocal Placoid Pigment Epitheliopathy (APMPPE).

A to F, This healthy 22-year-old woman developed blurred vision in both eyes 5 days before admission. Her past history was unremarkable. Visual acuity in the right eye was 20/200 and in the left eye was 20/20. Note the multifocal, flat, white lesions involving the RPE (A). The lesion superiorly had undergone partial resolution, and some details of the underlying choroid were visible. Note absence of serous detachment of the overlying retina. Early angiograms revealed absence of background fluorescence in the region of the active lesions (B). Some background fluorescence is visible in the partly resolved lesion superiorly. One hour after injection, the angiogram showed fluorescein staining of all lesions (C). Nine days later, her visual acuity had returned to 20/50. There was focal depigmentation of the RPE following the rapid resolution of the placoid lesions in both eyes (D and E). Seven months later, visual acuity was 20/20. Thirteen months after the onset of her disease she had recurrence of symptoms in the left eye with transient loss of vision. These lesions healed, and when last seen 40 months after the onset of her disease, visual acuity was 20/20. Note evidence of the more recent lesion superiorly (F).

G to J, This 45-year-old woman developed rapid loss of vision (10/200) in the left eye. Note the large centrally located lesion (G). Angiography revealed other lesions, all of which were nonfluorescent in the early phases of angiography (H) and which stained later (I). Twelve months later, her vision had returned to 20/20 (J). Thirty months after the onset of her disease she developed a similar large central lesion in the right eye and experienced an identical clinical course in that eye.

K and L, Severe bilateral acute posterior multifocal placoid pigment epitheliopathy in a 19-year-old woman who noted the onset of visual loss several days after an upper respiratory infection. Note the evidence of early resolution of the macular lesion (K). Vitreous cells were present. The patient's visual acuity was 20/200. A liver scan revealed hepatomegaly and abnormal uptake of radioisotopes in the left lobe. Her electrooculographic findings were normal. Her electroretinographic findings were subnormal. Six months later the visual acuity was 20/50 in the right eye and 20/25 in the left eye, despite the widespread alterations in the RPE throughout the posterior pole of both eyes (L).

(A to F from Gass.[590])

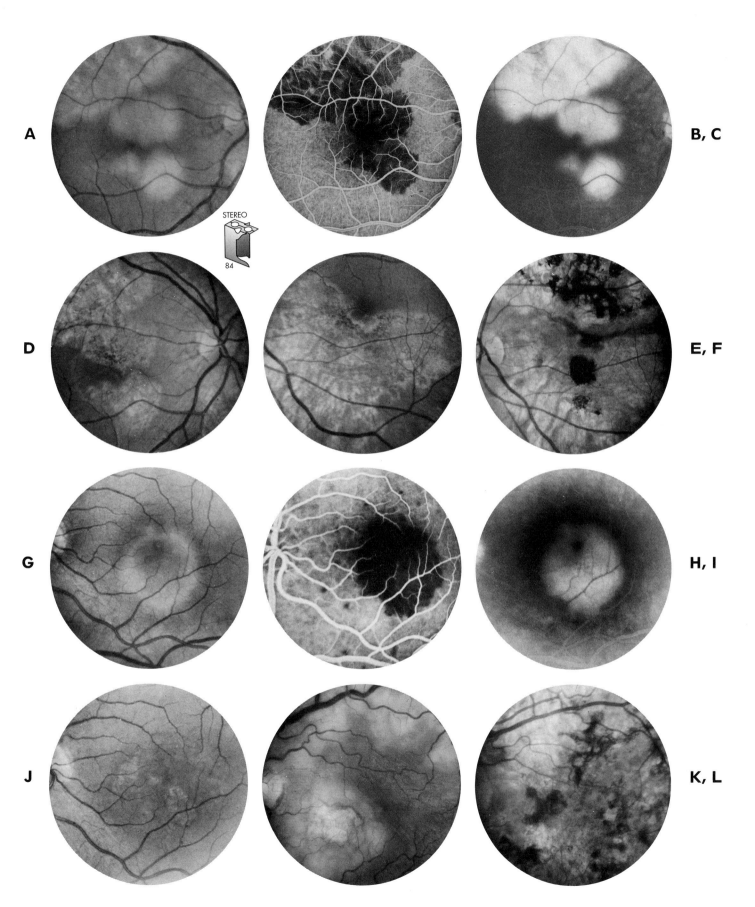

A

B, C

D

E, F

STEREO
84

G

H, I

J

K, L

669

Other ocular findings include perivenous exudation in the retina,[590,594] perichoroidal venous infiltration,[612] and dilation and tortuosity of the retinal veins, papilledema,[592] papillitis, optic neuritis,* episcleritis (Fig. 7-32, *A*),[591] iridocyclitis,[589,591] and central retinal vein occlusion (Dr. Lawrence A. Yannuzzi, personal communication). This latter may develop as a result of vasculitis and swelling within the optic nerve.

Infrequently, APMPPE occurs unilaterally. The second eye is usually involved within a few days or weeks after the first. In two patients the interval was 30 and 36 months (Fig. 7-31, *G* to *J*).[591] Recurrences are infrequent and usually occur in the first 6 months following the onset of symptoms (Fig. 7-31, *A* to *F*). Characteristic features of the disease are the rapid resolution of the fundus lesions and the delayed remarkable return of visual function usually to the level of approximately 20/30 or better (Fig. 7-31, *A* to *D*).[591] Within a few days following the onset of symptoms the acute gray-white lesions begin to fade centrally. Within 7 to 12 days they are completely replaced by areas of partly depigmented RPE (Fig. 7-31, *D* and *E*). Irregular clumping of pigment occurs, and day-to-day changes in its pattern develop over a period of months. The acute and subacute lesions superficially resemble those seen after photocoagulation.

During the acute phase of APMPPE the subretinal lesions block out most of the background choroidal fluorescence (Fig. 7-31, *B* and *H*, and 7-32, *C*). Mid- and late-phase angiograms demonstrate diffuse, even staining of the acute lesions (Fig. 7-31, *B*, *C*, *H*, and *I*). During the course of early resolution of these lesions, angiography demonstrates large choroidal vessels coursing through the center of the partly faded gray lesions before the development of staining in the later pictures (Fig. 7-31, *B*). During the later course of resolution, angiography demonstrates extensive alterations in the background choroidal fluorescence caused by changes in the content of the RPE but shows relatively little evidence of occlusion of the choriocapillaris. Subnormal electrooculographic findings have been reported during the acute stage of the disease. Most patients tested during the acute phases of the disease have normal electrooculograms and electroretinograms. One patient with severe involvement had normal electrooculographic findings with subnormal cone and rod electroretinographic findings (Fig. 7-31, *K* and *L*).

---

*References 592, 596, 597, 600, 609, 610, 615, 620.

FIG. 7-32 **Acute Posterior Multifocal Placoid Pigment Epitheliopathy (APMPPE).**

A, Episcleritis in a patient presenting with bilateral APMPPE.

B and **C,** APMPPE associated with a small subretinal hemorrhage *(arrow).*

D and **E,** Choroidal neovascularization *(arrows)* occurring several years after the patient recovered near normal visual acuity after bilateral APMPPE.

F to **I,** Schematic diagrams depicting probable histopathologic changes and fluorescein staining pattern in acute posterior multifocal placoid pigment epitheliopathy. The acute yellow-white focal lesion is probably composed of swollen retinal pigment epithelial *[RPE]* cells and damaged outer retinal segments between the arrows in **F, G,** and **H.** In the early phase angiograms the fluorescein *[black stippling]* has perfused the choroidal circulation (**F**), and quickly stains the choroid *[ch],* and is beginning to move into the base of the swollen RPE cells with cloudy cytoplasm (**G**). Loss of transparency of the RPE and outer retinal receptors totally obscures the fluorescein in the choroid. In the late stage of angiography (**H**) the dye has stained the affected cells, choroid *[ch],* and sclera *[S],* causing the acute lesion to appear hyperfluorescent. Healed stage of APMPPE, late phase of angiography (**I**) shows restoration of the outer retinal-blood barrier, patchy areas of depigmentation and hyperpigmentation of the RPE cells, and regrowth of the retinal outer segments, but some loss of receptor cells.

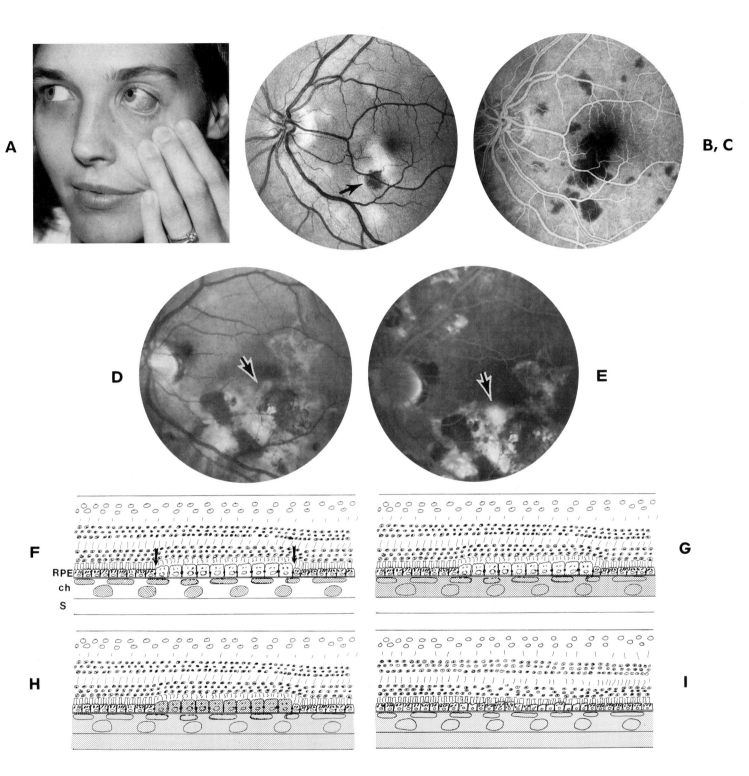

A

B, C

D

E

F

RPE

ch

S

G

H

I

671

The prognosis for visual recovery is good. Visual recovery can occur up to as long as 6 months. In an average followup of over 5 years in 30 patients seen at the Bascom Palmer Eye Institute, all but two eyes had 20/30 or better visual acuity at the last examination.[591] Many patients will identify small residual paracentral scotomata when carefully tested. Recurrences and the development of choroidal neovascularization occur infrequently (Fig. 7-32, *D* and *E*).[586,591,592,604]

The cause of this disease, which in many instances is associated with evidence of systemic involvement, is unknown. In the eye it appears to be an acute, self-limited disease, initially causing multifocal areas of color change in the RPE and perhaps retinal and receptor cells. The cell cytoplasm apparently becomes sufficiently cloudy that it blocks out all background choroidal fluorescence. The course and nature of the disease suggest the possibility of viral infection. Figure 7-32, *F* to *I,* illustrates schematically some of the presumed anatomic changes in this disease. Despite the extensive alterations in the pigment content, the RPE cells and most of the retinal receptors apparently recover and visual acuity usually returns to near normal. The end stage of this disease is similar in this respect to rubella.

FIG. 7-33 Atypical Acute Posterior Multifocal Placoid Pigment Epitheliopathy.

A to **F,** Acute loss of vision occurred in both eyes of this 49-year-old with multiple small, confluent subretinal lesions in both eyes (**A** and **B**). Angiography showed obstruction of choroidal fluorescence early (**C** and **D**) and later irregular and incomplete staining of the lesions (**E** and **F**). Seven months later her visual acuity was 20/30 right eye and 20/100 left eye.

G to **I,** Probable APMPPE causing acute loss of central vision in the left eye of a 50-year-old woman who had bilateral drusen (**F**). The findings, including the angiograms (**H** and **I**), were misinterpreted elsewhere as evidence of choroidal neovascularization. Four years later her visual acuity was 20/200 and there was a pattern of geographic thinning of the RPE corresponding with the acute lesion.

J to **L,** Probable APMPPE in the right eye of this 58-year-old man who had acute loss of vision in the right eye while recovering from an upper respiratory infection. He had bilateral familial macular drusen. The multifocal confluent gray lesions (**J**) were more apparent angiographically as nonfluorescent spots (**K**) when the patient was examined by his local physician. Nine months later his acuity in the right eye was 3/200. Note the atrophy of the RPE (**L**).

(**A** to **F,** courtesy of Dr Gerard L. Van Wesep.)

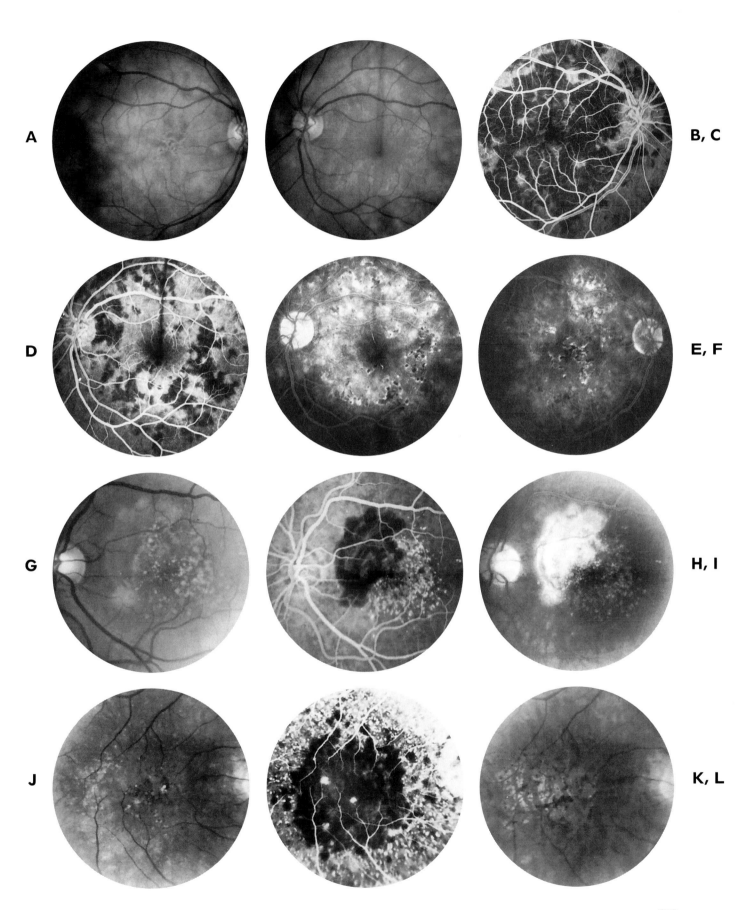

673

Most authors have favored choriocapillaris occlusion as the cause of the color change in the RPE and the early angiographic findings.[582-585,601,615,624] The following are difficult, however, to explain on the basis of choroidal vascular occlusion: (1) the variability in the size and shape of the lesions, which appear to have no relationship to the anatomy of the choriocapillaris; (2) the failure of the acute lesions to stain with fluorescein from the periphery inward, as would be expected to occur from neighboring normally perfused choriocapillaris; and (3) the frequency of recovery of visual function.[591] Demonstration of large fluorescent choroidal vessels coursing through the area of partly resolved acute lesions (Fig. 7-31, B) does not necessarily mean there is nonperfusion of the choriocapillaris in these areas. The RPE cells, which undoubtedly are still present in these areas, may be sufficiently opaque to attenuate the fluorescence arising from the choriocapillaris but not that in the large choroidal vessels. The findings with indocyanine green angiography are similar to that with fluorescein and in the author's opinion do not shed further light on the pathophysiology of APMPPE.[584]

Wolf et al. reported HLA-B7 antigens in 40% and HLA-DR2 antigens in 57% of patients with APMPPE vs 17% and 28%, respectively, in controls.[622]

There is no information concerning the relative value of systemic treatment with corticosteroids compared to no treatment of patients with APMPPE. The natural course of the disease suggests that the visual prognosis is favorable without treatment. Some might argue that corticosteroids should be given if for no other reason than to reduce the potential of CNS complications. It is unknown, however, whether this treatment is beneficial or harmful in this regard. Patients and their families should be alerted to the relatively low possibility of CNS complications and of the importance of promptly reporting any symptoms or signs suggesting CNS involvement. There is evidence that patients with idiopathic CNS angiitis do benefit from corticosteroid and cytotoxic therapy.[578]

It is important to differentiate APMPPE from serpiginous (geographic) choroiditis. Although the acute lesions in both diseases appear similar ophthalmoscopically and angiographically, the lesions of serpiginous choroiditis resolve more slowly and leave in their wake ophthalmoscopic and angiographic evidence of marked atrophy of the underlying choriocapillaris and larger choroidal vessels (see p. 160). Some patients reported as having APMPPE with atypical features, such as branch vein occlusion, may have had serpiginous choroiditis.[579,604] Serpiginous choroiditis is a chronic, recurring, often severe disease that may leave the patient with severe visual disability in one or both eyes. Table 7-1 outlines some of the important differences in these two diseases.

The multifocal white lesions in APMPPE must be differentiated from other causes of multifocal deep retinitis (e.g., diffuse unilateral subacute neuroretinitis) (Fig. 7-11, D and E), multiple evanescent white dot syndrome (Fig. 7-35, A and G), focal inflammatory cell infiltrates of the choroid (e.g., multifocal choroiditis with panuveitis [pseudo–presumed ocular histoplasmosis syndrome]), sarcoidosis,[575,585] secondary syphilis (Fig. 7-4, B), diffuse choroidal infiltration in Harada's disease that may be associated with multifocal ill-defined lesions at the level of the pigment epithelium (see Fig. 3-60, A),[580] sympathetic uveitis (see Fig. 3-62, D), multifocal zones of occlusion of the choriocapillaris (e.g., toxemia of pregnancy, see Fig. 3-67, D), primary or metastatic neoplastic infiltrates of the choroid or sub-RPE space (see Figs. 3-89, D and E, and 11-8, G and H), and multifocal areas of depigmentation of the choroid, such as occurs in vitiliginous chorioretinitis (see Fig. 7-49, A and B). Focal inflammatory cell infiltrates of the choroid are often smaller and slightly elevated, frequently persist for several weeks or more, and often cause secondary detachment of the overlying retina. They may completely resolve without leaving significant changes in the overlying RPE, or they may cause varying degrees of atrophy of the choroid and RPE. The author believes that the patients reported as having retinal detachment secondary to APMPPE showed features more typical of a diffuse underlying choroiditis, probably Harada's disease, rather than APMPPE (see Fig. 3-60, A).[573,623]

The syndrome of acute retinal pigment epithe-liitis is characterized by the development of clusters of small pigment spots surrounded by halos of depigmentation in young patients with a recent history of visual loss. These patients experience rapid recovery of vision (see p. 676). Photographs of the appearance of the fundus within the first few days after the onset of symptoms have not been published, and therefore it is possible that some of these patients may indeed have APMPPE. In general, however, the lesions in APMPPE are much larger than can be accounted for on the basis of the RPE findings in acute retinal pigment epitheliitis.

Extensive pigmentary changes remaining during the late stages of APMPPE (Fig. 7-31, L) may be mistaken for a widespread tapetoretinal dystrophy. The clinical history of rapid loss and recovery of vision, the normal appearing retinal vessels and optic nerve head, and usually normal electrophysiologic findings should differentiate retinal dystrophies from the late stages of APMPPE.

Priluck and associates have demonstrated the presence of urinary casts in three patients during the active phase of APMPPE.[606] The significance of this observation is unknown.

Although most patients with APMPPE present with multiple one-disc diameter–size white lesions randomly scattered in the posterior fundus, the size, shape, and distribution of the lesions may be variable (Figs. 7-31, G, and 7-33, A). In some cases the lesions are small, are confluent, and may show some persistence of nonfluorescence into the late stage of angiography (Fig. 7-33, A to F). I have seen what appears to be APMPPE occurring unilaterally in four patients in the sixth decade or beyond with multiple drusen in the macula (Fig. 7-33, F to L). In each case acute visual loss was attributed by the referring physician to senile macular degeneration. In two of the four cases visual acuity did not return to normal levels (Fig. 7-33, F to L). In several of these cases the lesions were uniformly small and closely spaced, similar to those which occurred in a 35-year-old man described as having diffuse punctate pigment epitheliopathy by Blinder et al.[574] Their patient failed to recover central vision.

▼ SERPIGINOUS CHOROIDITIS

See Chapter 3 for discussion of this acute multifocal choroiditis that may simulate APMPPE.

TABLE 7-1

DIFFERENTIAL DIAGNOSTIC FEATURES OF ACUTE POSTERIOR MULTIFOCAL PLACOID PIGMENT EPITHELIOPATHY (APMPPE) AND SERPIGINOUS CHOROIDITIS

	APMPPE	Serpiginous choroiditis
Age of onset	Second and third decades	Beyond third decade
Associated systemic disease	Upper respiratory infection, erythema nodosum, regional enteritis, hepatitis, episcleritis, cerebral vasculitis	None
Visual complaints at onset	Bilateral	Unilateral
Acute lesions	Flat, white, RPE lesions	Same
Lesion distribution	Postequatorial	Peripapillary
Lesion shape	Usually isolated	Usually contiguous
Vitritis	±	±
Choroidal atrophy	Minimal	Maximal
Proliferative subretinal scarring	None	Frequent
Visual recovery	Excellent	Poor
Recurrence	Rare	Typical
Choroidal neovascularization	Rare	30% of patients

▼ ACUTE IDIOPATHIC MACULOPATHY

Yannuzzi and coworkers reported 9 patients who after a flulike illness developed sudden severe unilateral central visual loss associated with vitreous cells; neurosensory macular detachment; retinal hemorrhages; an irregular white, gray, or yellow thickening of the RPE that was consistent with a subretinal infiltrate beneath a portion of the retinal detachment; and a neovascular process or acute swelling of the RPE cells (Fig. 7-34).[626] A peculiar pseudopodal extension of the subretinal exudation and subretinal hemorrhages were present in some cases. Irregular staining of the subretinal thickening angiographically simulated that occurring with subretinal neovascularization (Fig. 7-34, C and D). Complete staining occurred in late pictures. In spite of the appearance, the subretinal exudate disappeared and visual acuity returned to nearly normal. A characteristic "bull's-eye" pattern of pigment epithelial atrophy in the macula persisted. No patient had a recurrence. One patient had the late development of subretinal neovascularization. Fish and coworkers presented a similar case that in addition showed evidence of a pseudohypopyon in the macula during the acute phase of the disease.[625] In unpublished work Yannuzzi and coworkers have recently broadened the spectrum of this disorder to include eccentric macular lesions, fellow eye involvement, papillitis, and an association of the disorder with pregnancy and AIDS.

▼ ACUTE RETINAL PIGMENT EPITHELIITIS

Krill and Deutman[631] described the syndrome of acute retinal pigment epitheliitis, which is characterized by the rapid onset of visual disturbances in one or both eyes of young adults followed by gradual and almost complete recovery in 7 to 10 weeks.[627-630] One to 2 weeks after the onset of symptoms, these patients had multiple clusters of discrete, round, dark spots surrounded by depigmented halolike zones present at the level of the RPE in the macula and paramacular area (Fig. 7-34, E). These were usually one-fourth disc diameter in size. The fundus findings during the first week after the onset of symptoms have not been described. Fluorescein angiography demonstrates a halo of hyperfluorescence surrounding the dark spot seen ophthalmoscopically (Fig. 7-34, F). In some cases, angiography may be essentially normal. The loss of visual function is out of proportion to the changes seen in the macula. After

FIG. 7-34 Acute Idiopathic Maculopathy.

A to D, This healthy 38-year-old woman presented with a 2-day history of blurred vision into the right eye. Her visual acuity was 20/80. There was an exudative detachment of the retina in the macula associated with radiating retinal folds and cloudy subretinal exudate. The left eye was normal. The early-phase angiogram shows irregular mild hyperfluorescence corresponding to the area of detachment (**B**). Later there was intense staining of the subretinal fluid (*stereoangiograms,* **C** and **D**). Five days later her visual acuity was 20/30. Four years later her acuity was 20/20 in both eyes and the fundi were normal.

Acute Retinal Pigment Epitheliitis.

E to F, This 25-year-old woman noted photopsia, blurred vision, and multiple paracentral scotomata in the right eye 12 days before her examination at the Bascom Palmer Eye Institute. When examined by her local physician several days after the onset her acuity was 20/20 and the fundus was described as normal. One week later her acuity was 20/30 and some "yellow material was noted in the right macula." At the Bascom Palmer Eye Institute her acuity was 20/25. Multiple paracentral scotomata were demonstrable on the Amsler grid in the right eye. There were no vitreous cells. There were multiple, small, pigmented lesions surrounded by depigmented halos at the level of the RPE (*arrow,* **E**). The left fundus was normal. Angiography revealed small halos of hyperfluorescence corresponding with the lesions (*arrows,* **F**). She was last seen by her local physician 8 months after the onset of symptoms. Visual acuity was 20/20, and the fundus was normal.

recovery of central vision the RPE changes may be barely visible. The cause of this self-limited disorder is unknown.

The halolike lesions said to be the hallmark of this disease may be seen in patients with a variety of circumstances, including idiopathic central serous chorioretinopathy, drusen, adult-onset vitelliform foveomacular (pattern) dystrophy, and occult choroidal neovascularization, and in asymptomatic patients. Clumping of RPE surrounded by areas of depigmentation is a nonspecific reaction to a variety of insults and is a focus where fluid may escape temporarily into the subretinal space. Other possible causes of transient loss of vision in these young patients include mild cases of acute posterior multifocal placoid pigment epitheliopathy, multiple evanescent white dot syndrome, and acute macular neuroretinopathy. The author has never seen a patient with this disorder, which apparently occurs very uncommonly. Figure 7-34 depicts one of only a few cases coded as such in the files of the Bascom Palmer Eye Institute.

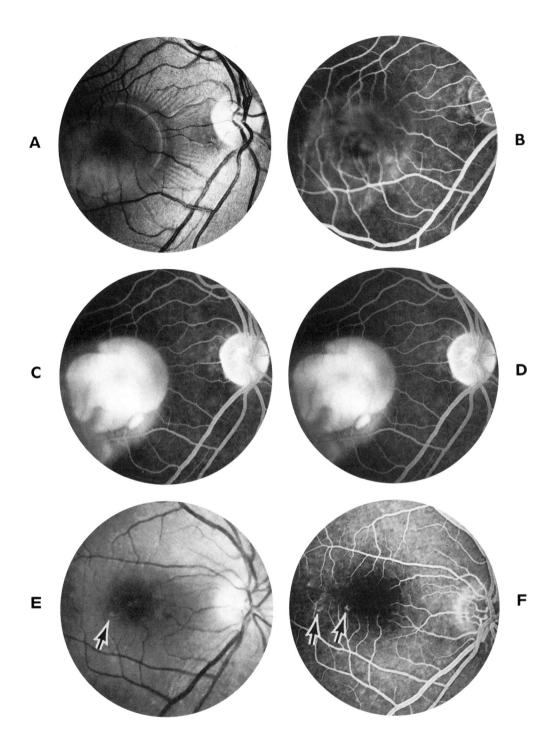

Chittum and Kalina reported eight patients with acute retinal pigment epitheliitis associated with a fine pattern of pigment stippling confined largely to the foveolar area.[627] These changes illustrated in their color fundus photographs appear similar to those seen in the foveolar area of patients with MEWDS (see next section).

▼ MULTIPLE EVANESCENT WHITE DOT SYNDROME

The following features characterize multiple evanescent white dot syndrome (MEWDS), which typically affects one eye of young females: (1) blurred vision, multiple paracentral scotomata, usually including a temporal scotoma, and photopsia occurring in approximately one-half of patients soon after a flulike illness; (2) vitreous cells; (3) multiple small, often poorly defined, gray-white patches at the level of the RPE and outer retina (Figs. 7-35, A, B, and G, 7-36, B and F); (4) a cluster of tiny white or light-orange dots in the foveola; (5) early punctate hyperfluorescence of the gray-white patches, which often show a cluster or wreath-shaped pattern (Fig. 7-35, C and D); (6) late fluorescein staining of these lesions, and in some cases staining of the optic nerve head (Fig. 7-35, E); (7) blind spot enlargement; (8) decrease in the electroretinogram a-wave and early receptor potential amplitudes; and (9) spontaneous recovery of visual function, normalization of the electroretinographic findings, and return of the ophthalmoscopic and angiographic findings toward normal in 7 to 10 weeks (Fig. 7-35, F).* The white spots in MEWDS, which are often small, ill defined, and located in the extramacular area, are easily overlooked. It is probable that most patients reported as having the acute idiopathic blind spot enlargement syndrome[641] probably had MEWDS, and that the white lesions were either overlooked or had faded at the time of their examination.[638,639,642,643,645,670]

---

*References 632, 634, 637, 644, 647, 648, 652, 654-657, 659, 661, 663-667.

FIG. 7-35 Multiple Evanescent White Dot Syndrome.

A to F, This 34-year-old woman noted multiple scotomata in the right eye of 1 day's duration. This was unassociated with other illness. Her visual acuity was 20/60. There were widely scattered gray-white patches at the level of the RPE throughout the posterior fundus (A and B). Each patch was composed of smaller, more intensely white dots. Angiographically, the lesions showed a wreathlike pattern of hyperfluorescent dots early and later staining and there was staining of the optic disc (C to E). The left eye was normal. Four weeks later the visual acuity was 20/25 in the right eye and the appearance of the right fundus was normal (F).

G to L, This 32-year-old pilot noted photopsia, temporal scotoma, and blurred vision in his left eye. His visual acuity was 20/20. He had a marked enlargement of the blind spot in the left eye. There were multiple focal outer retinal gray lesions in the perimacular and peripapillary region of the left eye (arrows, G and H). The optic disc margins were slightly blurred. There were several orange punctate lesions in the foveolar region. The right eye was normal. Angiography revealed faint multiple foci of staining (arrows, I) in the perimacular and peripapillary area as well as some staining of the optic disc. Within 10 weeks all of his symptoms resolved and the size of the blind spot decreased. One year later his only residual symptom was the presence of a temporal zone of "heat wave" distortion seen only in bright illumination.

(A to F from Mamalis and Daily.[657])

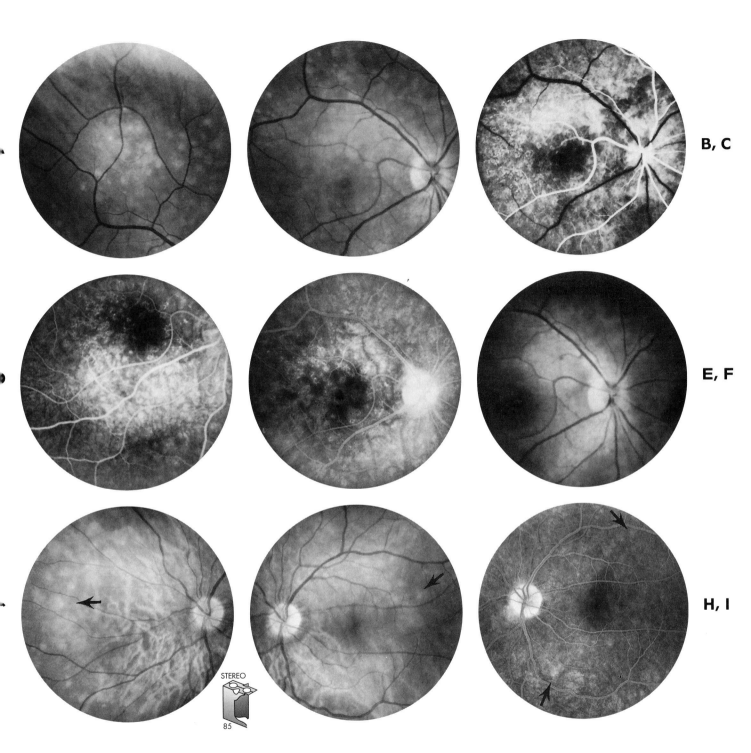

B, C

E, F

H, I

STEREO
85

679

Indocyanine green angiography demonstrates patchy hyperfluorescence at the level of the RPE as well as multiple, small, round, hypofluorescent lesions, some of which occurred in the absence of fundus changes.[646] Although fluorescein angiography often shows some staining of the optic disc during the acute phases of the disease, there is minimal evidence that damage to the retinal ganglion cells and optic nerve is responsible for visual loss.[639] Later in the course of the disease a zone of RPE depigmentation and hyperfluorescence corresponding with their enlarged blind spot or other field defect may develop (Fig. 7-36, E).[642,670] Subretinal neovascularization may occasionally occur.[658,672] Scanning laser densitometry demonstrates evidence of a focal defect in the visual pigment kinetics of the receptor cells in the macular area.[649,669] Evaluation for evidence of systemic disease is usually negative. Some visual field loss and color vision defect may persist.[662] The cause of the disease is unknown. Males may be affected, the disorder may occasionally affect both eyes, and late recurrences may occasionally occur.[633,648,659,663,668] In some cases the visual field defects do not resolve.[644]

Before or following MEWDS some patients develop evidence of pseudo–presumed ocular histoplasmosis syndrome, acute macular neuropathy, and acute onset of large visual field defects unassociated with visible changes in the fundi (Fig. 7-36).[636,643,650,658] Fig. 7-36, F to L, shows a patient who presented with findings typical for MEWDS in one eye and pseudo-presumed ocular histoplasmosis or punctate inner choroiditis in the fellow eye. There is evidence that MEWDS may be part of a spectrum of one disease or closely related diseases that include acute idiopathic blind spot enlargement,* acute zonal occult outer retinopathy (see discussion to follow), pseudo–presumed ocular histoplasmosis syndrome,† and acute macular neuroretinopathy,[635,643,665] All of the disorders affect predominantly young women and all may present with photopsia and zones of visual field loss caused by retinal receptor damage unexplained by biomicroscopic changes in the ocular fundi.[673]

---

*References 632, 636, 641, 651, 653, 665.
†References 636, 640, 660, 665, 671, 672.

FIG. 7-36   Multiple Evanescent White Dot Syndrome "Plus."

A to E, This 22-year-old woman noted the rapid onset of multiple scotomas and photopsia in the left eye. The visual acuity was 20/20 right eye, 20/30 left eye. There were multiple oval and round red-orange lesions at the level of the outer retina in the left macula (A). Angiography was normal. The diagnosis was acute macular neuroretinopathy. Fourteen months later the fundus and visual acuity were normal. Five years later she experienced the same but more severe symptoms in the left eye soon after an upper respiratory illness. Her visual acuity in the left eye was 20/80. She had an enlarged blind spot in the left eye. There were multiple outer retinal white lesions in the peripheral macular and juxtapapillary regions (B). Angiography revealed focal staining that in some areas corresponded with the lesions C and D. The visual acuity gradually improved to 20/20 over a period of 8 months. The enlarged blind spot and the photopsia persisted. Angiography demonstrated evidence of RPE depigmentation in a zone around the optic disc corresponding with her blind spot enlargement (E).

F to K, This 22-year-old woman had a 10-day history of decrease in vision in the left eye and 5 days before in the right eye associated with headache and myalgia. Visual acuity was 20/30, right eye, 20/70, left eye. She had a typical fundus and angiographic picture of MEWDS in the right eye (F and H), and punctate inner choroidopathy in the left eye (G and I). There were punctate yellow-orange dots in foveola bilaterally. There were no vitreous cells. There was some enlargement of the blind spot in the left eye. Indocyanine green angiography revealed multiple nonfluorescent lesions in the choroid in a pattern similar to the areas of staining in the fluorescein angiograms (J to L). Two years later her clinical and ICG findings were similar.

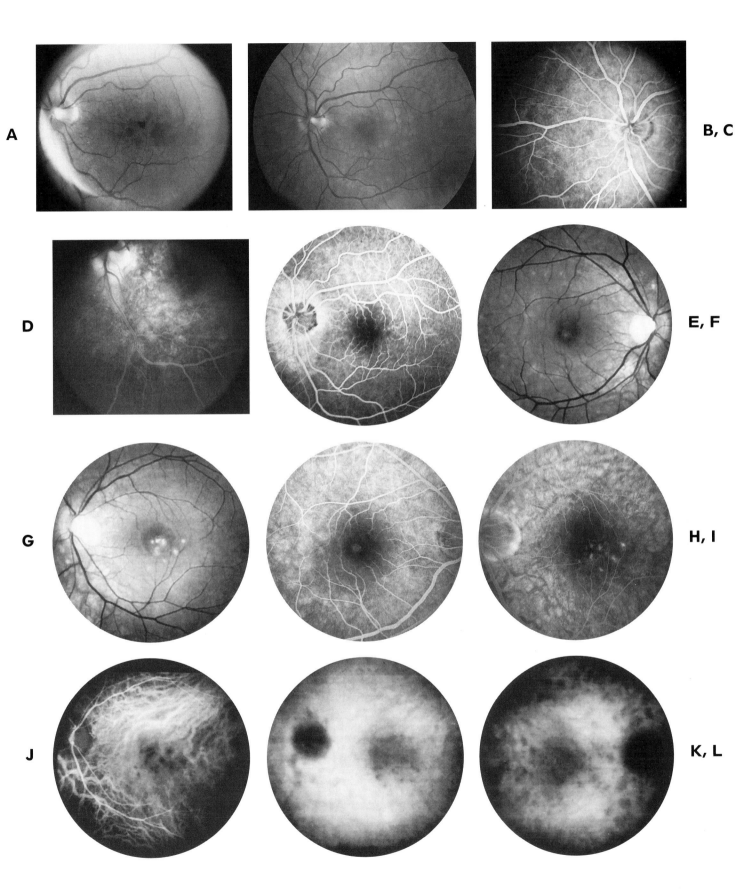

A

B, C

D

E, F

G

H, I

J

K, L

681

▼ ACUTE ZONAL OCCULT OUTER RETINOPATHY

In 1994 the author reported 13 patients, predominantly young women, with a syndrome characterized by rapid loss of one or more large zones of outer retinal function, photopsia, minimal funduscopic changes, usually mild vitritis, and electroretinographic abnormalities affecting one or both eyes (Fig. 7-37).[673] Progression of visual field loss occurred over a period of several weeks or months before either improving or stabilizing. Involvement of the second eye may be delayed for at least as long as 2 years (Fig. 7-37, A to I). All patients on followup examination had persistent visual field defects, and most had chronic photopsia and zones of pigment epithelial atrophy and retinal vascular narrowing, which in some cases mimicked that seen in retinitis pigmentosa and cancer-associated retinopathy (Fig. 7-37, J to L). In some patients large, permanent, visual field defects were unassociated with any visible changes in either the fundus or in fluorescein angiograms. The subtle nature of this presumed inflammatory disorder, which causes acute damage to broad zones of the outer retina without producing noticeable ophthalmoscopic changes, is responsible for the diagnostic confusion that usually results in extensive fruitless neurologic, medical, and ophthalmologic consultations and laboratory investigations. Demonstration during the early course of the disease of electroretinographic abnormalities is helpful in this regard. The ERGs in these patients show a pattern of visual dysfunction that is photoreceptor in origin, patchy in distribution, and asymmetric in the two eyes.[674] The cause of the acute damage to sharply defined zones of the retinal receptor cells in the absence of visible fundus changes in patients with acute zonal occult outer retinopathy (AZOOR) is unknown. There is no evidence to date for autoantibodies to any retinal cell type in patients with AZOOR.[674] Similar acute occult zones of visual field loss that are accompanied by ERG changes may occur in patients with MEWDS,[636,673] multifocal choroiditis and panuveitis (punctate inner choroiditis, pseudo-POHS),[636,650,665,673] and less often in patients with, or who previously have had, acute macular neuroretinopathy.[643,665] It is of interest that the initial reports of all of these syndromes, which affect primarily young adult women, have occurred since 1975. During the past 2 years the author has seen at least 10 other patients with evidence of overlap between MEWDS, pseudo-POHS, AZOOR, and acute idiopathic blind spot enlargement syndrome.

FIG. 7-37 Acute Zonal Outer Retinopathy, Occult Type.

A to C, This 24-year-old woman, while recovering from an upper respiratory infection, experienced rapid severe loss of vision over night in both eyes. Visual acuity in the right eye was 20/200, left eye 20/20. She had severe constriction of the visual field bilaterally. Both fundi and angiograms appeared normal (A and B). Seven months later she had bilateral photopsia; persistent, severe visual field defects; narrowing of the retinal vessels; and widespread hypopigmentation of the RPE (C). The visual field loss remained stable but she developed migration of pigment into the retina in a bone-corpuscle pattern peripherally.

D to I, Over a several month period this 36-year-old woman developed progressive loss of peripheral vision, photopsia, vitreous cells, narrowing of the retinal vessels, nonstaining cystoid macular edema (arrow, D), depigmentation of the RPE in the juxtapapillary area and ERG changes in the right eye (D and E). Visual field loss stabilized within 8 months. Twenty-six months after the onset of symptoms in the right eye she developed the same symptoms and signs in the left eye that previously was normal except for one focal scar (arrowhead, F). Compare F and G at the time of onset of symptoms in the left eye with H and I 1 year later, and note development of retinal vessel narrowing and depigmentation of the juxtapapillary RPE (arrowheads, I) The visual field stabilized in the left eye within 6 months. Both eyes have been unchanged for the past 3 years. Her visual acuity is 20/25 right eye and 20/20 left eye. She has mild macular edema bilaterally.

J to L, This 29-year-old woman noted the acute onset of photopsia and "shimmering heat wave" involving the superonasal field of the right eye. The fundi were normal. Medical and neurologic examinations were unremarkable. Her visual acuity was 20/20 in both eyes. Within 1 month she developed a zone of depigmentation and several foci of perivenous sheathing and staining (arrows, J and K) inferotemporally in the right eye. An ERG showed subnormal rod and cone amplitudes in the right eye. The fundi and visual fields remained unchanged over the subsequent 6 years except for migration of pigment into the retina (L) in the right eye and the development of several foci of perivascular sheathing in the left eye nasally. She is still troubled by the photopsia.

(A to L from Gass.[673])

I have seen no further patients linking these disorders with acute macular neuroretinopathy. Whereas occult visual field loss resulting from receptor cell damage is a common link among all these syndromes, we do not know the cause of any of these disorders or to what degree they are related pathogenetically and etiologically.

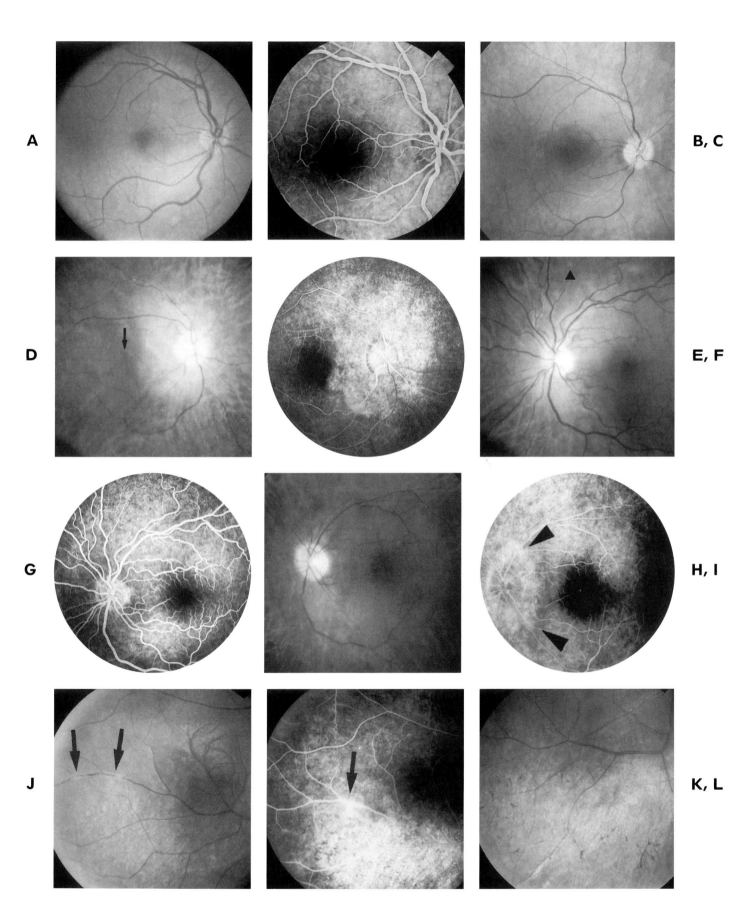

▼ ACUTE ANNULAR OCCULT OUTER RETINOPATHY

In a previous edition of this book the author presented the findings in an otherwise healthy young adult patient who presented with acute loss of a large zone of visual field associated with an unique funduscopic picture consisting of a large-diameter, thin, gray-white ring occupying most of the superior temporal fundus of the left eye (Fig. 7-38, *A* to *F*).[675] Except for slight narrowing of the retinal arteries within this zone, the retina and pigment epithelium had a normal ophthalmoscopic and fluorescein angiographic appearance (Fig. 7-38, *G*). There were no vitreous cells. There was a left afferent pupillary defect. For a period of approximately 3 weeks the ring and absolute visual field defect enlarged before stabilizing (Fig. 7-38, *C* to *F*). The ring disappeared. The visual acuity was normal throughout the course. The absence of angiographic changes suggested that the occult destructive process was affecting primarily the inner retina within the area of the ring and the disorder was termed "acute progressive zonal inner retinitis and degeneration." During followup over the following months and years, however, the patient developed, within the zone of visual field loss, depigmentation and migration of pigment epithelium into the overlying retina in a bone-corpuscular pattern, indicating that the original damage had in fact involved primarily the outer retinal receptors (Fig. 7-38, *H* and *I*).[676] During the 6 years of followup his visual acuity has remained 20/20 and the visual field loss is unchanged. Of interest, he no longer has an afferent pupillary defect. Luckie and coworkers recently reported a young woman with the identical findings and early clinical course in one eye.[677] She had serologic evidence of cytomegalovirus infection and they attributed her stabilization of field loss to treatment with acyclovir. The fact that their patient was immunocompetent suggests that her retinitis and clinical course may be unrelated to cytomegalovirus and her therapy.

FIG. 7-38   Acute Zonal Outer Retinopathy, Annular Occult Type.

A to *I*, A healthy 23-year-old man noticed the rapid onset of a large inferonasal scotoma in his left eye. His visual acuity was 20/20. When seen by his local ophthalmologist, the right eye was normal. The anterior chamber and vitreous were clear. In the left fundus there was a sharply defined, thin, gray, circular ring (*arrows*, **A** and **B**) occupying most of the superotemporal quadrant. The gray ring appeared to be within the retina but was external to the retinal vessels. It extended out to the equator but did not reach the ora serrata. The retina within the ring appeared normal. Visual field examination revealed a dense scotoma corresponding with the zone within the ring. Over the next week the scotoma progressively enlarged. When examined in Miami the gray ring was barely visible (*arrows*, **C** to **F**). The zone within the ring had enlarged (compare *arrows*, **A** and **B** with **C** and **D**) but did not reach the center of the macula. The diagram (**F**) illustrates the change in size of the ring. The retinal vessels within this zone were narrowed, and the surface retinal reflexes were attenuated. The RPE was unaffected. Fluorescein angiography confirmed the attenuation of the retinal vessels and the normality of the RPE (**G**). Over the subsequent several weeks the scotoma enlarged slightly and then stabilized. Within several years he developed depigmentation of the RPE and migration of pigment into the retina within the zone of visual field loss (*arrows*, **H** and **I**). His visual acuity 6.5 years later was 20/20. The right eye was normal.

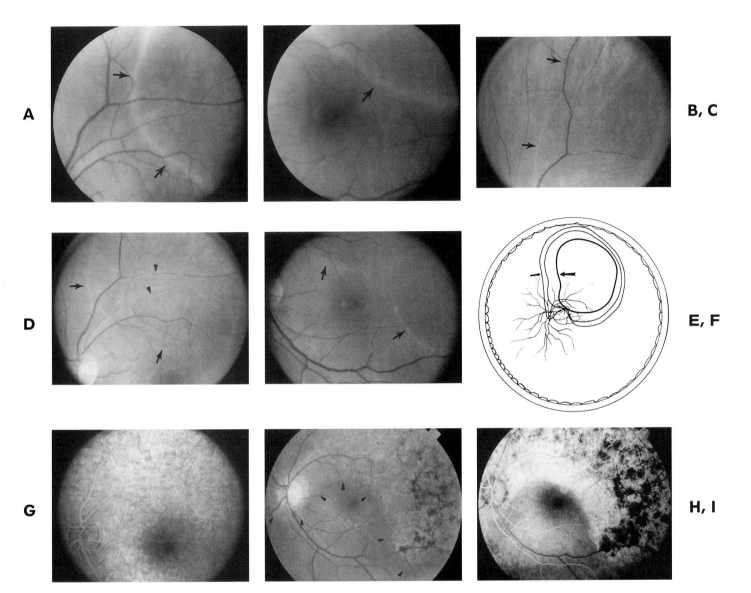

Except for the presence of the gray ring and the absence of a history of photopsia during the acute phase of the disease, the findings and course of the disease in these two patients are the same as those with acute zonal occult outer retinopathy (AZOOR). The cause of the zones of acute occult outer retinal damage in both groups of patients is unknown. An attractive, yet unsubstantiated, explanation for the fundus changes is that of a latent viral infection of selective zones of the outer retina that is somehow triggered into activity, causing acute inactivation of function and in some cases death of the retinal receptors within those zones without affecting retinal transparency (except for the ring) and without affecting either the outer or the inner blood–retinal barrier to fluorescein during the acute phase of the disease. The evanescent ring of retinal opacity occurs at the interface of the affected and unaffected outer retina and probably at the level of the outer plexiform layer and receptor cell nuclear layer, where it causes no angiographic abnormality. The ring may be the result of loss of transparency of the most recently affected retina, similar to that which may be seen in immune suppressed patients with cell-to-cell spread of cytomegalovirus retinopathy.[678] The ring may also be caused by a mild immune reaction taking place at the interface between the normal vascularized inner retina and the leading edge of the advancing infection in the outer avascularized retina, similar to that which may be observed in the cornea (Wesley ring). Neither explanation is completely satisfactory in view of the absence of detectable abnormality in either the inner or the outer blood–retinal barrier.

Figure 7-39 illustrates what may be a further variant of AZOOR in which the affected zone is associated with acute disruption of the RPE and variable degree of whitening of the outer retina and RPE.

FIG. 7-39   Acute Zonal Outer Retinopathy, Annular Overt Type.

A to **E,** This 50-year-old woman with the chronic fatigue syndrome noted the sudden onset of a large nasal scotoma in the left eye. Visual acuity was 20/20 right eye and 20/400 left eye. She had a dense scotoma corresponding with a large superotemporal zone of RPE depigmentation surrounded by a border of outer retinal whitening (**A** and **B**). This was associated with 2+ vitritis. Angiography revealed early nonfluorescence of the rim of the lesion and hyperfluorescence corresponding with its center (**C**), and late fluorescence of the entire lesion. Medical evaluation, including titers for syphilis and herpes viruses, was negative except for mild thrombocytosis and granulocytosis. She was hospitalized and received oral prednisone, acyclovir, and doxycycline. Visual acuity improved to 20/70 within 1 week. Over the following 5 weeks it decreased to 20/400 and the zone of RPE destruction continued to enlarge in a nasal direction (**D**). Five months after the onset of symptoms almost the entire fundus was affected (**E**), but the visual acuity had improved to 20/200 and continued to improve over the next year to 20/30. Four years later her condition was unchanged. The left eye was normal.

Acute Zonal Outer Retinopathy, Overt Type.

F to **J,** Soon after developing a sore throat this otherwise healthy 60-year-old man complained of progressive loss of the temporal field of vision in the left eye associated with "shimmering light" of 2 weeks' duration. Nine months previously he noted a similar but more peripheral temporal scotoma in the right eye associated with "shimmering." The symptoms in the right eye resolved spontaneously after several months. His visual acuity was 20/20 bilaterally. There was a 3+ afferent pupillary defect in the left eye. Visual field examination revealed a dense scotoma involving most of the peripheral and almost all of the temporal visual field of the left eye, and an enlarged blind spot in the right eye. In the right eye there were 2+ vitreous cells and a large well-demarcated zone of RPE atrophy involving the juxtapapillary and inferior and nasal areas out as far as the equator (**F**). This area was far larger than the zone of visual field loss. The optic disc and retinal vessels were normal bilaterally. Funduscopic examination of the left eye revealed 3+ vitreous cells and a sharply defined zone of disruption of the RPE involving most of the fundus but sparing much of the macular area (**G**). There was no gray-white demarcation line at the border of the RPE change. Temporal to the macula, however, there were several ill-defined areas of gray-white at the level of the RPE (**H**). In the left eye fluorescein angiography showed evidence of acute RPE damage but no evidence of involvement of the choriocapillaris (**J** and **K**). In the right eye there was mottled hyperfluorescence corresponding with the large area of old RPE damage (**I**). He received prednisone, 60 mg, and acyclovir, 4 g, daily by mouth. There was some progression of the visual loss and RPE changes in the left eye for several weeks before stabilization occurred (**L**).

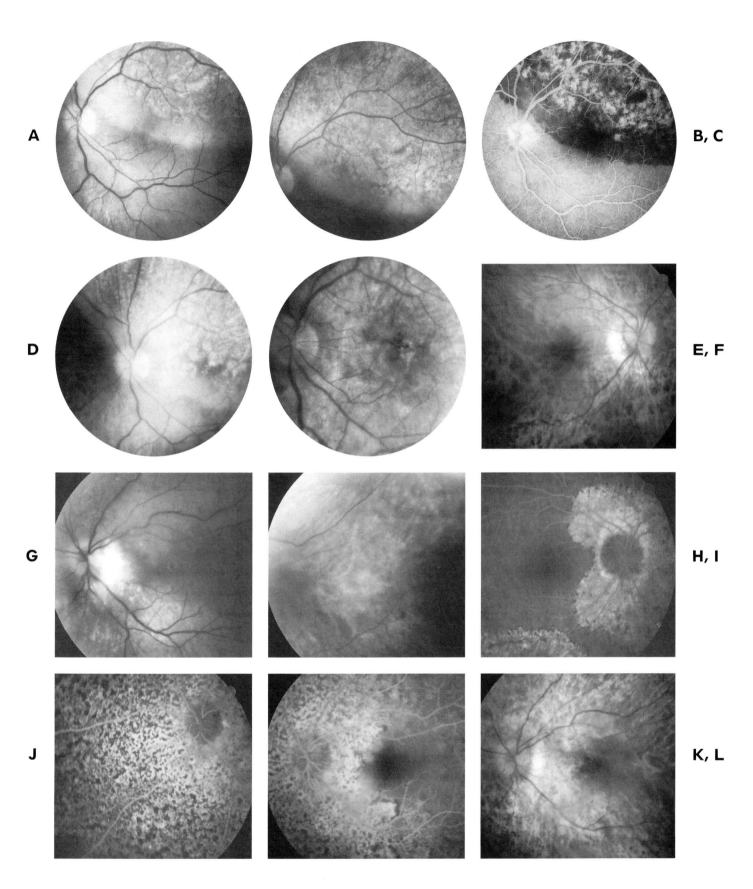

A

B, C

D

E, F

G

H, I

J

K, L

687

▼ DISORDERS SIMULATING THE PRESUMED OCULAR HISTOPLASMOSIS SYNDROME (PSEUDO-POHS)

The clinical features of POHS are described in Chapter 3. In recent years it has become apparent that there are other disorders, unrelated to infection with *Histoplasma,* that during their inactive stages may cause a pattern of chorioretinal scarring similar to POHS. Collectively referred to as pseudo-POHS there are at least two groups of patients that may simulate POHS.* They may or may not be pathogenetically related.

Multifocal choroiditis and panuveitis (MCP)

Nozik and Dorsch[686] and more recently Dreyer and Gass[681] and Tessler and Deutsch[694] described a syndrome of multifocal choroiditis and panuveitis MCP that simulates POHS with the following exceptions: (1) vitreous inflammation is present in one or both eyes; (2) anterior uveitis occurs in 50% of cases; (3) yellow and gray active choroidal lesions that angiographically may be nonfluorescent early and stain later are often observed or may develop during followup (Fig. 7-41, *A* to *C*); (4) the inactive lesions are in general smaller than those in the POHS (Figs. 7-40 and 7-41, *A* to *C*); (5) most patients come from areas nonendemic for histoplasmosis and have a negative histoplasmin skin test; (6) approximately one-half of eyes demonstrate subnormal electroretinographic findings (Figs. 7-40 and 7-41, *D* to *F*); (7) some patients develop acutely large visual field defects that are not explained on the basis of fundus findings and subsequently may develop large areas of RPE depigmentation, which may be associated with retinal vessel narrowing and migration of pigment epithelium into the retina; (8) patients with monocular involvement (25%) may develop severe involvement of the second eye months or years later (Fig. 7-40); (9) there is a female sex predilection; (10) the disorder may affect children or adults of any age; and (11) lack of HLA-DR2 specificity, which is often present in POHS.[691] The reader should realize that the presence of vitritis or iritis has been an important requirement for inclusion of patients in reports concerning MCP in order to exclude patients with POHS, and that some patients with MCP and with active choroidal lesions as well as multifocal scars may have no vitreous cells.

*References 660, 665, 680-683a, 686, 688-690, 694, 695.

FIG. 7-40   Multifocal Choroiditis and Panuveitis (Pseudo–Presumed Ocular Histoplasmosis Syndrome).

A to **I,** This healthy 39-year-old woman experienced floaters and blurred vision in the right eye. Her visual acuity was 20/200. There were 1+ cells in the anterior chamber and 2+ cells in the vitreous. There was mild papilledema and cystoid macular edema (**A**). In the equatorial area for 360 degrees there were hundreds of variably sized, round, chorioretinal scars (**B** and **C**). Angiography revealed cystoid macular edema and papilledema (**D**). There was late staining around some of the peripheral lesions (**E** and **F**). The left eye was normal. The scotopic electroretinographic responses were moderately abnormal in the right eye and borderline normal in the left eye. Over the subsequent 6½ years she experienced further loss of vision in the right eye related to subretinal neovascularization, before noting floaters in the left eye. At that time visual acuity in the right eye was 20/200 and in the left eye was 20/15. There were vitreous cells in both eyes. She had a disciform scar in the right macula (**G**). There were many focal chorioretinal lesions, some of which appeared active in the periphery of the left eye (**H** and **I**). Angiography revealed leaky capillaries in the optic disc and retina of both eyes.

J to **L,** This 31-year-old woman had a 1-year history of episodes of blurred vision and photophobia in the left eye. Visual acuity in the right eye was 20/20 and in the left eye was 20/300. The right fundus and vitreous were normal except for mild peripapillary scarring (**J**). In the left eye there were 2+ vitreous cells; multiple focal chorioretinal scars, some of which were stellate; and a subfoveal neovascular membrane (**K**). Ten months later, the visual acuity in the left eye was counting fingers, and there was massive subretinal fibrosis (**L**). The right eye was unchanged.

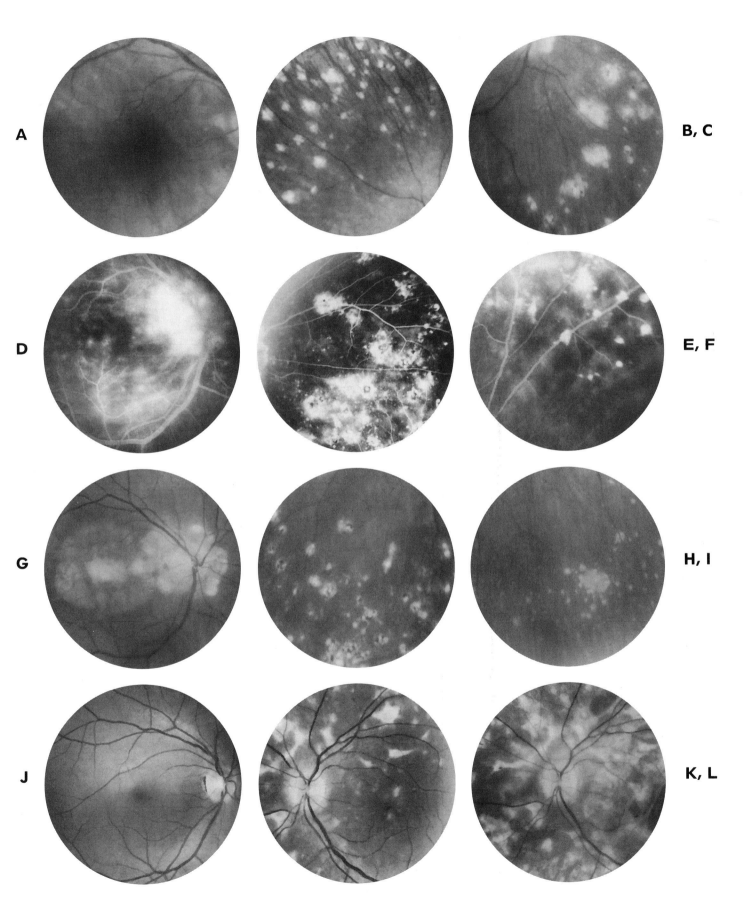

A

B, C

D

E, F

G

H, I

J

K, L

689

Features of MCP similar to POHS include punched-out peripheral and posterior pole chorioretinal scars that are occasionally arranged in a curvilinear pattern at the equator, juxtapapillary scarring, and the frequent development of juxtapapillary and macular subretinal neovascularization (Figs. 7-40 and 7-41).[679,682,693] I have seen three children with multifocal choroiditis and panuveitis in association with bilateral pars plana snow-bank exudation (see Fig. 7-47, *J* to *L*).[682] The cause of multifocal choroiditis and panuveitis is unknown. Features of MCP different from vitiliginous retinochoroiditis include (1) the punched-out nature of chorioretinal scars; (2) a lower median age (33 years); (3) a greater frequency of unilateral disease; (4) a greater frequency of panuveitis; (5) a lower incidence of optic disc pallor, nyctalopia, color vision deficit, and electroretinographic abnormalities; (6) a greater incidence of visual loss caused by choroidal neovascularization; and (7) lack of HLA-A29 specificity. The fundus of patients with unilateral involvement in MCP may simulate that in patients with diffuse unilateral subacute neuroretinitis. (See p. 622.) Visual loss in the latter disorder is usually unassociated with subretinal neovascularization and is more frequently accompanied by pallor of the optic disc, narrowing of the retinal vessels, and a markedly abnormal electroretinogram. Multifocal choroiditis may occasionally be a manifestation of sarcoidosis. Hershey et al. found focal granulomas on blind biopsy of the conjunctiva in a group of patients over 50 years of age with a fundus picture of pseudo-POHS and no other manifestations of sarcoidosis.[684]

FIG. 7-41 Multifocal Choroiditis and Panuveitis (Pseudo–Presumed Ocular Histoplasmosis Syndrome).

A to C, This 31-year-old woman had a 6-year history of loss of vision in the right eye caused by subfoveal neovascularization and recent blurring of vision in the left eye. In addition to widespread multifocal chorioretinal scars and vitritis in both eyes, there were active-appearing focal choroidal lesions in the macula, narrowing of the retinal vessels, and optic disc edema and pallor in the left eye (**A** and **B**). Angiography revealed that some of the chorioretinal lesions were nonfluorescent early (**C**) and stained later. Her visual fields were markedly constricted and the electroretinogram revealed severely abnormal rod and cone responses. Her father had subnormal vision that was attributed to working in a coal mine. Her FTA-ABS test was negative. It is of interest that coincident with the onset of visual symptoms, the patient had a jejunoileostomy for obesity and as a consequence lost 200 pounds. It is not known whether or not vitamin A deficiency played any role in her tapetoretinal dystrophy–like fundus changes.

D to F, This 30-year-old, healthy, mildly myopic woman noted blurred vision in the left eye of 1 week's duration. Visual acuity in the right eye was 20/20 and in the left eye was 20/200. There was a 1+ afferent pupillary reaction in the left eye. The right fundus was normal. A few vitreous cells were present in the left eye. There were multifocal active gray lesions in the macula and juxtapapillary area (**D**) as well as a few in the peripheral fundus. Angiography revealed late staining of many of these lesions. Medical evaluation for evidence of systemic disease including histoplasmosis was negative. The diagnosis was chorioretinitis and optic neuritis of unknown cause. Systemic and sub-Tenon's steroids were given. Two months later visual acuity had improved to 20/70. Most of the lesions appeared less active (**E**). Fourteen months later she returned because of visual loss in the left eye caused by serous detachment of the macula that resolved spontaneously. Nine years later the right eye was normal. The acuity in the left eye was 20/200. There was enlargement and hyperpigmentation of the chorioretinal scars, and several atrophic scars (*arrow;* **F**) were evident in areas of previously normal retina.

G to L, This young woman experienced the rapid onset of loss of temporal field and photopsia in her right eye. The fundi were normal (**G**). The gray spot (*arrow*) in **G** is an artifact. The scotoma partly resolved within several months, prior to her developing loss of central vision and an enlarged blind spot in the left eye that was associated with multiple active chorioretinal lesions (**H** and **I**). The diagnosis was punctate inner choroiditis. Six months later she developed blurred vision in the right eye associated with multiple foci of paracentral chorioretinitis (**J**). She soon developed evidence of subretinal neovascularization in the macular area of both eyes (**K** and **L**).

(**D** and **E** from Gass.[682])

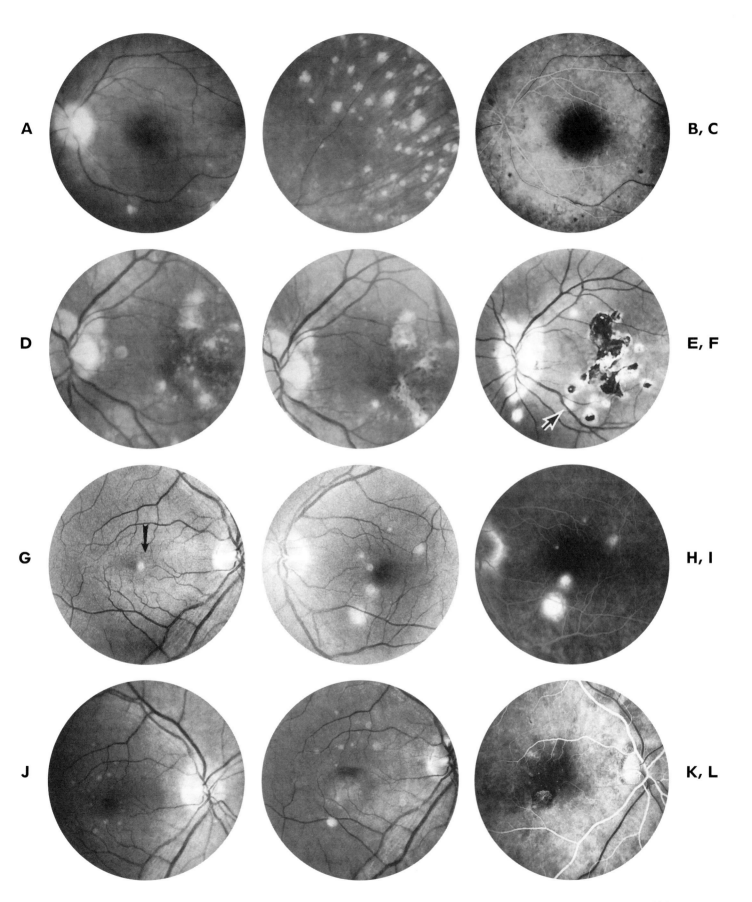

A

B, C

D

E, F

G

H, I

J

K, L

Punctate inner choroidopathy (PIC)

Watzke and associates[695] and Morgan and Schatz[660] reported a syndrome characterized by the following: (1) moderate myopia, blurred vision, photopsia, and scotomata in women; (2) multiple, yellow-white lesions of the inner choroid and retina that are largely confined to the posterior pole, and that after resolution leave atrophic pigmented scars simulating those in the presumed ocular histoplasmosis syndrome (Figs. 7-36, *G to L,* and 7-41, *D to L*); (3) frequent serous detachment of the retina that resolves spontaneously; (4) no signs of vitritis or anterior uveitis; (5) both eyes affected in most patients; (6) negative histoplasmin skin test (70%); (7) choroidal neovascularization in 40% of eyes; and (8) relatively good visual prognosis, with one-half of eyes retaining normal acuity. Doran and Hamilton[680] presented four similar cases. The macular lesions tend to be arranged in a linear or branching pattern in some cases. Figure 7-41, *D,* depicts such a pattern in the left eye of a 30-year-old myopic woman who also had mild vitritis and a few peripheral chorioretinal scars in the right eye.[682] The left eye was normal. This patient and others seen by the author suggest that the two syndromes (i.e., PIC and MCP) are probably the same disorder or have a similar pathogenesis.[690] The presence or absence of vitreous cells in these patients is probably a function of the size of the area of the fundus affected. Those with lesions confined to the posterior pole (PIC) are less likely to have vitreous cells than those with widespread lesions (MCP). Once the active lesions in both of these syndromes become inactive, and the vitritis and iritis resolve in the case of MCP, the fundus picture in many of these patients becomes indistinguishable from those with POHS. Just as the absence of vitreous cells does not entirely exclude the diagnosis of multifocal choroiditis and panuveitis, likewise, the presence of vitreous cells probably does not completely exclude POHS.

Some patients with MCP and PIC develop prominent subretinal fibrosis in the vicinity of the focal choroiditis (Fig. 7-40, *J* to *L*). This process of reactive fibrosis may be limited to small isolated areas around individual choroidal lesions or may form a large confluent interlacing network or plaque of subretinal fibrous tissue, either in the macula or in the peripheral fundus. Still others may develop massive widespread fibrous tissue mounds and severe visual loss. (See Fig. 3-57 and discussion of massive subretinal fibrosis in Chapter 3, p. 170.)[633a,687] The etiology, pathogenesis, and natural course of MCP and PIC are not known. Tiedeman and coworkers found serologic evidence to suggest that Epstein-Barr virus might be a causative factor.[465] This could not be confirmed by others.[692]

The multifocal features of these P-POHS disorders have obscured the fact that some of these patients develop large visual field defects that are usually overlooked, and that are not explained during the early stage of the disease by fundus changes (Fig. 7-41, *G* to *L*). These defects are probably caused by acute damage to zones of the retinal receptors that may or may not recover function. This loss of function may be confined to one or more small zones, particularly surrounding the optic disc, or to large peripheral zones. Loss of retinal receptors in large areas of the fundus is responsible for the narrowing of the retinal blood vessels and alterations in the retinal pigment epithelium that may simulate retinitis pigmentosa in some of these patients. This occult phase of these P-POHS disorders is similar to that which occurs in patients with acute zonal occult outer retinopathy (AZOOR), multiple evanescent white-dot syndrome (MEWDS), and acute idiopathic blind spot enlargement (AIBES).[772] (See previous discussion of MEWDS and AZOOR.)

Uncertain at this time is the frequency with which patients who have pseudo-POHS develop recurrent episodes of new lesions or visual loss, other than that which may occur from delayed development of subretinal neovascularization at the site of a focal scar. Although the author has observed delayed involvement of the second eye for up to 10 years, it is my impression that most of these patients experience a single acute or subacute event lasting for several months in one or both eyes, and that they are unlikely to have a recurrence of active disease in the same eye thereafter.

The predilection for pseudo-POHS, AZOOR, MEWDS, and AIBSE to occur primarily in women; the primary locus of the disease in these disorders at the level of the retinal receptors and pigment epithelium; and the similarity of the pathologic changes in eyes of patients with multifocal choroiditis and massive subretinal fibrosis to experimental uveitis induced in primates by interphotoreceptor retinoid-binding protein suggest that autoimmunity plays an important role in the pathogenesis of these disorders.[683a,685] (See Fig. 3-57 and discussion in Chapter 3.) The experimental model of Hirose and coworkers demonstrates some of the clinical features of pseudo-POHS, including multifocal choroidal lesions, that histologically were focal granulomas associated with widespread retinal receptor changes. Their model demonstrates that antigen localized specifically in the retina may cause widespread changes in the retinal receptors and also may initiate immunopathogenetic changes in the choroid as well. (See discussion in Chapter 3, p. 170.)

▼ ACUTE MACULAR NEURORETINOPATHY

Bos and Deutman[696] described peculiar cloverleaf, wedge-shaped, lesions that develop in the macular region of both eyes of young patients who complain of rapid loss of central and paracentral vision, usually following a flulike syndrome (Fig. 7-42, A to C).[696,699,703-705,707-713] The color of the fundus lesions is dependent upon the pigmentation of the fundus and varies from grayish to reddish brown. Visual acuity is usually reduced to 20/30 to 20/40. These patients can outline precisely on the Amsler grid negative scotomata corresponding with the fundus lesions (Fig. 7-42, G). In patients with the full-blown disease, dark, flower petal–shaped lesions are present in the central macular region (Fig. 7-42, A, B, and H). In other patients, however, the lesions are less prominent and may consist of multiple oval to round, faintly pinkish patches in the central or paracentral region (Fig. 7-42, D and E). They are seen most easily with red-free light. These lesions appear to lie at the level of the outer retinal layers,[699,707,708,712] rather than the superficial retina as suggested by Bos and Deutman. Only one eye may be involved. One or two small superficial, flame-shaped retinal hemorrhages may be present (Fig. 7-42, B).[699,707] The retinal vessels and optic disc are normal. There are no cells in the vitreous. Fluorescein angiography in well-developed cases shows a faint hypofluorescence corresponding with the lesions (Fig. 7-42, C and I). Resolution of the lesions and improvement in acuity and field loss occur slowly over a matter of weeks or months (Fig. 7-42, F).[709] The scotomas in some cases may be prolonged for many months or years.[703] Lesions identical to acute macular neuroretinopathy have occurred in patients with multiple evanescent white dot syndrome and acute blind spot enlargement (Fig. 7-36, A).[643,665]

Although most of these patients have noted the onset of symptoms within a week or two following a flulike illness, others develop identical appearing lesions and acute visual loss after receiving intravenous injections of sympathomimetics,[706] iodine-containing contrast agents,[701] or following anaphylactic shock after a bee sting (Fig. 7-42, G to I).[702] If examined immediately after the visual loss following the injections the lesions may have a gray-white appearance and later become more dark in color.

FIG. 7-42   Acute Macular Neuroretinopathy.

A to C, This 31-year-old Black woman gave a 2-week history of a flulike syndrome before the onset of blurred vision and paracentral scotomata in both eyes. She had some pain on ocular movement. Her visual acuity was 20/50 bilaterally. Note the petaloid dark areas in the macular region of both eyes (**A** and **B**) and the superficial retinal hemorrhage superior to the macula in the left eye (*arrow,* **B**). Angiography revealed only mild dilation of the retinal capillaries superior to the macula. There were no other changes in the fundi. Five months later visual acuity improved to 20/30 and J-1. The appearance of the macula had remained essentially unchanged. The patient was lost to followup.

D to F, This 26-year-old White woman noted multiple paracentral scotomata and photopsia in the left eye unassociated with a viral-like illness. The visual acuity was 20/25. She had multiple, small, variably sized, dark, round spots at the level of the outer retina (**D** and **E**). These corresponded with dense scotomata evident on the Amsler grid. Angiography, electroretinography, and electrooculography were normal. These spots and the scotomata faded over a period of many months. Visual acuity 7 years later was 20/25 (**F**).

G to I, In October 1988 this healthy 27-year-old woman noted multiple paracentral negative scotomas in the right eye. An optometrist noted multiple "hemorrhages" in the right macula. Five months later the scotomas persisted and were evident on Amsler grid testing (**G**). Visual acuity was 20/15 bilaterally. Funduscopic examination revealed a pattern of outer retinal red-orange lesions (**H**) that corresponded with the Amsler grid changes. The left eye was normal. Angiography revealed minimal changes (**I**). When she returned 6 years later the scotomas and visual acuity were unchanged but the fundus lesions were no longer present.

J and K, This healthy 28-year-old White woman had uterine bleeding after an elective cesarean delivery. She received 10 units of oxytocin (Pitocin) and epinephrine by intravenous push. She experienced severe headache, elevation of blood pressure, and extra systoles that were controlled with intravenous lidocaine and sodium pentothal anesthesia. On awakening she noted central scotomata and her visual acuity was 20/200. A "cherry-red spot and macular edema" were described. Her vision improved over the next few days. Six weeks later her visual acuity was 20/20. She had paracentral scotomata and the typical picture of acute macular neuroretinopathy in both macular areas (**J**). The reddish lesions involved the outer retina and they were slightly hypofluorescent angiographically (**K**). These lesions faded and were associated with subtle RPE changes, but they and their corresponding scotomas were still evident 5 years later.

L, This 24-year-old woman had an abdominal computed tomography (CT) scan performed with injection of 20 cc of iothalamate because of enlarged abdominal lymph nodes, probably caused by infectious mononucleosis. Because of development of urticaria, palpitations, and severe headache she was given an intravenous injection of 0.2 cc of epinephrine 1:1000 and 50 mg of Benadryl. Ten hours later on awaking she noted scotomas centrally. Macular abnormalities were noted. Three weeks later her visual acuity was 20/25, right eye, and 20/30, left eye. Similar reddish outer retinal lesions and corresponding scotomas were present in both maculas (**L,** left eye and **stereo color plate 86,** right eye). These lesions were associated with slight hypofluorescence angiographically. Three months later the visual acuity and fundi were unchanged. The scotomata were similar but less dense.

(**J** and **K** from O'Brien et al.[706]; **L** from Guzak et al.[701])

The fundus lesions, when they are reddish in color, may be mistaken for subretinal blood. This may have happened in the case reported by Weinberg and Nerney.[714] The milder forms of this disease (Fig. 7-42, *D* to *F*) may be misdiagnosed as acute retinal pigment epitheliitis since both diseases cause temporary loss of central vision, usually in young individuals (see p. 676). Early receptor potential changes may be evident electroretinographically and may persist for many months.[712] The pathology, pathogenesis, and course of these peculiar macular lesions are unknown. The sharply demarcated reddish lesions corresponding rather precisely to the visual field loss suggest that acute loss of the retinal outer receptor elements and to some degree the inner receptor elements in sharply delineated zones is responsible for well-demarcated zones of outer retinal thinning that cause the reddish appearance of the lesions. The mechanism of this focal damage is probably different in the patients who develop this disorder following a viral-like disorder than in the patients who develop it after intravenous injections that usually contain sympathomimetic drugs. In the latter patients, either transient choroidal ischemia or a toxic interaction between the drug and the receptor cells is a possible explanation for the damage. Other causes of sharply defined areas of retinal thinning, e.g., atrophy of the outer retina after resolution of Berlin's edema,[697] sickle cell hemoglobin macular infarcts,[698] cotton-wool infarcts,[700] and inner lamellar macular holes, may produce reddish lesions biomicroscopically.[697,698]

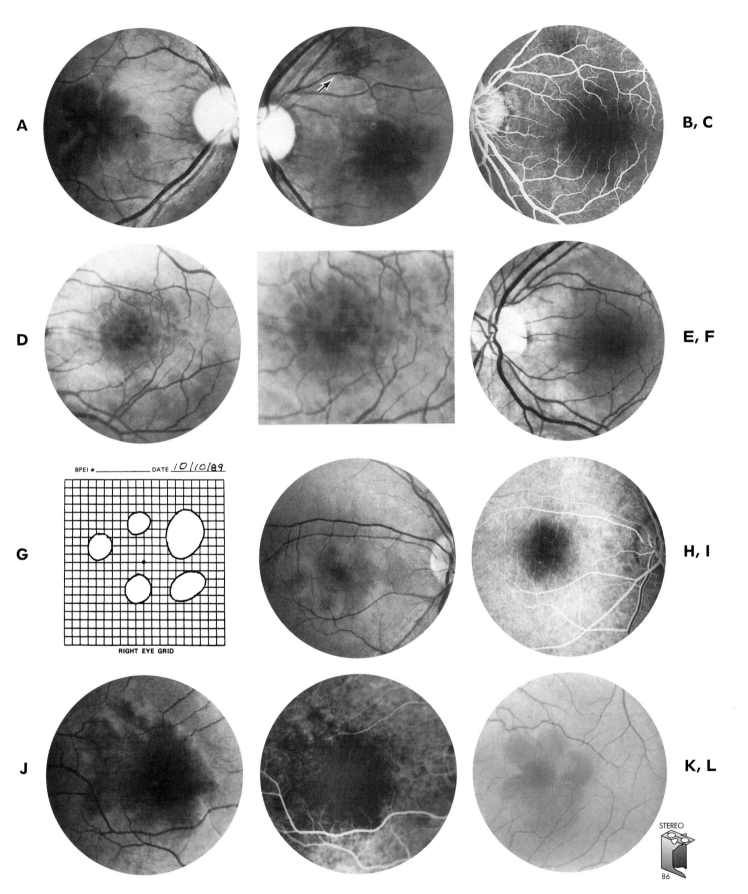

A

B, C

D

E, F

G

H, I

J

K, L

STEREO
86

695

▼ ACUTE EXUDATIVE POLYMORPHOUS VITELLIFORM MACULOPATHY

Gass and coworkers reported two young lightly pigmented White adults who presented because of the acute onset of headaches and visual loss associated with multiple yellow-white ill-defined subretinal lesions and serous retinal detachment in the macular area of both eyes (Fig. 7-43, *A, B,* and *H*).[715] The focal lesions demonstrated early hyperfluorescence and mild late staining (Fig. 7-42, *C, D,* and *I*). One patient had a few vitreous cells. Both patients were treated with oral corticosteroids. Over the following weeks gradual improvement of visual acuity was associated with development of prominent polymorphous deposits of subretinal yellow pigment that tended to gravitate to form a meniscus, giving an appearance similar to that in Best's vitelliform dystrophy (Fig. 7-42, *E, F, J,* and *K*). The visual acuity returned to normal levels and incomplete resolution of the yellow pigment occurred in both patients. It is probable that the yellow pigment is a product of damaged pigment epithelium and not a result of lipoproteins escaping from the choroidal vasculature. Both patients had subnormal electrooculographic findings, but neither had a family history of eye disease. The peculiar funduscopic and angiographic findings during the early stage of this disease are similar to those which occur in patients who present with bilateral acute visual loss and retinal detachment caused by bilateral melanocytic uveal melanocytic proliferation associated with an occult carcinoma. (See p. 237.) It is not known whether acute exudative polymorphous vitelliform maculopathy is an acquired inflammatory disease or an unusual manifestation of a genetically determined disorder, either Best's disease or some other as yet poorly defined RPE dystrophy.

FIG. 7-43   Acute Exudative Polymorphous Vitelliform Maculopathy.

A to **G,** In June 1982 this 24-year-old man presented with a 2-day history of headaches and progressive loss of vision in both eyes. His visual acuity was 20/50 right eye and 20/40 left eye. There was exudative detachment of the retina centrally, and numerous oval, round, and curvilinear yellow-white lesions underlying confluent blisterlike areas of serous retinal detachment bilaterally (**A** and **B**). Note the striking early hyperfluorescence of the yellow-white lesions (**C**) and minimal late staining (**D**). He received prednisone 80 mg daily and 1 week later visual acuity was 20/20, right eye, and 20/25, left eye. Accompanying resolution of the subretinal fluid was the development of large amounts of yellow subretinal material that showed a tendency to gravitate inferiorly (**E,** December 1982, and **F,** June 1983). When last seen in June 1984 visual acuity was 20/20 bilaterally and most of the yellow material had disappeared (**G**).

H to **L,** This 30-year-old presented with a 1-month history of visual loss and severe headaches. His findings and clinical course were similar to the previous patient. **H** and **I,** August 1984; **J** and **K,** April 1985; **L,** October 1985.

(**A** to **L** from Gass et al.[715])

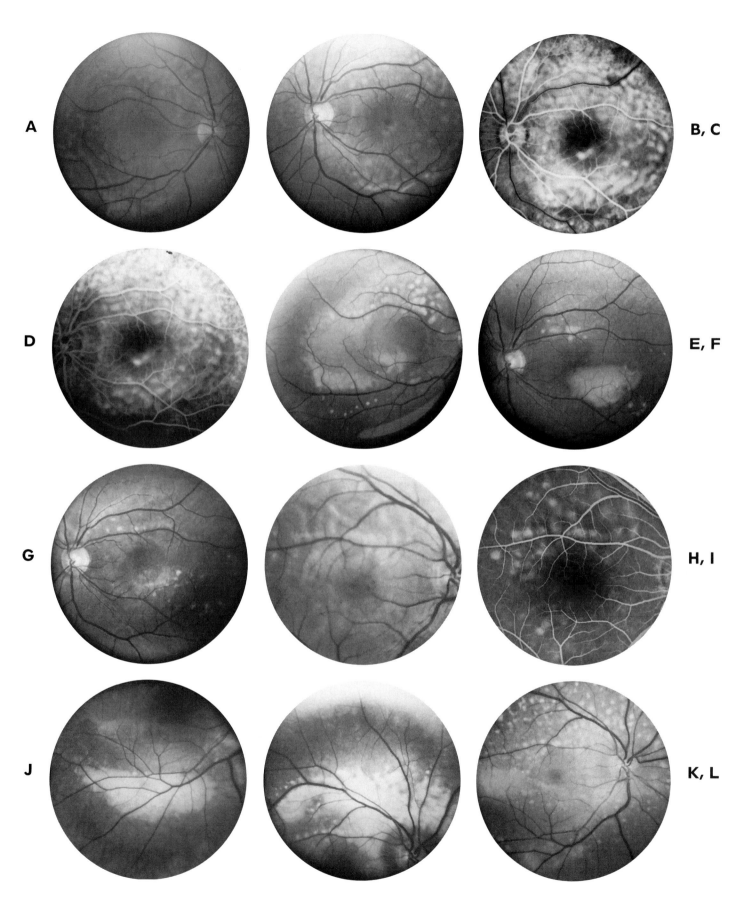

A

B, C

D

E, F

G

H, I

J

K, L

697

▼ RETINAL AND OPTIC NERVE SARCOIDOSIS

Sarcoidosis is a systemic noncaseating granulomatous disease of unknown cause. Although it has protean clinical manifestations it affects the pulmonary lymph nodes and eye most often.* Ocular involvement occurs in approximately 40% of patients with sarcoidosis and is more frequent in Blacks than in Whites. Anterior uveitis is more common than posterior fundus involvement. Fundus lesions more frequently involve the retina than the choroid and may occur in the absence of anterior uveitis and in patients with minimal or no other evidence of systemic disease. Characteristic funduscopic findings include perivenous exudation with candle wax–dripping exudate,[729,731,732,742] preretinal and intravitreal white nodules often arranged in a "string of pearls,"[731,732] focal superficial and deep retinal white nodules,[731,732] papilledema, nodular papillitis, optic neuritis, and occasionally large white masses on the inner surface of the retina and optic nerve head (Figs. 7-44 and 7-45).† All of these lesions are caused by epithelioid cell proliferation (Fig. 7-45).[721,723,726,729,731] Branch vein occlusion,[725,731,739] central retinal vein occlusion,[743] large areas of capillary nonperfusion, retinal neovascularization,[717,727,733,744] vitreous hemorrhage, and optic disc neovascularization[726,738] may occur as complications of the granulomatous periphlebitis and phlebitis (Fig. 7-45, A). The neovascularization may resolve after treatment with antiinflammatory agents.[738]

Focal granulomas may occur under the RPE (Fig. 7-45, C and D) and within the choroid. The predominance of T-helper lymphocytes in the choroid and retina infiltration suggests that sarcoidosis is a disease of heightened cellular immune response, particularly at the sites of organ and tissue involvement.[722,737] Patients with sarcoidosis confined to the choroid often experience loss of central vision caused by a solitary yellow-white choroidal mass in the paracentral region that may simulate metastatic carcinoma or an amelanotic melanoma (see Fig. 3-55, A to I). Patients with multifocal sarcoid choroiditis may simulate patients with multifocal choroiditis and panuveitis (pseudo-POHS) and bird-shot chorioretinitis.[684,720] Subretinal neovascularization and macular detachment occasionally complicate sarcoid choroiditis.[750] Sarcoidosis may cause widespread chorioretinal degeneration[728] and massive subretinal fibrosis (see Fig. 3-55, J to K).

---

*References 716, 734, 736, 749, 753, 757.
†References 721, 724, 730, 740, 741, 743, 745, 747.

FIG. 7-44 Sarcoidosis of the Retina, Optic Nerve, Skin, and Conjunctiva.

A to C, Macular star, optic disc swelling, and perivenous "candle wax–dripping" exudates in a 25-year-old Black man with biopsy-proven sarcoidosis. Angiography revealed evidence of perivenous leakage of dye in both eyes (B and C).

D, Perivenous exudation and macular star in a 32-year-old Black man with biopsy-proven sarcoidosis.

E and F, Typical sarcoid nodules of the right optic disc in a 21-year-old Black man with biopsy-proven sarcoidosis. Visual acuity in the left eye was 20/200. He was treated with systemic corticosteroids, and 6 months later most of the optic nerve head granulomas (E) had disappeared (F).

G, Preretinal nodules in a patient with sarcoidosis.

H, Sarcoid granulomas of the lid.

I, Sarcoid granuloma of the conjunctiva.

J and K, Sarcoidosis of the optic nerve head associated with prominent neovascularization.

L, Sarcoid periphlebitis and papillitis in a patient with sarcoid meningitis.

(L, courtesy of Dr. William F. Crosswell.)

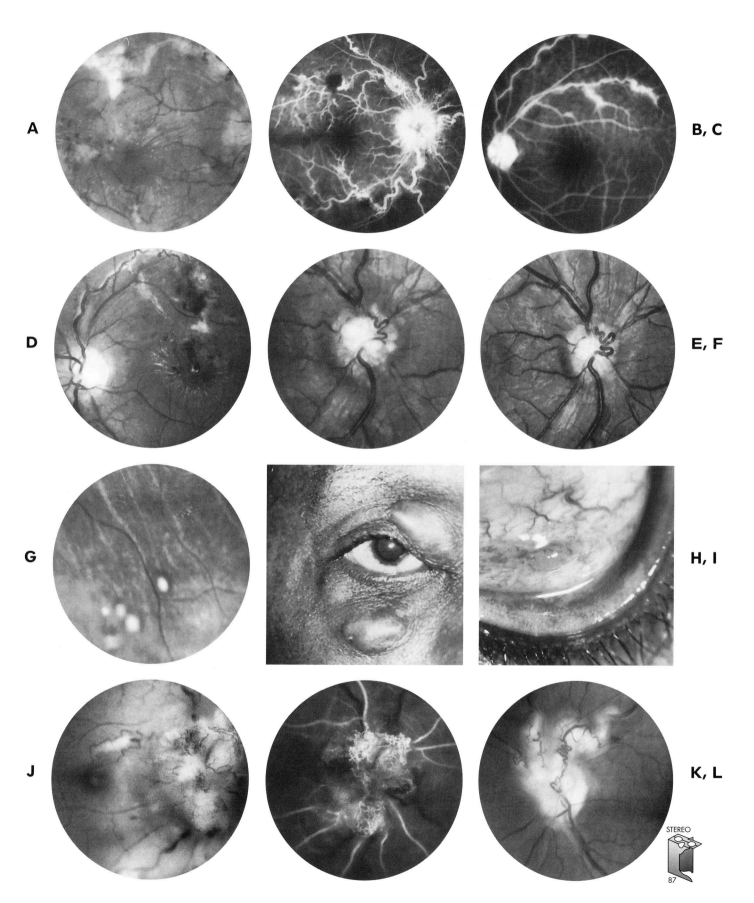

A

B, C

D

E, F

G

H, I

J

K, L

Approximately 20% to 30% of patients with retinal manifestations of sarcoidosis will have evidence of central nervous system involvement (Fig. 7-45).[731,732,748,751,754]

Candle wax–dripping exudation, usually accompanied by preretinal white exudates over the inferior fundus (Figs. 7-44, A and D, and 7-45, A, C, and D), and nodular papillitis (Figs. 7-44, E, F, and J, and 7-45, A) are two signs that should strongly suggest the diagnosis of sarcoidosis. The diagnosis can be confirmed by biopsy of affected lymph nodes, conjunctiva,[735,752,755] salivary glands,[746] and lacrimal gland. Fewer than 5% of patients with sarcoidosis show cutaneous reaction to tuberculin protein. The chest roentgenogram shows evidence of sarcoidosis in over 90% of cases. There is a high incidence of elevation of the angiotensin-converting enzyme in patients with sarcoidosis.[718,756,757] Gallium citrate uptake studies may be helpful in confirming the diagnosis.

All of the lesions of sarcoidosis usually respond to treatment with corticosteroids. Because of the chronic nature of the disease, corticosteroids should be employed judiciously, primarily for an immediate threat to loss of visual or other vital organ function. Occasionally, use of other agents such as cyclosporine is required to control the inflammation.[719] Neovascularization of the optic disc may show dramatic resolution following treatment with corticosteroids.[726] Photocoagulation may be helpful in controlling retinal neovascularization in the peripheral fundus.[717]

▼ ACUTE IDIOPATHIC MULTIFOCAL INNER RETINITIS AND NEURORETINITIS

These patients are typically children or young adults who soon after a viral-like illness develop loss of vision usually in one eye associated with one or more white foci of acute retinitis and neuroretinitis in one or both eyes.[758,759,761-765] The acute retinal lesions primarily involve the inner half of the retina and show some predilection for occurring adjacent to major retinal arteries and veins. In this latter location they may cause branch retinal artery or vein obstruction, which, together with optic nerve head involvement, are the major causes of symptoms in these patients (Fig. 7-2). At the time of eye examination the patient is usually afebrile. Blood cultures and medical evaluation are

FIG. 7-45 Ocular and Central Nervous System Sarcoidosis; Clinicopathologic Correlation.

This 38-year-old Black man had central nervous system sarcoidosis associated with bilateral retinal and optic nerve sarcoidosis. Fundus painting (A) showed granulomas on the optic disc, along the retinal veins, and in the vitreous inferiorly (inset). There was a branch vein occlusion in the inferotemporal quadrant. The patient died several months later, and histopathologic examination revealed multiple perivenous granulomas with extension of the granulomatous reaction into the overlying vitreous in the juxtapapillary area (B) and the peripheral retina (C and E). Note the granulomatous reaction surrounding the retinal veins (arrows, C and D) and extension of the granulomatous reaction beneath the RPE (C and D). There were multiple granulomas in the pre- and postlaminar parts of the optic nerve (F) and throughout the central nervous system.

(From Gass JDM, Olson CL: Sarcoidosis with optic nerve and retinal involvement: a clinicopathologic case report. Trans Am Acad Ophthalmol Otolaryngol 77: OP739, 1973.[731])

usually unremarkable. Some of these patients have a clinical history of a cat scratch and serologic evidence of cat-scratch disease.[13-22,24,25,760] (See discussion p. 604 and 996 and Figs. 7-2 and 13-11.) One patient had serologic evidence of influenza A infection.[765] Leptospira organisms were cultured from the spinal fluid of another patient.[18]

Within a week after involvement of the optic nerve head, a macular star figure usually becomes evident. Those presenting with branch retinal artery occlusion usually have a permanent scotoma, but most patients with retinal and optic nerve head involvement recover normal or nearly normal visual acuity spontaneously. A few may develop evidence of optic atrophy. The value of corticosteroid and antibiotic treatment is uncertain.

The fundus picture in patients with acute idiopathic multifocal inner retinitis and neuroretinitis may simulate that seen in patients with retinitis and neuroretinitis caused by pyogenic bacteria (Fig. 7-1), fungi, syphilis, and toxoplasmosis (Fig. 7-9, A to C). Patients with evidence of branch retinal artery occlusion may simulate patients with bilateral idiopathic recurrent branch retinal artery occlusion (see Fig. 6-11).

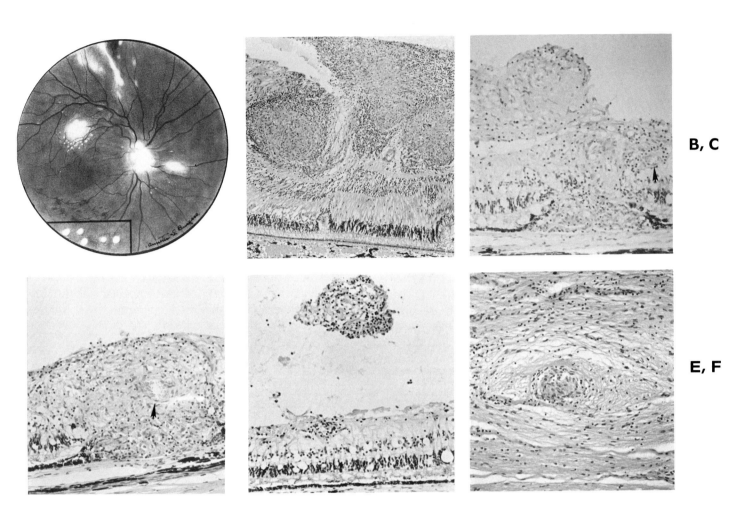

▼ BEHÇET'S DISEASE

Behçet's disease is a chronic systemic disease of unknown cause characterized clinically by aphthous ulcers of the mouth and genitalia (Fig. 7-46, *A* and *D*), intraocular inflammation, nondestructive seronegative arthritis, and cutaneous vasculitis including erythema nodosum (Fig. 7-46, *B*).* The criteria for diagnosis include oral aphthae or genital ulcers in association with any other two of the six major manifestations of the disease. The disease occurs most frequently in people of the Mediterranean basin and Japan. In approximately 80% of patients the ocular disease is bilateral, and it is twice as frequent in men.[783] Behçet's disease has been reported with less frequency in the United States, where the sex difference in regard to ocular involvement has been less pronounced.[774] Iritis and vitreous inflammatory cell infiltration are present in nearly all patients with ocular involvement. In most cases the iritis is nongranulomatous. Hypopyon occurs occasionally (Fig. 7-46, *C*). Edema of the macula and optic disc, patches of gray thickened retina, focal accumulations of yellow-white deep retinal exudates, scattered areas of delicate pigment clumping, perivasculitis, central and branch venous and arterial occlusions, papilledema, papillitis, and optic atrophy may occur (Fig. 7-46, *E, F, G,* and *L*). Visual loss is usually caused by long-standing retinitis, retinal arterial attenuation, cystoid macular edema, and, in some cases, retinitis proliferans and vitreous hemorrhage.[777,791] Whereas progressive optic atrophy may accompany the retinal changes, acute loss of vision caused by optic neuropathy without retinal involvement rarely occurs in patients with Behçet's disease.[784]

---

*References 767, 769, 770, 774-776, 780-783, 787-789, 792, 796, 800-803.

FIG. 7-46 Behçet's disease.

A, Aphthous ulcer *(arrow)*.

   B, Erythema nodosum of lower legs.

   C, Hypopyon.

   D to I, This 31-year-old woman with Behçet's disease had aphthous ulcers *(arrow,* **D**), multiple foci of retinitis causing branch retinal artery occlusion *(arrow,* **E**), and branch retinal vein occlusion *(arrow,* **F**) when she initially presented. One week later she developed another branch retinal artery occlusion *(arrow,* **G** to **I**) in the left eye.

   J to L, This 31-year-old man with aphthous stomatitis and hypopyon (**C**) in the right eye had bilateral vitritis, multiple retinal ischemic patches, and hemorrhages (**J**). His visual acuity was counting fingers in the right eye and 20/25 in the left eye. Angiography revealed perivascular leakage of fluorescein (**K**). Forty-two months later his acuity was 7/200. Note the pallor of the optic disc, marked narrowing and sheathing of the retinal vessels, and a macular scar (**L**).

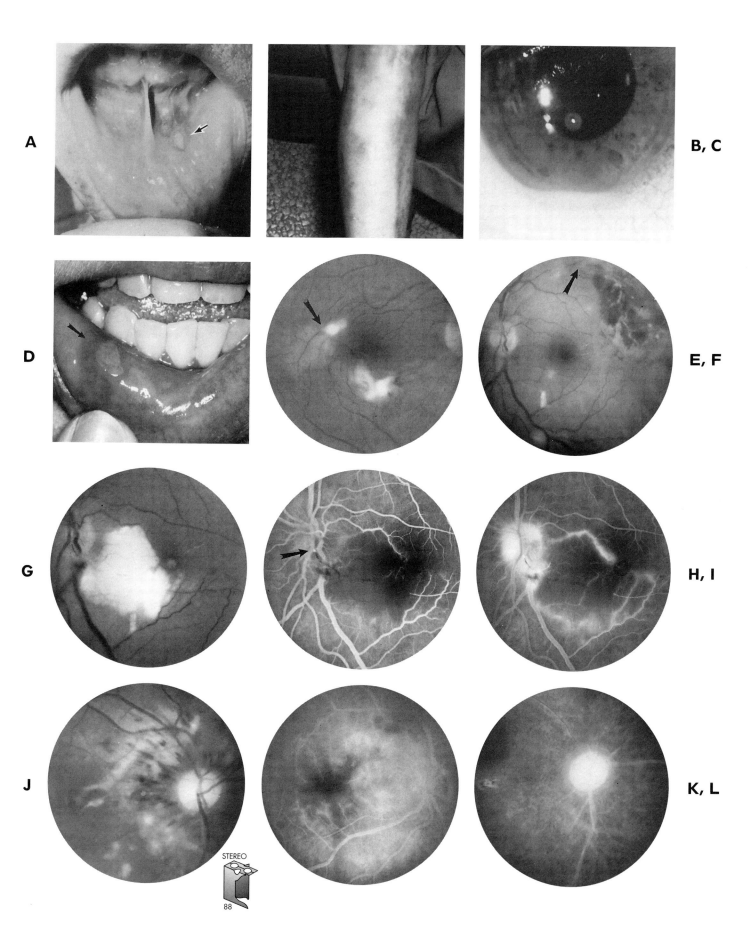

A

B, C

D

E, F

G

H, I

J

STEREO
88

K, L

703

During an acute attack the erythrocyte sedimentation rate, acute-phase proteins, and circulating immune complexes may be elevated along with dramatic alterations of serum complement levels.[766,778,787] Elevation of serum concentration of interleukin-2 receptor, C9, and complement-reactive protein may occur in all forms of the disease.[771,776,783,786,791] Antibodies against the vascular endothelial cells and mucosa can be demonstrated in some patients with Behçet's disease.[768,778,786,790,791] Antibody affinity to retinal S-antigen is lowered.[785]

A generalized vasculitis is responsible for the multiplicity of clinical manifestations. Activated T lymphocytes and hyalinized thickening are found in association with the retinal and optic nerve perivasculitis.[772] Although a virus was implicated early in the history of Behçet's disease,[799] the disease's cause is unknown. The increased incidence of HLA-B5 or -Bw51 antigens in patients with Behçet's disease in the Middle East and Japan suggests that susceptibility genes to the disease may have been spread by the old nomadic tribes or Turks via the silk route.[793,797] These antigens are found less frequently in the United States in patients with Behçet's disease.

Since Behçet's disease is a chronic disorder characterized by spontaneous remissions and exacerbations and since the course of the disease varies from one patient to another, the evaluation of therapy is difficult. Topical and oral corticosteroids constitute the first line of treatment in these patients. In severe cases these have been combined with cytotoxic agents, including azathioprine, chlorambucil, or cyclophosphamide.* These drugs may be used in concert with immunostimulation agents, including levamisole and colchicine.[779,785] Cyclosporine A, a specific anti–T cell medication, has been used successfully in some patients.[773,774,779,794,795] These latter agents should be employed only in severe cases because complications may be severe.[795,804] Plasma exchange may reduce ocular inflammation caused by Behçet's disease in patients unresponsive to standard medical therapy.[798] A controlled clinical trial demonstrated the safety and effectiveness of azathioprine in reducing the frequency of hypopyon uveitis, aphthous ulcers, and arthritis.[807]

The differential diagnosis includes sarcoidosis, the acute retinal necrosis syndrome, diffuse unilateral subacute neuroretinitis, idiopathic vitritis, pars planitis, vitiliginous chorioretinitis, and reticulum cell sarcoma.

---

*References 779, 788, 795, 803, 805, 806.

▼ DIFFUSE, CHRONIC NONNECROTIZING RETINITIS, VITRITIS, AND CYSTOID MACULAR EDEMA

The permeability of the retinal capillaries, particularly those in the macular region, may be affected by chronic diffuse inflammation involving the retina and vitreous. Although these patients may be categorized into several different syndromes, in none is the cause known and in none can it be established whether the primary tissue involved is the retina or the vitreous. The clinical features shared by these patients include complaints of floaters caused by inflammatory cell infiltration of the vitreous and loss of central vision caused by cystoid macular edema in eyes that externally show no signs of inflammation. Some degree of papilledema may be present. Bilateral involvement is the rule. A few retinal hemorrhages often occur peripherally. Evidence of peripheral retinal degeneration with some disturbance of the underlying RPE is seen eventually. Narrowing of the retinal vessels and pallor of the optic disc along with complaints of night blindness may occur in some cases. Retinal holes, retinal detachment, and preretinal vitreous membrane formation occur occasionally. The vitreous inflammation and cystoid macular edema often respond poorly to corticosteroids or other therapy.

These patients may be subdivided into three major clinical syndromes: (1) pars planitis, (2) idiopathic vitritis, and (3) vitiliginous (bird-shot) chorioretinitis.

Retinitis and vitritis with vitreous base organization (pars planitis,[850] peripheral uveitis,[817] or chronic cyclitis[838])

The term "pars planitis" has been used to describe patients with chronic vitritis who develop snow-bank exudates and vitreous condensation overlying the peripheral retina and pars plana, usually inferiorly in both eyes (Fig. 7-47).* These patients are typically children or young adults of both sexes in excellent general health when they develop floaters and blurred vision. The eyes are white. A few patients may have fine keratitic precipitates. Fine and coarse vitreous floaters are present and may be responsible for moderate loss of visual acuity. Snowball preretinal aggregates similar to those seen in sarcoidosis may be present (Fig. 7-47, H). Macular edema is the most common complication of the disease, and it may persist despite vigorous corticosteroid therapy (Fig. 7-47, B and C). Dilation of the major retinal vessels, particularly the veins; sheathing of the retinal veins; and varying degrees of papilledema often accompany the macular edema (Fig. 7-47, B and C). Other complications include secondary cataract, secondary glaucoma, sheathing and narrowing of the peripheral retinal vessels, traction and rhegmatogenous detachment of the peripheral retina,[815] retinoschisis,[814] subretinal neovascularization,[810] neovascularization of the optic disc[835] and retina (Fig. 7-47, E to G),[823] pseudogliomatous angiomatous formation,[823] vitreous hemorrhage, rhegmatogenous retinal detachment,[815] heterochromia irides, band keratopathy, and rarely phthisis bulbi. The disease is chronic but is subject to remissions and exacerbations. The amount of pars plana exudate generally correlates with the severity of vitreous inflammation and cystoid macular edema.[832] Most patients maintain useful vision in one or both eyes. Eyes with complete posterior vitreous separation may have a better visual prognosis.[833] There is some tendency for the disease to lessen in severity over a period of many years.[849]

Fluorescein angiography demonstrates a variable degree of permeability alterations of the capillaries of the retina and optic disc (Fig. 7-47, C).[825,847] In patients with macular edema there is usually angiographic evidence of widespread retinal edema, papilledema, and in some patients late staining of the larger retinal veins and venules (Fig. 7-47, C and G). Most patients have electroretinographic abnormalities, such as delayed b-wave implicit time, abnormal response to flicker, and reduced b-wave oscillations.[819]

The limited histopathologic data available suggest that this disease is a chronic nongranulomatous inflammation involving primarily the retina and vitreous.[812,824,836,845,851] The fluffy snow-bank opacities peripherally are probably caused primarily by cellular infiltrate within the vitreous. Later this fluffy appearance may be replaced by less elevated, white, organized scar tissue, which may be derived from glial elements of the peripheral retina.[851] Prominent perivenous and venous infiltration occurs with lymphocytes that are predominantly T-helper lymphocytes.[851] The uveal tract is relatively free of inflammation.[845]

The pathogenesis of pars planitis is unknown. The development of a migrating corneal endothelial rejection line (autoimmune endotheliopathy) in some patients with pars planitis suggests the possibility that the disorder may be an autoimmune process directed toward the vitreous.[837]

---

*References 809, 811, 812, 814-817, 819, 820, 822-825, 827-831, 836, 838, 841, 843, 845, 847-850, 852.

Some of these patients show improvement in visual function following oral corticosteroid therapy (Fig. 7-35, *B* to *D*). Many others, however, fail to respond to this therapy, which should be used sparingly because of the disease's chronic nature and its tendency to undergo remissions and exacerbations. In the presence of useful central vision it is probably unwise to treat these patients with long-term corticosteroids. The value of cyclodiathermy and cyclocryotherapy in treating the pars plana and peripheral retina is controversial.[809,821,829] These cyclodestructive procedures appear to be of most benefit in those patients unresponsive to corticosteroid therapy and who in addition have neovascularization in the region of the vitreous base.[821,834] The reason for accumulation of exudate over the pars plana predominantly in the inferior fundus is unknown; it is probably more a function of gravitational forces than locus of the disease. The value of vitrectomy in treating cystoid macular edema is also uncertain.[842] Although some success has been reported utilizing combination therapy of corticosteroids with antimetabolites, the value of this treatment in the long-term management of these patients is uncertain.[829-831,844] There are significant risks in such treatment, and therefore it should be employed only in patients with severe involvement.

The differential diagnosis includes sarcoidosis, peripheral toxoplasmosis, Behçet's syndrome, *Toxocara canis,* acute recurring cyclitis, and the pseudo–presumed ocular histoplasmosis syndrome. I have seen three children with this latter syndrome who in addition had dense white pars plana exudate and who developed loss of macular function secondary to choroidal neovascularization and disciform detachment.[825,826] Lyme disease may be associated with pars planitis and anterior uveitis (see Fig. 7-3, *C* to *H*).

Pars planitis has occurred in multiple members of at least eight families.[811,820,822,828,851] Pars planitis has occurred in patients developing evidence of

FIG. 7-47 Pars planitis.

A, Fundus drawing showing usual distribution of snow-bank exudates over the pars plana inferiorly.

B to D, This 17-year-old woman with pars planitis noted loss of vision because of cystoid macular edema (**B** and **C**). Four months later, after systemic corticosteroid therapy, the edema had resolved (**D**).

E to G, Retinitis proliferans *(arrows)* in the macular area of a 31-year-old man with pars planitis. Angiography demonstrated leakage of fluorescein from these vessels and cystoid macular edema (**F** and **G**).

H and I, Preretinal nodules (**H**) and cystoid macular edema (**I**) were present bilaterally in this 52-year-old woman with snow-bank exudates on the pars plana.

J to L, Pars planitis associated with multifocal choroiditis, macular edema, papilledema, vitritis and anterior uveitis in a 13-year-old male with 3-year history of photophobia, floaters, and visual loss. General physical examination was negative except for axillary lymphadenopathy. Biopsy of the nodes revealed granulomatous inflammation of unknown cause. Serologic tests for toxoplasmosis, syphilis, and Lyme disease were negative. Treatment with systemic corticosteroids and doxycycline produced minimal improvement.

(**A** from Welch RB, Maumenee AE, Wahlen HE: *Arch Ophthalmol* 64:540, 1960; copyright 1960, American Medical Association.[850])

demyelinating disease.* A long-term followup of patients with pars planitis revealed that optic neuritis developed in four patients (7.4%) and multiple sclerosis in an additional eight patients (14.8%).[839] This same group found an association of HLA-DR2 in 67.5% of patients with pars planitis (28% controls), and they cited others who had found HLA-DR2 in 50% to 75% of North Americans and Europeans with multiple sclerosis (20% to 25% controls).[818,840]

---

*References 813, 818, 827, 839, 840, 843, 846.

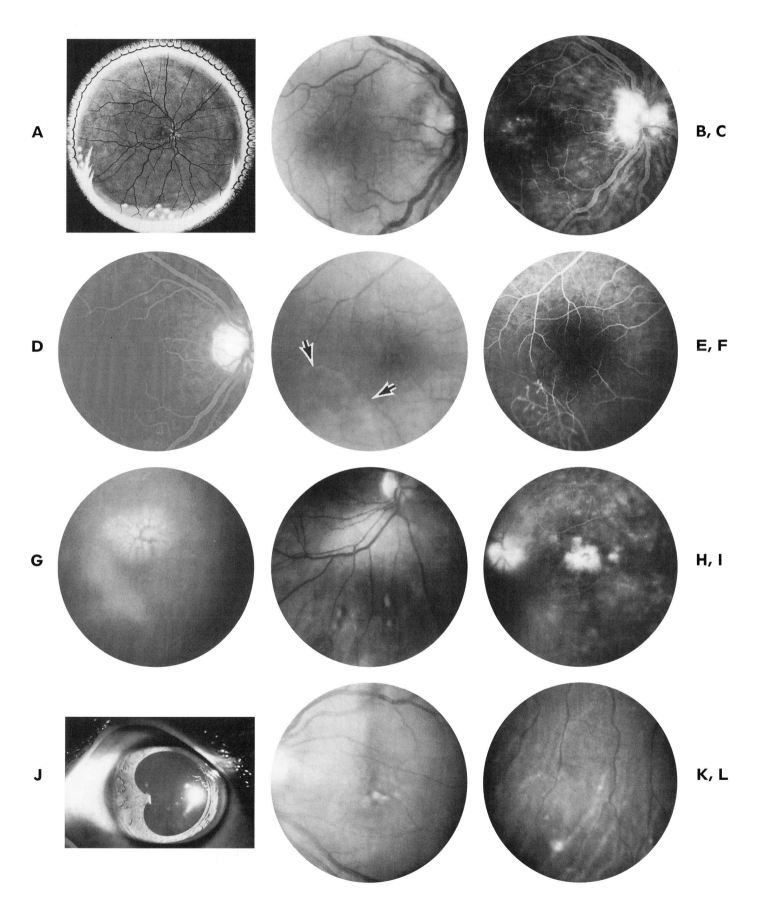

A

B, C

D

E, F

G

H, I

J

K, L

Idiopathic diffuse nonnecrotizing retinitis without vitreous base organization (idiopathic senile vitritis)

The most frequently encountered group of patients with floaters or loss of vision secondary to chronic vitritis and diffuse retinitis are healthy middle-aged or elderly patients, most frequently women, who develop cystoid macular as well as diffuse retinal edema, in some cases papilledema, and cellular infiltrate of the vitreous without any evidence of snow-bank pars plana deposits (Fig. 7-48).[854,857] Cellophane maculopathy caused by an epiretinal membrane is frequently present in the macular areas. Externally the eyes are quiet. The peripheral fundi often show evidence of narrowing and sheathing of the retinal vessels as well as irregular derangement of the RPE. Retinal edema and vitritis often respond poorly to corticosteroids or other therapy. The cause is unknown. I have seen idiopathic vitritis in identical twins (Fig. 7-48, *E* to *I*).[857] Bennett and coworkers reported a large family with autosomal dominant adult-onset vitreous inflammation, selective loss of the ERG b-wave, mild anterior chamber inflammation, and later retinal scarring, pigmentation, peripheral retinal vascular closure, peripheral retinal neovascularization, vitreous hemorrhage, and cystoid macular edema.[853]

Patients with idiopathic vitritis share many features in common with patients with vitiliginous chorioretinitis (see next subsection). Differentiating patients with idiopathic vitritis from patients with genetically determined retinitis pigmentosa sine pigmenti is difficult. The electroretinographic abnormalities are usually less severe in patients with idiopathic vitritis. Other disorders that may simulate idiopathic vitritis include Whipple's disease (see p. 714), large-cell non-Hodgkin's lymphoma (see p. 880), metastatic carcinoma and melanoma to the vitreous (see p. 893) and lymphocytic infiltration of the vitreous associated with X-linked immunodeficiency with increased IgM.[858]

FIG. 7-48   Diffuse Nonnecrotizing Retinitis, Vitritis, and Cystoid Macular Edema Without Pars Plana Exudation (Idiopathic Vitritis).

A to **D,** This 70-year-old woman noted floaters and visual loss in both eyes at 65 years of age. Visual acuity was 20/200 in the right eye and 20/50 in the left eye. She had bilateral vitritis, cystoid macular edema, and diffuse retinal edema. Note angiographic evidence of irregular focal scars in the periphery and the multiloculated fluorescein staining pattern in the extramacular as well as the macular area (**B** to **D**). She has been observed for 22 years, and her acuity and findings are unchanged.

E and **F,** Cystoid macular edema, mild papilledema, and vitritis in a 59-year-old woman whose visual acuity was 20/40 in the right eye and 20/400 in the left eye.

G to **I,** The identical twin sister of patient illustrated in **E** and **F** with the same condition in both eyes. Note the marked retinal capillary dilation (**H**) and the extramacular and macular polycystic edema (**I**). Both twins noted the onset of floaters and blurred vision at 50 years of age. Both have markedly subnormal rod and cone electroretinographic responses.

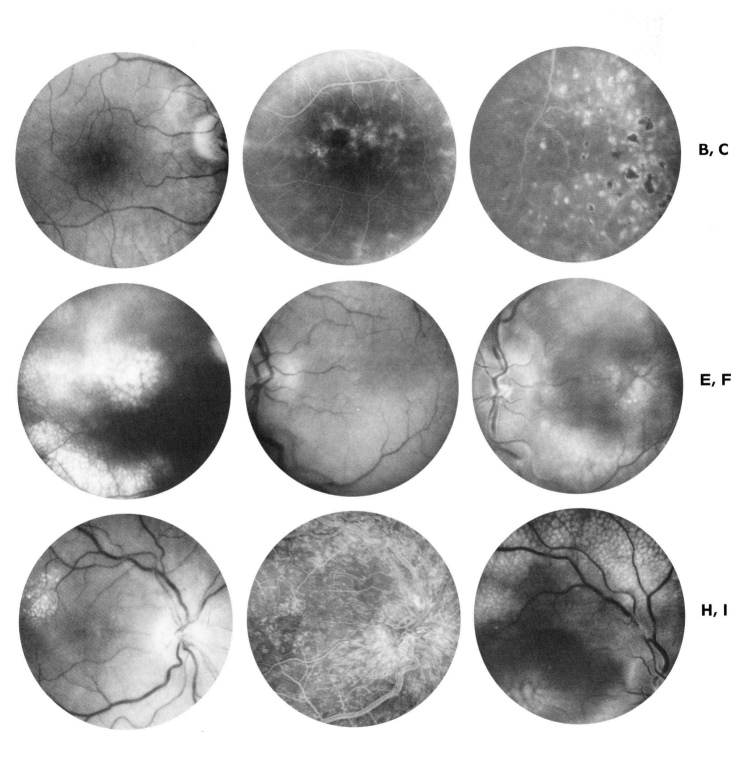

B, C

E, F

H, I

Vitiliginous chorioretinitis (bird-shot retinochoroidopathy)

The syndrome of vitiliginous chorioretinitis or bird-shot retinochoroidopathy is characterized by (1) onset, in apparently healthy patients, usually women in the fifth to seventh decade of life, of floaters, photopsia, and blurred vision, often followed later by night blindness and color blindness; (2) vitreous inflammation; (3) multifocal patches of depigmentation first occurring in the choroid and later the RPE in the postequatorial fundi; (4) varying degrees of retinal edema and papilledema, and narrowing of the retinal vessels and mild optic atrophy; (5) moderate to severe electroretinographic abnormalities; (6) a variable rate of progression and severity but with a tendency toward stabilization and preservation of good central vision in at least one eye; and (7) strong association with HLA-A29.*

Before the initial publication of this syndrome, called bird-shot retinochoroidopathy by Ryan and Maumenee, the name "vitiliginous chorioretinitis" had been used at the Bascom Palmer Eye Institute to describe patients with this syndrome. The author chose this name for this syndrome because of the similarity in the appearance and evolution of the patches of choroidal depigmentation to those occurring in the skin of patients with vitiligo.[868] These orange or yellow ill-defined patches, which may not be present when the patient is seen initially with vitreous cells and macular edema, are typically scattered in the postequatorial portion of the fundus (Figs. 7-49 and 7-50). They are most numerous in a broad area surrounding the nasal two-thirds of the optic disc and early in the course of the disease are often absent in the macular area. The patches vary in size and shape. Many of the patches are round to oval. Some are irregular or elongated, often in a pattern that radiates toward the peripheral fundus (Fig. 7-49, A and B). Striking and characteristic features of these patches are the absence of hyperpigmentation within or at their margins and the absence of slit-lamp evidence of thinning of either the retina or the choroid in the area of depigmentation. Large choroidal blood vessels are often visible within these lesions, and the overlying retinal vessels appear normal. During the early stages of depigmentation, particularly when associated with severe vitreous inflammation, absence of visible choroidal vessels within these lesions may then give the appearance of nonelevated choroidal inflammatory infiltrates. Angio-

*References 863, 866, 868-870, 872, 873, 875, 878, 879, 881, 882.

FIG. 7-49   Vitiliginous Chorioretinitis.

A to C, This 58-year-old woman complained of floaters and had a visual acuity of 20/20. There were 2+ vitreous cells. A similar pattern of multifocal areas of yellowish depigmentation of the choroid was present in both eyes (**A** and **B**). Note relative sparing of the macular areas, and elongation of the more peripheral lesions. Early phases of angiography showed no abnormality in the region of these patches (compare **B** and **C**).

D to F, This 50-year-old man experienced floaters and mild loss of vision. Only a few small vitiliginous patches were evident in the juxtapapillary area (**D**). He had angiographic evidence of cystoid macular edema (**E**). Two years later, his visual acuity was 20/400 and he had many large vitiliginous patches throughout both fundi (**F**).

G and H, This 49-year-old woman complained of floaters, blurred vision, and metamorphopsia in both eyes when she was initially examined in February of 1980. Bilateral serous detachment of the macula was present. This resolved spontaneously. When seen at Bascom Palmer Eye Institute 2 years later she complained of nyctalopia and loss of color vision. She had vitreous cells, pigment mottling of the macula, and widespread vitiliginous patches throughout the postequatorial fundi with relatively sparing of the macular areas (**G** and **H**).

(**A to F** from Gass JDM: *Arch Ophthalmol* 99:1778, 1981; copyright 1981, American Medical Association.[868])

graphically in their early evolution these patches show no abnormality (Fig. 7-49, *C*). The lesions are usually symmetrically distributed in both eyes. In time the patches enlarge and may be associated with biomicroscopic and angiographic evidence of depigmentation and atrophy of the overlying RPE and retina. Hyperpigmentation may occur in some lesions in the late stages of the disease. Loss of central vision may be caused by cystoid macular edema (Fig. 7-49, *E*), by atrophy of the retina associated with the depigmentation of the RPE and choroid (Fig. 7-49, *F*), and occasionally by serous macular detachment (Fig. 7-49, *G* and *H*) or by choroidal neovascularization (Fig. 7-50, *H* and *I*).[863,880] Proliferation of new vessels from the optic disc and retina may occasionally occur and cause vitreous hemorrhage (Fig. 7-50, *J* to *L*). Rare associations with vitiliginous chorioretinitis include hearing loss[870] and Lyme disease.[883]

Fluorescein angiography may show evidence of delay in the retinal artery appearance time, increased retinal circulation time, and varying degrees of unexplained quenching of fluorescence of the retinal vessels during the course of angiography.[868] Electroretinography shows moderately to

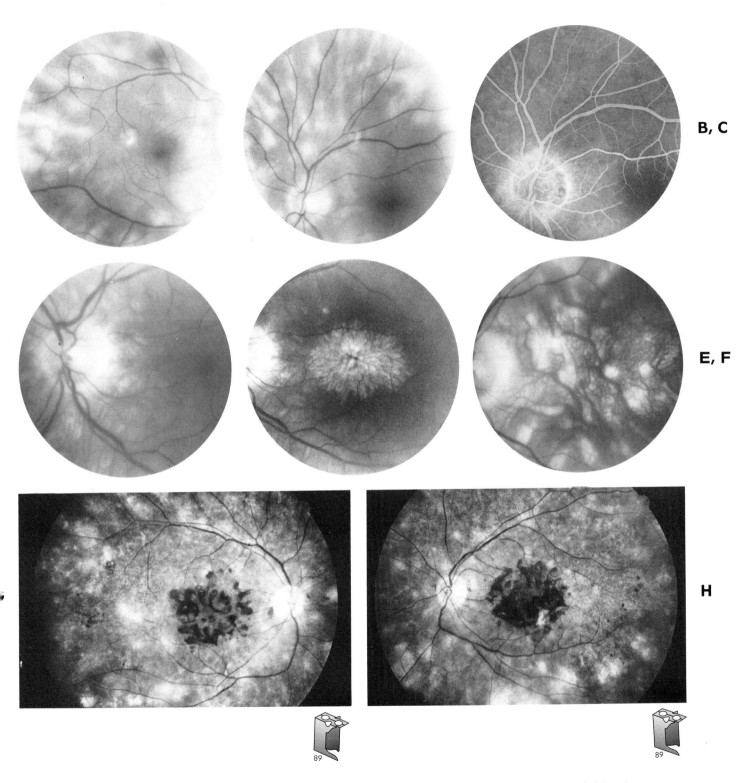

B, C

E, F

H

severely abnormal rod and cone function in both eyes of most patients.[871,876] The electrooculogram may be either normal or subnormal. Dark-adaptation studies may show subnormal rod function. Although I have observed multiple depigmented spots on the arms and legs of several

patients with vitiliginous chorioretinitis, these appear to be more closely related to idiopathic guttate hypomelanosis than vitiligo. This former disease is a common skin change of unknown origin and similar in both its clinical and histopathologic appearance to vitiligo.[864] Albert and associates[859]

711

observed five patients with cutaneous vitiligo and a fundus picture that appeared similar to vitiliginous chorioretinitis. Depigmentation of the choroid and RPE similar to that seen in vitiliginous choroiditis may occur in patients with other ocular diseases that may be associated with vitiligo (Vogt-Koyanagi-Harada disease, sympathetic uveitis, and acute Vogt-Koyanagi-Harada-like uveitis caused by metastatic cutaneous melanoma). This suggests the possibility of a common autoimmune mechanism.[859-861,867,885] Progressive degeneration of the peripheral retina, retinal artery narrowing, and optic disc pallor and night blindness are features that may occur in all four diseases. Vitiliginous chorioretinitis is usually a chronic, slowly progressive disease that is subject to remissions and exacerbations. Most patients retain useful central vision in at least one eye for many years. Most respond poorly to corticosteroid therapy. Low-dose cyclosporine (2.5 to 5 mg/kg daily), with or without other corticosteroid-sparing immunosuppressive agents, has been used as an alternative to long-term corticosteroids.[884]

Antigen HLA-A29 is found in approximately 90% of patients with vitiliginous chorioretinitis.[873,874,877,878] Vitiliginous chorioretinitis has occurred in monozygotic twins.[865] Over 50% of patients may demonstrate evidence of an in vitro mitotic immune response to purified retinal S-antigen.[874] These findings suggest that this disease has a genetic predisposition and that retinal autoimmunity plays a role in its manifestations.

The differential diagnosis before the development of the typical hypopigmented fundus lesions includes pars planitis, idiopathic vitritis, reticulum cell sarcoma, papillitis, and papilledema. Irregular dilation of the retinal veins and scattered retinal hemorrhages (Fig. 7-50, E and F) suggested a diagnosis of macroglobulinemia in one case. Several patients with papilledema were thought initially to have an intracranial tumor (Fig. 7-50, G). Once the typical hypopigmented fundus lesions develop, the appearance and course of this disease differentiate it from other diseases that have white spots in the fundus associated with vitreous inflammation, such as serpiginous choroiditis, acute posterior multifocal placoid pigment epitheliopathy, diffuse unilateral subacute neuroretinitis, sarcoidosis, Behcet's disease, reticulum cell sarcoma, and Whipple's disease.

FIG. 7-50 Vitiliginous Chorioretinitis.

A to D, This healthy middle-aged woman complained of floaters and blurred vision. Note blurring of the margins of the pale optic disc and narrowing of the retinal arteries (A and B). Angiography revealed increased retinal circulation time and widespread leakage of fluorescein in the retinal vessels (C and D).

E and F, Irregular dilation of retinal veins and retinal hemorrhages in this 51-year-old man who had only a few depigmented patches in his left eye when initially examined (E). Three years later he had developed prominent vitiliginous patches in both eyes (F).

G, This 47-year-old woman had experienced "graying of vision" 5 months previously. Bilateral papilledema was diagnosed, and a neurologic evaluation was negative. Soon afterward her ophthalmologist noted evidence of vitreous inflammation and she was referred to Bascom Palmer Eye Institute for evaluation. Visual acuity was 20/20 in the right eye and 20/15 in the left eye. There were 2+ vitreous cells, papilledema, and choroidal lesions typical of vitiliginous chorioretinitis bilaterally (G). The electroretinogram in both eyes showed severely abnormal rod and cone functions.

H and I, This 54-year-old woman with vitiliginous chorioretinitis developed loss of central vision in both eyes because of choroidal neovascularization.

J to L, This man with vitiliginous chorioretinitis developed retinal and optic disc neovascularization that required panretinal photocoagulation and vitrectomy.

(E and F from Gass JDM: *Arch Ophthalmol* 99:1778, 1981; copyright 1981, American Medical Association.[868])

Vitiliginous chorioretinitis shares some features in common with the multifocal choroiditis and panuveitis (pseudo–presumed ocular histoplasmosis syndrome) (see p. 688). Unlike the latter syndrome, vitiliginous chorioretinitis rarely affects children and young adults; is infrequently associated with anterior uveitis, punched-out chorioretinal scars, or choroidal neovascularization; and is associated with HLA-A29.

The relationship of patients with vitiliginous chorioretinitis and the more frequently encountered patients, most commonly middle-aged or older women, with chronic vitritis and macular edema but without evidence of the typical vitiliginous lesions is unknown (see p. 708).

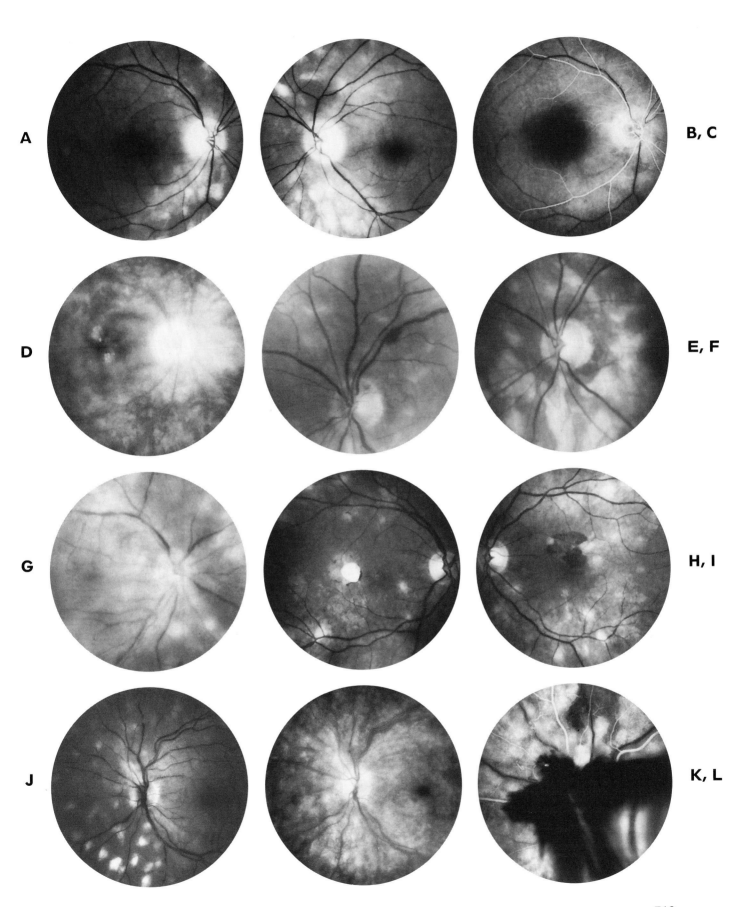

A

B, C

D

E, F

G

H, I

J

K, L

713

▼ VITRITIS AND RETINITIS IN WHIPPLE'S DISEASE

Whipple's disease is a chronic multisystemic disease characterized by fever, diarrhea, weight loss, steatorrhea, polyserositis, and arthralgia and impaired intestinal absorption. Other features include mesenteric and peripheral adenopathy; cutaneous pigmentation; heart murmur; neurologic signs and symptoms including personality changes, dementia, and memory defect; myoclonus; ataxia; supranuclear ophthalmoplegia; and seizure disorders.[886-896] Ocular findings include vitreous opacities,[887,889,890] exudative material overlying the pars plana,[887] retinal hemorrhages, cotton-wool patches, scattered white exudates, chorioretinitis,[886] retinal vasculitis and uveitis,[887,895] papilledema,[894] and glaucoma. One patient studied with fluorescein angiography showed multifocal areas of retinal capillary closure, diffuse retinal vasculitis, and choroidal folds.[886]

Histopathologically, foamy macrophages with many periodic acid–Schiff (PAS) positive intercellular granules are found in many of the organs of the body including the brain and eye (Fig. 7-51).[888,889] Jejunal biopsy is the usual method of diagnosis. Vitrectomy has been employed in some cases.[887] Electron microscopy reveals degenerated rod-shaped bacteria within and adjacent to macrophages. This gram-negative actinomycete with distinct morphologic characteristics is named *Tropheryma whippelii*. The organism cannot be cultured, but it can be identified by polymerase chain reaction assay, as was done in the vitreous aspirate from a woman with uveitis and only minimal symptoms of Whipple's disease.[894] Margo and coworkers found macrophages filled with PAS-positive particles similar to those in Whipple's disease in the vitreous aspirate removed from the eye of a patient with coryneform bacterial endophthalmitis and no evidence of Whipple's disease.[893]

Treatment of patients with Whipple's disease with antibiotics results in remission of symptoms and reduction in the PAS-positive macrophages. Whipple's disease should be considered in the differential diagnosis of patients with evidence of vitritis and retinitis and signs and symptoms of neurologic disease. The differential diagnosis includes reticulum cell sarcoma, Behcet's disease, sarcoidosis, and other causes of vitritis.

FIG. 7-51 Whipple's Disease.

A, Photomicrograph showing clusters of macrophages within the inner retinal layers and in the vitreous *(arrow)*.

B, Higher-power photomicrograph showing clusters of macrophages within the retina *(arrows)*.

(From Font et al.[888])

▼ CROHN'S DISEASE

Crohn's disease (regional ileitis) is a granulomatous enterocolitis of unknown etiology that usually affects young adults. Approximately 10% of patients develop ocular complications.[900] These include corneal infiltrates, conjunctivitis, corneal ulceration, episcleritis, scleritis, choroidal folds, acute anterior nongranulomatous and less often chronic posterior granulomatous uveitis, acute iritis, macular edema, central serous chorioretinopathy, proptosis, papilledema, retinal vasculitis and neuroretinitis.[900-903,905-907] I have seen one patient with Crohn's disease associated with erythema nodosum and typical acute posterior multifocal placoid pigment epitheliopathy (APMPPE).[899] Others have reported multifocal choroidal infiltrates similar to APMPPE but associated with serous retinal detachment in Crohn's disease.[898] Systemic manifestations include low-grade fever, abdominal pain, diarrhea, anemia, weight loss, arthritis, psoriasis, erythema nodosum, and hepatitis. Ocular complications are more likely to occur during the active phase of the disease, and at least 50% of these patients will have evidence of arthritis.[897,900] Patients with colitis and ileocolitis are more likely to have ocular involvement than patients with only small bowel involvement.[897] There is a higher than normal prevalence of HLA-B27-type leukocytes in patients with Crohn's disease.[904]

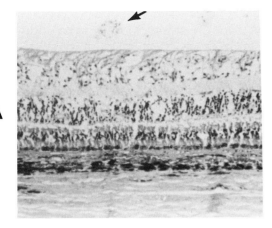 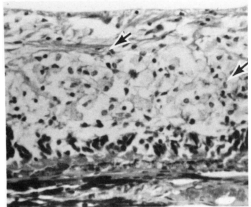

REFERENCES
Pyogenic Chorioretinitis

1. Blodi BA, Johnson MW, McLeish WM, Gass JDM: Presumed choroidal tuberculosis in a human immunodeficiency virus infected host. *Am J Ophthalmol* 108:605-607, 1989.
2. Davis JL, Nussenblatt RB, Bachman DM, et al: Endogenous bacterial retinitis in AIDS. *Am J Ophthalmol* 107:613-623, 1989.
3. Duane TD, Osher RH, Green WR: White centered hemorrhages: Their significance. *Ophthalmology* 87:66-69, 1980.
4. Herschorn BJ, Brucker AJ: Embolic retinopathy due to *Corynebacterium minutissimum* endocardititis. *Br J Ophthalmol* 69:29-31, 1985.
5. Kennedy JE, Wise GN: Clinicopathological correlation of retinal lesions; subacute bacterial endocarditis. *Arch Ophthalmol* 74:658-662, 1965.
6. Litten M: Ueber die bei der acuten malignen Endocarditis und anderen septischen Erkrankungen vorkommenden Retinalveränderungen. *Ber Ophthalmol Ges* 10:140-143, 1877.
7. Munier F, Othenin-Girard P: Subretinal neovascularization secondary to choroidal septic metastasis from acute bacterial endocarditis. *Retina* 12:108-112, 1992.
8. Neudorfer M, Barnea Y, Geyer O, Siegman-Igra Y: Retinal lesions in septicemia. *Am J Ophthalmol* 116:728-734, 1993.
9. Packer AJ, Weingeist TA, Abrams GW: Retinal periphlebitis as an early sign of bacterial endophthalmitis. *Am J Ophthalmol* 96:66-71, 1983.
10. Roth M: Beiträge zur Kenntniss der varicösen Hypertrophie der Nervenfasern. *Arch Pathol Anat Physiol* 55:197-217, 1872.
11. Roth M: Ueber Netzhautaffection bei Wundfiebern. *Dtsch Z Chir* 1:471, 1872.

Cat-Scratch Disease (CSD)

12. Angritt P, Tuur SM, Macher AM, et al: Epithelioid angiomatosis in HIV infection: Neoplasm or cat-scratch disease? *Lancet* 1:996, 1988.
13. Bar S, Segal M, Shapira R, Savir H: Neuroretinitis associated with cat scratch disease. *Am J Ophthalmol* 110:703-705, 1990.
14. Carithers HA, Margileth AM: Cat-scratch disease; acute encephalopathy and other neurologic manifestations. *Am J Dis Child* 145:98-101, 1991.

15. Chrousos GA, Drack AV, Young M, et al: Neuroretinitis in cat scratch disease. *J Clin Neuro-Ophthalmol* 10:92-94, 1990.
15a. Dalton MJ, Robinson LE, Cooper J et al.: Use of *Bartonella* antigens for serologic diagnosis of cat-scratch disease at a national referral center. *Arch Intern Med* 155(15):1670-1676, 1995.
16. Fish RH, Hogan RN, Nightingale SD, Anand R: Peripapillary angiomatosis associated with cat-scratch neuroretinitis. *Arch Ophthalmol* 110:323, 1992.
17. Gass JDM: *Stereoscopic atlas of macular diseases; diagnosis and treatment,* ed 2, St. Louis, 1977, CV Mosby, p. 376.
18. Gass JDM: *Stereoscopic atlas of macular diseases; diagnosis and treatment,* ed 3, St. Louis, 1987, CV Mosby, pp. 746-751.
19. Golnik KC, Marotto ME, Fanous MM, et al: Ophthalmic manifestations of *Rochalimaea* species. *Am J Ophthalmol* 118:145-151, 1994.
20. Grossniklaus HE: The cat scratch disease-bacillary angiomatosis puzzle. *Am J Ophthalmol* 118:246-248, 1994.
21. LeBoit PE, Berger TG, Egbert BM, et al: Epithelioid haemangioma-like vascular proliferation in AIDS: Manifestation of cat scratch disease or bacillus infection? *Lancet* 1:960-963, 1988.
22. Schlossberg D, Morad Y, Krouse TB, et al: Culture-proved disseminated cat-scratch disease in acquired immunodeficiency syndrome. *Arch Intern Med* 149:1437-1439, 1989.
23. Stoler MH, Bonfiglio TA, Steigbigel RT, Pereira M: An atypical subcutaneous infection associated with acquired immune deficiency syndrome. *Am J Clin Pathol* 80:714-718, 1983.
24. Ulrich GG, Waecker NJ Jr, Meister SJ, et al: Cat scratch disease associated with neuroretinitis in a 6-year-old girl. *Ophthalmology* 99:246-249, 1992.
25. Wear DJ, Margileth AM, Hadfield TL, et al: Cat scratch disease: a bacterial infection. *Science* 221:1403-1405, 1983.
26. Weiss AH, Beck RW: Neuroretinitis in childhood. *J Pediatr Ophthalmol Strabismus* 26:198-203, 1989.

Luetic Chorioretinitis

27. Arruga J, Valentines J, Mauri F, et al: Neuroretinitis in acquired syphilis. *Ophthalmology* 92:262-270, 1985.
28. Belin MW, Baltch AL, Hay PB: Secondary syphilitic uveitis. *Am J Ophthalmol* 92:210-214, 1981.

29. Berger JR: Diagnosing neurosyphilis; the value of the cerebrospinal fluid VDRL or lack thereof. *J Clin Neuro-Ophthalmol* 9:234-235, 1989.

30. Crouch ER Jr, Goldberg MF: Retinal periarteritis secondary to syphilis. *Arch Ophthalmol* 93:384-387, 1975.

31. DeLuise VP, Clark SW III, Smith JL, Collart P: Syphilitic retinal detachment and uveal effusion. *Am J Ophthalmol* 94:757-761, 1982.

32. de Souza EC, Jalkh AE, Trempe CL, et al: Unusual central chorioretinitis as the first manifestation of early secondary syphilis. *Am J Ophthalmol* 105:271-276, 1988.

33. Duke-Elder S, Dobree JH: *System of ophthalmology,* vol. 10. *Diseases of the retina,* St. Louis, 1967, CV Mosby, pp. 100, 172, 221, 252, 530.

34. Duke-Elder S, Perkins ES: *System of ophthalmology,* vol. 9. *Diseases of the uveal tract,* St. Louis, 1966, CV Mosby, p. 292.

35. Folk JC, Weingeist TA, Corbett JJ, et al: Syphilitic neuro-retinitis. *Am J Ophthalmol* 95:480-486, 1983.

36. Friberg TR: Photo essay. Syphilitic chorioretinitis. *Arch Ophthalmol* 107:1676-1677, 1989.

37. Gass JDM, Braunstein RA, Chenoweth RG: Acute syphilitic posterior placoid chorioretinitis. *Ophthalmology* 97:1288-1297, 1990.

38. Halperin LS, Berger AS, Grand MG: Photoessay. Syphilitic disc edema and periphlebitis. *Retina* 10:223-225, 1990.

39. Halperin LS, Lewis H, Blumenkranz MS, et al: Choroidal neovascular membrane and other chorioretinal complications of acquired syphilis. *Am J Ophthalmol* 108:554-562, 1989.

40. Kranias G, Schneider D, Raymond LA: A case of syphilitic uveitis. *Am J Ophthalmol* 91:261-263, 1981.

41. Levy JH, Liss RA, Maguire AM: Neurosyphilis and ocular syphilis in patients with concurrent human immunodeficiency virus infection. *Retina* 9:175-180, 1989.

42. Lobes LA Jr, Folk JC: Syphilitic phlebitis simulating branch vein occlusion. *Ann Ophthalmol* 13:825-827, 1981.

43. McLeish WM, Pulido JS, Holland S, et al: The ocular manifestations of syphilis in the human immunodeficiency virus type 1-infected host. *Ophthalmology* 97:196-203, 1990.

44. Mendelsohn AD, Jampol LM: Syphilitic retinitis; a cause of necrotizing retinitis. *Retina* 4:221-224, 1984.

45. Moore JE: Syphilitic iritis; a study of 249 patients. *Am J Ophthalmol* 14:110-122, 1931.

46. Morgan CM, Webb RM, O'Connor GR: Atypical syphilitic chorioretinitis and vasculitis. *Retina* 4:225-231, 1984.

47. Passo MS, Rosenbaum JT: Ocular syphilis in patients with human immunodeficiency virus infection. *Am J Ophthalmol* 106:1-6, 1988.

48. Ryan SJ, Hardy PH, Hardy JM, Oppenheimer EH: Persistence of virulent *Treponema pallidum* despite penicillin therapy in congenital syphilis. *Am J Ophthalmol* 73:258-261, 1972.

49. Saari M: Disciform detachment of the macula. III. Secondary to inflammatory diseases. *Acta Ophthalmol* 56:510-517, 1978.

50. Sacks JG, Osher RH, Elconin H: Progressive visual loss in syphilitic optic atrophy. *J Clin Neuro-Ophthalmol* 3:5-8, 1983.

51. Savir H, Kurz O: Fluorescein angiography in syphilitic retinal vasculitis. *Ann Ophthalmol* 8:713-716, 1976.

52. Schlaegel TF Jr, Kao SF: A review (1970-1980) of 28 presumptive cases of syphilitic uveitis. *Am J Ophthalmol* 93:412-414, 1982.

53. Shimuzu R, Numaga T, Kimura Y, Horiuchi T: Acute syphilitic retinochoroiditis. *Jpn J Clin Ophthalmol* 43:13-19, 1989.

54. Stoumbos VD, Klein ML: Syphilitic retinitis in a patient with acquired immunodeficiency syndrome-related complex. *Am J Ophthalmol* 103:103-104, 1987.

55. Walsh FB, Hoyt WF: *Clinical neuro-ophthalmology,* ed. 3, Baltimore, 1969, Williams & Wilkins, p. 1551.

56. Yagasaki T, Akiyama K, Nomura H, Awaya S: Two cases of acquired syphilis with acute central chorioretinitis as initial manifestation. *Jpn J Ophthalmol* 36:301-309, 1992.

Lyme Borreliosis

57. Aaberg TM: The expanding ophthalmologic spectrum of Lyme disease. *Am J Ophthalmol* 107:77-80, 1989.

58. Berglöff J, Gasser R, Feigl B: Ophthalmic manifestations of Lyme Borreliosis; a review. *J Neuro-Ophthalmol* 14:15-20, 1994.

59. Bialasiewicz AA, Ruprecht KW, Naumann GOH, Blenk H: Bilateral diffuse choroiditis and exudative retinal detachments with evidence of Lyme disease. *Am J Ophthalmol* 105:419-420, 1988.

60. Breeveld J, Rothova A, Kuiper H: Intermediate uveitis and Lyme borreliosis. *Br J Ophthalmol* 76:181-182, 1992.

61. Jacobson DM, Frens DB: Pseudotumor cerebri syndrome associated with Lyme disease. *Am J Ophthalmol* 107:81-82, 1989.

62. Lesser RL, Kornmehl EW, Pachner AR, et al: Neuro-ophthalmologic manifestations of Lyme disease. *Ophthalmology* 97:699-706, 1990.

63. Schönherr U, Lang GE, Meythaler FH: Bilaterale Lebersche Neuroretinitis stellata bei *Borrelia burgdorferi*-Serokonversion. *Klin Monatsbl Augenheilkd* 198:44-47, 1991.

64. Smith JL, Crumpton BC, Hummer J: The Bascom Palmer Eye Institute Lyme/syphilis survey. *J Clin Neuro-Ophthalmol* 10:255-260, 1990.

65. Smith JL, Parsons TM, Paris-Hamlin AJ, Porschen RK: The prevalence of Lyme disease in a nonendemic area; a comparative serologic study in a south Florida eye clinic population. *J Clin Neuro-Ophthalmol* 9:148-155, 1989.

66. Smith JL, Winward KE, Nicholson DF, Albert DW: Retinal vasculitis in Lyme borreliosis. *J Clin Neuro-Ophthalmol* 11:7-15, 1991.

67. Suttorp-Schulten MSA, Luyendijk L, van Dam AP, et al: Birdshot chorioretinopathy and Lyme borreliosis. *Am J Ophthalmol* 115:149-153, 1993.

68. Winward KE, Smith JL, Culbertson WW, Paris-Hamelin A: Ocular Lyme borreliosis. *Am J Ophthalmol* 108:651-657, 1989.

Candida Retinochoroiditis

69. Aguilar GL, Blumenkranz MS, Egbert PR, McCulley JP: *Candida* endophthalmitis after intravenous drug abuse. *Arch Ophthalmol* 97:96-100, 1979.

70. Axelrod AJ, Peyman GA, Apple DJ: Toxicity of intravitreal injection of amphotericin B. *Am J Ophthalmol* 76:578-583, 1973.

71. Barrie T: The place of elective vitrectomy in the management of patients with *Candida* endophthalmitis. *Graefes Arch Clin Exp Ophthalmol* 225:107-113, 1987.

72. Brod RD, Flynn HW Jr, Clarkson JG, et al: Endogenous *Candida* endophthalmitis; management without intravenous amphotericin B. *Ophthalmology* 97:666-674, 1990.

73. Brownstein S, Mahoney-Kinsner J, Harris R: Ocular *Candida* with pale-centered hemorrhages. *Arch Ophthalmol* 101:1745-1748, 1983.

74. Chess J, Kaplan S, Rubinstein A, et al: *Candida* retinitis in bare lymphocyte syndrome. *Ophthalmology* 93:696-698, 1986.

75. Daily MJ, Dickey JB, Packo KH: Endogenous *Candida* endophthalmitis after intravenous anesthesia with propofol. *Arch Ophthalmol* 109:1081-1084, 1991.

76. Dellon AL, Stark WJ, Chretien PB: Spontaneous resolution of endogenous *Candida* endophthalmitis complicating intravenous hyperalimentation. *Am J Ophthalmol* 79:648-654, 1975.

77. Donahue SP, Greven CM, Zuravleff JJ, et al: Intraocular candidiasis in patients with candidemia; clinical implications derived from a prospective multicenter trial. *Ophthalmology* 101:1302-1309, 1994.

78. Dunn ET, Mansour AM: Retinal striae as a sign of resolving candidal chorioretinitis. *Graefes Arch Clin Exp Ophthalmol* 226:591-592, 1988.

79. Edwards JE Jr, Foos RY, Montgomerie JZ, Guze LB: Ocular manifestations of *Candida* septicemia: review of seventy-six cases of hematogenous *Candida* endophthalmitis. *Medicine* 53:47-75, 1974.

80. Elliott JH, O'Day DM, Gutow GS, et al: Mycotic endophthalmitis in drug abusers. *Am J Ophthalmol* 88:66-72, 1979.

81. Fisher JF, Taylor AT, Clark J, et al: Penetration of amphotericin B into the human eye. *J Infect Dis* 147:164, 1983.

82. Fishman LS, Griffin JR, Sapico FL, Hecht R: Hematogenous *Candida* endophthalmitis—a complication of candidemia. *N Engl J Med* 286:675-681, 1972.

83. Fleming KO: *Candida albicans* abscess of retina. *Can J Ophthalmol* 7:132-135, 1972.

84. Griffin JR, Pettit TH, Fishman LS, Foos RY: Blood-borne *Candida* endophthalmitis; a clinical and pathologic study of 21 cases. *Arch Ophthalmol* 89:450-456, 1973.

85. Henderson DK, Edwards JE Jr, Montgomerie JZ: Hematogenous *Candida* endophthalmitis in patients receiving parenteral hyperalimentation fluids. *J Infect Dis* 143:655-661, 1981.

86. Jones DB: Chemotherapy of experimental endogenous *Candida albicans* endophthalmitis. *Trans Am Ophthalmol Soc* 78:846-895, 1980.

87. McDonald HR, De Bustros S, Sipperley JO: Vitrectomy for epiretinal membrane with *Candida* chorioretinitis. *Ophthalmology* 97:466-469, 1990.

88. McDonnell PJ, McDonnell JM, Brown RH, Green WR: Ocular involvement in patients with fungal infections. *Ophthalmology* 92:706-709, 1985.

89. Morinelli EN, Dugel PU, Lee M, et al: Opportunistic intraocular infections in AIDS. *Trans Am Ophthalmol Soc* 90:97-109, 1992.

90. Palmer EA: Endogenous *Candida* endophthalmitis in infants. *Am J Ophthalmol* 89:388-395, 1980.

91. Parke DW II, Jones DB, Gentry LO: Endogenous endophthalmitis among patients with candidemia. *Ophthalmology* 89:789-796, 1982.

92. Perraut LE Jr, Perraut LE, Bleiman B, Lyons J: Successful treatment of *Candida albicans* endophthalmitis with intravitreal amphotericin B. *Arch Ophthalmol* 99:1565-1567, 1981.

93. Snip RC, Michels RG: Pars plana vitrectomy in the management of endogenous *Candida* endophthalmitis. *Am J Ophthalmol* 82:699-704, 1976.

94. Stern GA, Fetkenhour CL, O'Grady RB: Intravitreal amphotericin B treatment of *Candida* endophthalmitis. *Arch Ophthalmol* 95:89-93, 1977.

95. Van Buren JM: Septic retinitis due to *Candida albicans*. *AMA Arch Pathol* 65:137-146, 1958.

Aspergillosis

96. Bodoia RD, Kinyoun JL, Qingli L, Bunt-Milam AH: *Aspergillus* necrotizing retinitis; a clinico-pathologic study and review. *Retina* 9:226-231, 1989.

97. Doft BH, Clarkson JG, Rebell G, Forster RK: Endogenous *Aspergillus* endophthalmitis in drug abusers. *Arch Ophthalmol* 98:859-862, 1980.

98. Gross JG: Endogenous aspergillus-induced endophthalmitis; successful treatment without systemic antifungal medication. *Retina* 12:341-345, 1992.

99. Halperin LS, Roseman RL: Successful treatment of a subretinal abscess in an intravenous drug abuser. *Arch Ophthalmol* 106:1651-1652, 1988.

100. Lance SE, Friberg TR, Kowalski RP: *Aspergillus flavus* endophthalmitis and retinitis in an intravenous drug abuser; a therapeutic success. *Ophthalmology* 95:947-949, 1988.

101. McDonnell PJ, McDonnell JM, Brown RH, Green WR: Ocular involvement in patients with fungal infections. *Ophthalmology* 92:706-709, 1985.

101a.Weishaar PD, Flynn HW Jr, Murray TG, et al: Endogenous *Aspergillus* endophthalmitis: clinical features and treatment outcomes. ARVO Abstracts. *Invest Ophthalmol Vis Sci* 36:789, 1995.

Sporotrichosis

102. Font RL, Jakobiec FA: Granulomatous necrotizing retinochoroiditis caused by *Sporotrichum schenkii;* report of a case including immunofluorescence and electron microscopical studies. *Arch Ophthalmol* 94:1513-1519, 1976.

Trichosporonosis

103. Walsh TJ, Orth DH, Shapiro CM, et al: Metastatic fungal chorioretinitis developing during trichosporon sepsis. *Ophthalmology* 89:152-156, 1982.

Histoplasmosis Retinochoroiditis in Immune Incompetent Patients

104. Klintworth GK, Hollingsworth AS, Lusman PA, Bradford WD: Granulomatous choroiditis in a case of disseminated histoplasmosis; histologic demonstration of *Histoplasma capsulatum* in choroidal lesions. *Arch Ophthalmol* 90:45-48, 1973 (Correspondence 91:237, 1974).

105. Macher A, Rodriguez MM, Kaplan W, et al: Disseminated bilateral chorioretinitis due to *Histoplasma capsulatum* in a patient with the acquired immunodeficiency syndrome. *Ophthalmology* 92:1159-1164, 1985.

106. Morinelli EN, Dugel PU, Riffenburgh R, Rao NA: Infectious multifocal choroiditis in patients with acquired immune deficiency syndrome. *Ophthalmology* 100:1014-1021, 1993.

107. Specht CS, Mitchell KT, Bauman AE, Gupta M: Ocular histoplasmosis with retinitis in a patient with acquired immune deficiency syndrome. *Ophthalmology* 98:1356-1359, 1991.

Toxoplasmosis Retinitis

108. Acers TE: Toxoplasmic retinochoroiditis: a double blind therapeutic study. *Arch Ophthalmol* 71:58-62, 1964.

109. Aouizerate F, Cazenave J, Poirier L, et al: Detection of *Toxoplasma gondii* in aqueous humour by the polymerase chain reaction. *Br J Ophthalmol* 77:107-109, 1993.

110. Asbell PA, Vermund SH, Hofeldt AJ: Presumed toxoplasmic retinochoroiditis in four siblings. *Am J Ophthalmol* 94:656-663, 1982.

111. Awan KJ: Congenital toxoplasmosis: Chances of occurrence in subsequent siblings. *Ann Ophthalmol* 10:459-465, 1978.

112. Berger BB, Egwuagu CE, Freeman WR, Wiley CA: Miliary toxoplasmic retinitis in acquired immunodeficiency syndrome. *Arch Ophthalmol* 111:373-376, 1993.

113. Bottoni F, Gonnella P, Autelitano A, Orzalesi N: Diffuse necrotizing retinochoroiditis in a child with AIDS and toxoplasmic encephalitis. *Graefes Arch Clin Exp Ophthalmol* 228:36-39, 1990.

114. Braunstein RA, Gass JDM: Branch artery obstruction caused by acute toxoplasmosis. *Arch Ophthalmol* 98:512-513, 1980.

115. Chan C-C, Palestine AG, Li Q, Nussenblatt RB: Diagnosis of ocular toxoplasmosis by the use of immunocytology and the polymerase chain reaction. *Am J Ophthalmol* 117:803-805, 1994.

116. Cochereau-Massin I, LeHoang P, Lautier-Frau M, et al: Ocular toxoplasmosis in human immunodeficiency virus-infected patients. *Am J Ophthalmol* 114:130-135, 1992.

117. Colin J, Harie JC: Chororétinites présumées toxoplasmiques: Étude comparative des traitements par pyriméthamine et sulfadiazine ou clindamycine. *J Fr Ophtalmol* 12:161-165, 1989.

118. Cotliar AM, Friedman AH: Subretinal neovascularisation in ocular toxoplasmosis. *Br J Ophthalmol* 66:524-529, 1982.

119. Culbertson WW, Tabbara KF, O'Connor GR: Experimental ocular toxoplasmosis in primates. *Arch Ophthalmol* 100:321-323, 1982.

120. de Abreu MT, Belfort R Jr, Hirata PS: Fuchs' heterochromic cyclitis and ocular toxoplasmosis. *Am J Ophthalmol* 93:739-744, 1982.

121. Doft BH, Gass JDM: Punctate outer retinal toxoplasmosis. *Arch Ophthalmol* 103:1332-1336, 1985.

122. Engstrom RE Jr, Holland GN, Nussenblatt RB, Jabs DA: Current practices in the management of ocular toxoplasmosis. *Am J Ophthalmol* 111:601-610, 1991.

123. Fine SL, Owens SL, Haller JA, et al: Choroidal neovascularization as a late complication of ocular toxoplasmosis. *Am J Ophthalmol* 91:318-322, 1981.

124. Fish RH, Hoskins JC, Kline LB: Toxoplasmosis neuroretinitis. *Ophthalmology* 100:1177-1182, 1993.

125. Folk JC, Lobes LA: Presumed toxoplasmic papillitis. *Ophthalmology* 91:64-67, 1984.

126. Gagliuso DJ, Teich SA, Friedman AH, Orellana J: Ocular toxoplasmosis in AIDS patients. *Trans Am Ophthalmol Soc* 88:63-86, 1990.

127. Gass JDM: Fluorescein angiography in endogenous intraocular inflammation. *In:* Aronson SB, Gamble CN, Goodner EK, O'Connor GR, editors: *Clinical methods in uveitis: the Fourth Sloan Symposium on Uveitis,* St. Louis, 1968, CV Mosby, pp. 202-229.

128. Gass JDM: *Stereoscopic atlas of macular diseases; diagnosis and treatment,* ed. 2, St. Louis, 1977, CV Mosby, pp. 296-297.

129. Gass JDM: *Stereoscopic atlas of macular diseases; diagnosis and treatment,* ed. 3, St. Louis, 1987, CV Mosby, pp. 465-467.

130. Gaynon MW, Boldrey EE, Strahlman ER, Fine SL: Retinal neovascularization and ocular toxoplasmosis. *Am J Ophthalmol* 98:585-589, 1984.

131. Ghartey KN, Brockhurst RJ: Photocoagulation of active toxoplasmic retinochoroiditis. *Am J Ophthalmol* 89:858-864, 1980.

132. Gilbert HD: Unusual presentation of acute ocular toxoplasmosis. *Albrecht von Graefes Arch Klin Exp Ophthalmol* 215:53-58, 1980.

133. Glasner PD, Silveira C, Kruszon-Moran D, et al: An unusually high prevalence of ocular toxoplasmosis in southern Brazil. *Am J Ophthalmol* 114:136-144, 1992.

134. Greven CM, Teot LA: Cytologic identification of *Toxoplasma gondii* from vitreous fluid. *Arch Ophthalmol* 112:1086-1088, 1994.

135. Grossniklaus HE, Specht CS, Allaire G, Leavitt JA: *Toxoplasma gondii* retinochoroiditis and optic neuritis in acquired immune deficiency syndrome. *Ophthalmology* 97:1342-1346, 1990.

136. Hogan MJ: Ocular toxoplasmosis; clinical and laboratory diagnosis; evaluation of immunologic tests; treatment. *Arch Ophthalmol* 55:333-345, 1956.

137. Hogan MJ, Zimmerman LE: *Ophthalmic pathology; an atlas and textbook,* ed. 2, Philadelphia, 1962, WB Saunders, pp. 488-491.

138. Holland GN, Engstrom RE Jr, Glasgow BJ, et al: Ocular toxoplasmosis in patients with the acquired immunodeficiency syndrome. *Am J Ophthalmol* 106:653-667, 1988.

139. Jampel HD, Schachat AP, Conway B, et al: Retinal pigment epithelial hyperplasia assuming tumor-like proportions; report of two cases. *Retina* 6:105-112, 1986.

140. Kasp E, Whiston R, Dumonde D, et al: Antibody affinity to retinal S-antigen in patients with retinal vasculitis. *Am J Ophthalmol* 113:697-701, 1992.

141. Kennedy JE, Wise GN: Retinochoroidal vascular anastomosis in uveitis. *Am J Ophthalmol* 71:1221-1225, 1971.

142. Kyrieleis W: Über atypische Gefässtuberkulose der Netzhaut (Periarteriitis "nodosa" tuberculosa). *Arch Augenheilkd* 107:182-190, 1933.

143. La Hey E, Rothova A, Baarsma GS, et al: Fuchs' heterochromic iridocyclitis is not associated with ocular toxoplasmosis. *Arch Ophthalmol* 110:806-811, 1992.

144. Lou P, Kazdan J, Basu PK: Ocular toxoplasmosis in three consecutive siblings. *Arch Ophthalmol* 96:613-614, 1978.

145. Manschot WA, Daamen CBF: Connatal ocular toxoplasmosis. *Arch Ophthalmol* 74:48-54, 1965.

146. Matthews JD, Weiter JJ: Outer retinal toxoplasmosis. *Ophthalmology* 95:941-946, 1988.

147. Moorthy RS, Smith RE, Rao NA: Progressive ocular toxoplasmosis in patients with acquired immunodeficiency syndrome. *Am J Ophthalmol* 115:742-747, 1993.

148. Morgan CM, Gragoudas ES: Photo essay: branch retinal artery occlusion associated with recurrent toxoplasmic retinochoroiditis. *Arch Ophthalmol* 105:130-131, 1987.

149. Morinelli EN, Dugel PU, Lee M, et al: Opportunistic intraocular infections in AIDS. *Trans Am Ophthalmol Soc* 90:97-109, 1992.

150. Nicholson DH, Wolchok EB: Ocular toxoplasmosis in an adult receiving long-term corticosteroid therapy. *Arch Ophthalmol* 94:248-254, 1976.

151. O'Connor GR, Frenkel JK: Dangers of steroid treatment in toxoplasmosis; periocular injections and systemic therapy. *Arch Ophthalmol* 94:213, 1976.

152. Opremcak EM, Scales DK, Sharpe MR:Trimethoprim-sulfamethoxazole therapy for ocular toxoplasmosis. *Ophthalmology* 99:920-925, 1992.

153. Owens PL, Goldberg MF, Busse BJ: Prospective observation of vascular anastomoses between the retina and choroid in recurrent toxoplasmosis. *Am J Ophthalmol* 88:402-405, 1979.

154. Parke DW II, Font RL: Diffuse toxoplasmic retinochoroiditis in a patient with AIDS. *Arch Ophthalmol* 104:571-575, 1986.

155. Pauleikhoff D, Messmer E, Beelen DW, et al: Bone-marrow transplantation and toxoplasmic retinochoroiditis. *Graefes Arch Clin Exp Ophthalmol* 225:239-243, 1987.

156. Perkins ES, Smith CH, Schofield PB: Treatment of uveitis with pyrimethamine (Daraprim). *Br J Ophthalmol* 40:577-586, 1956.

157. Rao NA, Font RL: Toxoplasmic retinochoroiditis; electron-microscopic and immunofluorescence studies of formalin-fixed tissue. *Arch Ophthalmol* 95:273-277, 1977.

158. Rothova A: Ocular involvement in toxoplasmosis. *Br J Ophthalmol* 77:371-377, 1993; "correction" p. 683.

159. Rothova A, Buitenhuis HJ, Meenken C, et al: Therapy of ocular toxoplasmosis. *Int Ophthalmol* 13:415-419, 1989.

160. Rothova A, Meenken C, Buitenhuis HJ, et al: Therapy for ocular toxoplasmosis. *Am J Ophthalmol* 115:517-523, 1993.

161. Rothova A, van Knapen F, Baarsma GS, et al: Serology in ocular toxoplasmosis. *Br J Ophthalmol* 70:615-622, 1986.

162. Ryan SJ Jr, Smith RE: Ocular toxoplasmosis. *In:* Ryan SJ Jr, Smith RE, editors: *Selected topics on the eye in systemic disease,* New York, 1974, Grune & Stratton, pp. 259-273.

163. Saari M, Miettinen R, Nieminen H, Räisänen S: Retinochoroidal vascular anastomosis in toxoplasmic chorioretinitis; report of a case. *Acta Ophthalmol* 53:44-51, 1975.

164. Saari M, Vuorre I, Neiminen H, Räisänen S: Acquired toxoplasmic chorioretinitis. *Arch Ophthalmol* 94:1485-1488, 1976.

165. Sabates R, Pruett RC, Brockhurst RJ: Fulminant ocular toxoplasmosis. *Am J Ophthalmol* 92:497-503, 1981.

166. Schlaegel TF Jr, Weber JC: The macula in ocular toxoplasmosis. *Arch Ophthalmol* 102:697-698, 1984.

167. Schuman JS, Weinberg RS, Ferry AP, Guerry RK: Toxoplasmic scleritis. *Ophthalmology* 95:1399-1403, 1988.

168. Schwab IR: The epidemiologic association of Fuchs' heterochromic iridocyclitis and ocular toxoplasmosis. *Am J Ophthalmol* 111:356-362, 1991.

169. Schwartz PL: Segmental retinal periarteritis as a complication of toxoplasmosis. *Ann Ophthalmol* 9:157-162, 1977.

170. Scott EH: New concepts in toxoplasmosis. *Surv Ophthalmol* 18:255-274, 1974.

171. Silveira C, Belfort R Jr, Burnier M Jr, Nussenblatt R: Acquired toxoplasmic infection as the cause of toxoplasmic retinochoroiditis in families. *Am J Ophthalmol* 106:362-364, 1988.

172. Silveira C, Belfort R Jr, Nussenblatt R, et al: Unilateral pigmentary retinopathy associated with ocular toxoplasmosis. *Am J Ophthalmol* 107:682-684, 1989.

173. Singer MA, Hagler WS, Grossniklaus HE: *Toxoplasma gondii* retinochoroiditis after liver transplantation. *Retina* 13:40-45, 1993.

174. Spalter HF, Campbell CJ, Noyori KS, et al: Prophylactic photocoagulation of recurrent toxoplasmic retinochoroiditis; a preliminary report. *Arch Ophthalmol* 75:21-31, 1966.

175. Tetz M, Holz FG, Gallasch G, Völcker HE: Segmentale retinale Arteriitis und Retinochorioiditis. *Ophthalmologe* 89:71-76, 1992.

176. Webb RM, Tabbara KF, O'Connor GR: Retinal vasculitis in ocular toxoplasmosis in nonhuman primates. *Retina* 4:182-188, 1984.

177. Weiss A, Margo CE, Ledford DK, et al: Toxoplasmic retinochoroiditis as an initial manifestation of the acquired immune deficiency syndrome. *Am J Ophthalmol* 101:248-250, 1986.

178. Weiss MJ, Velazquez N, Hofeldt AJ: Serologic tests in the diagnosis of presumed toxoplasmic retinochoroiditis. *Am J Ophthalmol* 109:407-411, 1990.

179. Willerson D Jr, Aaberg TM, Reeser F, Meredith TA: Unusual ocular presentation of acute toxoplasmosis. *Br J Ophthalmol* 61:693-698, 1977.

180. Yeo JH, Jakobiec FA, Iwamoto T, et al: Opportunistic toxoplasmic retinochoroiditis following chemotherapy for systemic lymphoma; a light and electron microscopic study. *Ophthalmology* 90:885-898, 1983.

Malaria

181. Lewallen S, Taylor TE, Molyneux ME, et al: Ocular fundus findings in Malawian children with cerebral malaria. *Ophthalmology* 100:857-861, 1993.

Diffuse Unilateral Subacute Neuroretinitis (DUSN)

181a. Bowman DD, personal communication, 1996.

182. Carney MD, Combs JL: Diffuse unilateral subacute neuroretinitis. *Br J Ophthalmol* 75:633-635, 1991.

183. Cunha de Souza E, Lustosa da Cunha S, Gass JDM: Diffuse unilateral subacute neuroretinitis in South America. *Arch Ophthalmol* 110:1261-1263, 1992.

183a. Cunha de Souza E, Nakashima Y: Diffuse unilateral subacute neuroretinitis; report of transvitreal surgical removal of a subretinal nematode. *Ophthalmology* 102:1183-1186,1995.

184. Fox AS, Kazacos KR, Gould NS, et al: Fatal eosinophilic meningoencephalitis and visceral larva migrans caused by the raccoon ascarid, *Baylisascaris procyonis. N Engl J Med* 312: 1619-1623, 1985.

185. Gass JDM: *Stereoscopic atlas of macular diseases; diagnosis and treatment,* ed. 3, 1987, St. Louis, CV Mosby, pp.474-475.

186. Gass JDM, Braunstein RA: Further observations concerning the diffuse unilateral subacute neuroretinitis syndrome. *Arch Ophthalmol* 101:1689-1697, 1983.

187. Gass JDM, Callanan DG, Bowman B: Oral therapy in diffuse unilateral subacute neuroretinitis. *Arch Ophthalmol* 110:675-680, 1992.

188. Gass JDM, Gilbert WR Jr, Guerry RK, Scelfo R: Diffuse unilateral subacute neuroretinitis. *Ophthalmology* 85:521-545, 1978.

189. Gass JDM, Scelfo R: Diffuse unilateral subacute neuroretinitis. *J R Soc Med* 71:95-111, 1978.

190. Goldberg MA, Kazacos KR, Boyce WM, et al: Diffuse unilateral subacute neuroretinitis; morphometric, serologic, and epidemiologic support for *Baylisascaris* as a causative agent. *Ophthalmology* 100:1695-1701, 1993.

191. Huff DS, Neafie RC, Binder MJ, et al: The first fatal *Baylisascaris* infection in humans: an infant with eosinophilic meningoencephalitis. *Pediatr Pathol* 2:345-352, 1984.

192. John T, Barsky HJ, Donnelly JJ, Rockey JH: Retinal pigment epitheliopathy and neuroretinal degeneration in ascarid-infected eyes. *Invest Ophthalmol Vis Sci* 28:1583-1598, 1987.

193. Kazacos KR, Raymond LA, Kazacos EA, Vestre WA: The raccoon ascarid; a probable cause of human ocular larva migrans. *Ophthalmology* 92:1735-1743, 1985.

194. Kazacos KR, Reed WM, Kazacos EA, Thacker HL: Fatal cerebrospinal disease caused by *Baylisascaris procyonis* in domestic rabbits. *J Am Vet Med Assoc* 183:967-971, 1983.

195. Kazacos KR, Vestre WA, Kazacos EA, Raymond LA: Diffuse unilateral subacute neuroretinitis syndrome: probable cause. *Arch Ophthalmol* 102:967-968, 1984.

196. Kazacos KR, Wirtz WL: Experimental cerebrospinal nematodiasis due to *Baylisascaris procyonis* in chickens. *Avian Dis* 27:55-65, 1983.

197. Kazacos KR, Wirtz WL, Burger PP, Christmas CS: Raccoon ascarid larvae as a cause of fatal central nervous system disease in subhuman primates. *J Am Vet Med Assoc* 179:1089-1094, 1981.

198. Kelsey JH: Diffuse unilateral subacute neuroretinitis. *J R Soc Med* 71:303-304, 1978.

199. Küchle M, Knorr HLJ, Medenblik-Frysch S, et al: Diffuse unilateral subacute neuroretinitis syndrome in a German most likely caused by the raccoon roundworm, *Baylisascaris procyonis. Graefes Arch Clin Exp Ophthalmol* 231:48-51, 1993.

200. Kuhnt H: Extraction eines neuen Entozoon zus dem Glaskörper des Menschen. *Arch Augenheilkd* 24:205-229, 1892.

201. Lewis RA: Discussion of Kazacos KR, Raymond LA, Kazacos EA, Vestre WA: The raccoon ascarid; a probable cause of human ocular larva migrans. *Ophthalmology* 92:1743-1744, 1985.

202. Nichols RL: The etiology of visceral larva migrans. II. Comparative larval morphology of *Ascaris lumbricoides, Necator americanus, Strongyloides stercoralis,* and *Acylostoma caninum. Parasitol* 42:363-399, 1956.

203. Oppenheim S, Rogell G, Peyser R: Diffuse unilateral subacute neuroretinitis. *Ann Ophthalmol* 17:336-338, 1985.

204. Parsons HE: Nematode chorioretinitis; report of a case, with photographs of a viable worm. *Arch Ophthalmol* 47:799-800, 1952.

205. Price JA Jr, Wadsworth JAC: An intraretinal worm; report of a case of macular retinopathy caused by invasion of the retina by a worm. *Arch Ophthalmol* 83:768-770, 1970.

206. Raymond LA, Gutierrez Y, Strong LE, et al: Living retinal nematode (filarial-like) destroyed with photocoagulation. *Ophthalmology* 85:944-949, 1978.

207. Rubin ML, Kaufman HE, Tierney JP, Lucas HC: An intraretinal nematode (a case report). *Trans Am Acad Ophthalmol Otolaryngol* 72:855-866, 1968.

208. Sivalingam A, Goldberg RE, Augsburger J, Frank P: Diffuse unilateral subacute neuroretinitis. *Arch Ophthalmol* 109:1028, 1991.

Onchocerciasis

209. Anderson J, Font RL: Ocular onchocerciasis. *In:* Binford CH, Connor DH, editors: *Pathology of tropical and extraordinary diseases,* Washington, D.C., 1976, Armed Forces Institute of Pathology, pp. 373-381.

210. Bird AC, Anderson J, Fuglsang H: Morphology of posterior segment lesions of the eye in patients with onchocerciasis. *Br J Ophthalmol* 60:2-20, 1976.

211. Bird AC, El Sheikh H, Anderson J, Fuglsang H: Changes in visual function and in the posterior segment of the eye during treatment of onchocerciasis with diethylcarbamazine citrate. *Br J Ophthalmol* 64:191-200, 1980.

212. Chan C-C, Nussenblatt RB, Kim MK, et al: Immunopathology of ocular onchocerciasis. 2. Anti-retinal autoantibodies in serum and ocular fluids. *Ophthalmology* 94:439-443, 1987.

213. Dadzie KY, Bird AC, Awadzi K, et al: Ocular findings in a double-blind study of ivermectin versus diethycarbamazine versus placebo in the treatment of onchocerciasis. *Br J Ophthalmol* 71:78-85, 1987.

214. Murphy RP, Taylor H, Greene BM: Chorioretinal damage in onchocerciasis. *Am J Ophthalmol* 98:519-521, 1984.

215. Neumann E, Gunders AE: Pathogenesis of the posterior segment lesion of ocular onchocerciasis. *Am J Ophthalmol* 75:82-89, 1973.

216. Newland HS, White AT, Greene BM, et al: Ocular manifestations of onchocerciasis in a rain forest area of West Africa. *Br J Ophthalmol* 75:163-169, 1991.

217. Rodger FC: The pathogenesis and pathology of ocular onchocerciasis. Part IV. The pathology. *Am J Ophthalmol* 49:327-337, 1960.

218. Semba RD, Murphy RP, Newland HS, et al: Longitudinal study of lesions of the posterior segment in onchocerciasis. *Ophthalmology* 97:1334-1341, 1990.

219. Taylor HR: Ivermectin treatment of ocular onchocerciasis. *Acta Leidensia* 59:201-206, 1990.

220. Taylor HR, Greene BM: Ocular changes with oral and transepidermal diethylcarbamazine therapy of onchocerciasis. *Br J Ophthalmol* 65:494-502, 1981.

221. Taylor HR, Murphy RP, Newland HS, et al: Treatment of onchocerciasis; the ocular effects of ivermectin and diethylcarbamazine. *Arch Ophthalmol* 104:863-870, 1986.

222. Van der Lelij A, Rothova A, Stilma JS, et al: Cell-mediated immunity against human retinal extract, S-antigen, and interphotoreceptor retinoid binding protein in onchocercal chorioretinopathy. *Invest Ophthalmol Vis Sci* 31:2031-2036, 1990.

223. Winter FC: The control of onchocerciasis. *Am J Ophthalmol* 108:84-85, 1989.

Dirofilariasis

224. Frieling E, Fritz E, Schmidt U, et al: Vitreoretinale Dirofilariose. *Klin Monatsbl Augenheilkd* 196:233-236, 1990.

225. Gutierrez Y: *Diagnostic pathology of parasitic infections with clinical correlations,* Philadelphia, 1990, Lea & Febiger, pp. 323-324.

226. Kerkenezov N: Intra-ocular filariasis in Australia. *Br J Ophthalmol* 46:607-615, 1962.

227. Moorhouse DE: Dirofilaria immitis: A cause of human intra-ocular infection. *Infection* 6:192-193, 1978.

228. Vodovozov AM, Jarulin GR, Djakonowa SW: *Dirofilaria im Glaskörper des Menschen. Ophthalmologica* 166:88-93, 1973.

Gnathostomiasis

229. Bathrick ME, Mango CA, Mueller JF: Intraocular gnathostomiasis. *Ophthalmology* 88:1293-1295, 1981.

230. Funata M, Custis P, De La Cruz Z, et al: Intraocular gnathostomiasis. *Retina* 13:240-244, 1993.

231. Hernández Ortiz G, Nesme Kuri J, Flores Castañón, Hernández Cuesta PE: Gnatostomiasis humana. Manifestaciones oculares. *An Soc Mex Oftalmol* 56:65-73, 1982.

232. Kittiponghansa S, Prabriputaloong A, Pariyanonda S, Ritch R: Intracameral gnathostomiasis: a cause of anterior uveitis and secondary glaucoma. *Br J Ophthalmol* 71:618-622, 1987.

Other Nematode Infections of the Eye

233. Goodart RA, Riekhof FT, Beaver PC: Subretinal nematode; an unusual etiology for uveitis and retinal detachment. *Retina* 5:87-90, 1985.

Ophthalmomyiasis

234. Anderson WB: Ophthalmomyiasis interna; case report and review of the literature. *Trans Am Acad Ophthalmol Otolaryngol* 39:218-238, 1934.

234a.Baird CR: Development of *Cuterebra jellisoni* (diptera: cuterebridae) in six species of rabbits and rodents. *J Med Entomol* 8:615-622, 1971.

235. Cameron JA, Shoukrey NM, Al-Garni AA: Conjunctival ophthalmomyiasis by the sheep nasal botfly (*Oestrus ovis.*) *Am J Ophthalmol* 112:331-334, 1991.

236. Campbell RJ, Steele JC, Cox TA, et al: Pathologic findings in the retinal pigment epitheliopathy associated with the amyotrophic lateral sclerosis/Parkinsonism-dementia complex of Guam. *Ophthalmology* 100:37-42, 1993.

237. Chodosh J, Clarridge J: Ophthalmomyiasis: a review with special reference to *Cochliomyia hominivorax. Clin Infect Dis* 14:444-449, 1992.

238. Cox TA, McDarby JV, Lavine L, et al: A retinopathy on Guam with high prevalence in Lytico-Bodig. *Ophthalmology* 96:1731-1735, 1989.

239. Custis PH, Pakalnis VA, Klintworth GK, et al: Posterior

internal ophthalmomyiasis; identification of a surgically re-moved *Cuterebra* larva by scanning electron microscopy. *Ophthalmology* 90:1583-1590, 1983.

240. DeBoe MP: Dipterous larva passing from the optic nerve into the vitreous chamber. *Arch Ophthalmol* 10:824-825, 1933.

241. Dixon JM, Winkler CH, Nelson JH: Ophthalmomyiasis interna caused by *Cuterebra* larva. *Trans Am Ophthalmol Soc* 67:110-115, 1969.

242. Edwards KM, Meredith TA, Hagler WS, Healy GR: Oph-thalmomyiasis interna causing visual loss. *Am J Ophthalmol* 97:605-610, 1984.

243. Fitzgerald CR, Rubin ML: Intraocular parasite destroyed by photocoagulation. *Arch Ophthalmol* 91:162-164, 1974.

244. Forman AR, Cruess AF, Benson WE: Ophthalmomyiasis treated by argon-laser photocoagulation. *Retina* 4:163-165, 1984.

245. Gass JDM, Lewis RA: Subretinal tracks in ophthalmomyiasis. *Arch Ophthalmol* 94:1500-1505, 1976.

245a. Glasgow BJ, Maggiano JM: *Cuterebra* ophthalmomyiasis. *Am J Ophthalmol* 119:512-514, 1995.

246. Hanlon SD, Steele JC: An unusual retinal pigment epitheli-opathy endemic to the island of Guam. *Optom Vis Sci* 70:854-859, 1993.

247. Haut J, Ullern M, Marre JM, et al: Présentation d'un nouveau cas de parasitose endoculaire: Myiase. *Bull Soc Ophtalmol Fr* 77:929-930, 1977.

248. Hunt EW Jr: Unusual case of ophthalmomyiasis interna posterior. *Am J Ophthalmol* 70:978-980, 1970.

249. Kearney MS, Nilssen AC, Lyslo A, et al: Ophthalmomyiasis caused by the reindeer warble fly larva. *J Clin Pathol* 44:276-284, 1991.

250. Kersten RC, Shoukrey NM, Tabbara KF: Orbital myiasis. *Ophthalmology* 93:1228-1232, 1986.

251. Mason GI: Bilateral ophthalmomyiasis interna. *Am J Oph-thalmol* 91:65-70, 1981.

252. O'Brien CS, Allen JH: Ophthalmomyiasis interna anterior; report of *Hypoderma* larva in anterior chamber. *Am J Ophthalmol* 22:996-998, 1939.

253. Perry HD, Donnenfeld ED, Font RL: Intracorneal ophthal-momyiasis. *Am J Ophthalmol* 109:741-742, 1990.

254. Potgieter F, Scheuer JA: Oftalmomiïase met subretinale spore; 'n gevalbespreking. *S Afr Med J* 55:957-958, 1979.

255. Rapoza PA, Michels RG, Semeraro RJ, Green WR: Vitrec-tomy for excision of intraocular larva (*Hypoderma* species). *Retina* 6:99-104, 1986.

256. Savino DF, Margo CE, McCoy ED, Friedl FE: Dermal myiasis of the eyelid. *Ophthalmology* 93:1225-1227, 1986.

257. Slusher MM, Holland WD, Weaver RG, Tyler ME: Ophthal-momyiasis interna posterior; subretinal tracks and intraocular larvae. *Arch Ophthalmol* 97:885-887, 1979.

258. Steahly LP, Peterson CA: Ophthalmomyiasis. *Ann Ophthal-mol* 14:137-139, 1982.

259. Syrdalen P, Nitter T, Mehl R: Ophthalmomyiasis interna posterior: report of case caused by the reindeer warble fly larva and review of previous reported cases. *Br J Ophthalmol* 66:589-593, 1982.

260. Syrdalen P, Stenkula S: Ophthalmomyiasis interna posterior. *Graefes Arch Clin Exp Ophthalmol* 225:103-106, 1987.

261. Vine AK, Schatz H: Bilateral posterior internal ophthal-momyiasis. *Ann Ophthalmol* 13:1041-1043, 1981.

262. Ziemianski MC, Lee KY, Sabates FN: Ophthalmomyiasis interna. *Arch Ophthalmol* 98:1588-1589, 1980.

263. Zumpt F: Ophthalmomyiasis in man, with special reference to the situation in Southern Africa. *S Afr Med J* 37:425-428, 1963.

Echinococcosis

264. Litricin O: Echinococcus cyst of the eye ball. *Arch Ophthalmol* 50:506-509, 1953.

265. Sinav S, Demirci A, Sinav B, et al: A primary intraocular hydatid cyst. *Acta Ophthalmol* 69:802-804, 1991.

Intraocular Trematoda

266. Dickinson AJ, Rosenthal AR, Nicholson KG: Inflammation of the retinal pigment epithelium: a unique presentation of ocular schistosomiasis. *Br J Ophthalmol* 74:440-442, 1990.

267. Freeman RS, Stuart PF, Cullen JB, et al: Fatal human infection with *Alaria americanus. Am J Trop Med Hyg* 25:803, 1976.

268. McDonald HR, Kazacos KR, Schatz H, Johnson RN: Two cases of intraocular infection with *Alaria mesocercaria* (Trematoda). *Am J Ophthalmol* 117:447-455, 1994.

269. Shea M, Maberley AL, Walters J, et al: Intraretinal larval trematode. *Trans Am Acad Ophthalmol Otolaryngol* 77: OP784-OP791, 1973.

Retinopathy Associated with Rickettsial Diseases

270. Chamberlain WP Jr: Ocular findings in scrub typhus. *Arch Ophthalmol* 48:313-321, 1952.

271. Cherubini TD, Spaeth GL: Anterior nongranulomatous uveitis associated with Rocky Mountain spotted fever; first report of a case. *Arch Ophthalmol* 81:363-365, 1969.

272. Duffey RJ, Hammer ME: The ocular manifestations of Rocky Mountain spotted fever. *Ann Ophthalmol* 19:301-306, 1987.

273. Haynes RE, Sanders DY, Cramblett HG: Rocky Mountain spotted fever in children. *J Pediatr* 76:685-693, 1970.

274. Manor E, Politi F, Marmor A, Cohn DF: Papilledema in endemic typhus. *Am J Ophthalmol* 84:559-562, 1977.

275. Marcus DM, Frederick AR Jr, Hodges T, et al: Photo essay. Typhoidal tularemia. *Arch Ophthalmol* 108:118-119, 1990.

276. Presley GD: Fundus changes in Rocky Mountain spotted fever. *Am J Ophthalmol* 67:263-267, 1969.

277. Raab EL, Leopold IH, Hodes HL: Retinopathy in Rocky Mountain spotted fever. *Am J Ophthalmol* 68:42-46, 1969.

278. Scheie HG: Ocular changes associated with scrub typhus; a study of four hundred and fifty-one patients. *Arch Ophthalmol* 40:245-267, 1948.

279. Smith TW, Burton TC: The retinal manifestations of Rocky Mountain spotted fever. *Am J Ophthalmol* 84:259-262, 1977.

280. Sulewski ME, Green WR: Ocular histopathologic features of a presumed case of Rocky Mountain spotted fever. *Retina* 6:125-130, 1986.

Herpes Simplex Retinochoroiditis

281. Bloom JN, Katz JI, Kaufman HE: Herpes simplex retinitis and encephalitis in an adult. *Arch Ophthalmol* 95:1798-1799, 1977.

282. Cibis GW, Flynn JT, Davis EB: Herpes simplex retinitis. *Arch Ophthalmol* 96:299-302, 1978.

283. Cogan DG, Kuwabara T, Young GF, Knox DL: Herpes simplex retinopathy in an infant. *Arch Ophthalmol* 72:641-645, 1964.

284. el Azazi M, Malm G, Forsgren M: Late ophthalmologic manifestations of neonatal herpes simplex virus infection. *Am J Ophthalmol* 109:1-7, 1990.

285. Grutzmacher RD, Henderson D, McDonald PJ, Coster DJ: Herpes simplex chorioretinitis in a healthy adult. *Am J Ophthalmol* 96:788-796, 1983.

286. Huang J-S, Russack V, Flores-Aguilar M, et al: Evaluation of cytologic specimens obtained during experimental vitreous biopsy. *Retina* 13:160-165, 1993.

287. Johnson BL, Wisotzkey HM: Neuroretinitis associated with herpes simplex encephalitis in an adult. *Am J Ophthalmol* 83:481-489, 1977.

288. Lewis ML, Culbertson WW, Post JD, et al: Herpes simplex virus type 1; a cause of the acute retinal necrosis syndrome. *Ophthalmology* 96:875-878, 1989.

289. Martin DF, Chan C-C, deSmet MD, et al: The role of chorioretinal biopsy in the management of posterior uveitis. *Ophthalmology* 100:705-714, 1993.

290. Minckler DS, McLean EB, Shaw CM, Hendrickson A: *Herpesvirus hominis* encephalitis and retinitis. *Arch Ophthalmol* 94:89-95, 1976.

291. Nahmias AJ, Hagler WS: Ocular manifestations of herpes simplex in the newborn (neonatal ocular herpes). *Int Ophthalmol Clin* 12(2):191-213, 1972.

292. Nahmias AJ, Josey WE, Naib ZM, et al: Perinatal risk associated with maternal genital herpes simplex virus infection. *Am J Obstet Gynecol* 110:825-837, 1971.

293. Partamian LG, Morse PH, Klein HZ: Herpes simplex type 1 retinitis in an adult with systemic herpes zoster. *Am J Ophthalmol* 92:215-220, 1981.

294. Pepose J, Kreiger AE, Tomiyasu U, et al: Immunocytologic localization of herpes simplex type 1 viral antigens in herpetic retinitis and encephalitis in an adult. *Ophthalmology* 92:160-166, 1985.

295. Reynolds JD, Griebel M, Mallory S, Steele R: Congenital herpes simplex retinitis. *Am J Ophthalmol* 102:33-36, 1986.

296. Tarkkanen A, Laatikainen L: Late ocular manifestations in neonatal herpes simplex infection. *Br J Ophthalmol* 61:608-616, 1977.

297. Thompson WS, Culbertson WW, Smiddy WE, et al: Acute retinal necrosis caused by reactivation of herpes simplex virus type 2. *Am J Ophthalmol* 118:205-211, 1994.

298. Uninsky E, Jampol LM, Kaufman S, Naraqi S: Disseminated herpes simplex infection with retinitis in a renal allograft recipient. *Ophthalmology* 90:175-178, 1983.

299. Whittum JA, McCulley JP, Niederkorn JY, Streilein JW: Ocular disease induced in mice by anterior chamber inoculation of herpes simplex virus. *Invest Ophthalmol Vis Sci* 25:1065-1073, 1984.

Herpesvirus B

300. Centers for Disease Control. B-virus infection in humans: Pensacola, Florida. *MMWR Morb Mortal Wkly Rep* 36:289-290; 295-296, 1987.

301. Kelly SP, Rosenthal AR, Nicholson KG, Woodward CG: Retinochoroiditis in acute Epstein-Barr virus infection. *Br J Ophthalmol* 73:1002-1003, 1989.

302. Nanda M, Curtin VT, Hilliard JK, et al: Ocular histopathologic findings in a case of human herpes B virus infection. *Arch Ophthalmol* 108:713-716, 1990.

303. Roth AM, Purcell TW: Ocular findings associated with encephalomyelitis caused by *Herpesvirus simiae*. *Am J Ophthalmol* 84:345-348, 1977.

Cytomegalovirus Retinochoroiditis and Optic Neuritis

304. Aaberg TM, Cesarz TJ, Rytel MW: Correlation of virology and clinical course of cytomegalovirus retinitis. *Am J Ophthalmol* 74:407-415, 1972.

305. Anand R, Font RL, Fish RH, Nightingale SD: Pathology of cytomegalovirus retinitis treated with sustained release intravitreal ganciclovir. *Ophthalmology* 100:1032-1039, 1993.

306. Astle JN, Ellis PP: Ocular complications in renal transplant patients. *Ann Ophthalmol* 6:1269-1274, 1974.

307. Augsburger JJ, Henry RY: Retinal aneurysms in adult cytomegalovirus retinitis. *Am J Ophthalmol* 86:794-797, 1978.

308. Bachman DM, Bruni LM, DiGioia RA, et al: Visual field testing in the management of cytomegalovirus retinitis. *Ophthalmology* 99:1393-1399, 1992.

309. Bachman DM, Rodrigues MM, Chu FC, et al: Culture-proven cytomegalovirus retinitis in a homosexual man with the acquired immunodeficiency syndrome. *Ophthalmology* 89:797-804, 1982.

310. Berger BB, Weinberg RS, Tessler HH, et al: Bilateral cytomegalovirus panuveitis after high-dose corticosteroid therapy. *Am J Ophthalmol* 88:1020-1025, 1979.

311. Boniuk I: The cytomegaloviruses and the eye. *Int Ophthalmol Clin* 12(2):169-190, 1972.

312. Broughton WL, Cupples HP, Parver LM: Bilateral retinal detachment following cytomegalovirus retinitis. *Arch Ophthalmol* 96:618-619, 1978.

313. Burns RP: Cytomegalic inclusion disease uveitis; report of a case with isolation from aqueous humor of the virus in tissue culture. *Arch Ophthalmol* 61:376-387, 1959.

314. Cantrill HL, Henry K, Melroe NH, et al: Treatment of cytomegalovirus retinitis with intravitreal ganciclovir; long-term results. *Ophthalmology* 96:367-374, 1989.

315. Chawla HB, Ford MJ, Munro JF, et al: Ocular involvement in cytomegalovirus infection in a previously healthy adult. *Br Med J* 2:281-282, 1976.

316. Christensen L, Beeman HW, Allen A: Cytomegalic inclusion disease. *Arch Ophthalmol* 57:90-99, 1957.

317. Chumbley LC, Robertson DM, Smith TF, Campbell RJ: Adult cytomegalovirus inclusion retino-uveitis. *Am J Ophthalmol* 80:807-816, 1975.

318. CMV Retinitis Trial: Announcement. *Retina* 10:323-324, 1990.

319. Cochereau-Massin I, Lehoang P, Lautier-Frau M, et al: Efficacy and tolerance of intravitreal ganciclovir in cytomegalovirus retinitis in acquired immune deficiency syndrome. *Ophthalmology* 98:1348-1353, 1991.

320. Cox F, Meyer D, Hughes WT: Cytomegalovirus in tears from patients with normal eyes and with acute cytomegalovirus chorioretinitis. *Am J Ophthalmol* 80:817-824, 1975.

321. DeVenecia G, Zu Rhein GM, Pratt MV, Kisken W: Cytomegalic inclusion retinitis in an adult; a clinical, histopathologic, and ultrastructural study. *Arch Ophthalmol* 86:44-57, 1971.

322. Digre KB, Blodi CF, Bale JF: Cytomegalovirus infection in a healthy adult associated with recurrent branch retinal artery occlusion. *Retina* 7:230-232, 1987.

323. Dugel PU, Liggett PE, Lee MB, et al: Repair of retinal detachment caused by cytomegalovirus retinitis in patients with the acquired immunodeficiency syndrome. *Am J Ophthalmol* 112:235-242, 1991.

324. Faber DW, Crapotta JA, Wiley CA, Freeman WR: Retinal calcifications in cytomegalovirus retinitis. *Retina* 13:46-49, 1993.

325. Faber DW, Wiley CA, Lynn GB, et al: Role of HIV and CMV in the pathogenesis of retinitis and retinal vasculopathy in AIDS patients. *Invest Ophthalmol Vis Sci* 33:2345-2353, 1992.

326. Fay MT, Freeman WR, Wiley CA, et al: Atypical retinitis in patients with the acquired immunodeficiency syndrome. *Am J Ophthalmol* 105:483-490, 1988.

327. Felsenstein D, D'Amico DJ, Hirsch MS, et al: Treatment of cytomegalovirus retinitis with 9-[2-hydroxy-1-(hydroxymethyl) ethoxymethyl]guanine. *Ann Intern Med* 103:377-380, 1985.

328. Flores-Aquilar M, Kuppermann BD, Quiceno JI, et al: Pathophysiology and treatment of clinically resistant cytomegalovirus retinitis. *Ophthalmology* 100:1022-1031, 1993.

329. Freeman WR: Editorial: Intraocular antiviral therapy. *Arch Ophthalmol* 107:1737-1739, 1989.

330. Freeman WR, Friedberg DN, Berry C, et al: Risk factors for development of rhegmatogenous retinal detachment in patients with cytomegalovirus retinitis. *Am J Ophthalmol* 116:713-720, 1993.

331. Freeman WR, Quiceno JI, Crapotta JA, et al: Surgical repair of rhegmatogenous retinal detachment in immunosuppressed patients with cytomegalovirus retinitis. *Ophthalmology* 99:466-474, 1992.

332. Gangan PA, Besen G, Munguia D, Freeman WR: Macular serous exudation in patients with acquired immunodeficiency syndrome and cytomegalovirus retinitis. *Am J Ophthalmol* 118:212-219, 1994.

333. Geier SA, Nasemann J, Klauss V, et al: Frosted branch angiitis associated with cytomegalovirus retinitis. *Am J Ophthalmol* 114:514-515, 1992.

334. Geier SA, Nasemann J, Klauss V, et al: Frosted branch angiitis in a patient with the acquired immunodeficiency syndrome. *Am J Ophthalmol* 113:203-205, 1992.

335. Gross JG, Bozzette SA, Mathews WC, et al: Longitudinal study of cytomegalovirus retinitis in acquired immune deficiency syndrome. *Ophthalmology* 97:681-686, 1990.

336. Gross JG, Sadun AA, Wiley CA, Freeman WR: Severe visual loss related to isolated peripapillary retinal and optic nerve head cytomegalovirus infection. *Am J Ophthalmol* 108:691-698, 1989.

337. Heinemann M-H: Long-term intravitreal gancyclovir therapy for cytomegalovirus retinopathy. *Arch Ophthalmol* 107:1767-1772, 1989.

338. Henderly DE, Freeman WR, Causey DM, Rao NA: Cytomegalovirus retinitis and response to therapy with ganciclovir. *Ophthalmology* 94:425-434, 1987.

339. Holland GN: Editorial: The management of retinal detachments in patients with acquired immunodeficiency syndrome. *Arch Ophthalmol* 109:791-793, 1991.

340. Holland GN, Sidikaro Y, Kreiger AE, et al: Treatment of cytomegalovirus retinopathy with ganciclovir. *Ophthalmology* 94:815-823, 1987.

341. Holland GN, Sison RF, Jatulis DE, et al: Survival of patients with the acquired immune deficiency syndrome after development of cytomegalovirus retinopathy. *Ophthalmology* 97:204-211, 1990.

342. Jabs DA, Enger C, Bartlett JG: Cytomegalovirus retinitis and acquired immunodeficiency syndrome. *Arch Ophthalmol* 107:75-80, 1989.

343. Jabs DA, Enger C, Haller J, deBustros S: Retinal detachments in patients with cytomegalovirus retinitis. *Arch Ophthalmol* 109:794-799, 1991.

344. Jabs DA, Newman C, DeBustros S, Polk BF: Treatment of cytomegalovirus retinitis with ganciclovir. *Ophthalmology* 94:824-830, 1987.

345. Keefe KS, Freeman WR, Peterson TJ, et al: Atypical healing of cytomegalovirus retinitis; significance of persistent border opacification. *Ophthalmology* 99:1377-1384, 1992.

346. Kuppermann BD, Flores-Aguilar M, Quiceno JI, et al: Combination gancyclovir and foscarnet in the treatment of clinically resistant cytomegalovirus retinitis in patients with acquired immunodeficiency syndrome. *Arch Ophthalmol* 111:1359-1366, 1993.

347. Kuppermann BD, Petty JG, Richman DD, et al: Correlation between CD4+ counts and prevalence of cytomegalovirus retinitis and human immunodeficiency virus-related noninfectious retinal vasculopathy in patients with acquired immunodeficiency syndrome. *Am J Ophthalmol* 115:575-582, 1993.

348. Lee S, Ai E: Disc neovascularization in patients with AIDS and cytomegalovirus retinitis. *Retina* 11:305-308, 1991.

349. Lehoang P, Girard B, Robinet M, et al: Foscarnet in the treatment of cytomegalovirus retinitis in acquired immune deficiency syndrome. *Ophthalmology* 96:865-874, 1989.

350. Meredith TA, Aaberg TM, Reeser FH: Rhegmatogenous retinal detachment complicating cytomegalovirus retinitis. *Am J Ophthalmol* 87:793-796, 1979.

351. Morinelli EN, Dugel PU, Lee M, et al: Opportunistic intraocular infections in AIDS. *Trans Am Ophthalmol Soc* 90:97-109, 1992.

352. Orellana J, Teich SA, Lieberman RM, et al: Treatment of retinal detachments in patients with the acquired immune deficiency syndrome. *Ophthalmology* 98:939-943, 1991.

353. Pepose JS, Newman C, Bach MC, et al: Pathologic features of cytomegalovirus retinopathy after treatment with the antiviral agent ganciclovir. *Ophthalmology* 94:414-424, 1987.

354. Porter R: Acute necrotizing retinitis in a patient receiving immunosuppressive therapy. *Br J Ophthalmol* 56:555-558, 1972.

355. Rabb MF, Jampol LM, Fish RH, et al: Retinal periphlebitis in patients with acquired immunodeficiency syndrome with cytomegalovirus retinitis mimics acute frosted retinal periphlebitis. *Arch Ophthalmol* 110:1257-1260, 1992.

356. Rahhal FM, Rosberger DF, Polsky B, et al: Cytomegalovirus retinitis in a patient with a normal helper T-cell (CD4) count. *Arch Ophthalmol* 111:1325-1326, 1993.

357. Robinson MR, Teitelbaum C, Taylor-Findlay C: Thrombocytopenia and vitreous hemorrhage complicating ganciclovir treatment. *Am J Ophthalmol* 107:560-561, 1989.

358. Rowe WP, Hartley JW, Waterman S, et al: Cytopathogenic agent resembling human salivary gland virus recovered from tissue cultures of human adenoids. *Proc Soc Exp Biol Med* 92:418-424, 1956.

359. Sanborn GE, Anand R, Torti RE, et al: Sustained-release ganciclovir therapy for treatment of cytomegalovirus retinitis; use of an intravitreal device. *Arch Ophthalmol* 110:188-195, 1992.

360. Secchi AG, Tognon MS, Turrini B, Carniel G: Acute frosted retinal periphlebitis associated with cytomegalovirus retinitis. *Retina* 12:245-247, 1992.

361. Sidikaro Y, Silver L, Holland GN, Kreiger AE: Rhegmatogenous retinal detachments in patients with AIDS and necrotizing retinal infections. *Ophthalmology* 98:129-135, 1991.

362. Sison RF, Holland GN, MacArthur LJ, et al: Cytomegalovirus retinopathy as the initial manifestation of the acquired immunodeficiency syndrome. *Am J Ophthalmol* 112:243-249, 1991.

363. Skolnik PR, Pomerantz RJ, de la Monte SM, et al: Dual infection of retina with human immunodeficiency virus type 1 and cytomegalovirus. *Am J Ophthalmol* 107:361-372, 1989.

364. Smith ME: Retinal involvement in adult cytomegalic inclusion disease. *Arch Ophthalmol* 72:44-49, 1964.

365. Smith ME, Zimmerman LE, Harley RD: Ocular involvement in congenital cytomegalic inclusion disease. *Arch Ophthalmol* 76:696-699, 1966.

366. Smith TJ, Pearson PA, Blandford DL, et al: Intravitreal sustained-release ganciclovir. *Arch Ophthalmol* 110:255-258, 1992.

367. Spaide RF, Vitale AT, Toth IR, Oliver JM: Frosted branch angiitis associated with cytomegalovirus retinitis. *Am J Ophthalmol* 113:522-528, 1992.

368. Stevens G Jr, Palestine AG, Rodriguez MM, et al: Failure of argon laser to halt cytomegalovirus retinitis. *Retina* 6:119-122, 1986.

369. Studies of Ocular Complications of AIDS Research Group in Collaboration with the AIDS Clinical Trials Group: Foscarnet-Ganciclovir cytomegalovirus trial. 4. Visual outcomes. *Ophthalmology* 101:1250-1261, 1994.

370. To KW, Nadel AJ: Atypical presumed CMV retinitis. *Graefes Arch Clin Exp Ophthalmol* 227:535-537, 1989.

371. Wyhinny GJ, Apple DJ, Guastella FR, Vygantas CM: Adult cytomegalic inclusion retinitis. *Am J Ophthalmol* 76:773-781, 1973.

Herpes Zoster Retinochoroiditis, Optic Neuritis, and the Acute Retinal Necrosis Syndrome

372. Amanat LA, Cant JS, Green FD: Acute phthisis bulbi and external ophthalmoplegia in herpes zoster ophthalmicus. *Ann Ophthalmol* 17:46-51, 1985.

373. Amano Y, Ohashi Y, Haruta Y, et al: A new fundus finding in patients with zoster ophthalmicus. *Am J Ophthalmol* 102:532-533, 1986.

374. Ando F, Kato M, Goto S, et al: Platelet function in bilateral acute retinal necrosis. *Am J Ophthalmol* 96:27-32, 1983.

375. Bando K, Kinoshita A, Mimura Y: Six cases of so called "Kirisawa type" uveitis. *Jpn J Clin Ophthalmol* 33:1515-1521, 1979.

376. Bartlett RE, Mumma CS, Irvine AR: Herpes zoster ophthalmicus with bilateral hemorrhagic retinopathy. *Am J Ophthalmol* 34:45-48, 1951.

377. Bloom SM, Snady-McCoy L: Multifocal choroiditis uveitis occurring after herpes zoster ophthalmicus. *Am J Ophthalmol* 108:733-735, 1989.

378. Blumenkranz M, Clarkson J, Culbertson WW, et al: Visual results and complications after retinal reattachment in the acute retinal necrosis syndrome; the influence of operative technique. *Retina* 9:170-174, 1989.

379. Blumenkranz M, Clarkson J, Culbertson WW, et al: Vitrectomy for retinal detachment associated with acute retinal necrosis. *Am J Ophthalmol* 106:426-429, 1988.

380. Blumenkranz MS, Culbertson WW, Clarkson JG, Dix R: Treatment of the acute retinal necrosis syndrome with intravenous acyclovir. *Ophthalmology* 93:296-300, 1986.

381. Blumenkranz MS, Kaplan HJ, Clarkson JG, et al: Acute multifocal hemorrhagic retinal vasculitis. *Ophthalmology* 95:1663-1672, 1988.

382. Brown RM, Mendis U: Retinal arteritis complicating herpes zoster ophthalmicus. *Br J Ophthalmol* 57:344-346, 1973.

383. Capone A Jr, Meredith TA: Central visual loss caused by chickenpox retinitis in a 2-year-old child. *Am J Ophthalmol* 113:592-593, 1992.

384. Carney MD, Peyman GA, Goldberg MF, et al: Acute retinal necrosis. *Retina* 6:85-94, 1986.

385. Cho N, Han H: Central retinal artery occlusion after varicella. *Am J Ophthalmol* 113:591-592, 1992.

386. Clarkson JG, Blumenkranz MS, Culbertson WW, et al: Retinal detachment following the acute retinal necrosis syndrome. *Ophthalmology* 91:1665-1668, 1984.

387. Copenhaver RM: Chickenpox with retinopathy. *Arch Ophthalmol* 75:199-200, 1966.

388. Culbertson WW, Blumenkranz MS: The acute retinal necrosis syndrome. *In:* Blodi FC, editor: *Herpes simplex infections of the eye,* New York, 1984, Churchill Livingstone, pp. 77-89.

389. Culbertson WW, Blumenkranz MS, Haines H, et al: The acute retinal necrosis syndrome. Part 2: Histopathology and etiology. *Ophthalmology* 89:1317-1325, 1982.

390. Culbertson WW, Blumenkranz MS, Pepose JS, et al: Varicella zoster virus is a cause of the acute retinal necrosis syndrome. *Ophthalmology* 93:559-569, 1986.

391. Culbertson WW, Brod RD, Flynn HW Jr, et al: Chickenpox-associated acute retinal necrosis syndrome. *Ophthalmology* 98:1641-1645, 1991.

392. Diddie KR, Schanzlin DJ, Mausolf FA, et al: Necrotizing retinitis caused by opportunistic virus infection in a patient with Hodgkin's disease. *Am J Ophthalmol* 88:668-673, 1979.

393. Duker JS, Shakin EP: Rapidly progressive outer retinal necrosis in the acquired immunodeficiency syndrome. *Am J Ophthalmol* 111:255-256, 1991.

394. Edgerton AE: Herpes zoster ophthalmicus; report of cases and review of literature. *Arch Ophthalmol* 34:114-153, 1945.

395. el Azaza M, Samuelsson A, Linde A, Forsgren M: Intrathecal antibody production against viruses of the herpesvirus family in acute retinal necrosis syndrome. *Am J Ophthalmol* 112:76-82, 1991.

396. Engstrom RE Jr, Holland GN, Margolis TP, et al: The progressive outer retinal necrosis syndrome; a variant of necrotizing herpetic retinopathy in patients with AIDS. *Ophthalmology* 101:1488-1502, 1994.

397. Fisher JP, Lewis ML, Blumenkranz M, et al: The acute retinal necrosis syndrome. Part I: Clinical manifestations. *Ophthalmology* 89:1309-1316, 1982.

398. Forster DJ, Dugel PU, Frangieh GT, et al: Rapidly progressive outer retinal necrosis in the acquired immunodeficiency syndrome. *Am J Ophthalmol* 110:341-348, 1990.

399. Freeman WR, Thomas EL, Rao NA, et al: Demonstration of herpes group virus in acute retinal necrosis syndrome. *Am J Ophthalmol* 102:701-709, 1986.

400. Freeman WR, Wiley CA, Gross JG, et al: Endoretinal biopsy in immunosuppressed and healthy patients with retinitis; indications, utility, and techniques. *Ophthalmology* 96:1559-1565, 1989.

401. Friberg TR, Jost BF: Acute retinal necrosis in an immunosuppressed patient. *Am J Ophthalmol* 98:515-517, 1984.

402. Friedberg MA, Micale AJ: Monocular blindness from central retinal artery occlusion associated with chickenpox. *Am J Ophthalmol* 117:117-118, 1994.

403. Gartry DS, Spalton DJ, Tilzey A, Hykin PG: Acute retinal necrosis syndrome. *Br J Ophthalmol* 75:292-297, 1991.

404. Gass JDM: Acute herpetic thrombotic retinal angiitis and necrotizing neuroretinitis ("acute retinal necrosis syndrome"). *In: Symposium on medical and surgical diseases of the retina and vitreous; transactions of the New Orleans Academy of Ophthalmology,* St. Louis, 1983, CV Mosby, pp. 97-107.

405. Gass JDM: Giant cell reaction surrounding Bruch's membrane and internal limiting membrane. Presented at the Eastern Ophthalmic Pathology Society Meeting, 1991.

406. Gilbert GJ: Herpes zoster ophthalmicus and delayed contralateral hemiparesis; relationship of the syndrome to central nervous system granulomatous angiitis. *JAMA* 229:302-304, 1974.

407. Gorman BD, Nadel AJ, Coles RS: Acute retinal necrosis. *Ophthalmology* 89:809-814, 1982.

408. Green WR, Zimmerman LE: Granulomatous reaction to Descemet's membrane. *Am J Ophthalmol* 64:555-558, 1967.

409. Grossniklaus HE, Aaberg TM, Purnell EW, et al: Retinal necrosis in X-linked lymphoproliferative disease. *Ophthalmology* 101:705-709, 1994.

410. Han DP, Abrams GW, Williams GA: Regression of disc neovascularization by photocoagulation in the acute retinal necrosis syndrome. *Retina* 8:244-246, 1988.

411. Han DP, Lewis H, Williams GA, et al: Laser photocoagulation in the acute retinal necrosis syndrome. *Arch Ophthalmol* 105:1051-1054, 1987.

412. Hayreh MMS, Kreiger AE, Straatsma BR, et al: Acute retinal necrosis. ARVO Abstracts. *Invest Ophthalmol Vis Sci* 19 (Suppl):48, 1980.

413. Hayreh SS: Acute retinal necrosis. *Am J Ophthalmol* 97:661-662, 1984.

414. Hedges TR III, Albert DM: The progression of the ocular abnormalities of herpes zoster; histopathologic observations of nine cases. *Ophthalmology* 89:165-177, 1982.

415. Hesse RJ: Herpes zoster ophthalmicus associated with delayed retinal thrombophlebitis. *Am J Ophthalmol* 84:329-331, 1977.

416. Holland GN, Cornell PJ, Park MS, et al: An association between acute retinal necrosis syndrome and HLA-DQw7 and phenotype Bw62,DR4. *Am J Ophthalmol* 108:370-374, 1989.

417. Holland GN, Executive Committee of the American Uveitis Society: Standard diagnostic criteria for the acute retinal necrosis syndrome. *Am J Ophthalmol* 117:663-666, 1994.

418. Hugkulstone CE, Watt LL: Branch retinal arteriolar occlusion with chicken-pox. *Br J Ophthalmol* 72:78-80, 1988.

419. Jabs DA, Schachat AP, Liss R, et al: Presumed varicella zoster retinitis in immunocompromised patients. *Retina* 7:9-13, 1987.

420. Jampol LM: Acute retinal necrosis. *Am J Ophthalmol* 93:254-255, 1982.

421. Jensen J: A case of herpes zoster ophthalmicus complicated with neuroretinitis. *Acta Ophthalmol* 26:551-555, 1948.

422. Johnston WH, Holland GN, Engstrom RE Jr, Rimmer S: Recurrence of presumed varicella-zoster virus retinopathy in patients with acquired immunodeficiency syndrome. *Am J Ophthalmol* 116:42-50, 1993.

423. Kelly SP, Rosenthal AR: Chickenpox chorioretinitis. *Br J Ophthalmol* 74:698-699, 1990.

424. Knox DL, King J Jr: Retinal arteritis, iridocyclitis, and giardiasis. *Ophthalmology* 89:1303-1308, 1982.

425. Kometani J, Asayama T: A case of specific uveitis occurring acutely in the right eye. *Folia Ophthalmol Jpn* 29:1397-1401, 1978.

426. Lambert SR, Taylor D, Kriss A, et al: Ocular manifestations of the congenital varicella syndrome. *Arch Ophthalmol* 107:52-56, 1989.

427. Lightman S: Editorial: Acute retinal necrosis. *Br J Ophthalmol* 75:449, 1991.

428. Linnemann CC Jr, Alvira MM: Pathogenesis of varicella-zoster angiitis in the CNS. *Arch Neurol* 37:239-240, 1980.

429. Margo CE: (PORN) Progressive outer retinal necrosis syndrome. Presented at the Verhoeff Society Meeting, 1994.

430. Margolis T, Irvine AR, Hoyt WF, Hyman R: Acute retinal necrosis syndrome presenting with papillitis and arcuate neuroretinitis. *Ophthalmology* 95:937-940, 1988.

431. Margolis TP, Lowder CY, Holland GN, et al: Varicella-zoster virus retinitis in patients with the acquired immunodeficiency syndrome. *Am J Ophthalmol* 112:119-131, 1991.

432. Martenet A-C: Fréquence et aspects cliniques des complications rétiniennes de l'uvéite intermédiaire. *Bull Mem Soc Fr Ophtalmol* 92:40-42, 1980.

433. Matsuo T, Date S, Tsuji T, et al: Immune complex containing herpesvirus antigen in a patient with acute retinal necrosis. *Am J Ophthalmol* 101:368-371, 1986.

434. Matsuo T, Koyama M, Matsuo N: Acute retinal necrosis as a novel complication of chickenpox in adults. *Br J Ophthalmol* 74:443-444, 1990.

435. Matsuo T, Morimoto K, Matsuo N: Factors associated with poor visual outcome in acute retinal necrosis. *Br J Ophthalmol* 75:450-454, 1991.

436. Matsuo T, Nakayama T, Koyama T, et al: A proposed mild type of acute retinal necrosis syndrome. *Am J Ophthalmol* 105:579-583, 1988.

437. McDonald HR, Lewis H, Kreiger AE, et al: Surgical management of retinal detachment associated with acute retinal necrosis syndrome. *Br J Ophthalmol* 75:455-458, 1991.

438. Naumann G, Gass JDM, Font RL: Histopathology of herpes zoster ophthalmicus. *Am J Ophthalmol* 65:533-541, 1968.

439. Nishi M, Hanashiro R, Mori S, et al: Polymerase chain reaction for the detection of the varicella-zoster genome in ocular samples from patients with acute retinal necrosis. *Am J Ophthalmol* 114:603-609, 1992.

440. Okinami S, Tsukahara I: Acute severe uveitis with retinal vasculitis and retinal detachment. *Ophthalmologica* 179:276-285, 1979.

441. Palay DA, Sternberg P Jr, Davis J, et al: Decrease in the risk of bilateral acute retinal necrosis by acyclovir therapy. *Am J Ophthalmol* 112:250-255, 1991.

442. Pepose JS, Flowers B, Stewart JA, et al: Herpesvirus antibody levels in the etiologic diagnosis of the acute retinal necrosis syndrome. *Am J Ophthalmol* 113:248-256, 1992.

443. Peyman GA, Goldberg MF, Uninsky E, et al: Vitrectomy and intravitreal antiviral drug therapy in acute retinal necrosis syndrome; report of two cases. *Arch Ophthalmol* 102:1618-1621, 1984.

444. Price FW Jr, Schlaegel TF Jr: Bilateral acute retinal necrosis. *Am J Ophthalmol* 89:419-424, 1980.

445. Rabinovitch T, Nozik RA, Varenhorst MP: Bilateral acute retinal necrosis syndrome. *Am J Ophthalmol* 108:735-736, 1989.

446. Reese LT, Shafer DM, Zweifach P: Acute acquired toxoplasmosis. *Ann Ophthalmol* 13:467-470, 1981.

447. Regillo CD, Sergott RC, Ho AC, et al: Hemodynamic alterations in the acute retinal necrosis syndrome. *Ophthalmology* 100:1171-1176, 1993.

448. Rummelt V, Wenkel H, Rummelt C, et al: Detection of varicella zoster virus DNA and viral antigen in the late stage of bilateral acute retinal necrosis syndrome. *Arch Ophthalmol* 110:1132-1136, 1992.

449. Saari KM, Böke W, Manthey KF, et al: Bilateral acute retinal necrosis. *Am J Ophthalmol* 93:403-411, 1982.

450. Schwartz JN, Cashwell F, Hawkins HK, Klintworth GK: Necrotizing retinopathy with herpes zoster ophthalmicus; a light and electron microscopical study. *Arch Pathol Lab Med* 100:386-391, 1976.

451. Sergott RC, Anand R, Belmont JB, et al: Acute retinal necrosis neuropathy; clinical profile and surgical therapy. *Arch Ophthalmol* 107:692-696, 1989.

452. Soushi S, Ozawa H, Matsuhashi M, et al: Demonstration of varicella-zoster virus antigens in the vitreous aspirates of patients with acute retinal necrosis syndrome. *Ophthalmology* 95:1394-1398, 1988.

453. Sternberg P Jr, Han DP, Yeo JH, et al: Photocoagulation to prevent retinal detachment in acute retinal necrosis. *Ophthalmology* 95:1389-1393, 1988.

454. Sternberg P Jr, Knox DL, Finkelstein D, et al: Acute retinal necrosis syndrome. *Retina* 2:145-151, 1982.

455. Taylor D, Day S, Tiedemann K, et al: Chorioretinal biopsy in a patient with leukaemia. *Br J Ophthalmol* 65:489-493, 1981.

456. Topilow HW, Nussbaum JJ, Freeman HM, et al: Bilateral acute retinal necrosis; clinical and ultrastructural study. *Arch Ophthalmol* 100:1901-1908, 1982.

457. Urayama A, Yamada N, Sasaki T, et al: Unilateral acute uveitis with retinal periarteritis and detachment. *Jpn J Clin Ophthalmol* 25:607-619, 1971.

458. Willerson D Jr, Aaberg TM, Reeser FH: Necrotizing vaso-occlusive retinitis. *Am J Ophthalmol* 84:209-219, 1977.

459. Womack LW, Liesegang TJ: Complications of herpes zoster ophthalmicus. *Arch Ophthalmol* 101:42-45, 1983.

460. Yeo JH, Pepose JS, Stewart JA, et al: Acute retinal necrosis syndrome following herpes zoster dermatitis. *Ophthalmology* 93:1418-1422, 1986.

461. Young NJA, Bird AC: Bilateral acute retinal necrosis. *Br J Ophthalmol* 62:581-590, 1978.

Epstein-Barr Virus

462. Kelly SP, Rosenthal AR, Nicholson KG, Woodward CG: Retinochoroiditis in acute Epstein-Barr virus infection. *Br J Ophthalmol* 73:1002-1003, 1989.

463. Purtilo DT: Epstein-Barr virus: The spectrum of its manifestations in human beings. *South Med J* 80:943-947, 1987.

464. Raymond LA, Wilson CA, Linnemann CC Jr, et al: Punctate outer retinitis in acute Epstein-Barr virus infection. *Am J Ophthalmol* 104:424-426, 1987.

465. Tiedeman JS: Epstein-Barr viral antibodies in multifocal choroiditis and panuveitis. *Am J Ophthalmol* 103:659-663, 1987.

466. Wong KW, D'Amico DJ, Hedges TR III, et al: Ocular involvement associated with chronic Epstein-Barr virus disease. *Arch Ophthalmol* 105:788-792, 1987.

Human Immunodeficiency Virus (HIV) and Acquired Immune Deficiency Syndrome (AIDS)

467. Boyer DS: Discussion of paper by Holland GN, Pepose JS, Pettit TH, et al: Acquired immune deficiency syndrome; ocular manifestations. *Ophthalmology* 90:872-873, 1983.

468. Broder S, Gallo RC: A pathogenic retrovirus (HTLV-III) linked to AIDS. *N Engl J Med* 311:1292-1297, 1984.

469. Brodie SE, Friedman AH: Retinal dysfunction as an initial ophthalmic sign in AIDS. *Br J Ophthalmol* 74:49-51, 1990.

470. Brooks HL Jr, Downing J, McClure JA, Engel HM: Orbital Burkitt's lymphoma in a homosexual man with acquired immune deficiency. *Arch Ophthalmol* 102:1533-1537, 1984.

471. Cantrill HL, Henry K, Jackson B, et al: Recovery of human immunodeficiency virus from ocular tissues in patients with acquired immune deficiency syndrome. *Ophthalmology* 95: 1458-1462, 1988.

472. Centers for Disease Control: Kaposi's sarcoma and *Pneumocystis* pneumonia among homosexual men—New York City and California. *MMWR Morb Mortal Wkly Rep* 30:305-308, 1981.

472a. Centers for Disease Control: Guidelines for prophylaxis against *Pneumocystis carinii* pneumonia for adults and children infected with human immunodeficiency virus. *MMWR* 41(RR-4):1-11, 1992.

473. Centers for Disease Control: *Pneumocystis* pneumonia—Los Angeles. *MMWR Morb Mortal Wkly Rep* 30:250-252, 1981.

474. Centers for Disease Control: Provisional Public Health Service inter-agency recommendations for screening donated blood and plasma for antibody to the virus causing acquired immunodeficiency syndrome. *MMWR Morb Mortal Wkly Rep* 34:1-5, 1985.

475. Cole EL, Meisler DM, Calabrese LH, et al: Herpes zoster ophthalmicus and acquired immune deficiency syndrome. *Arch Ophthalmol* 102:1027-1029, 1984.

476. Croxatto JO, Mestre C, Puente S, Gonzalez G: Nonreactive tuberculosis in a patient with acquired immune deficiency syndrome. *Am J Ophthalmol* 102:659-660, 1986.

477. Davis JL, Nussenblatt RB, Bachman DM, et al: Endogenous bacterial retinitis in AIDS. *Am J Ophthalmol* 107:613-623, 1989.

478. Dennehy PJ, Warman R, Flynn JT, et al: Ocular manifestations in pediatric patients with acquired immunodeficiency syndrome. *Arch Ophthalmol* 107:978-982, 1989.

479. Drew WL, Buhles W, Erlich KS: Herpesvirus infections (cytomegalovirus, herpes simplex virus, varicella-zoster virus); how to use ganciclovir (DHPG) and acyclovir. *Infect Dis Clin North Am* 2(2):495-509, 1988.

480. Engstrom RE Jr, Holland GN, Hardy WD, Meiselman HJ: Hemorheologic abnormalities in patients with human immunodeficiency virus infection and ophthalmic microvasculopathy. *Am J Ophthalmol* 109:153-161, 1990.

481. Forster DJ, Dugel PU, Frangieh GT, et al: Rapidly progressive outer retinal necrosis in the acquired immunodeficiency syndrome. *Am J Ophthalmol* 110:341-348, 1990.

482. Freeman WR, Chen A, Henderly DE, et al: Prevalence and significance of acquired immunodeficiency syndrome-related retinal microvasculopathy. *Am J Ophthalmol* 107:229-235, 1989.

483. Freeman WR, Lerner CW, Mines JA, et al: A prospective study of the ophthalmologic findings in the acquired immune deficiency syndrome. *Am J Ophthalmol* 97:133-142, 1984.

484. Fujikawa LS, Salahuddin SZ, Ablashi D, et al: HTLV-III in the tears of AIDS patients. *Ophthalmology* 93:1479-1481, 1986.

485. Fujikawa LS, Salahuddin SZ, Ablashi D, et al: Human T-cell leukemia/lymphotropic virus type III in the conjunctival epithelium of a patient with AIDS. *Am J Ophthalmol* 100:507-509, 1985.

486. Gal A, Pollack A, Oliver M: Ocular findings in the acquired immunodeficiency syndrome. *Br J Ophthalmol* 68:238-241, 1984.

487. Geier SA, Schielke E, Klauss V, et al: Retinal microvasculopathy and reduced cerebral blood flow in patients with acquired immunodeficiency syndrome. *Am J Ophthalmol* 113:100-101, 1992.

488. Glascow BJ, Weisberger AK: A quantitative and cartographic study of retinal microvasculopathy in acquired immunodeficiency syndrome. *Am J Ophthalmol* 118:46-56, 1994.

489. Holland GN, Gottlieb MS, Foos RY: Retinal cotton-wool patches in acquired immunodeficiency syndrome. *N Engl J Med* 307:1704, 1982.

490. Holland GN, Pepose JS, Pettit TH, et al: Acquired immune deficiency syndrome; ocular manifestations. *Ophthalmology* 90:859-872, 1983.

491. Hummer J, Gass JDM, Huang AJW: Conjunctival Kaposi's sarcoma treated with interferon alpha-2a. *Am J Ophthalmol* 116:502-503, 1993.

492. Jabs DA, Green WR, Fox R, et al: Ocular manifestations of acquired immune deficiency syndrome. *Ophthalmology* 96: 1092-1099, 1989.

493. Jensen OA, Gerstoft J, Thomsen HK, Marner K: Cytomegalovirus retinitis in the acquired immunodeficiency syndrome (AIDS); light-microscopical, ultrastructural and immunohistochemical examination of a case. *Acta Ophthalmol* 62:1-9, 1984.

494. Kestelyn P, Van de Perre P, Rouvroy D, et al: A prospective study of the ophthalmologic findings in the acquired immune deficiency syndrome in Africa. *Am J Ophthalmol* 100:230-238, 1985.

495. Khadem M, Kalish SB, Goldsmith J, et al: Ophthalmologic findings in acquired immune deficiency syndrome (AIDS). *Arch Ophthalmol* 102:201-206, 1984.

496. Kwok S, O'Donnell JJ, Wood IS: Retinal cotton-wool spots in a patient with *Pneumocystis carinii* infection. *N Engl J Med* 307:184-185, 1982.

496a. Lifson AR, Rutherford GW, Jaffe HW: The natural history of human immunodeficiency virus infection. *J Infect Dis* 158:1360-1367, 1988.

497. Macher A, Rodriguez MM, Kaplan W, et al: Disseminated bilateral chorioretinitis due to *Histoplasma capsulatum* in a patient with the acquired immunodeficiency syndrome. *Ophthalmology* 92:1159-1164, 1985.

498. Mansour AM, Jampol LM, Logani S, et al: Cotton-wool spots in acquired immunodeficiency syndrome compared with diabetes mellitus, systemic hypertension, and central retinal vein occlusion. *Arch Ophthalmol* 106:1074-1077, 1988.

499. Morinelli EN, Dugel PU, Lee M, et al: Opportunistic intraocular infections in AIDS. *Trans Am Ophthalmol Soc* 90:97-109, 1992.

500. Newsome DA, Green WR, Miller ED, et al: Microvascular aspects of acquired immune deficiency syndrome retinopathy. *Am J Ophthalmol* 98:590-601, 1984.

501. Nussenblatt RB, Palestine AG: Editorial: Human immunodeficiency virus, herpes zoster, and the retina. *Am J Ophthalmol* 112:206-207, 1991.

502. Palestine AG, Frishberg B: Macular edema in acquired immunodeficiency syndrome-related microvasculopathy. *Am J Ophthalmol* 111:770-771, 1991.

503. Palestine AG, Rodrigues MM, Macher AM, et al: Ophthalmic involvement in acquired immunodeficiency syndrome. *Ophthalmology* 91:1092-1099, 1984.

504. Pepose JS, Hilborne LH, Cancilla PA, Foos RY: Concurrent herpes simplex and cytomegalovirus retinitis and encephalitis in the acquired immune deficiency syndrome (AIDS). *Ophthalmology* 91:1669-1677, 1984.

505. Pepose JS, Holland GN, Nestor MS, et al: Acquired immune deficiency syndrome; pathogenic mechanisms of ocular disease. *Ophthalmology* 92:472-484, 1985.

506. Qavi HB, Green MT, SeGall GK, Font RL: Demonstration of HIV-1 and HHV-6 in AIDS-associated retinitis. *Curr Eye Res* 8:379-387, 1989.

507. Quiceno JI, Capparelli E, Sadun AA, et al: Visual dysfunction without retinitis in patients with acquired immunodeficiency syndrome. *Am J Ophthalmol* 113:8-13, 1992.

508. Rodrigues MM, Palestine A, Nussenblatt R, et al: Unilateral cytomegalovirus retinochoroiditis and bilateral cytoid bodies in a bisexual man with the acquired immunodeficiency syndrome. *Ophthalmology* 90:1577-1582, 1983.

509. Rosenberg PR, Uliss AE, Friedland GH, et al: Acquired immunodeficiency syndrome; ophthalmic manifestations in ambulatory patients. *Ophthalmology* 90:874-878, 1983.

510. Schuman JS, Friedman AH: Retinal manifestations of the acquired immune deficiency syndrome (AIDS): Cytomegalovirus, *Candida albicans, Cryptococcus,* toxoplasmosis, and *Pneumocystis carinii. Trans Ophthalmol Soc UK* 103:177-190, 1983.

511. Tanenbaum M, Russell S, Richmond P, Gass JDM: Calcified cytoid bodies in acquired immunodeficiency syndrome. *Retina* 7:84-88, 1987.

512. Tenhula WN, Xu S, Madigan MC, et al: Morphometric comparisons of optic nerve axon loss in acquired immunodeficiency syndrome. *Am J Ophthalmol* 113:14-20, 1992.

513. Welch K, Finkbeiner W, Alpers CE, et al: Autopsy findings in the acquired immune deficiency syndrome. *JAMA* 252:1152-1159, 1984.

514. Whitcup SM, Butler KM, Caruso R, et al: Retinal toxicity in human immunodeficiency virus-infected children treated with 2′,3′-dideoxyinosine. *Am J Ophthalmol* 113:1-7, 1992.

515. Winward KE, Hamed LM, Glaser JS: The spectrum of optic nerve disease in human immunodeficiency virus infection. *Am J Ophthalmol* 107:373-380, 1989.

Human T-Lymphotropic Virus Type 1

516. Hayasaka S, Takatori Y, Noda S, et al: Retinal vasculitis, in a mother and her son with human T-lymphotropic virus type 1 associated myelopathy. *Br J Ophthalmol* 75:566-567, 1991.

517. Mochizuki M, Watanabe T, Yamaguchi K, et al: Uveitis associated with human T-cell lymphotropic virus type I. *Am J Ophthalmol* 114:123-129, 1992.

518. Ohba N, Matsumoto M, Sameshima M, et al: Ocular manifestations in patients infected with human T-lymphotropic virus type I. *Jpn J Ophthalmol* 33:1-12, 1989.

519. Sasaki K, Morooka I, Inomata H, et al: Retinal vasculitis in human T-lymphotropic virus type I associated myelopathy. *Br J Ophthalmol* 73:812-815, 1989.

520. Spalton DJ, Nicholson F: Mini review: HTLV-I infection in human disease. *Br J Ophthalmol* 75:174-175, 1991.

Rubella Retinitis

521. Alfano JE: Ocular aspects of the maternal rubella syndrome. *Trans Am Acad Ophthalmol Otolaryngol* 70:235-266, 1966.

522. Boniuk M, Zimmerman LE: Ocular pathology in the rubella syndrome. *Arch Ophthalmol* 77:455-472, 1967.

523. Collis WJ, Cohen DN: Rubella retinopathy; a progressive disorder. *Arch Ophthalmol* 84:33-35, 1970.

524. Deutman AF, Grizzard WS: Rubella retinopathy and subretinal neovascularization. *Am J Ophthalmol* 85:82-87, 1978.

525. Franceschetti A, Dieterle P, Schwarz A: Rétinite pigmentaire à virus: Relation entre tableau clinique et électrorétinogramme (ERG). *Ophthalmologica* 135:545-554, 1958.

526. Frank KE, Purnell EW: Subretinal neovascularization following rubella retinopathy. *Am J Ophthalmol* 86:462-466, 1978.

527. Gass JDM: *Stereoscopic atlas of macular diseases; diagnosis and treatment,* ed. 2, St. Louis, 1977, CV Mosby, pp. 40, 92, 210.

528. Givens KT, Lee DA, Jones T, Ilstrup DM: Congenital rubella syndrome: Ophthalmic manifestations and associated systemic disorders. *Br J Ophthalmol* 77:358-363, 1993.

529. Gregg NM: Discussion of Marks EO: Pigmentary abnormality in children congenitally deaf following maternal German measles. *Trans Ophthalmol Soc Aust* 6:124, 1946.

530. Hertzberg R: Twenty-five-year follow-up of ocular defects in congenital rubella. *Am J Ophthalmol* 66:269-271, 1968.

531. Krill AE: The retinal disease of rubella. *Arch Ophthalmol* 77:445-449, 1967.

532. Krill AE: Retinopathy secondary to rubella. *Int Ophthalmol Clin* 12(2):89-103, 1972.

533. Menser MA, Dods L, Harley JD: A twenty-five-year follow-up of congenital rubella. *Lancet* 2:1347-1350, 1967.

534. Slusher MM, Tyler ME: Rubella retinopathy and subretinal neovascularization. *Ann Ophthalmol* 14:292-294, 1982.

535. Wolff SM: The ocular manifestations of congenital rubella. *Trans Am Ophthalmol Soc* 70:577-614, 1972.

Subacute Sclerosing Panencephalitis (Dawson's Encephalitis)

536. Cochereau-Massin I, Gaudric A, Reinert P, et al: Altérations du fond d'oeil au cours de la panencéphalite sclérosante subaiguë. *J Fr Ophtalmol* 15:255-261, 1992.

537. David P, Elia M, Mariotti P, Macchi G: Adult onset of subacute sclerosing panencephalitis; a case report. *Riv Neurol* 60:83-87, 1990.

538. Font RL, Jenis EH, Tuck KD: Measles maculopathy associated with subacute sclerosing panencephalitis; immunofluorescent and immuno-ultrastructural studies. *Arch Pathol* 96:168-174, 1973.

539. Gravina RF, Nakanishi AS, Faden A: Subacute sclerosing panencephalitis. *Am J Ophthalmol* 86:106-109, 1978.

540. Green SH, Wirtschafter JD: Ophthalmoscopic findings in subacute sclerosing panencephalitis. *Br J Ophthalmol* 57:780-787, 1973.

541. Haltia M, Tarkkanen A, Vaheri A, et al: Measles retinopathy during immunosuppression. *Br J Ophthalmol* 62:356-360, 1978.

542. Karel I, Otradovec J, Peleška M, Nevšímal O: Fluoroangiographic picture of the macular lesion in subacute sclerosing leukoencephalitis van Bogaert. *Ophthalmologica* 162:348-354, 1971.

543. Kovács B, Vastag O: Fluoroangiographic picture of the acute stage of the retinal lesion in subacute sclerosing panencephalitis. *Ophthalmologica* 177:264-269, 1978.

544. Landers MB III, Klintworth GK: Subacute sclerosing panencephalitis (SSPE); a clinicopathologic study of the retinal lesions. *Arch Ophthalmol* 86:156-163, 1971.

545. Nelson DA, Weiner A, Yanoff M, dePeralta J: Retinal lesions in subacute sclerosing panencephalitis. *Arch Ophthalmol* 84:613-621, 1970.

546. Robb RM, Watters GV: Ophthalmic manifestations of subacute sclerosing panencephalitis. *Arch Ophthalmol* 83:426-435, 1970.

547. Schulz E: Ophthalmologische Frühmanifestation einer subakuten sklerosierenden Panencephalitis; diagnostische und mögliche therapeutische Aspekte. *Ophthalmologica* 180:281-287, 1980.

548. Zagami AS, Lethlean AK: Chorioretinitis as a possible very early manifestation of subacute sclerosing panencephalitis. *Aust NZ J Med* 21:350-352, 1991.

Mumps Neuroretinitis

549. Foster RE, Lowder CY, Meisler DM, et al: Mumps neuroretinitis in an adolescent. *Am J Ophthalmol* 110:91-93, 1990.

550. Riffenburgh RS: Ocular manifestations of mumps. *Arch Ophthalmol* 66:739-743, 1961.

Rift Valley Fever Retinitis

551. Cohen C, Luntz MH: Rift-Valley-Fieber und Rickettsianretinitis einschliesslich Fluoresceinangiographie. *Klin Monatsbl Augenheilkd* 169:685-699, 1976.

552. Deutman AF, Klomp HJ: Rift Valley fever retinitis. *Am J Ophthalmol* 92:38-42, 1981.

553. Freed I: Rift Valley fever in man complicated by retinal changes and loss of vision. *S Afr Med J* 25:930-932, 1951.

554. Schrire L: Macular changes in Rift Valley fever. *S Afr Med J* 25:926-930, 1951.

555. Siam AL, Meegan JM, Gharbawi KF: Rift Valley fever ocular manifestations: Observations during the 1977 epidemic in Egypt. *Br J Ophthalmol* 64:366-374, 1980.

Retinal Vasculitis, Postviral and Other

556. Browning DJ: Mild frosted branch periphlebitis. *Am J Ophthalmol* 114:505-506, 1992.

557. Gass JDM: Fluorescein angiography in endogenous intraocular inflammation. *In:* Aronson SB, Gamble CN, Goodner EK, O'Connor GR, editors: *Clinical methods in uveitis: the Fourth Sloan Symposium on Uveitis,* St. Louis, 1968, CV Mosby, pp. 202-229.

558. Gass JDM: *Stereoscopic atlas of macular diseases; diagnosis and treatment,* ed. 2, St. Louis, 1977, CV Mosby, pp 310-311.

559. Ito Y, Nakano M, Kyu N, Takeuchi M: Frosted-branch angiitis in a child. *Jpn J Clin Ophthalmol* 30:797-803, 1976.

560. Karel I, Peleška M, Divišová G: Fluorescence angiography in retinal vasculitis in children's uveitis. *Ophthalmologica* 166:251-264, 1973.

561. Kasp E, Whiston R, Dumonde D, et al: Antibody affinity to retinal S-antigen in patients with retinal vasculitis. *Am J Ophthalmol* 113:697-701, 1992.

562. Kleiner RC, Kaplan HJ, Shakin JL, et al: Acute frosted retinal periphlebitis. *Am J Ophthalmol* 106:27-34, 1988.

563. Lim JI, Tessler HH, Goodwin JA: Anterior granulomatous uveitis in patients with multiple sclerosis. *Ophthalmology* 98:142-145, 1991.

564. Rabon RJ, Louis GJ, Zegarra H, Gutman FA: Acute bilateral posterior angiopathy with influenza A viral infection. *Am J Ophthalmol* 103:289-293, 1987.

565. Rucker CW: Sheathing of the retinal veins in multiple sclerosis. *JAMA* 127:970-973, 1945.

566. Sugin SL, Henderly DE, Friedman SM, et al: Unilateral frosted branch angiitis. *Am J Ophthalmol* 111:682-685, 1991.

567. Vander JF, Masciulli L: Unilateral frosted branch angiitis. *Am J Ophthalmol* 112:477-478, 1991.

568. Watanabe Y, Takeda N, Adachi-Usami E: A case of frosted branch angiitis. *Br J Ophthalmol* 71:553-558, 1987.

Retinochoroidal Degeneration Associated with Progressive Iris Necrosis

569. Margo CE, Friedman SM, Purdy EP, Mcleod EK: Retinochoroidal degeneration associated with progressive iris necrosis. *Arch Ophthalmol* 108:989-992, 1990.

Acute Posterior Multifocal Placoid Pigment Epitheliopathy (APMPPE)

570. Althaus C, Unsöld R, Figge C, Sundmacher R: Cerebral complications in acute posterior multifocal placoid pigment epitheliopathy. *Ger J Ophthalmol* 2:150-154, 1993.

571. Annesley WH, Tomer TL, Shields JA: Multifocal placoid pigment epitheliopathy. *Am J Ophthalmol* 76:511-518, 1973.

572. Azar P Jr, Gohd RS, Waltman D, Gitter KA: Acute posterior multifocal placoid pigment epitheliopathy associated with an adenovirus type 5 infection. *Am J Ophthalmol* 80:1003-1005, 1975.

573. Bird AC, Hamilton AM: Placoid pigment epitheliopathy presenting with bilateral serous retinal detachment. *Br J Ophthalmol* 56:881-886, 1972.

574. Blinder KJ, Peyman GA, Paris CL: Diffuse posterior punctate pigment epitheliopathy. *Retina* 14:31-35, 1994.

575. Bodiguel E, Benhamou A, Le Hoang P, Gautier JC: Infarctus cerebral, epitheliopathie en plaques et sarcoidose. *Rev Neurol* 148:746-751, 1992.

576. Bodine SR, Marino J, Camisa TJ, Salvate AJ: Multifocal choroiditis with evidence of Lyme disease. *Ann Ophthalmol* 24:169, 1992.

577. Bullock JD, Fletcher RL: Cerebrospinal fluid abnormalities in acute posterior multifocal placoid pigment epitheliopathy. *Am J Ophthalmol* 84:45-49, 1977.

578. Calabrese LH, Mallek JA: Primary angiitis of the central nervous system; report of 8 new cases, review of the literature, and proposal for diagnostic criteria. *Medicine* 67:20-39, 1988.

579. Charteris DG, Khanna V, Dhillon B: Acute posterior multifocal placoid pigment epitheliopathy complicated by central retinal vein occlusion. *Br J Ophthalmol* 73:765-768, 1989.

580. Charteris DG, Lee WR: Multifocal posterior uveitis: Clinical and pathological findings. *Br J Ophthalmol* 74:688-693, 1990.

581. DeLaey JJ: Fluoro-angiographic study of the choroid in man. *Doc Ophthalmol* 45:113-139, 1978.

582. Deutman AF, Lion F: Choriocapillaris nonperfusion in acute multifocal placoid pigment epitheliopathy. *Am J Ophthalmol* 84:652-657, 1977.

583. Deutman AF, Oosterhuis JA, Boen-Tan TN, Aan de Kerk AL: Acute posterior multifocal placoid pigment epitheliopathy; pigment epitheliopathy or choriocapillaritis. *Br J Ophthalmol* 56:863-874, 1972.

584. Dhaliwal RS, Maguire AM, Flower RW, Arribas NP: Acute posterior multifocal placoid pigment epitheliopathy; an indocyanine green angiographic study. *Retina* 13:317-325, 1993.

585. Dick DJ, Newman PK, Richardson J, et al: Acute posterior multifocal placoid pigment epitheliopathy and sarcoidosis. *Br J Ophthalmol* 72:74-77, 1988.

586. Espinasse-Berrod MA, Gotte D, Parent de Cruzon H, et al: Un cas d'épithéliopathie en plaques associé à des néovaisseaux sous-rétiniens. *J Fr Ophtalmol* 11:191-194, 1988.

587. Fishman GA, Baskin M, Jednock N: Spinal fluid pleocytosis in acute posterior multifocal placoid pigment epitheliopathy. *Ann Ophthalmol* 33-36, 1977.

588. Fishman GA, Rabb MF, Kaplan J: Acute posterior multifocal placoid pigment epitheliopathy. *Arch Ophthalmol* 92:173-177, 1974.

589. Fitzpatrick PJ, Robertson DM: Acute posterior multifocal placoid pigment epitheliopathy. *Arch Ophthalmol* 89:373-376, 1973.

590. Gass JDM: Acute posterior multifocal placoid pigment epitheliopathy. *Arch Ophthalmol* 80:177-185, 1968.

591. Gass JDM: Acute posterior multifocal placoid pigment epitheliopathy: a long-term follow-up study. *In:* Fine SL, Owens SL, editors: *Management of retinal vascular and macular disorders,* Baltimore, 1983, Williams & Wilkins, pp. 176-181.

592. Gass JDM: *Stereoscopic atlas of macular diseases; diagnosis and treatment,* ed. 3, St. Louis, 1987, CV Mosby, pp. 504-510.

593. Hammer ME, Grizzard WS, Travies D: Death associated with acute posterior multifocal placoid pigment epitheliopathy. *Arch Ophthalmol* 107:170-171, 1989.

594. Hector RE: Acute posterior multifocal placoid pigment epitheliopathy. *Am J Ophthalmol* 86:424-425, 1978.

595. Holt WS, Regan CDJ, Trempe C: Acute posterior multifocal placoid pigment epitheliopathy. *Am J Ophthalmol* 81:403-412, 1976.

596. Jacklin HN: Acute posterior multifocal placoid pigment epitheliopathy and thyroiditis. *Arch Ophthalmol* 95:995-997, 1977.

597. Jenkins RB, Savino PJ, Pilkerton AR: Placoid pigment epitheliopathy with swelling of the optic disks. *Arch Neurol* 29:204-205, 1973.

598. Kawaguchi Y, Hara M, Hirose T, et al: A case of systemic lupus erythematosus complicated with multifocal posterior pigment epitheliopathy. *Ryumachi* 30:396-400, 1990.

599. Kersten DH, Lessell S, Carlow TJ: Acute posterior multifocal placoid pigment epitheliopathy and late-onset meningoencephalitis. *Ophthalmology* 94:393-396, 1987.

600. Kirkham TH, Ffytche TJ, Sanders MD: Placoid pigment epitheliopathy with retinal vasculitis and papillitis. *Br J Ophthalmol.* 56:875-880, 1972.

601. Laatikainen LT, Erkkilä H: Clinical and fluorescein angiographic findings of acute multifocal central subretinal inflammation. *Acta Ophthalmol* 51:645-655, 1973.

602. Laatikainen LT, Immonen IJR: Acute posterior multifocal placoid pigment epitheliopathy in connection with acute nephritis. *Retina* 8:122-124, 1988.

603. Lewis RA, Martonyi CL: Acute posterior multifocal placoid pigment epitheliopathy; a recurrence. *Arch Ophthalmol* 93:235-238, 1975.

604. Lyness AL, Bird AC: Recurrences of acute posterior multifocal placoid pigment epitheliopathy. *Am J Ophthalmol* 98:203-207, 1984.

605. McGuinness R, Mitchell P: A case of acute posterior multifocal placoid pigment epitheliopathy associated with erythema nodosum. *Aust J Ophthalmol* 5:48-51, 1977.

606. Priluck IA, Robertson DM, Buettner H: Acute posterior multifocal placoid pigment epitheliopathy; urinary findings. *Arch Ophthalmol* 99:1560-1562, 1981.

607. Reuscher A: Zur Pathogenese der sogenannten akuten hinteren multifokalen placoiden Pigmentepitheliopathie. *Klin Monatsbl Augenheilkd* 165:775-784, 1974.

608. Ryan SJ, Maumenee AE: Acute posterior multifocal placoid pigment epitheliopathy. *Am J Ophthalmol* 74:1066-1074, 1972.

609. Savino PJ, Weinberg RJ, Yassin JG, Pilkerton AR: Diverse manifestations of acute posterior multifocal placoid pigment epitheliopathy. *Am J Ophthalmol* 77:659-662, 1974.

610. Sigelman J, Behrens M, Hilal S: Acute posterior multifocal placoid pigment epitheliopathy associated with cerebral vasculitis and homonymous hemianopia. *Am J Ophthalmol* 88:919-924, 1979.

611. Smith CH, Savino PJ, Beck RW, et al: Acute posterior multifocal placoid pigment epitheliopathy and cerebral vasculitis. *Arch Neurol* 40:48-50, 1983.

612. Spaide RF, Yannuzzi LA, Slakter J: Choroidal vasculitis in acute posterior multifocal placoid pigment epitheliopathy. *Br J Ophthalmol* 75:685-687, 1991.

613. Stoll G, Reiners K, Schwartz A, et al: Acute posterior multifocal placoid pigment epitheliopathy with cerebral involvement. *J Neurol Neurosurg Psychiatr* 54:77-79, 1991.

614. Tönjes W, Mielke U, Schmidt HJ, et al: Akute multifokale plakoide Pigmentepitheliopathie mit entzündlichem Liquorbefund; sonderform einer Borreliose? *Dtsch Med Wochenschr* 114:793-795, 1989.

615. Van Buskirk EM, Lessell S, Friedman E: Pigmentary epitheliopathy and erythema nodosum. *Arch Ophthalmol* 85:369-372, 1971.

616. Weinstein JM, Bresnick GH, Bell CL, et al: Acute posterior multifocal placoid pigment epitheliopathy associated with cerebral vasculitis. *J Clin Neuro-Ophthalmol* 8:195-201, 1988.

617. Williams DF, Mieler WF: Long-term follow-up of acute multifocal posterior placoid pigment epitheliopathy. *Br J Ophthalmol* 73:985-990, 1989.

618. Wilson CA, Choromokos EA, Sheppard R: Acute posterior multifocal placoid pigment epitheliopathy and cerebral vasculitis. *Arch Ophthalmol* 106:796-800, 1988.

619. Wolf MD, Alward WLM, Folk JC: Long-term visual function in acute posterior multifocal placoid pigment epitheliopathy. *Arch Ophthalmol* 109:800-803, 1991.

620. Wolf MD, Folk JC, Goeken NE: Acute posterior multifocal pigment epitheliopathy and optic neuritis in a family. *Am J Ophthalmol* 110:89-90, 1990.

621. Wolf MD, Folk JC, Nelson JA, Peeples ME: Acute, posterior, multifocal, placoid, pigment epitheliopathy and Lyme disease. *Arch Ophthalmol* 110:750, 1992.

622. Wolf MD, Folk JC, Panknen CA, Goeken NE: HLA-B7 and HLA-DR2 antigens and acute posterior multifocal placoid pigment epitheliopathy. *Arch Ophthalmol* 108:698-700, 1990.

729

623. Wright BE, Bird AC, Hamilton AM: Placoid pigment epitheliopathy and Harada's disease. *Br J Ophthalmol* 62:609-621, 1978.

624. Young NJA, Bird AC, Sehmi K: Pigment epithelial diseases with abnormal choroidal perfusion. *Am J Ophthalmol* 90:607-618, 1980.

Acute Idiopathic Maculopathy

625. Fish RH, Territo C, Anand R: Pseudohypopyon in unilateral acute idiopathic maculopathy. *Retina* 13:26-28, 1993.

626. Yannuzzi LA, Jampol LM, Rabb MF, et al: Unilateral acute idiopathic maculopathy. *Arch Ophthalmol* 109:1411-1416, 1991.

Acute Retinal Pigment Epitheliitis

627. Chittum ME, Kalina RE: Acute retinal pigment epitheliitis. *Ophthalmology* 94:1114-1119, 1987.

628. Deutman AF: Acute retinal pigment epitheliitis. *Am J Ophthalmol* 78:571-578, 1974.

629. Eifrig DE, Knobloch WH, Moran JA: Retinal pigment epitheliitis. *Ann Ophthalmol* 9:639-642, 1977.

630. Friedman MW: Bilateral recurrent acute retinal pigment epitheliitis. *Am J Ophthalmol* 79:567-570, 1975.

631. Krill AE, Deutman AF: Acute retinal pigment epitheliitis. *Am J Ophthalmol* 74:193-205, 1972.

Multiple Evanescent White Dot Syndrome

632. Aaberg TM: Multiple evanescent white dot syndrome. *Arch Ophthalmol* 106:1162-1163, 1988.

633. Aaberg TM, Campo RV, Joffe L: Recurrences and bilaterality in the multiple evanescent white-dot syndrome. *Am J Ophthalmol* 100:29-37, 1985.

634. Borruat F-X, Othenin-Girard P, Safran AB: Multiple evanescent white dot syndrome. *Klin Monatsbl Augenheilkd* 198:453-456, 1991.

635. Bos PJM, Deutman AF: Acute macular neuroretinopathy. *Am J Ophthalmol* 80:573-584, 1975.

636. Callanan D, Gass JDM: Multifocal choroiditis and choroidal neovascularization associated with the multiple evanescent white dot and acute idiopathic blind spot enlargement syndrome. *Ophthalmology* 99:1678-1685, 1992.

637. Chung Y-M, Yeh T-S, Liu J-H: Increased serum IgM and IgG in the multiple evanescent white-dot syndrome. *Am J Ophthalmol* 104:187-188, 1987.

638. Cooper ML, Lesser RL: Prolonged course of bilateral acute idiopathic blind spot enlargement. *J Clin Neuro-Ophthalmol* 12:173-177, 1992.

639. Dodwell DG, Jampol LM, Rosenberg M, et al: Optic nerve involvement associated with the multiple evanescent white-dot syndrome. *Ophthalmology* 97:862-868, 1990.

640. Dreyer RF, Gass JDM. Multifocal choroiditis and panuveitis; a syndrome that mimics ocular histoplasmosis. *Arch Ophthalmol* 102:1776-1784, 1984.

641. Fletcher WA, Imes RK, Goodman D, Hoyt WF: Acute idiopathic blind spot enlargement; a big blind spot syndrome without optic disc edema. *Arch Ophthalmol* 106:44-49, 1988.

642. Gass JDM: Editorial: Retinal causes of the big blind spot syndrome. *J Clin Neuro-Ophthalmol* 9:144-145, 1989.

643. Gass JDM, Hamed LM: Acute macular neuroretinopathy and multiple evanescent white dot syndrome occurring in the same patients. *Arch Ophthalmol* 107:189-193, 1989.

644. Hamed LM, Glaser JS, Gass JDM, Schatz NJ: Protracted enlargement of the blind spot in multiple evanescent white dot syndrome. *Arch Ophthalmol* 107:194-198, 1989.

645. Hamed LM, Schatz NJ, Glaser JS, Gass JDM: Acute idiopathic blind spot enlargement without optic disc edema. *Arch Ophthalmol* 106:1030-1031, 1988.

646. Ie D, Glaser BM, Murphy RP, et al: Indocyanine green angiography in multiple evanescent white-dot syndrome. *Am J Ophthalmol* 117:7-12, 1994.

647. Jampol LM, Sieving PA, Pugh D, et al: Multiple evanescent white dot syndrome. I. Clinical findings. *Arch Ophthalmol* 102:671-674, 1984.

648. Jost BF, Olk RJ, McGaughey A: Bilateral symptomatic multiple evanescent white-dot syndrome. *Am J Ophthalmol* 101:489-490, 1986.

649. Keunen JEE, van Norren D: Foveal densitometry in the multiple evanescent white-dot syndrome. *Am J Ophthalmol* 105:561-562, 1988.

650. Khorram KD, Jampol LM, Rosenberg MA: Blind spot enlargement as a manifestation of multifocal choroiditis. *Arch Ophthalmol* 109:1403-1407, 1991.

651. Kimmel AS, Folk JC, Thompson HS, Strnad LS: The multiple evanescent white-dot syndrome with acute blind spot enlargement. *Am J Ophthalmol* 107:425-426, 1989.

652. Laatikainen L, Immonen I: Multiple evanescent white dot syndrome. *Graefes Arch Clin Exp Ophthalmol* 226:37-40, 1988.

653. Laatikainen L, Mustonen E: Asymmetry of retinitis pigmentosa-related to initial optic disc vasculitis. *Acta Ophthalmol* 70:543-548, 1992.

654. Lefrançois A, Hamard H, Corbe C, et al: A propos d'un cas de MEWDS. "Syndrome des taches blanches rétiniennes fugaces." *J Fr Ophtalmol* 12:103-109, 1989.

655. Leys A, Leys M, Jonckheere P, De Laey JJ: Multiple evanescent white dot syndrome (MEWDS). *Bull Soc Belge Ophtalmol* 236:97-108, 1990.

656. Leys M, Van Slycken S, Koller J, Van de Sompel W: Acute macular neuropathy after shock. *Bull Soc Belge Ophtalmol* 241:95-104, 1991.

657. Mamalis N, Daily MJ: Multiple evanescent white-dot syndrome; a report of eight cases. *Ophthalmology* 94:1209-1212, 1987.

658. McCollum CJ, Kimble JA: Peripapillary subretinal neovascularization associated with multiple evanescent white-dot syndrome. *Arch Ophthalmol* 110:13-15, 1992.

659. Meyer RJ, Jampol LM: Recurrences and bilaterality in the multiple evanescent white-dot syndrome. *Am J Ophthalmol* 101:388-389, 1986.

660. Morgan CM, Schatz H: Recurrent multifocal choroiditis. *Ophthalmology* 93:1138-1147, 1986.

661. Nakao K, Isashiki M: Multiple evanescent white dot syndrome. *Jpn J Ophthalmol* 30:376-384, 1986.

662. Nishimuta M, Kubota M, Kandatsu A, Kitahara K: Color vision defect in multiple evanescent white dot syndrome. *Folia Ophthalmol Jpn* 39:211-217, 1988.

663. Noske W, Danisevskis M, Priesnitz M, Foerster MH: Multiple evanescent white dot-syndrome. *Klin Monatsbl Augenheilkd* 201:107-109, 1992.

664. Sieving PA, Fishman GA, Jampol LM, Pugh D: Multiple evanescent white dot syndrome. II. Electrophysiology of the photoreceptors during retinal pigment epithelial disease. *Arch Ophthalmol* 102:675-679, 1984.

665. Singh K, de Frank MP, Shults WT, Watzke RC: Acute idiopathic blind spot enlargement; a spectrum of disease. *Ophthalmology* 98:497-502, 1991.

666. Slusher MM, Weaver RG: Multiple evanescent white dot syndrome. *Retina* 8:132-135, 1988.

667. Takeda M, Kimura S, Tamiya M: Acute disseminated retinal

pigment epitheliopathy. *Folia Ophthalmol Jpn* 35:2613-2620, 1984.

668. Tsai L, Jampol LM, Pollock SC, Olk J: Chronic recurrent multiple evanescent white dot syndrome. *Retina* 14:160-163, 1994.

669. van Meel GJ, Keunen JEE, van Norren D, van de Kraats J: Scanning laser densitometry in multiple evanescent white dot syndrome. *Retina* 13:29-35, 1993.

670. Wakakura M, Furuno K: Bilateral slowly progressive big blind spot syndrome. *J Neuro-Ophthalmol* 9:141-143, 1989.

671. Watzke RC, Packer AJ, Folk JC, et al: Punctate inner choroidopathy. *Am J Ophthalmol* 98:572-584, 1984.

672. Wyhinny GJ, Jackson JL, Jampol LM, Caro NC: Subretinal neovascularization following multiple evanescent white-dot syndrome. *Arch Ophthalmol* 108:1384, 1990.

Acute Zonal Occult Outer Retinopathy

673. Gass JDM: Acute zonal occult outer retinopathy. *J Clin Neuro-Ophthalmol* 13:79-97, 1993.

674. Jacobson SG, Morales DS, Sun XK, et al: Pattern of retinal dysfunction in acute zonal occult outer retinopathy. *Ophthalmology* 102:1187-1198, 1995.

Acute Annular Zonal Outer Retinopathy

675. Gass JDM: *Stereoscopic atlas of macular diseases; diagnosis and treatment,* ed. 3, St. Louis, 1987, CV Mosby, pp. 514-515.

676. Gass JDM, Stern C: Acute annular outer retinopathy as a variant of acute zonal occult outer retinopathy. *Am J Ophthalmol* 119:330-334, 1995.

677. Luckie A, Ai E, Del Piero E: Progressive zonal outer retinitis. *Am J Ophthalmol* 118:583-588, 1994.

678. Salem M, Ismail L: Immune complex deposition lines in a case of retinal vasculitis. *Graefes Arch Clin Exp Ophthalmol* 231:56-57, 1993.

Disorders Simulating the Presumed Ocular Histoplasmosis Syndrome (Pseudo-POHS)

679. Bottoni FG, Deutman AF, Aandekerk AL: Presumed ocular histoplasmosis syndrome and linear streak lesions. *Br J Ophthalmol* 73:528-535, 1989.

680. Doran RML, Hamilton AM: Disciform macular degeneration in young adults. *Trans Ophthalmol Soc UK* 102:471-480, 1982.

681. Dreyer RF, Gass JDM: Multifocal choroiditis and panuveitis; a syndrome that mimics ocular histoplasmosis. *Arch Ophthalmol* 102:1776-1784, 1984.

682. Gass JDM: *Stereoscopic atlas of macular diseases; diagnosis and treatment,* ed. 2, St Louis, 1977, CV Mosby, pp. 220, 360.

683. Gass JDM: *Stereoscopic atlas of macular diseases; diagnosis and treatment,* ed. 3, St. Louis, 1987, CV Mosby, pp. 534-549.

683a. Gass JDM, Margo CE, Levy MH: Progressive subretinal fibrosis and blindness in patients with multifocal granulomatous chorioretinitis. *Am J Ophthalmol* 122:76-85, 1996.

684. Hershey JM, Pulido JS, Folberg R, et al: Non-caseating conjunctival granulomas in patients with multifocal choroiditis and panuveitis. *Ophthalmology* 101:596-601, 1994.

685. Hirose S, Kuwabara T, Nussenblatt RB, et al: Uveitis induced in primates by interphotoreceptor retinoid-binding protein. *Arch Ophthalmol* 104:1698-1702, 1986.

686. Nozik RA, Dorsch W: A new chorioretinopathy associated with anterior uveitis. *Am J Ophthalmol* 76:758-762, 1973.

687. Palestine AG, Nussenblatt RB, Parver LM, Knox DL: Progressive subretinal fibrosis and uveitis. *Br J Ophthalmol* 68:667-673, 1984.

688. Saraux H, Pelosse B, Guigui A: Choroïdite multifocale interne: Pseudohistoplasmose. Forme européenne de l'histo-

plasmose présumée américaine. *J Fr Ophtalmol* 9:645-651, 1986.

689. Scheider A: Multifocal inner choroiditis. *Ger J Ophthalmol* 2:1-9, 1993.

690. Singerman LJ: Discussion of Morgan CM, Schatz H: Recurrent multifocal choroiditis. *Ophthalmology* 93:1143-1147, 1986.

691. Spaide RF, Skerry JE, Yannuzzi LA, DeRosa JT: Lack of the HLA-DR2 specificity in multifocal choroiditis and panuveitis. *Br J Ophthalmol* 74:536-537, 1990.

692. Spaide RF, Sugin S, Yannuzzi LA, DeRosa JT: Epstein-Barr virus antibodies in multifocal choroiditis and panuveitis. *Am J Ophthalmol* 112:410-413, 1991.

693. Spaide RF, Yannuzzi LA, Freund KB: Linear streaks in multifocal choroiditis and panuveitis. *Retina* 11:229-231, 1991.

694. Tessler HH, Deutsch TA: Multifocal choroiditis (inflammatory pseudo-histoplasmosis). *In:* Saari KM, editor: *Uveitis update: proceedings of the First International Symposium on Uveitis held in Hanasaari, Espoo, Finland on May 16-19, 1984,* Amsterdam, 1984, Excerpta Medica, pp. 221-226.

695. Watzke RC, Packer AJ, Folk JC, et al: Punctate inner choroidopathy. *Am J Ophthalmol* 98:572-584, 1984.

Acute Macular Neuroretinopathy

696. Bos PJM, Deutman AF: Acute macular neuroretinopathy. *Am J Ophthalmol* 80:573-584, 1975.

697. Campo RV, Flindall RJ: Traumatic macular atrophy. *Ocular Ther* 2(1):2-7, 1985.

698. Gass JDM, Hamed LM: Acute macular neuroretinopathy and multiple evanescent white dot syndrome occurring in the same patients. *Arch Ophthalmol* 107:189-193, 1989.

699. Gass JDM: *Stereoscopic atlas of macular diseases; diagnosis and treatment,* ed. 2, St. Louis, 1977, CV Mosby, p. 304.

700. Goldbaum MH: Retinal depression sign indicating a small retinal infarct. *Am J Ophthalmol* 86:45-55, 1978.

701. Guzak SV, Kalina RE, Chenoweth RG: Acute macular neuroretinopathy following adverse reaction to intravenous contrast media. *Retina* 3:312-317, 1983.

702. Leys M, Van Slycken S, Koller J, Van de Sompel W: Acute macular neuropathy after shock. *Bull Soc Belge Ophtalmol* 241:95-104, 1991.

703. Miller MH, Spalton DJ, Fitzke FW, Bird AC: Acute macular neuroretinopathy. *Ophthalmology* 96:265-269, 1989.

704. Nagasawa N, Hommura S: A case of acute macular neuroretinopathy—an optical consideration on the peculiar features of fundus oculi. *Acta Soc Ophthalmol Jpn* 86:2044-2049, 1982.

705. Neetens A, Burvenich H: Presumed inflammatory maculopathies. *Trans Ophthalmol Soc UK* 98:160-166, 1978.

706. O'Brien DM, Farmer SG, Kalina RE, Leon JA: Acute macular neuroretinopathy following intravenous sympathomimetics. *Retina* 9:281-286, 1989.

707. Priluck IA, Buettner H, Robertson DM: Acute macular neuroretinopathy. *Am J Ophthalmol* 86:775-778, 1978.

708. Putteman A, Toussaint D, Deutman AF: Neuroretinopathie maculaire aigue. *Bull Soc Belge Ophtalmol* 199-200:35-41, 1982.

709. Rait JL, O'Day J: Acute macular neuroretinopathy. *Aust NZ J Ophthalmol* 15:337-340, 1987.

710. Rush JA: Acute macular neuroretinopathy. *Am J Ophthalmol* 83:490-494, 1977.

711. Sanders MD: Diagnostic difficulties in optic nerve disease and in papilloedema and disc oedema. *Trans Ophthalmol Soc UK* 96:386-394, 1976.

712. Sieving PA, Fishman GA, Salzano T, Rabb MF: Acute macular neuroretinopathy: Early receptor potential change suggests photoreceptor pathology. *Br J Ophthalmol* 68:229-234, 1984.

713. Van Herck M, Leys A, Missotten L: Acute macular neuroretinopathy. *Bull Soc Belge Ophtalmol* 210:119-125, 1984.

714. Weinberg RJ, Nerney JJ: Bilateral submacular hemorrhages associated with an influenza syndrome. *Ann Ophthalmol* 15:710-712, 1983.

Acute Exudative Polymorphous Vitelliform Maculopathy

715. Gass JDM, Chuang EL, Granek H: Acute exudative polymorphous vitelliform maculopathy. *Trans Am Ophthalmol Soc* 86:354-363, 1988.

Retinal and Optic Nerve Sarcoidosis

716. Aaberg TA: Editorial: The role of the ophthalmologist in the management of sarcoidosis. *Am J Ophthalmol* 103:99-100, 1987.

717. Asdourian GK, Goldberg MF, Busse BJ: Peripheral retinal neovascularization in sarcoidosis. *Arch Ophthalmol* 93:787-791, 1975.

718. Baarsma GS, La Hey E, Glasius E, et al: The predictive value of serum angiotensin converting enzyme and lysozyme levels in the diagnosis of ocular sarcoidosis. *Am J Ophthalmol* 104:211-217, 1987.

719. Bielory L, Frohman LP: Low-dose cyclosporine therapy of granulomatous optic neuropathy and orbitopathy. *Ophthalmology* 98:1732-1736, 1991.

720. Brod RD: Presumed sarcoid choroidopathy mimicking birdshot retinochoroidopathy. *Am J Ophthalmol* 109:357-358, 1990.

721. Brownstein S, Jannotta FS: Sarcoid granulomas of the optic nerve and retina; report of a case. *Can J Ophthalmol* 9:372-378, 1974.

722. Chan C-C, Wetzig RP, Palestine AG, et al: Immunohistopathology of ocular sarcoidosis; report of a case and discussion of immunopathogenesis. *Arch Ophthalmol* 105:1398-1402, 1987.

723. Chumbley LC, Kearns TP: Retinopathy of sarcoidosis. *Am J Ophthalmol* 73:123-131, 1972.

724. DeBroff BM, Donahue SP: Bilateral optic neuropathy as the initial manifestation of systemic sarcoidosis. *Am J Ophthalmol* 116:108-111, 1993.

725. Denis P, Nordmann J-P, Laroche L, Saraux H: Branch retinal vein occlusion associated with a sarcoid choroidal granuloma. *Am J Ophthalmol* 113:333-334, 1992.

726. Doxanas MT, Kelley JS, Prout TE: Sarcoidosis with neovascularization of the optic nerve head. *Am J Ophthalmol* 90:347-351, 1980.

727. Duker JS, Brown GC, McNamara JA: Proliferative sarcoid retinopathy. *Ophthalmology* 95:1680-1686, 1988.

728. Fiore PM, Friedman AH: Unusual chorioretinal degeneration associated with sarcoidosis. *Am J Ophthalmol* 106:490-491, 1988.

729. Franceschetti A, Babel J: La chorio-rétinite en "taches de bougie," manifestation de la maladie de Besnier-Boeck. *Ophthalmologica* 118:701-710, 1949.

730. Galetta S, Schatz NJ, Glaser JS: Acute sarcoid optic neuropathy with spontaneous recovery. *J Clin Neuro-Ophthalmol* 9:27-32, 1989.

731. Gass JDM, Olson CL: Sarcoidosis with optic nerve and retinal involvement; a clinicopathologic case report. *Trans Am Acad Ophthalmol Otolaryngol* 77:OP739-OP750, 1973.

732. Gould HL, Kaufman HE: Boeck's sarcoid of the ocular fundus; historical review and report of a case. *Am J Ophthalmol* 52:633-637, 1961.

733. Graham EM, Stanford MR, Shilling JS, Sanders MD: Neovascularisation associated with posterior uveitis. *Br J Ophthalmol* 71:826-833, 1987.

734. Jabs DA, Johns CJ: Ocular involvement in chronic sarcoidosis. *Am J Ophthalmol* 102:297-301, 1986.

735. Karcioglu ZA, Brear R: Conjunctival biopsy in sarcoidosis. *Am J Ophthalmol* 99:68-73, 1985.

736. Karma A: Ophthalmic changes in sarcoidosis. *Acta Ophthalmol Suppl* 141, 1979.

737. Karma A, Taskinen E, Kainulainen H, Partanen M: Phenotypes of conjunctival inflammatory cells in sarcoidosis. *Br J Ophthalmol* 76:101-106, 1992.

738. Kelly PJ, Weiter JJ: Resolution of optic disk neovascularization associated with intraocular inflammation. *Am J Ophthalmol* 90:545-548, 1980.

739. Kimmel AS, McCarthy MJ, Blodi CF, Folk JC: Branch retinal vein occlusion in sarcoidosis. *Am J Ophthalmol* 107:561-562, 1989.

740. Krohel GB, Charles H, Smith RS: Granulomatous optic neuropathy. *Arch Ophthalmol* 99:1053-1055, 1981.

741. Laties AM, Scheie HG: Evolution of multiple small tumors in sarcoid granuloma of the optic disk. *Am J Ophthalmol* 74:60-67, 1972.

742. Letocha CE, Shields JA, Goldberg RE: Retinal changes in sarcoidosis. *Can J Ophthalmol* 10:184-192, 1975.

743. Lustgarten JS, Mindel JS, Yablonski ME, Friedman AH: An unusual presentation of isolated optic nerve sarcoidosis. *J Clin Neuro-Ophthalmol* 3:13-18, 1983.

744. Madigan JC Jr, Gragoudas ES, Schwartz PL, Lapus JV: Peripheral retinal neovascularization in sarcoidosis and sickle cell anemia. *Am J Ophthalmol* 83:387-391, 1977.

745. Mansour AM: Sarcoid optic disc edema and optociliary shunts. *J Clin Neuro-Ophthalmol* 6:47-52, 1986.

746. Nessan VJ, Jacoway JR: Biopsy of minor salivary glands in the diagnosis of sarcoidosis. *N Engl J Med* 301:922-924, 1979.

747. Noble KG: Ocular sarcoidosis occurring as a unilateral optic disk vascular lesion. *Am J Ophthalmol* 87:490-493, 1979.

748. Obenauf CD, Shaw HE, Sydnor CF, Klintworth GK: Sarcoidosis and its ophthalmic manifestations. *Am J Ophthalmol* 86:648-655, 1978.

749. Ohara K, Okubo A, Sasaki H, Kamata K: Intraocular manifestations of systemic sarcoidosis. *Jpn J Ophthalmol* 36:452-457, 1992.

750. Pellegrini V, Ohno S, Hirose S, et al: Subretinal neovascularisation and snow banking in a case of sarcoidosis: case report. *Br J Ophthalmol* 70:474-477, 1986.

751. Sanders MD, Shilling JS: Retinal, choroidal, and optic disc involvement in sarcoidosis. *Trans Ophthalmol Soc UK* 96:140-144, 1976.

752. Spaide RF, Ward DL: Conjunctival biopsy in the diagnosis of sarcoidosis. *Br J Ophthalmol* 74:469-471, 1990.

753. Spalton DJ, Sanders MD: Fundus changes in histologically confirmed sarcoidosis. *Br J Ophthalmol* 65:348-358, 1981.

754. Tang RA, Grotta JC, Lee KF, Lee YE: Chiasmal syndrome in sarcoidosis. *Arch Ophthalmol* 101:1069-1073, 1983.

755. Weinreb RN: Diagnosing sarcoidosis by transconjunctival biopsy of the lacrimal gland. *Am J Ophthalmol* 97:573-576, 1984.

756. Weinreb RN, Kimura SJ: Uveitis associated with sarcoidosis and angiotensin converting enzyme. *Am J Ophthalmol* 89:180-185, 1980.

757. Weinreb RN, Tessler H: Laboratory diagnosis of ophthalmic sarcoidosis. *Surv Ophthalmol* 28:653-664, 1984.

Acute Idiopathic Multifocal Inner Retinitis and Neuroretinitis

758. Carroll DM, Franklin RM: Leber's idiopathic stellate retinopathy. *Am J Ophthalmol* 93:96-101, 1982.

759. Cohen SM, Davis JL, Gass JDM: Branch retinal arterial occlusions in multifocal retinitis with optic nerve edema. *Arch Ophthalmol* 113:1271-1276, 1995.

760. Dreyer RF, Hopen G, Gass JDM, Smith JL: Leber's idiopathic stellate neuroretinitis. *Arch Ophthalmol* 102:1140-1145, 1984.

761. Foster RE, Gutman FA, Meyers SM, Lowder CY: Acute multifocal inner retinitis. *Am J Ophthalmol* 111:673-681, 1991.

762. Gass JDM: Fluorescein angiography in endogenous intraocular inflammation. *In:* Aronson SB, Gamble CN, Goodner EK, O'Connor GR, editors: *Clinical methods in uveitis: the Fourth Sloan Symposium on Uveitis,* St. Louis, 1968, CV Mosby, pp. 214-215.

763. Goldstein BG, Pavan PR: Retinal infiltrates in six patients with an associated viral syndrome. *Retina* 5:144-150, 1985.

764. Maitland CG, Miller NR: Neuroretinitis. *Arch Ophthalmol* 102:1146-1150, 1984.

765. Rabon RJ, Louis GJ, Zegarra H, Gutman FA: Acute bilateral posterior angiopathy with influenza A viral infection. *Am J Ophthalmol* 103:289-293, 1987.

Behçet's Disease

766. Adinolfi M, Lehner T: Acute phase proteins and C9 in patients with Behçet's syndrome and aphthous ulcers. *Clin Exp Immunol* 25:36-39, 1976.

767. Atmaca LS: Fundus changes associated with Behçet's disease. *Graefes Arch Clin Exp Ophthalmol* 227:340-344, 1989.

768. Aydıntug AO, Tokgöz G, D'Cruz DP, et al: Antibodies to endothelial cells in patients with Behçet's disease. *Clin Immunol Immunopathol* 67:157-162, 1993.

769. Barra C, Belfort R Jr, Abreu MT, et al: Behçet's disease in Brazil—a review of 49 cases with emphasis on ophthalmic manifestations. *Jpn J Ophthalmol* 35:339-346, 1991.

770. BenEzra D, Cohen E: Treatment and visual prognosis in Behçets disease. *Br J Ophthalmol* 70:589-592, 1986.

771. BenEzra D, Maftzir G, Kalichman I, Barak V: Serum levels of interleukin-2 receptor in ocular Behçet's disease. *Am J Ophthalmol* 115:26-30, 1993.

772. Charteris DG, Champ C, Rosenthal AR, Lightman SL: Behçet's disease: Activated T lymphocytes in retinal perivasculitis. *Br J Ophthalmol* 76:499-501, 1992.

773. Chavis PS, Antonios SR, Tabbara KF: Cyclosporin effects on optic nerve and retinal vasculitis in Behçet's disease. *Doc Ophthalmol* 80:133-142, 1992.

774. Colvard DM, Robertson DM, O'Duffy JD: The ocular manifestations of Behçet's disease. *Arch Ophthalmol* 95:1813-1817, 1977.

775. D'Alessandro LP, Forster DJ, Rao NA: Anterior uveitis and hypopyon. *Am J Ophthalmol* 112:317-321, 1991.

776. Graham EM, Stanford MR, Sanders MD, et al: A point prevalence study of 150 patients with idiopathic retinal vasculitis: 1. Diagnostic value of ophthalmological features. *Br J Ophthalmol* 73:714-721, 1989.

777. Graham EM, Stanford MR, Shilling JS, Sanders MD: Neovascularisation associated with posterior uveitis. *Br J Ophthalmol* 71:826-833, 1987.

778. Gupta RC, O'Duffy JD, McDuffie FC, et al: Circulating immune complexes in active Behçet's disease. *Clin Exp Immunol* 34:213-218, 1978.

779. Hijikata K, Masuda K: Visual prognosis in Behçet's disease: Effects of cyclophosphamide and colchicine. *Jpn J Ophthalmol* 22:506, 1978.

780. International Study Group for Behçet's disease: Criteria for diagnosis of Behçet's disease. *Lancet* 335:1078-1080, 1990.

781. James DG: Editorial: Behçet's syndrome. *N Engl J Med* 301:431-432, 1979.

782. James DG: 'Silk route disease' (Behçet's disease). *West J Med* 148:433-437, 1988.

783. James DG, Spiteri MA: Behçet's disease. *Ophthalmology* 89:1279-1284, 1982.

784. Kansu T, Kirkali P, Kansu E, Zileli T: Optic neuropathy in Behçet's disease. *J Clin Neuro-Ophthalmol* 9:277-280, 1989.

785. Kasp E, Whiston R, Dumonde D, et al: Antibody affinity to retinal S-antigen in patients with retinal vasculitis. *Am J Ophthalmol* 113:697-701, 1992.

786. Lehner T: Behçet's syndrome and autoimmunity. *Br Med J* 1:465-467, 1967.

787. Levinsky RJ, Lehner T: Circulating soluble immune complexes in recurrent oral ulceration and Behçet's syndrome. *Clin Exp Immunol* 32:193-198, 1978.

788. Mamo JG: Treatment of Behçet disease with chlorambucil; a follow-up report. Arch Ophthalmol 94:580-583, 1976.

789. Mamo JG, Baghdassarian A: Behçet's disease; a report of 28 cases. *Arch Ophthalmol* 71:4-14, 1964.

790. Michelson JB, Chisari FV, Kansu T: Antibodies to oral mucosa in patients with ocular Behçet's disease. *Ophthalmology* 92:1277-1281, 1985.

791. Michelson JB, Michelson PE, Chisari FV: Subretinal neovascular membrane and disciform scar in Behçet's disease. *Am J Ophthalmol* 90:182-185, 1980.

792. Mishima S, Masuda K, Izawa Y, et al: Behçet's disease in Japan: ophthalmologic aspects. *Trans Am Ophthalmol Soc* 77:225-279, 1979.

793. Mizuki N, Inoko H, Ando H, et al: Behçet's disease associated with one of the HLA-B51 subantigens, HLA-B* 5101. *Am J Ophthalmol* 116:406-409, 1993.

794. Müftüoglu AÜ, Pazarli H, Yurdakul S, et al: Short term cyclosporin A treatment of Behçet's disease. *Br J Ophthalmol* 71:387-390, 1987.

795. Nussenblatt RB, Palestine AG, Chan C-C: Cyclosporin A therapy in the treatment of intraocular inflammatory disease resistant to systemic corticosteroids and cytotoxic agents. *Am J Ophthalmol* 96:275-282, 1983.

796. O'Duffy JD, Carney JA, Deodhar S: Behçet's disease; report of 10 cases, 3 with new manifestations. *Ann Intern Med* 75:561-570, 1971.

797. Ohno S, Ohguchi M, Hirose S, et al: Close association of HLA-Bw51 with Behçet's disease. *Arch Ophthalmol* 100:1455-1458, 1982.

798. Raizman MB, Foster CS: Plasma exchange in the therapy of Behçet's disease. *Graefes Arch Clin Exp Ophthalmol* 227:360-363, 1989.

799. Sezer FN: The isolation of a virus as the cause of Behçet's disease. *Am J Ophthalmol* 36:301-315, 1953.

800. Shimizu K: Fluorescein fundus angiography in Behçet's syndrome. Mod Probl Ophthalmol 10:224-228, 1972.

801. Shimizu T: Clinical and immunological studies on Behçet's syndrome. *Folia Ophthalmol Jpn* 22:801-810, 1971.

802. Shimizu T: Clinicopathological studies on Behçet's disease. *In:* Dilşen N, Koniçe M, Övül C, editors: *Behçet's disease: proceedings of an International Symposium on Behçet's Disease, Istanbul, 29-30 September 1977,* Amsterdam, 1979, Excerpta Medica, pp. 9-43.

803. Smulders FM, Oosterhuis JA: Treatment of Behçet's disease with chlorambucil. *Ophthalmologica* 171:347-352, 1975.

804. Tabbara KF: Chlorambucil in Behçet's disease; a reappraisal. *Ophthalmology* 90:906-908, 1983.

805. Tessler HH, Jennings T: High-dose short-term chlorambucil for intractable sympathetic ophthalmia and Behçet's disease. *Br J Ophthalmol* 74:353-357, 1990.

806. Whitcup SM, Salvo EC Jr, Nussenblatt RB: Combined cyclosporine and corticosteroid therapy for sight-threatening uveitis in Behçet's disease. *Am J Ophthalmol* 118:39-45, 1994.

807. Yazici H, Pazarli H, Barnes CG, et al: A controlled trial of azathioprine in Behçet's syndrome. *N Engl J Med* 322:281-285, 1990.

Retinitis and Vitritis with Vitreous Base Organization (Par Planitis, Peripheral Uveitis, or Chronic Cyclitis)

808. Aaberg TM: Editorial: The enigma of pars planitis. *Am J Ophthalmol* 103:828-830, 1987.

809. Aaberg TM, Cesarz TJ, Flickinger RR: Treatment of peripheral uveoretinitis by cryotherapy. *Am J Ophthalmol* 75:685-688, 1973.

810. Arkfeld DF, Brockhurst RJ: Peripapillary subretinal neovascularization in peripheral uveitis. *Retina* 5:157-160, 1985.

811. Augsburger JJ, Annesley WH Jr, Sergott RC, et al: Familial pars planitis. *Ann Ophthalmol* 13:553-557, 1981.

812. Bec P, Arne JL, Philippot V, et al: L'uvéo-rétinite basale (uvéite périphérique, cyclite postérieure chronique, pars planite, vitrite, hyalo-rétinite) et les autres inflammations de la périphérie rétinienne. *Arch Ophthalmol (Paris)* 37:169-196, 1977.

813. Breger BC, Leopold IH: The incidence of uveitis in multiple sclerosis. *Am J Ophthalmol* 62:540-545, 1966.

814. Brockhurst RJ: Retinoschisis; complication of peripheral uveitis. *Arch Ophthalmol* 99:1998-1999, 1981.

815. Brockhurst RJ, Schepens CL: Uveitis. IV. Peripheral uveitis: the complication of retinal detachment. *Arch Ophthalmol* 80:747-753, 1968.

816. Brockhurst RJ, Schepens CL, Okamura ID: Uveitis. II. Peripheral uveitis: clinical description, complications and differential diagnosis. *Am J Ophthalmol* 49:1257-1266, 1960.

817. Brockhurst RJ, Schepens CL, Okamura ID: Uveitis. III. Peripheral uveitis: pathogenesis, etiology and treatment. *Am J Ophthalmol* 51:19-26, 1961.

818. Calder V, Owen S, Watson C, et al: MS: A localized immune disease of the central nervous system. *Immunol Today* 10:99-103, 1989.

819. Cantrill HL, Ramsay RC, Knobloch WH, Purple RL: Electrophysiologic changes in chronic pars planitis. *Am J Ophthalmol* 91:505-512, 1981.

820. Culbertson WW, Giles CL, West C, Stafford T: Familial pars planitis. *Retina* 3:179-181, 1983.

821. Devenyi RG, Mieler WF, Lambrou FH, et al: Cryopexy of the vitreous base in the management of peripheral uveitis. *Am J Ophthalmol* 106:135-138, 1988.

822. Doft BH: Pars planitis in identical twins. *Retina* 3:32-33, 1983.

823. Felder KS, Brockhurst RJ: Neovascular fundus abnormalities in peripheral uveitis. *Arch Ophthalmol* 100:750-754, 1982.

824. Gärtner J: The fine structure of the vitreous base of the human eye and pathogenesis of pars planitis. *Am J Ophthalmol* 71:1317-1327, 1971.

825. Gass JDM: Fluorescein angiography in endogenous intraocular inflammation. *In:* Aronson SB, Gamble CN, Goodner EK, O'Connor GR, editors: *Clinical methods in uveitis: the Fourth Sloan Symposium on Uveitis,* St. Louis, 1968, CV Mosby, pp. 202-229.

826. Gass JDM: *Stereoscopic atlas of macular diseases; diagnosis and treatment,* ed. 2, St. Louis, 1977, CV Mosby, p. 306.

827. Giles CL: Peripheral uveitis in patients with multiple sclerosis. *Am J Ophthalmol* 70:17-19, 1970.

828. Giles CL, Tanton JH: Peripheral uveitis in three children of one family. *J Pediatr Ophthalmol Strabismus* 17:297-299, 1980.

829. Gills JP Jr: Combined medical and surgical therapy for complicated cases of peripheral uveitis. *Arch Ophthalmol* 79:723-728, 1968.

830. Godfrey WA, Epstein WV, O'Connor GR, et al: The use of chlorambucil in intractable idiopathic uveitis. *Am J Ophthalmol* 78:415-428, 1974.

831. Green WR: Discussion of Godfrey WA, Smith RE, Kimura SJ: Chronic cyclitis: corticosteroid therapy. *Trans Am Ophthalmol Soc* 74:187-188, 1976.

832. Henderly DE, Haymond RS, Rao NA, Smith RE: The significance of the pars plana exudate in pars planitis. *Am J Ophthalmol* 103:669-671, 1987.

833. Hikichi T, Trempe CL: Role of the vitreous in the prognosis of peripheral uveitis. *Am J Ophthalmol* 116:401-405, 1993.

834. Josephberg RG, Kanter ED, Jaffee RM: A fluorescein angiographic study of patients with pars planitis and peripheral exudation (snowbanking) before and after cryopexy. *Ophthalmology* 101:1262-1266, 1994.

835. Kalina PH, Pach JM, Buettner H, Robertson DM: Neovascularization of the disc in pars planitis. *Retina* 10:269-273, 1990.

836. Kenyon KR, Pederson JE, Green WR, Maumenee AE: Fibroglial proliferation in pars planitis. *Trans Ophthalmol Soc UK* 95:391-397, 1975.

837. Khodadoust AA, Karnama Y, Stoessel KM, Puklin JE: Pars planitis and autoimmune endotheliopathy. *Am J Ophthalmol* 102:633-639, 1986.

838. Kimura SJ, Hogan MJ: Chronic cyclitis. *Trans Am Ophthalmol Soc* 61:397-417, 1963.

839. Malinowski SM, Pulido JS, Folk JC: Long-term visual outcome and complications associated with pars planitis. *Ophthalmology* 100:818-825, 1993.

840. Malinowski SM, Pulido JS, Goeken NE, et al: The association of HLA-B8, B51, DR2, and multiple sclerosis in pars planitis. *Ophthalmology* 100:1199-1205, 1993.

841. Maumenee AE: Clinical entities in "uveitis": an approach to the study of intraocular inflammation. *Am J Ophthalmol* 69:1-27, 1970.

842. Mieler WF, Will BR, Lewis H, Aaberg TM: Vitrectomy in the management of peripheral uveitis. *Ophthalmology* 95:859-864, 1988.

843. Nissenblatt MJ, Masciulli L, Yarian DL, Duvoisin P: Pars planitis—a demyelinating disease? *Arch Ophthalmol* 99:697, 1981.

844. Nussenblatt RB, Palestine AG: Cyclosporin (Sandimmun®) therapy: Experience in the treatment of pars planitis and present therapeutic guidelines. *Dev Ophthalmol* 23:177-184, 1992.

845. Pederson JE, Kenyon KR, Green WR, Maumenee AE: Pathology of pars planitis. *Am J Ophthalmol* 86:762-774, 1978.

846. Porter R: Uveitis in association with multiple sclerosis. *Br J Ophthalmol* 56:478-481, 1972.

847. Pruett RC, Brockhurst RJ, Letts NF: Fluorescein angiography of peripheral uveitis. *Am J Ophthalmol* 77:448-453, 1974.

848. Shorb SR, Irvine AR, Kimura SJ, Morris BW: Optic disk neovascularization associated with chronic uveitis. *Am J Ophthalmol* 82:175-178, 1976.

849. Smith RE, Godfrey WA, Kimura SJ: Chronic cyclitis. I. Course and visual prognosis. *Trans Am Acad Ophthalmol Otolaryngol* 77:OP760-OP768, 1973.

850. Welch RB, Maumenee AE, Wahlen HE: Peripheral posterior segment inflammation, vitreous opacities, and edema of the posterior pole; pars planitis. *Arch Ophthalmol* 64:540-549, 1960.

851. Wetzig RP, Chan C-C, Nussenblatt RB, et al: Clinical and immunopathological studies of pars planitis in a family. *Br J Ophthalmol* 72:5-10, 1988.

852. Yokoyama MM, Matsui Y, Yamashiroya HM, et al: Humoral and cellular immunity studies in patients with Vogt-Koyanagi-Harada syndrome and pars planitis. *Invest Ophthalmol Vis Sci* 20:364-370, 1981.

Idiopathic Diffuse Nonnecrotizing Retinitis and Vitritis Without Vitreous Base Organization (Idiopathic Senile Vitritis)

853. Bennett SR, Folk JC, Kimura AE, et al: Autosomal dominant neovascular inflammatory vitreoretinopathy. *Ophthalmology* 97:1125-1136, 1990.

854. Brinton GS, Osher RH, Gass JDM: Idiopathic vitritis. *Retina* 3:95-98, 1983.

855. Dugel PU, Rao NA, Ozler S: Pars plana vitrectomy for intraocular inflammation-related cystoid macular edema unresponsive to corticosteroids; a preliminary study. *Ophthalmology* 99:1535-1541, 1992.

856. Gass JDM: Fluorescein angiography in endogenous intraocular inflammation. *In:* Aronson SB, Gamble CN, Goodner EK, O'Connor GR, editors: *Clinical methods in uveitis: the Fourth Sloan Symposium on Uveitis,* St. Louis, 1968, CV Mosby, pp. 202-229.

857. Gass JDM: *Stereoscopic atlas of macular diseases; diagnosis and treatment,* ed. 3, St. Louis, 1987, CV Mosby, pp. 526-527.

858. Johns KJ, Hummell DS, McCurley TL, Lawton AR III: Cellular infiltration of the vitreous in a patient with X-linked immunodeficiency with increased IgM. *Am J Ophthalmol* 113:183-186, 1992.

Vitiliginous Chorioretinitis (Bird-Shot Retinochoroidopathy)

859. Albert DM, Nordlund JJ, Lerner AB: Ocular abnormalities occurring with vitiligo. *Ophthalmology* 86:1145-1158, 1979.

860. Albert DM, Sober AJ, Fitzpatrick TB: Iritis in patients with cutaneous melanoma and vitiligo. *Arch Ophthalmol* 96:2081-2084, 1978.

861. Albert DM, Wagoner MD, Pruett RC, et al: Vitiligo and disorders of the retinal pigment epithelium. *Br J Ophthalmol* 67:153-156, 1983.

862. Brod RD: Presumed sarcoid choroidopathy mimicking bird-shot retinochoroidopathy. *Am J Ophthalmol* 109:357-358, 1990.

863. Brucker AJ, Deglin EA, Bene C, Hoffman ME: Subretinal choroidal neovascularization in birdshot retinochoroidopathy. *Am J Ophthalmol* 99:40-44, 1985.

864. Cummings KI, Cottel WI: Idiopathic guttate hypomelanosis. *Arch Dermatol* 93:184-186, 1966.

865. Fich M, Rosenberg T: Birdshot retinochoroidopathy in monozygotic twins. *Acta Ophthalmol* 70:693-697, 1992.

866. Fuerst DJ, Tessler HH, Fishman GA, et al: Birdshot retinochoroidopathy. *Arch Ophthalmol* 102:214-219, 1984.

867. Gass JDM: Acute Vogt-Koyanagi-Harada-like syndrome occurring in a patient with metastatic cutaneous melanoma. *In:* Saari KM, editor: *Uveitis update: proceedings of the First International Symposium on Uveitis held in Hanasaari, Espoo, Finland on May 16-19, 1984,* Amsterdam, 1984, Excerpta Medica, pp. 407-408.

868. Gass JDM: Vitiliginous chorioretinitis. *Arch Ophthalmol* 99:1778-1787, 1981.

869. Godel V, Baruch E, Lazar M: Late development of chorioretinal lesions in birdshot retinochoroidopathy. *Ann Ophthalmol* 21:49-52, 1989.

870. Heaton JM, Mills RP: Sensorineural hearing loss associated with birdshot retinochoroidopathy. *Arch Otolaryngol Head Neck Surg* 119:680-681, 1993.

871. Hirose T, Katsumi O, Pruett RC, et al: Retinal function in birdshot retinochoroidopathy. *Acta Ophthalmol* 69:327-337, 1991.

872. Kaplan HJ, Aaberg TM: Birdshot retinochoroidopathy. *Am J Ophthalmol* 90:773-782, 1980.

873. LeHoang P, Ozdemir N, Benhamou A, et al: HLA-A29.2 subtype associated with birdshot retinochoroidopathy. *Am J Ophthalmol* 113:33-35, 1992.

874. Nussenblatt RB, Mittal KK, Ryan S, et al: Birdshot retinochoroidopathy associated with HLA-A29 antigen and immune responsiveness to retinal S-antigen. *Am J Ophthalmol* 94:147-158, 1982.

875. Oosterhuis JA, Baarsma GS, Polak BCP: Birdshot chorioretinopathy—vitiliginous chorioretinitis. *Int Ophthalmol* 5:137-144, 1982.

876. Priem HA, De Rouck A, De Laey J-J, Bird AC: Electrophysiological studies in birdshot chorioretinopathy. *Am J Ophthalmol* 106:430-436, 1988.

877. Priem HA, Kijlstra A, Noens L, et al: HLA typing in birdshot chorioretinopathy. *Am J Ophthalmol* 105:182-185, 1988.

878. Priem HA, Oosterhuis JA: Birdshot chorioretinopathy: clinical characteristics and evolution. *Br J Ophthalmol* 72:646-659, 1988.

879. Rosenberg PR, Noble KG, Walsh JB, Carr RE: Birdshot retinochoroidopathy. *Ophthalmology* 91:304-306, 1984.

880. Ryan SJ, Maumenee AE: Birdshot retinochoroidopathy. *Am J Ophthalmol* 89:31-45, 1980.

881. Soubrane G, Bokobza R, Coscas G: Late developing lesions in birdshot retinochoroidopathy. *Am J Ophthalmol* 109:204-210, 1990.

882. Soubrane G, Coscas G, Binaghi M, et al: Birdshot retinochoroidopathy and subretinal new vessels. *Br J Ophthalmol* 67:461-467, 1983.

883. Suttorp-Schulten MSA, Luyendijk L, van Dam AP, et al: Birdshot chorioretinopathy and Lyme borreliosis. *Am J Ophthalmol* 115:149-153, 1993.

884. Vitale AT, Rodriguez A, Foster CS: Low-dose cyclosporine therapy in the treatment of birdshot retinochoroidopathy. *Ophthalmology* 101:822-831, 1994.

885. Wagoner MD, Albert DM, Lerner AB, et al: New observations on vitiligo and ocular disease. *Am J Ophthalmol* 96:16-26, 1983.

Vitritis and Retinitis in Whipple's Disease

886. Avila MP, Jalkh AE, Feldman E, et al: Manifestations of Whipple's disease in the posterior segment of the eye. *Arch Ophthalmol* 102:384-390, 1984.

887. Durant WJ, Flood T, Goldberg MF, et al: Vitrectomy and Whipple's disease. *Arch Ophthalmol* 102:848-851, 1984.

888. Font RL, Rao NA, Issarescu S, McEntee WJ: Ocular involvement in Whipple's disease; light and electron microscopic observations. *Arch Ophthalmol* 96:1431-1436, 1978.

889. Gärtner J: Whipple's disease of the central nervous system, associated with ophthalmoplegia externa and severe asteroid hyalitis: a clinicopathologic study. *Doc Ophthalmol* 49:155-187, 1980.

890. Knox DL, Bayless TM, Yardley JH, Charache P: Whipple's disease presenting with ocular inflammation and minimal intestinal symptoms. *Johns Hopkins Med J* 123:175-182, 1968.

891. Krücke W, Stochdroph O: Über Veränderungen im Zentralnervensystem bei Whipple'scher Krankheit. *Verh Dtsch Ges Pathol* 46:198-202, 1962.

892. Leland TM, Chambers JK: Ocular findings in Whipple's disease. *South Med J* 71:335-337, 1978.

893. Margo CE Pavan PR, Groden LR: Chronic vitritis with macrophagic inclusions; a sequela of treated endophthalmitis due to a coryneform bacterium. *Ophthalmology* 95:156-161, 1988.

894. Rickman LS, Freeman WR, Green WR, et al: Brief report: Uveitis caused by *Tropheryma whippelii* (Whipple's bacillus). *N Engl J Med* 332:363-366, 1995.

895. Selsky EJ, Knox DL, Maumenee AE, Green WR: Ocular involvement in Whipple's disease. *Retina* 4:103-106, 1984.

896. Switz DM, Casey TR, Bogaty GV: Whipple's disease and papilledema; an unreported presentation. *Arch Intern Med* 123:74-77, 1969.

Crohn's Disease

897. Duker JS, Brown GC, Brooks L: Retinal vasculitis in Crohn's disease. *Am J Ophthalmol* 103:664-668, 1987.

898. Ernst BB, Lowder CY, Meisler DM, Gutman FA: Posterior segment manifestations of inflammatory bowel disease. *Ophthalmology* 98:1272-1280, 1991.

899. Gass JDM: *Stereoscopic atlas of macular disease; diagnosis and treatment.* ed. 3, St. Louis, 1987, CV Mosby, p. 538.

900. Hopkins DJ, Horan E, Burton IL, et al: Ocular disorders in a series of 332 patients with Crohn's disease. *Br J Ophthalmol* 58:732-737, 1974.

901. Johnson LA, Wirostko E, Wirostko WJ: Crohn's disease uveitis; parasitization of vitreous leukocytes by mollicute-like organisms. *Am J Clin Pathol* 91:259-264, 1989.

902. Knox DL, Schachat AP, Mustonen E: Primary, secondary and coincidental ocular complications of Crohn's disease. *Ophthalmology* 91:163-173, 1984.

903. Macoul KL: Ocular changes in granulomatous ileocolitis. *Arch Ophthalmol* 84:95-97, 1970.

904. Mallas EG, Mackintosh P, Asquith P, Cooke WT: Histocompatibility antigens in inflammatory bowel disease; their clinical significance and their association with arthropathy with special reference to HLA-B27 (W27). *Gut* 17:906-910, 1976.

905. Ruby AJ, Jampol LM: Crohn's disease and retinal vascular disease. *Am J Ophthalmol* 110:349-353, 1990.

906. Salmon JF, Wright JP, Bowen RM, Murray AD: Granulomatous uveitis in Crohn's disease; a clinicopathologic case report. *Arch Ophthalmol* 107:718-719, 1989.

907. Salmon JF, Wright JP, Murray ADN: Ocular inflammation in Crohn's disease. *Ophthalmology* 98:480-484, 1991.

8

Traumatic Retinopathy

▼ BERLIN'S EDEMA (COMMOTIO RETINAE)

After a blunt contusion to the front of the eye, a patient may experience acute visual loss caused by Berlin's edema (commotio retinae). In this condition the retina develops a gray-white color that affects primarily the outer retina[3,4,7,13,14] and that may be confined to the macular area (Fig. 8-1, *A* and *E*) or may involve extensive areas of the peripheral retina (Fig. 8-1, *B*). In some cases the whitening may be accompanied by retinal or preretinal hemorrhages (Fig. 8-2, *A* and *B*) or subretinal blood and choroidal rupture. The retinal whitening in the macular area may clear completely, and central vision may be restored (Fig. 8-1, *F*). In other instances, loss of central vision may be permanent and may be associated with either no visible fundus change, mottling of the retinal pigment epithelium (RPE), migration of pigment into the overlying retina, or partial- or full-thickness macular hole formation (Figs. 8-2, *D, G,* and *H,* and 8-4). The whitening in the peripheral retina may be followed initially by pigment mottling and later by atrophy of the RPE and migration of pigment into the overlying retina, producing a peripheral change that clinically and histopathologically simulates retinitis pigmentosa (Fig. 8-2, *E* and *F*).[1,6]

FIG. 8-1 Berlin's Edema (Commotio Retinae).

A to **D,** This 10-year-old boy was struck in the left eye by a rock. Visual acuity was 20/70. Note the zone of whitening involving the outer retinal layer in the macula (*arrows,* **A**). There was a large area of retinal whitening in the far periphery of the same eye (**B**). Angiography was normal and showed no evidence of retinal vascular abnormalities (**C** and **D**).

E and **F,** Berlin's edema of the left macula in a 20-year-old woman (**E**). Three days later the edema had disappeared and the macular function had returned to normal (**F**).

G to **I,** Photomicrographs of normal monkey retina (**G**), retina 4 hours (**H**), and retina 48 hours (**I**) after blunt trauma. Note disruption of photoreceptor cells outer segments (*arrow,* **H**), pyknotic nuclei in the outer nuclear layer *(ONL)* (**H** and **I**), and vacuolization of inner segment layer of photoreceptors (*arrow,* **I,** paraphenylenediamine dye).

(**G** and **H** from Sipperly JO, Quigley HA, Gass JDM: *Arch Ophthalmol* 96:2267, 1978; copyright 1978, American Medical Association.[13])

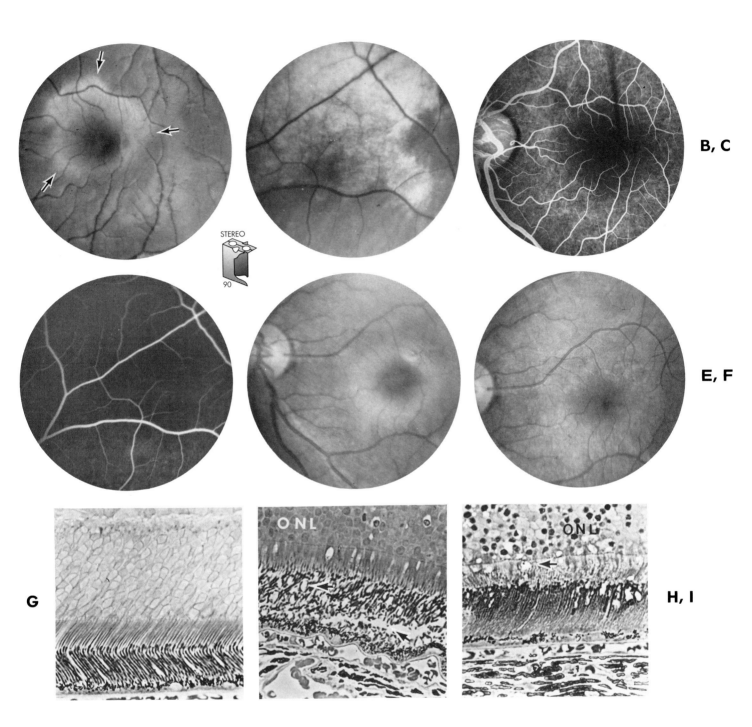

B, C

E, F

G

H, I

Fluorescein angiography typically shows no evidence of retinal vascular or choroidal permeability alterations in the area of Berlin's edema (Fig. 8-1, C and D).[1,7-9] Angiography occasionally shows a transient leakage of dye from the retinal arterioles in the posterior pole or staining at the level of the RPE (Fig. 8-2, C).[2] Following resolution of the outer retinal whitening, angiography may or may not show evidence of window defects in the RPE. Vitreous fluorophotometry usually shows no evidence of breakdown of the blood–retinal barrier.[12] Light and electron microscopic studies of Berlin's edema in humans as well as that produced experimentally in animals have shown that the outer retinal whitening is caused by fragmentation of the photoreceptor outer segments and acute damage to the receptor cells (Fig. 8-1, G and H).[9,11,13] This loss of transparency is associated with no or minimal extracellular or intracellular edema in the retinal cells and with minimal damage to the choriocapillaris.[4,5,11,13] Other changes may include breakdown of the outer blood–retinal barrier at the level of the RPE that is usually reestablished between 7 and 14 days.[5] If only the outer segments of the receptor cells are involved, these will regenerate rapidly and the retina may regain its normal appearance and function. A more severe contusion may cause contusion necrosis and atrophy of the outer retina (Fig. 8-2, G and H). The contusion damage to the retinal receptor cells is probably caused by mechanical distortion of the retina by deformation of the vitreous as well as hydraulic forces.[11]

Subretinal hemorrhage caused by choroidal rupture may occasionally accompany Berlin's edema (see Chapter 3). Trauma similar to that which causes Berlin's edema may also cause acute damage to the RPE and serous detachment of the macula (Fig. 8-2, C, and see Fig. 3-72, A to C), as well as acute tears in the retinal pigment epithelium.[10]

FIG. 8-2   Contusion Necrosis of the RPE and Retina.

A to C, This man sustained blunt trauma and visual loss in the right eye. Note outer retinal whitening and retinal and preretinal blood (**A** and **B**). Angiography (**C**) showed extensive staining caused by necrosis of the RPE, as well as evidence of curvilinear choroidal rupture underlying the blood.

D, Postcontusion macular hole *(arrow)* and retinal and RPE atrophy in a 19-year-old man previously struck in the eye with a baseball.

E and **F,** Peripheral retinal and RPE degeneration caused by blunt trauma. Note narrowing of the retinal vessels and migration of pigment into the retina *(arrow)* similar to that seen in retinitis pigmentosa.

G, Photomicrograph of the foveal area showing focal loss of receptor cells, cystic degeneration, and chorioretinal adhesions *(arrows)* following trauma. The separation of retina from the RPE is probably artifactitious.

H, Photomicrograph of the foveal area showing more severe postcontusion atrophy of the retina and RPE.

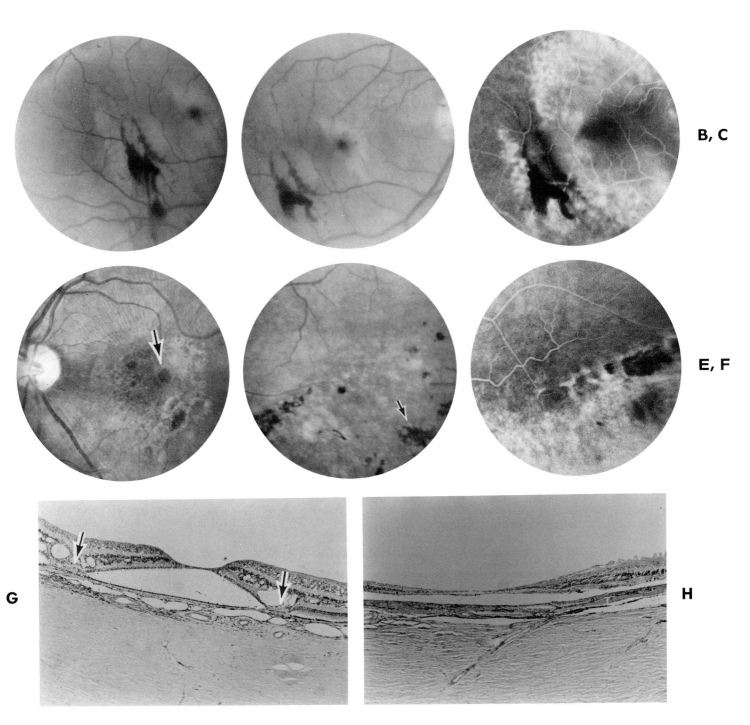

B, C

E, F

G

H

741

▼ POSTERIOR CHOROIDAL RUPTURE

See Chapter 3.

▼ MACULAR COMPLICATIONS OF PERIPHERAL CHORIORETINAL CONTUSION AND RUPTURE (SCLOPETARIA)

Contusion and rupture of the peripheral choroid and retina caused by a high-velocity missile striking or passing close to but not penetrating the globe (sclopetaria) is an infrequent manifestation of nonpenetrating ocular trauma.[15-17] A large, often ragged retinal and choroidal break associated with surrounding retinal whitening and varying amounts of blood are the cardinal funduscopic features (Fig. 8-3, *A* to *F*). The white sclera may be visible within the break. In spite of the break in the retina, rhegmatogenous detachment occurs infrequently. Loss of macular function may occur acutely because of extension of the damage posteriorly (Fig. 8-3, *A*), or it may develop many months after the injury as the result of vascular proliferative and exudative changes occurring within the peripheral scar (Fig. 8-3, *G* to *L*).

FIG. 8-3   Contusion Injury to the Peripheral Retina and Choroid.

A to **F,** Sclopetaria with rupture of the peripheral choroid and retina caused by a bullet passing adjacent to the eye wall. Note the stellate choroidal ruptures, scarring, and subretinal blood extending into the macula (**A**) from the peripheral site of chorioretinal rupture (**B**). Six months later note the extensive scarring posteriorly (**C** and **D**) and peripherally in the area of retinal (**E**) and chorioretinal dehiscence (**F**).

G to **K,** Delayed loss of vision occurred in this young woman who developed an exudative retinal detachment (**G**) caused by a peripheral fibrovascular subretinal mass (**H**) several years following a contusion injury to the retina inferotemporally. The subretinal exudate resolved following transscleral cryopexy (**I** and **J**). Six months later she noted mild metamorphopsia caused by traction of an epiretinal membrane that over a period of several months partly peeled from the retinal surface (**J** and **K**).

L, A large zone of retinal and RPE atrophy with bone corpuscular pigmentation *(arrows)* developed over a period of several years following an inferotemporal contusion injury to the right eye.

(**L,** courtesy Dr. Maurice F. Rabb.)

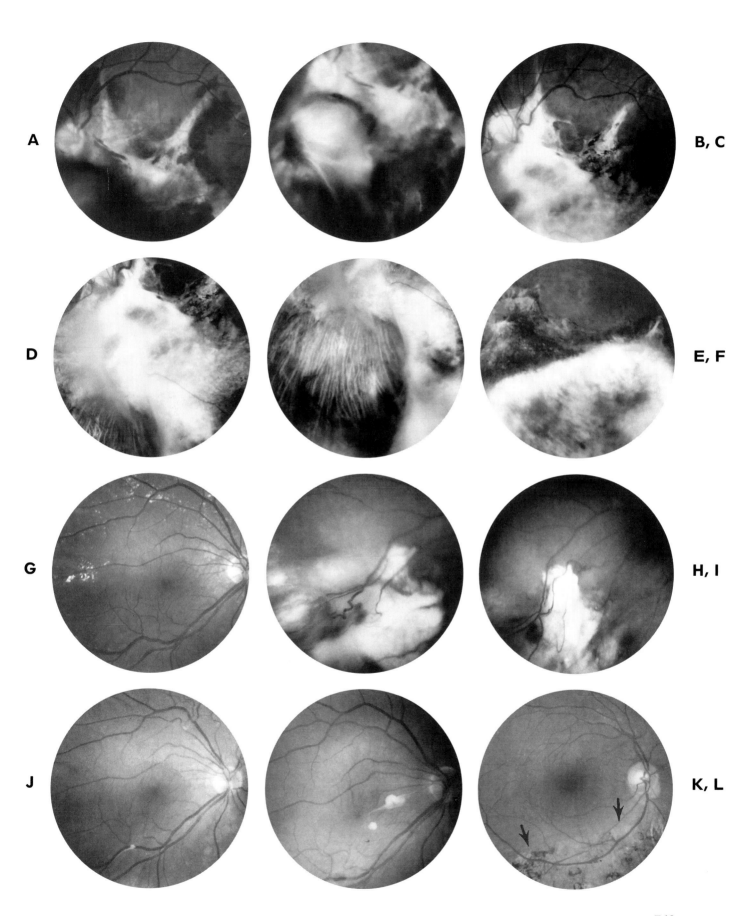

A

B, C

D

E, F

G

H, I

J

K, L

743

▼ POSTTRAUMATIC MACULAR HOLE AND FOVEOLAR PIT

The foveolar part of the retina is extremely thin, and blunt trauma may cause a full-thickness macular hole by either one or a combination of mechanisms: (1) contusion necrosis, (2) subfoveal hemorrhage, and (3) vitreous traction. A macular hole may accompany or soon develop in patients with severe Berlin's edema, with a subretinal hemorrhage caused by choroidal rupture (Fig. 8-4), or in a whiplash separation of the vitreous from the retina (see Chapter 12 for additional discussion of the pathogenesis of macular hole).

Central macular pits identical to those seen in patients following sun gazing have been described following blunt trauma to the eye and whiplash injuries (Fig. 8-4, *H*).[20-22] Loss of visual function occurs infrequently as the result of whiplash.[18] The syndrome of whiplash maculopathy consists of a history of flexion–extension of the head and neck trauma without direct eye injury, immediate mild reduction in acuity of no more than 20/30 in one or both eyes, gray swelling of the foveal zone, and the development of a 50- to 100-μm-diameter foveolar pit. The retinal opacity disappears, and the acuity usually returns to 20/20, but the pit and its whitish borders remain. There may be a slight posterior vitreous detachment, and there may be a micro-operculum. Fluorescein angiography either is normal or may show a tiny focal area of early hyperfluorescence.[22] Grey described a similar pit developing in three patients who experienced direct trauma to the eye and postulated that any agent, either physical or toxic, that causes selective central photoreceptor loss will give rise to the appearance of a central foveolar pit.[21] Small prefoveal vitreous wisps, opercula, and full-thickness macular holes are other changes that may be caused by trauma-induced alterations at the vitreous–macular interface.[19,20] Patients with trauma–induced macular holes unassociated with a large rim of retinal detachment, or if accompanied by pigment epithelial atrophy are probably not good candidates for macular hole surgery because of contusion damage to the retina surrounding the hole (see discussion of macular hole, Chapter 12).

FIG. 8-4 Traumatic Macular Hole.

A and **B**, Subretinal hemorrhage, macular hole (*arrow,* **A**) and choroidal rupture (*arrow,* **B**) caused by a blunt injury to the eye.

C, Macular hole and choroidal rupture *(arrow)* in a 7-year-old boy previously struck in the left eye.

D to **G**, Large macular hole and broad choroidal rupture in a 35-year-old woman (**D**). Angiography revealed absence of choriocapillaris but preservation of some of the large choroidal vessels (*arrow,* **E**) in the region of the hole. Late angiograms showed fluorescein staining in the region of the choroidal rupture as well as at several areas of the hole (**F**). Thirty-six months later the macular hole had enlarged and two additional holes had developed superior to the macula (*arrows,* **G**).

H to **K**, Small lamellar macular hole or pit *(arrow)* in the right eye simulating solar maculopathy (**H**), and full-thickness macular hole in the left eye (**I**) of a 46-year-old chronic alcoholic who had sustained multiple episodes of trauma to both eyes. Angiography revealed evidence of focal choroidal fluorescence in both eyes (**J** and **K**).

▼ POSTCONTUSION NEURORETINOPATHY

Blunt trauma to the eye or periorbital region may cause acute visual loss associated with a swollen optic disc, and optic disc and retinal hemorrhages that are usually confined to the posterior fundus. Some of the blood is derived from the deep plexus of retinal blood vessels and it may extend into the outer plexiform layer of Henle to form a radiating pattern centrally. The fundus picture may simulate that seen in patients with papillophlebitis, with Terson's syndrome, and following epidural injections (see Fig. 8-6, *H* to *J*). A sudden elevation in the central retinal venous pressure caused by the trauma is presumed to be important in the pathogenesis of the optic disc and retinal hemorrhages. A similar pattern of inner and outer retinal hemorrhages occasionally occurs unilaterally in healthy patients with no explanation for them (see Fig. 8-6, *K* and *L*).

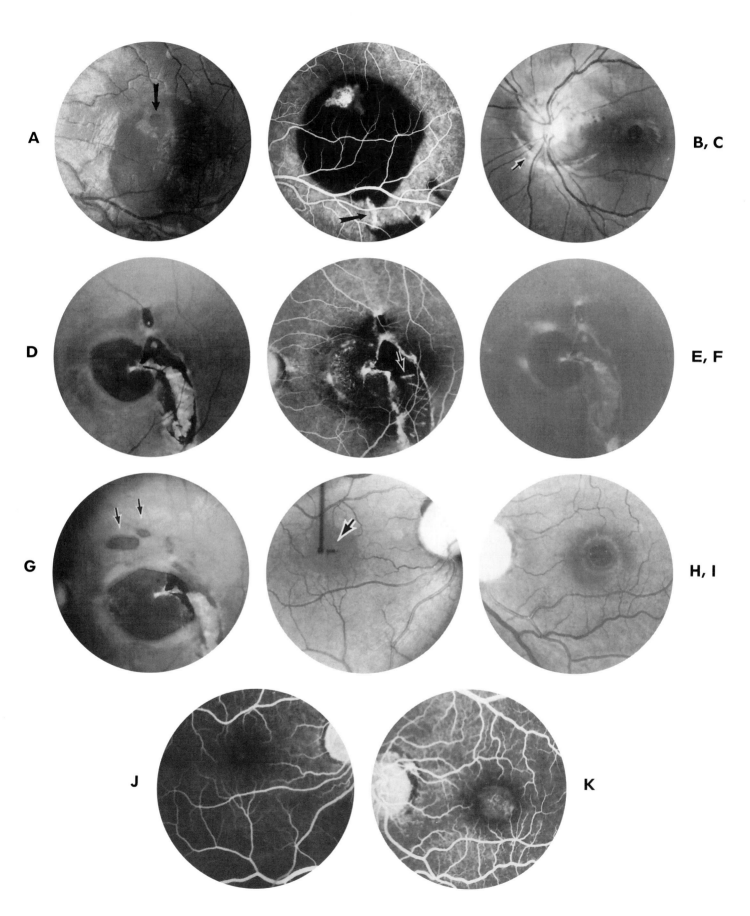

A

B, C

D

E, F

G

H, I

J

K

▼ PURTSCHER'S RETINOPATHY

Following severe compression injury to the head or trunk, the patient may experience visual loss associated with a peculiar retinopathy in one or both eyes.[23-32] The characteristic ophthalmoscopic findings in Purtscher's retinopathy include multiple patches of superficial retinal whitening and retinal hemorrhages surrounding the optic nerve head, which usually appears normal (Fig. 8-5, *A* and *B*). The white patches are located mainly in the area surrounding the optic disc and often do not extend into the center of the macula. Part of the retinal whitening appears to lie anterior to the retinal vessels. In some cases there may be confluence of the white patches (Fig. 8-5, *G*). Fluorescein angiography in milder cases may show leakage of dye from the retinal arterioles, capillaries, and venules in the area of the white retinal lesions[27] and, in more severe cases, may show evidence of arteriolar obstruction and leakage in the region of the white patches (Fig. 8-5, *C* and *D*).[24,25] These patches and hemorrhages disappear, but the patient may be left with some loss of central vision and optic atrophy (Fig. 8-5, *E* and *F*).

The pathogenesis of Purtscher's retinopathy is controversial. The white patches that are often referred to as exudates are probably focal areas of ischemic retinal whitening. Angiographic findings of retinal arteriolar leakage in some cases of Berlin's edema[23] as well as in some cases of Purtscher's retinopathy[24,27] suggest that acute endothelial damage related to trauma may predispose the retinal vascular tree to intravascular coagulopathy or granulocytic aggregation[26] that may be the cause of multiple arteriolar obstructions. Air embolism in patients with chest compression[24] and fat embolism in patients with long-bone fractures[32] have been implicated as causative factors in some cases of Purtscher's retinopathy. The white retinal infarcts, however, in fat embolism are usually smaller and are often situated more peripherally in the retina.[28,29]

Histopathologic examination of an eye 34 months after development of Purtscher's retinopathy has demonstrated inner retinal atrophy compatible with retinal arterial occlusion.[30]

A funduscopic picture virtually identical to that of Purtscher's retinopathy may occur in patients with central retinal artery obstruction, acute pancreatitis, lupus erythematosus, dermatomyositis, scleroderma, and amniotic fluid embolism (see discussion in Chapter 6 and Figs. 6-7; 6-8; 6-13, *H*; and 8-11, *J*).

FIG. 8-5 Purtscher's Retinopathy.

A to **F**, This 45-year-old man noted blurred vision after falling out of a racing boat going at high speed. Visual acuity was 20/30. Note patchy swelling of the retina surrounding the optic nerve head (**A**). The white material appeared to lie mostly anterior to the retinal vessels. It was associated with superficial hemorrhage. Note relative sparing of the macula (**B**). There were no lesions in the peripheral fundus. Arteriovenous-phase angiograms showed lack of filling and obscuration of the capillary bed in the region of the white lesions (**C**) and later showed evidence of fluorescein leakage into the retina (**D**). Ten days later there had been considerable clearing of the retinopathy (**E**). Five months later there was mild temporal pallor (**F**). Visual acuity was 20/30.

G to **I**, This 28-year-old man was thrown from his car and sustained a basilar and ethmoidal fracture. Note the large area of ischemic whitening and hematomas that probably lie beneath the internal limiting membrane (**G** and **H**). The left eye was normal. Note the superficial retinal scar (*arrow,* **I**) and traction lines extending through the macula approximately 5 weeks later.

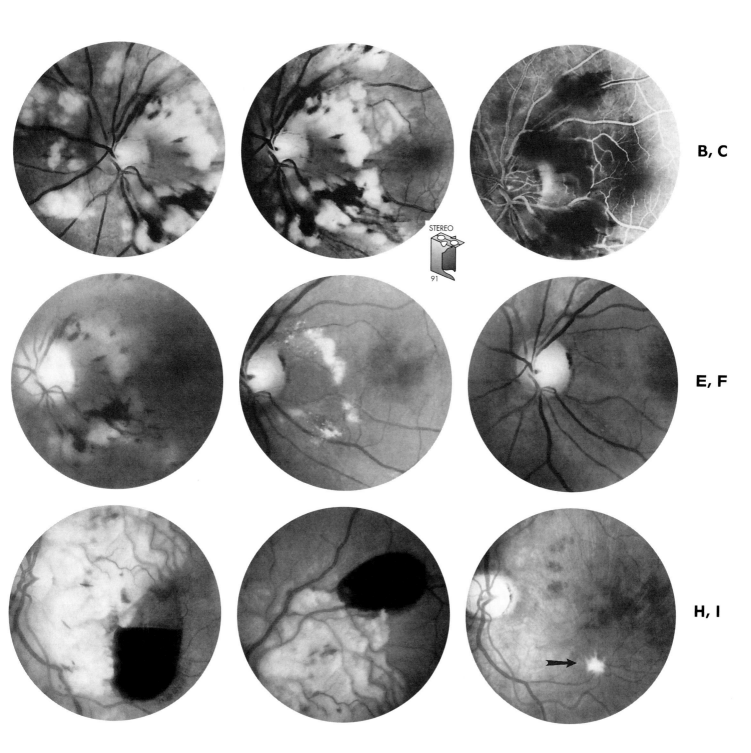

B, C

STEREO
91

E, F

H, I

▼ RETINAL AND VITREOUS HEMORRHAGE ASSOCIATED WITH SUBARACHNOID AND SUBDURAL HEMORRHAGE (TERSON'S SYNDROME)

Terson described vitreous hemorrhage occurring in patients with subarachnoid hemorrhage and attributed it to a sudden increase in venous pressure that ruptures epipapillary and peripapillary capillaries.[37,42,43] Others have attributed the intraocular hemorrhages to a rapid increase in intracranial pressure causing compression of the central retinal vein and its choroidal anastomotic channels.[37] Approximately 20% of patients suffering either spontaneous or posttraumatic subarachnoid or subdural hemorrhages develop intraocular hemorrhages that in most cases are confined to the juxtapapillary and macular areas (Fig. 8-6, *A* to *D*).[41,45] Intraretinal and subretinal bleeding occurs primarily from the optic disc and retinal blood vessels. Elevated mounds of blood either beneath the internal limiting membrane of the retina or in the subhyaloid space may occur.[38,46] In most cases these hemorrhages clear spontaneously and visual function is unaffected. Occasionally the vitreous hemorrhage fails to clear and vitrectomy may be necessary to restore vision.[33,34,40] The surgeon may find some evidence of the retinal blood vessel and RPE damage (Fig. 8-6, *E* and *F*). The amount of blood in the eye is not necessarily related to the severity of the subarachnoid hemorrhage.[35] A perimacular retinal fold may develop after resolution of the subinternal limiting membrane hematoma in some patients.[36] Epiretinal membrane in the macula is the most common sequela of Terson's syndrome but is unassociated with visual morbidity.[39] Because severe proliferative vitreoretinopathy occasionally develops, patients should be monitored periodically with ultrasonography while awaiting clearance of the vitreous blood.[44]

▼ HEMORRHAGIC MACULOPATHY CAUSED BY SUBARACHNOID AND EPIDURAL INJECTIONS

Patients may develop multiple scotomas caused by retinal hemorrhages in one or both eyes immediately after the injection of oxygen into the subarachnoid space during the course of myelography,[49] or following epidural injection of corticosteroids for relief of back pain (Fig. 8-6, *G*).[47,48] These hemorrhages often occur as the result of bleeding from the deep retinal capillary plexus and cause a petaloid pattern of blood with tapered

FIG. 8-6   Terson's Syndrome.

A to **D**, This 45-year-old woman noted visual blurring in both eyes soon after admission to the hospital because of a subarachnoid hemorrhage. Note the multiple darker superficial subinternal limiting membrane retinal hemorrhages (*arrow*), lighter subretinal hemorrhages, and optic disc edema in both eyes (**A** to **C**). Fluorescein angiography revealed evidence of optic disc edema (**D**).

E and **F**, This 50-year-old man experienced an acute hypertensive crisis, headache, neck pain, and coma. Fresh superficial globular juxtapapillary hemorrhages were noted in both eyes. Six days later he had bilateral dense vitreous hemorrhages. Over the subsequent 6 years his vision was hand motions only because of the persistence of the vitreous blood. When seen at the Bascom Palmer Eye Institute neither fundus could be visualized because of old vitreous blood. He had a vitrectomy in both eyes. Postoperatively, his visual acuity in the right eye was 20/25 and in the left eye was 20/40. The right fundus was normal except for hypertensive retinal arterial narrowing and two white choroidal vessels in the macular area (**E**). In the left fundus, similar choroidal vessels were associated with a zone of RPE atrophy in the macula (**F**).

Hemorrhagic Maculopathy Caused by Epidural Injections

G, Multiple, primarily deep retinal hemorrhages and sudden visual loss were associated with an epidural injection of corticosteroids. Note the similarity of the distribution of the hemorrhages to that in patients **H, I,** and **K**.

Postcontusion Hemorrhagic Neuroretinopathy

H to **J**, This young woman experienced loss of vision after being shoved against a wall. Note the swollen optic disc, and superficial and deep retinal hemorrhages, which gradually cleared. Mild optic atrophy was associated with 20/50 acuity.

Idiopathic Unilateral Deep Retinal Hemorrhages

K and **L**, Unilateral visual loss and multiple deep retinal hemorrhages occurred in the left eye of this otherwise healthy young adult who gave no history of trauma or illness. Note the petaloid arrangement of the hemorrhages that probably are located in the outer plexiform layer.

(**G** from Kushner and Olson[47]; **K** and **L**, courtesy Dr. Maurice Rabb.)

edges centrally surrounding the center of the macula. Sudden elevation of the cerebrospinal fluid pressure and elevation of retinal venous pressure are the most likely explanation for the hemorrhages, some of which may occur from the superficial as well as the deep retinal capillaries in a pattern similar to that seen in Terson's syndrome. The prognosis for the spontaneous return of normal visual function is good.

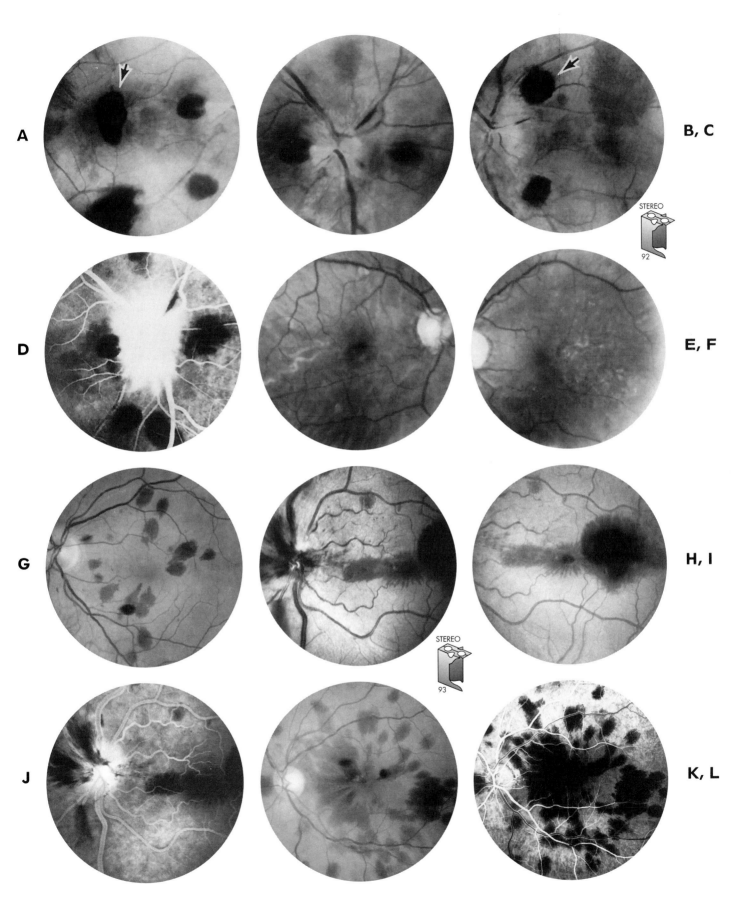

A

B, C

D

E, F

G

H, I

J

K, L

749

▼ SHAKEN BABY SYNDROME

Shaken baby syndrome results from severe shaking of infants, often as a form of punishment. The signs and symptoms are nonspecific and may mimic infection, intoxication, or metabolic abnormalities. These include (1) bradycardia, apnea, and hypothermia; (2) lethargy, irritability, seizures, hypotonia, full or bulging fontanelle, and increased head size; (3) scattered superficial retinal hemorrhages, dome-shaped subinternal limiting membrane or subhyaloid hematomas, and cotton-wool patches; and (4) skin bruises.[50-53,55-59,63,65-67] A history of a recent minor accident or shaking in an effort to resuscitate may be obtained in some cases. The retinopathy may simulate that seen in Terson's syndrome, Purtscher's retinopathy, or central retinal vein occlusion (Fig. 8-7). Late funduscopic changes include a circular retinal fold that may create a craterlike depression in the macula and traumatic retinoschisis.[52,54,56,57,62] The circular retinal fold may be a product of abrupt vitreoretinal traction associated with shaking,[54] vitreous traction after partial separation of the vitreous in the central macular region,[62] or contraction of the internal limiting membrane or the posterior hyaloid membrane after resolution of a subinternal limiting membrane or subhyaloid hematoma. Laboratory findings include bloody cerebrospinal fluid and subdural tap and, in almost all cases, computed tomographic evidence of at least one of the following: subdural hemorrhage, subarachnoid hemorrhage, or cerebral contusion.[61] The prognosis is poor, and many children are left with severe neurologic and developmental defects, including visual deficits and in some cases blindness.

The histopathologic findings in the eyes of these patients reveal evidence of intraretinal blood, subhyaloid and subinternal limiting membrane

FIG. 8-7   Shaken Baby Syndrome.

A and **B,** Shaken baby syndrome with multiple superficial retinal hemorrhages (*arrow,* **A**) in a 6-month-old infant.

C, Photomicrograph of subinternal limiting membrane hemorrhage in an infant who died of complications of shaken baby syndrome.

D and **E,** Photograph of gross findings in a 42-week-old infant with extensive intraretinal hemorrhages and papilledema (**D**) and blood in the perineural sheath of the optic nerve (*arrow,* **E**). Similar changes were present in both eyes.

F and **G,** Photomicrographs of another physically abused infant with gross findings similar to **D** and **E** in both eyes. Note peripapillary subretinal blood (*upper arrow,* **F**) and hemorrhagic infarction of the retina (**G**). There was blood in the subarachnoid and subdural space (*lower arrow,* **F**) in both eyes.

hematomas, as well as blood in the subdural and subarachnoid spaces around the optic nerve (Fig. 8-7, *C* to *G*).* The subdural and subarachnoid hemorrhage in the optic nerve may be subtle and the only manifestation of the shaken baby syndrome. Special stains for iron may be helpful in detecting evidence of previous blood in these areas occurring many months before the eyes are obtained at autopsy.

The finding of retinal hemorrhages in a child with suspected injury is more likely to be caused by shaking than by blunt trauma,[50,51,64] and it is an important predictor of neurologic injury.[68]

*References 50, 52, 60, 62-64.

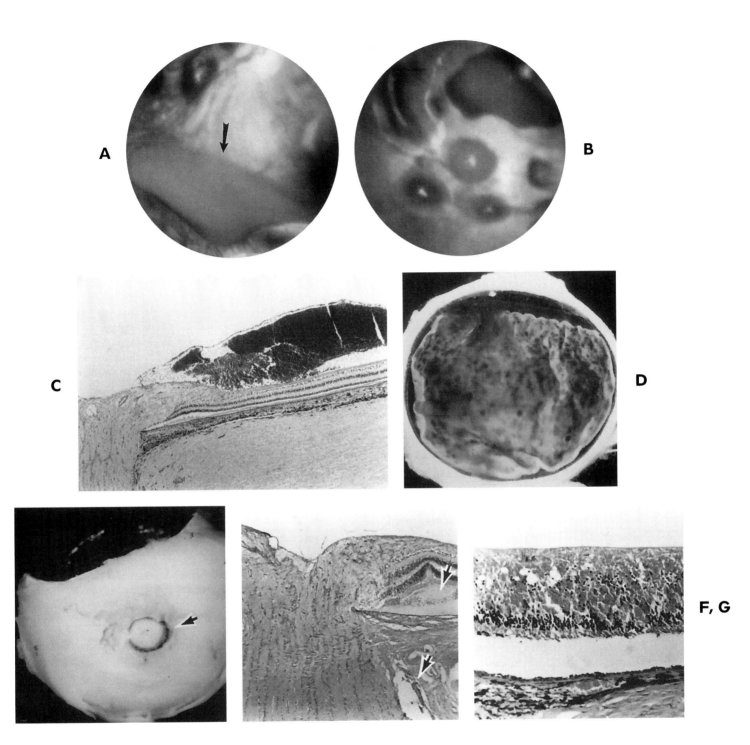

751

▼ RETINAL VESSEL RUPTURE ASSOCIATED WITH PHYSICAL EXERTION (VALSALVA RETINOPATHY)

A sudden rise in intrathoracic or intraabdominal pressure, particularly against a closed glottis (Valsalva's maneuver) during lifting, bowel movement, coughing, or vomiting, may cause a rapid rise of intravenous pressure within the eye and spontaneous rupture of superficial retinal capillaries in otherwise normal eyes or in eyes associated with acquired retinal vascular abnormalities (diabetic or hypertensive retinal angiopathy) or congenital retinal vascular disease (retinal telangiectasis and congenital retinal artery tortuosity) (Fig. 8-8).[69,71,72,74,75] Sudden loss of vision may result from hemorrhagic detachment of the internal limiting membrane, vitreous hemorrhage, or, if bleeding occurs near the foveal region, dissection of blood beneath the retina. These patients typically have a circumscribed, round or dumbbell-shaped, bright red mound of blood beneath the internal limiting membrane in or near the central macular area (Fig. 8-8, *A, D, F, H* and *J*). A glistening light reflex is present on the surface. A few fine striae indicative of wrinkling of the internal limiting membrane may be present on the surface of the hematoma. Part of the blood turns yellow after several days. The shape and color of these lesions may suggest an intraocular parasite (Fig. 8-8, *D* and *E*). A fluid level caused by settling of the formed blood elements may develop soon after the hemorrhage (Fig. 8-8, *H* and *J*). As the blood resolves, the serous detachment of the internal limiting membrane may persist for several days or weeks (Fig. 8-8, *I*). Spontaneous reattachment occurs, and the appearance of the macula and visual acuity usually return to normal.

Occasionally, a small (less than one disc diameter), round, preretinal hemorrhage centered in the foveal area occurs.[69,74] The surface may show multiple yellow-white dots simulating that of a strawberry (see Figs. 6-14, *D,* and 8-8, *D*). Its surface usually does not show a reflex suggestive of the presence of an internal limiting membrane. It may represent a small amount of blood lying between the internal limiting membrane and the posterior hyaloid interface. In addition, patients with these small central lesions often have a thin layer of blood lying beneath the retina in the paramacular area. Complete recovery of vision usually occurs spontaneously. In unusual circumstances where a subinternal limiting membrane hematoma is responsible for visual loss in the

FIG. 8-8   Valsalva Retinopathy.

A to C, This healthy 24-year-old woman developed sudden onset of blurring of vision of the left eye during a bout of tenesmus. Note the subinternal limiting membrane hemorrhage that extends down into the central foveolar area. Fluorescein angiography showed no retinal abnormality. Two months later the hemorrhage had cleared completely and the visual acuity was 20/20 **(D).**

D and E, This young man, who was on a respirator because of acute respiratory distress syndrome of unknown cause, experienced loss of central vision in the left eye. He was referred to the eye clinic because of a suspected intraocular parasite. Note the superficial retinal blood that probably lies beneath the internal limiting membrane **(D).** Angiography revealed no retinal or choroidal vascular abnormality **(E).** The blood cleared, and the visual acuity returned to normal.

F and G, This 56-year-old man was lifting a heavy box when he suddenly lost central vision in his right eye 3 months before examination at Bascom Palmer Eye Institute. His local physician suspected an intraocular *Cysticercus* larva. Visual acuity was 20/200. Note the parasite-like shape of the subinternal limiting membrane blood **(F).** Angiography revealed no evidence of retinal vascular change **(G).**

H and I, Serous and hemorrhagic detachment of the internal limiting membrane of the retina in a 33-year-old man who experienced sudden loss of vision during a bout of vomiting **(H).** Visual acuity was 20/80. There was no other evidence of retinal vascular disease. Three months later a shallow serous detachment of the internal limiting membrane remained **(I).** Visual acuity was 20/15.

J and K, This 30-year-old woman had a cardiac arrest during surgery on her hand. Cardiac resuscitation was successful and, when she regained consciousness 2 days later, she noted blurred vision in the right eye. Three weeks later her visual acuity in the right eye was 20/40. She had a subinternal limiting membrane hematoma in the macula and blood in the vitreous inferiorly in the right eye **(J).** The left eye was normal. Within 4 months her acuity returned to 20/20 **(K).**

L, This woman noted the sudden loss of vision in the right eye during labor. This photograph was made several days after delivery of a normal infant.

patient's only normally functioning eye, neodymium-YAG laser disruption of the internal limiting membrane allowing the blood to gravitate into the inferior vitreous cavity may restore central vision more promptly.[70]

Subinternal limiting membrane hemorrhage and preretinal hemorrhage identical to that just described occasionally occur in the normal individual in the absence of a clear-cut history of unusual exertion or Valsalva's maneuver.[76,77] Some pa-

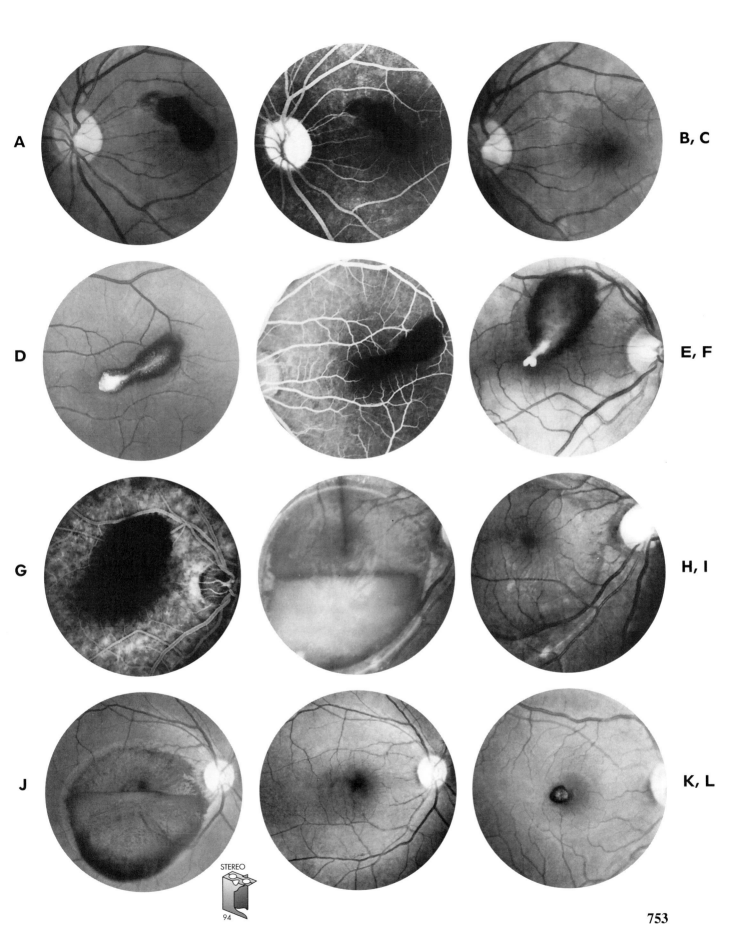

A

B, C

D

E, F

G

H, I

J

STEREO
94

K, L

753

tients may have evidence of retinal vascular disease, for example, diabetes or hypertension (Fig. 6-15, G to J). Other apparently healthy patients may give a history of multiple previous episodes of loss of central or paracentral vision secondary to spontaneous retinal hemorrhages. Their family members may give a similar history.[73] Tortuosity of the second- and third-order retinal arterioles may or may not be present in these patients with a familial history (see Fig. 6-1, A to C). No specific hematologic disorder has been described in this condition, which is probably inherited as an autosomal dominant trait. Recovery of vision is the rule.

▼ EVULSION OF THE OPTIC DISC

A forceful backward dislocation of the optic nerve from the scleral canal can occur under several circumstances, including (1) extreme rotation and forward displacement of the globe, (2) penetrating orbital injury causing a backward pull on the optic nerve, or (3) sudden increase in intraocular pressure causing a rupture of the lamina cribrosa.[78-81] This latter mechanism might be more appropriately termed "expulsion" rather than "evulsion." In all cases a tear in the lamina cribrosa and nerve fibers at the disc margin occurs. This tear may be partial or complete and may be associated with massive intraocular hemorrhage (Fig. 8-9, G and H) or only minimal bleeding (Fig. 8-9, A to C, E, and F).[82] In the latter case the dark, pitlike deformity caused by a partial evulsion may simulate an optic pit (Fig. 8-9, A).[79,80] Visual loss from these injuries is usually great. Over a period of weeks or months, fibroglial proliferation obliterates the cavity caused by the evulsion (Fig. 8-8, D).

A penetrating injury of the optic nerve head may simulate a partial evulsion (Fig. 8-9, I).

FIG. 8-9   Evulsion of the Optic Nerve Head.

A to **D,** Partial evulsion of the optic nerve head in a man who sustained sudden loss of vision in the left eye during a brawl. His visual acuity was 8/200. There was a large, gray, optic pit–like depression (*arrows,* **A**) involving the temporal half of the optic disc. There was juxtapapillary retinal and subretinal blood. Angiography showed an intact cilioretinal artery in the area of the partly evulsed optic disc (**B** and **C,** *stereo).* Eleven years later extensive fibroglial proliferation obscured the optic nerve head from view (**D**).

E and **F,** Contusion necrosis and partial evulsion of the inferior half of the optic nerve head in an 8-year-old boy immediately after the injury (**E**) and 4 months later (**F**).

G and **H,** Severe evulsion of the optic nerve head and contusion necrosis of the surrounding retina. Angiography showed intense staining in area of nerve head (**H**).

I, Perforating wound of the eye simulating a partial evulsion of the optic nerve head in a 6-year-old boy who was hit in the eye with a homemade safety pin dart that entered the eye adjacent to the inferior limbus, missed the lens, and perforated the juxtapapillary eye wall (*arrow).* The child withdrew the dart himself. His visual acuity was 20/200. Two months later he developed cells, flare, and keratitic precipitates in the opposite eye.

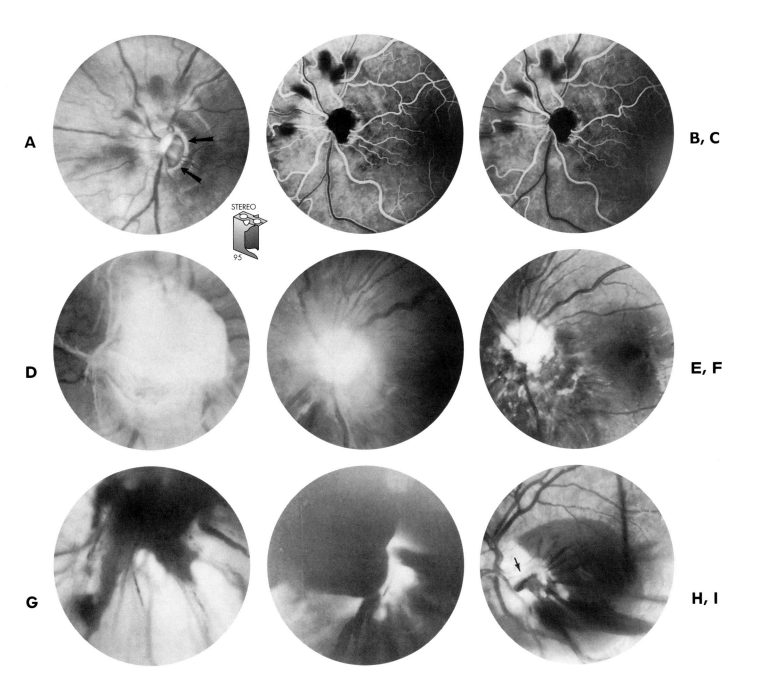

A

B, C

D

E, F

G

H, I

STEREO
9.5

▼ OCULAR DECOMPRESSION RETINOPATHY

Some patients following glaucoma surgery will develop superficial and deep retinal hemorrhages as a result of the pressure lowering.[83] Some of the hemorrhages may be white centered. This is most likely to occur in patients with high preoperative pressures. The visual acuity is typically unaffected by these changes.

▼ INTRAOCULAR FOREIGN BODIES

A great variety of foreign bodies may penetrate the ocular wall and become lodged within the choroid and retina. In most instances their identity is known and measures for removal are often undertaken promptly. In some cases, however, the invasion of the foreign body may not be recognized until months or years later, when the patient experiences signs or symptoms related to breakdown of the foreign body (e.g., siderosis or chalcosis; Fig. 8-10, *B, C, I,* and *J*) or when a mass lesion in the fundus is discovered on routine eye examination (Fig. 8-10, *B* to *E*). Occasionally it may simulate a melanoma and result in removal of the eye (Fig. 8-10, *B* to *E*).[79,85,87,88] The use of ultrasonography, radiography, and electroretinography in mass lesions of uncertain etiology can reduce the chances of this mistake (Fig. 8-10, *B*). The late development of subretinal neovascularization occurring at a foreign body impact site may occur.[84]

FIG. 8-10   Intraocular Foreign Bodies.

A, Metallic foreign body lying on the inner retinal surface.

B, Juxtapapillary pigmented tumor that was suspected to be a melanoma. An orbital roentgenogram, however, revealed a metallic foreign body within the pigmented mass.

C to **E,** A juxtapapillary pigmented mass that was diagnosed as a choroidal melanoma and the eye was enucleated. Gross photographs show the mass (*arrows,* **C**). Photomicrographs show the juxtapapillary mass that lies within the sclera and choroid beneath the atrophic retina (**D**). It stained positively for iron and calcium, and polarization (**E**) revealed evidence of hemosiderin. These changes probably resulted from the impact and subsequent disintegration of an unsuspected iron foreign body.

F to **H,** Intraocular iron foreign body sustained while hammering on metal. Stereoscopic angiogram shows elevation at the site of the imbedded foreign body that was still present following an attempt to remove it after pars plana vitrectomy and lensectomy.

I and **J,** Chalcosis in a 40-year-old schizophrenic man who had visual acuity of 20/25, a mild sunflower cataract (**I**), mild vitritis, and a yellow mass in the superotemporal quadrant of the left eye (**J**). There was no history of a foreign body injury, and no site of entry was found. Orbital roentgenogram revealed a foreign body that proved to be brass after removal via the pars plana.

(**D** to **F** from Rones B, Zimmerman LE: *Arch Ophthalmol* 70:30, 1963; copyright 1963, American Medical Association.[88])

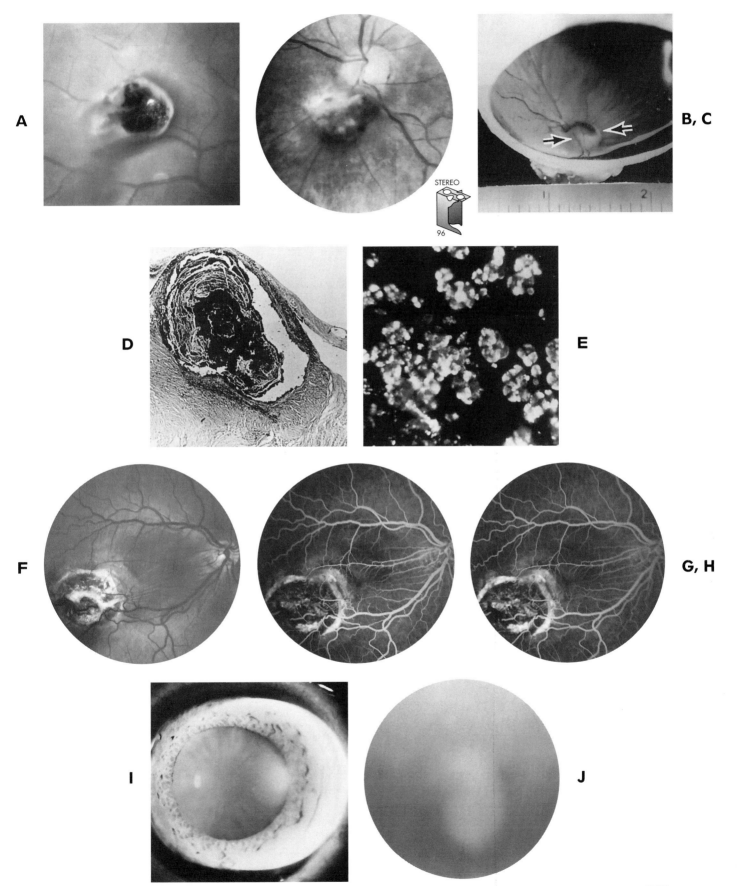

STEREO
96

▼ CHORIORETINOPATHY AND OPTIC NEUROPATHY ASSOCIATED WITH RETROBULBAR INJECTIONS

Acute visual loss may be associated with retrobulbar local anesthetic injections. There are a variety of mechanisms causing visual loss. These include: penetration of the eye wall,[92,94-96,101-103,105] penetration of the optic nerve,[96,102,103] compression of the optic nerve, intraarterial injection of anesthesia,[103] and spasm of the central retinal artery (Fig. 8-11).[99] In cases of perforation of the eye the site of exit is often visible in the posterior pole and is associated with variable amounts of intraretinal, subretinal and vitreous blood (Fig. 8-11, *A* and *B*). Retinal detachment, vitreous traction, and subretinal neovascularization may occur as late complications (Fig. 8-11, *A* to *D*). Penetration of the optic nerve sheaths may be associated with intrasheath injection, brainstem anesthesia, respiratory arrest,[89-91,93,97,100] and anterior extension of the anesthetic into the subretinal space.[102,103] Intrasheath injection as well as injection into the optic nerve may cause occlusion of the central retinal artery and vein,[102,103,104] or severe ischemic optic neuropathy (Fig. 8-11, *E* to *L*). Risk factors include: sharp needles, needles longer than 1.25 inches, axial myopia, multiple injections, injections by nonophthalmologists, enophthalmos, previous scleral buckling procedure, traditional superonasal gaze position during the injection, and poor patient cooperation.[94,98,105] Use of blunted retrobulbar needles 1.25 inches or less in length and injection with the eye in the straight-ahead position may be helpful in preventing visual loss.[98,102]

Penetration of the anterior ocular coats during peribulbar anesthetic injections, particularly with sharp, small-gauge needles, may occur and often is unassociated with permanent visual loss.[92] The author has seen one patient who sustained immediate loss of vision associated with subretinal injection of Xylocaine and epinephrine local anesthetic (see Fig. 9-10, *I* to *L*).

FIG. 8-11   Complications of Retrobulbar Anesthesia.

A to **D,** Ocular perforation with a needle occurred during local anesthesia in this elderly woman scheduled for cataract extraction. She noted a dark violaceous spot at the time of the retrobulbar injection and poor central vision postoperatively. Three weeks later her visual acuity in the left eye was 20/300. There was an entrance site inferiorly and an exit site just superior to the center of the macula (*arrows,* **A** and **B**). Ten months later her visual acuity in the right eye was 5/200. There was evidence of subretinal neovascularization surrounding the exit site (**C** and **D**).

E and **F,** Combined central retinal artery and central retinal vein occlusion was present on the first day after cataract surgery under local anesthesia.

G and **H,** This patient noted marked visual loss on the first postoperative day after cataract extraction done several months before these photographs were taken. Note pallor of the optic disc and narrowing and cuffing of the inferior branch retinal arteries. Angiography revealed a large inferior zone of capillary nonperfusion (**H**).

I, Subretinal and intravitreal depo-prednisolone following a scleral buckling procedure.

J and **K,** This hypertensive woman noted loss of vision in this eye during the course of cataract extraction. On the first postoperative day her visual acuity was light perception only and the fundus showed a picture simulating Purtscher's retinopathy (**J**). The visual function gradually improved and several months later her visual acuity was 20/30. There was mild optic atrophy (**K**).

L, This 48-year-old man, whose preoperative visual acuity was 20/60, had an apparently uneventful cataract extraction in this eye. On the first postoperative day his visual acuity was no light perception. Note the pale swelling of the optic disc and evidence of the cilioretinal artery occlusion (**L**). Four days later his findings were unchanged.

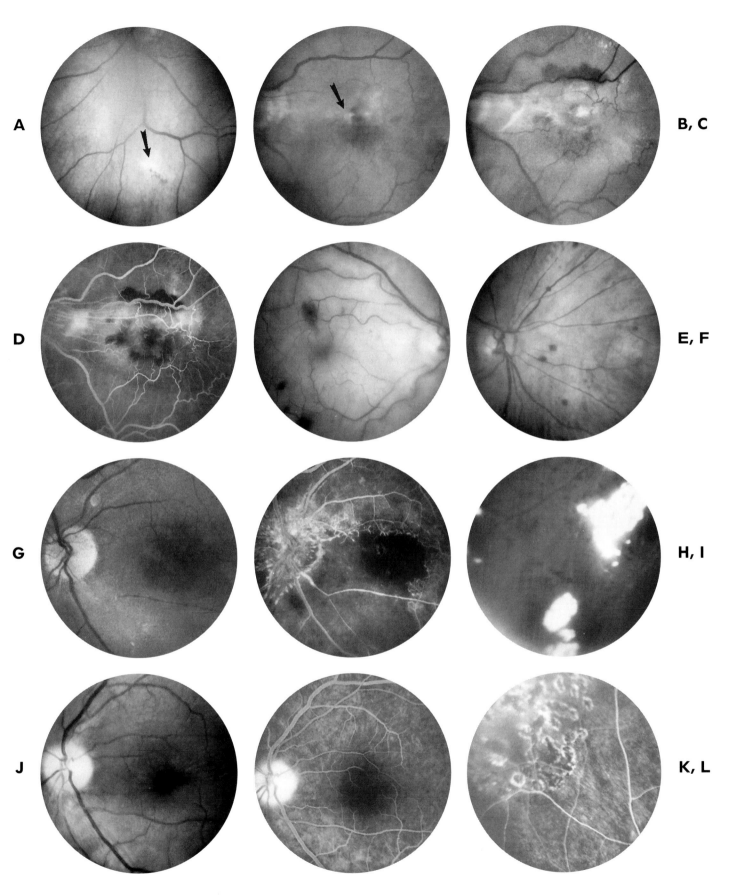

A

B, C

D

E, F

G

H, I

J

K, L

759

▼ PHOTIC MACULOPATHY

Light may cause damage to retinal tissues by means of three basic mechanisms: photochemical, photocoagulative, and mechanical.[106,202] Photochemical damage occurs when light of the visible spectrum, particularly the blue end, causes photochemical changes and retinal injury without significantly raising the tissue temperature. Photocoagulation occurs when light generates a temperature of more than 10°F above body temperature and causes coagulation of retinal proteins. Mechanical injury is caused by acoustic waves or gaseous formation after rapid tissue absorption of light. Many factors, including pigmentation, clarity and nature of the media, wavelength of light, dose rate, and body temperature, are important in determining the nature of the injury.

Solar retinopathy

The terms "solar retinopathy," "eclipse burns," and "foveomacular retinitis," which by most authors are believed to be synonymous, refer to a specific foveolar lesion that occurs (1) in certain patients following viewing of an eclipse[121,181]; (2) after direct sun gazing by lookouts,[170] sunbathers,[135] malingerers,[126,129] or schizophrenics[108]; (3) as part of a religious ritual[119,149]; (4) in young people under the influence of hallucinogenic agents, particularly LSD (Figs. 8-12 and 8-13)[125,132,187]; and (5) in patients, typically children or young adults who deny a history of unusual exposure to sun.[120,134] Those who admit to sun gazing often develop, soon after exposure, a central scotoma, chromatopsia, metamorphopsia, and headache. The visual acuity is reduced to 20/40 to 20/70. In most cases visual acuity returns to between 20/20 and 20/40 within a period of 3 to 6 months.[181]

During the first few days after exposure a small yellow-white spot with a surrounding faint gray zone develops in the center of the foveolar area (Fig. 8-12, *A*). This spot fades after several days and is replaced by a reddish spot with a pigment halo. After approximately 10 to 14 days this often fades from view and is usually replaced by a small (25 to 50 μm), reddish, sharply circumscribed, often irregularly shaped, faceted lamellar hole or depression in the foveolar area (Fig. 8-12, *B* to *F*). This defect may lie immediately beneath or just adjacent to the foveal reflex that is typically present. It is unassociated with an overlying operculum or evidence of posterior vitreous separation. Occasionally the diameter of this pit may be 100 to 200 μm (Fig. 8-12, *E* and *F*). This pit is probably caused by focal loss of the retinal receptors.[134,150] It is permanent and is highly suggestive of previous sun gazing. Similar lesions, however, may occur after spontaneous vitreous separation, usually in patients 50 years or older (see discussion of macular holes, Chapter 12), and in some patients after whiplash-like injuries (see p. 745).[137,156]

FIG. 8-12   Solar Maculopathy.

A to D, This 16-year-old boy noted blurred vision in both eyes soon after having gazed at the sun. When seen initially, his visual acuity was 20/30 in the right eye and 20/100 in the left eye. He had a small yellow spot in the foveal center of both eyes (**A**). Fluorescein angiography was normal. Thirteen weeks later, visual acuity was 20/20 in the right eye and 20/100 in the left eye. In the center of both foveae there was a sharply circumscribed inner lamellar hole (**B** and **C**). Two months later the pits had enlarged slightly (**D**) and they remained unchanged 7 years later when his visual acuity was 20/15 in the right eye and 20/20 in the left eye.

E and **F,** Large foveolar pits many years after sun gazing. The patient's visual acuity was 20/30.

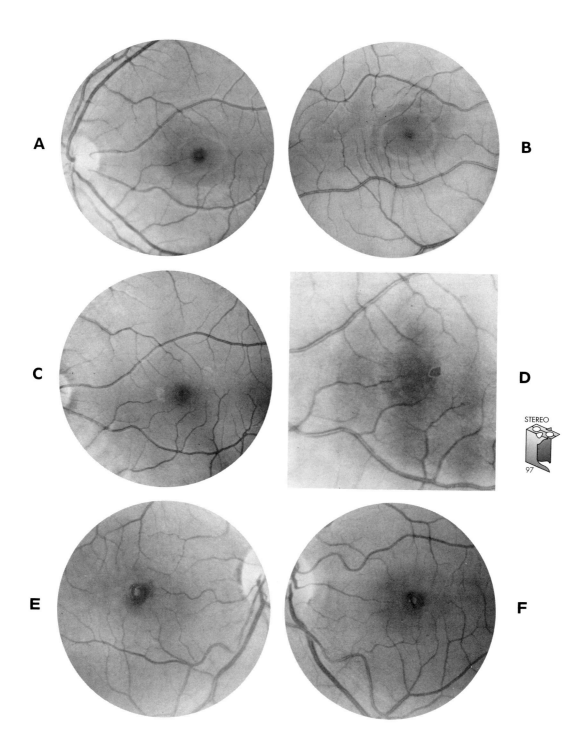

A

B

C

D

STEREO
97

E

F

761

In some patients sustaining prolonged or repeated exposures, particularly those under the influence of hallucinogenic agents, a larger lesion with mottling of the RPE may occur (Fig. 8-13, *A*).[132,134,187] Possible factors predisposing to macular damage from the sun include younger age (lens clearer), pupil dilation, relative emmetropia, high body temperature, and geophysical conditions allowing increase in the atmospheric transmission of UV-B radiation to the Earth's surface.[201]

Fluorescein angiography in most patients shows no abnormality during either the early or the late phases of the disease. In a few patients seen within the first 48 hours, a small focal area of staining may be present. Days to weeks later there may be a small spot of hyperfluorescence caused by a window defect in the RPE. The presence of xanthophyll pigment in the foveal area may be responsible for the difficulty in demonstrating angiographic evidence of minor RPE damage in these cases.

There is experimental evidence to suggest that the blue wavelengths of light are chiefly responsible for producing a photochemical injury that during the first 48 hours manifests itself primarily as damage to the apical melanosomes of the RPE followed by macrophage phagocytosis of the melanosomes in the subretinal space. Between 48 hours and 5 days after exposure, disruption of the receptor elements becomes more apparent. Much of this damage is reversible and thus explains why many patients regain good acuity.[139-143,165,166,194] In severe cases, depigmentation of the RPE and permanent loss of the receptor elements may occur (Fig. 8-13).[134] There is also evidence to suggest that there is great individual variation in susceptibility for developing solar retinopathy. Some patients with minimal exposure to the sun (e.g., during sunbathing) may develop a macular lesion,[120,135] whereas others, even after purposely staring at the sun as long as an hour, may develop only a minimal lesion.[194] Most patients recover normal or nearly normal acuity, and no treatment has been proved to be of value.

FIG. 8-13 Clinicopathologic Correlation of a Probable Solar Macular Burn.

A 20-year-old Air Force enlisted man with a 2-week history of blurred vision in the right eye and a 1-week history of blurred vision in the left eye. He admitted being under the influence of LSD but denied sun gazing. Visual acuity in the right eye was 20/200 and in the left eye was 20/60. In the right eye he had a large oval area of RPE derangement centered in the macula (**A**). In the left macula he had a small yellow lesion identical to that depicted in Fig. 8-12, *A*. Fluorescein angiography showed evidence of a window defect in the RPE in the right macula (**B**). It showed no abnormality in the left eye. Seven days later the visual acuity in the left eye had improved to 20/30. Approximately 6 months later he was killed in an automobile accident, and his eyes were obtained at autopsy. Histopathologic examination of the eye depicted in **A** showed focal loss of the rod and cone nuclei and receptor elements in the central macular area (*arrows*, **C**). There was focal thinning and depigmentation of the otherwise viable RPE cells in the foveal region (**D**). Arrow indicates the juncture between the normal and depigmented RPE. Note that Bruch's membrane, the choriocapillaris, and the remaining choroidal vessels are normal. Serial sections of the left eye failed to reveal a definite abnormality in the foveal area.

It is probable that acute visual loss in naval personnel attributed to foveomacular retinitis was caused primarily by sun gazing.[157] It is also probable that some reported cases of idiopathic foveolar lesions, identical to solar maculopathy, occurred in patients who for a variety of reasons may have denied sun gazing.[120] The possibility still exists, however, that there are other as yet unidentified causes for this clinical picture.

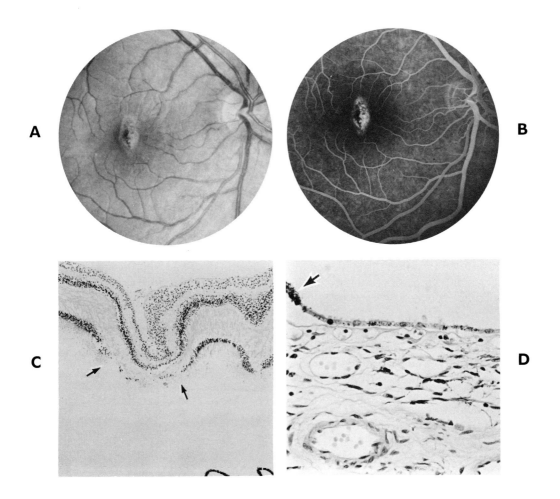

Welding arc maculopathy

Exposure to a welding arc commonly causes keratoconjunctivitis, but only rarely does it cause visual loss. In certain instances, however, there is some evidence that prolonged exposure over a period of minutes or more may cause facial burn, decreased pupillary response to light, decreased acuity with a central scotoma, a concentric peripheral field loss, and biomicroscopic changes in the macula that appear almost identical to those seen following exposure to the sun (Fig. 8-14, *A* to *D*).* Depending on the severity of the disease, visual acuity usually returns to normal in a matter of days or weeks. The course of visual recovery and fundus changes closely parallels solar maculopathy. As in the case of solar maculopathy, there is evidence to suggest that the retinal damage secondary to a welding arc is probably explained on a photochemical rather than a thermal basis and is primarily caused by the wavelengths at the blue end of the visible spectrum.[175] Similar photochemical macular burns may occur after brief exposure to the flash associated with short circuiting a high-tension electric current (Fig. 8-14, *E* to *I*).[133] Dolphin and Lincoff reported homonymous, oval, white, retinal lesions in a patient exposed to a 700-volt electric discharge that occurred when two electric rails generated an arc of light.[123]

Unusual fundus lesions reported in two patients exposed to electric arc welding appear to be unrelated RPE detachments in one patient and nonspecific chorioretinal scars in the other.[111,115] There is one report of a macular hole occurring after exposure to electric welding arc.[200]

---

*References 134, 178, 183, 191, 197.

FIG. 8-14   Photic Maculopathy.

A to **D,** Photic maculopathy caused by welding in this 19-year-old man who developed marked pain in the eyes and progressive visual loss soon after spending 2 hours "tacking" with a helium welder 2 weeks before his initial examination at the Bascom Palmer Eye Institute. He had symmetric, small, yellow, foveolar lesions at the level of the RPE (**A** and **B**). His visual acuity in the right eye was 20/100 and in the left eye was 20/200. Angiography in both eyes showed a small focal window defect in the RPE centrally (**C**). Ten months later the patient's visual acuity had returned in the right eye to 20/30+ and in the left eye to 20/50+. Note the slight enlargement of the area of depigmentation in the center of the macular area (**D**).

E to **I,** Photic maculopathy and facial burns caused by electric arc flash occurred in this workman (**E**) when he drove a spike into a high-voltage line. Forty-eight hours after the injury, his visual acuity in the left eye was 20/50. He had a yellow spot in the center of the fovea (**F**). Two weeks after injury his acuity was 20/40 and the spot was less prominent (**G**). Eight months after injury his visual acuity was 20/20. There was a circular zone of depigmentation of the RPE (**H**) that was readily apparent as a ring of hyperfluorescence angiographically (**I**).

(**E** to **I** from Gardner et al.[133])

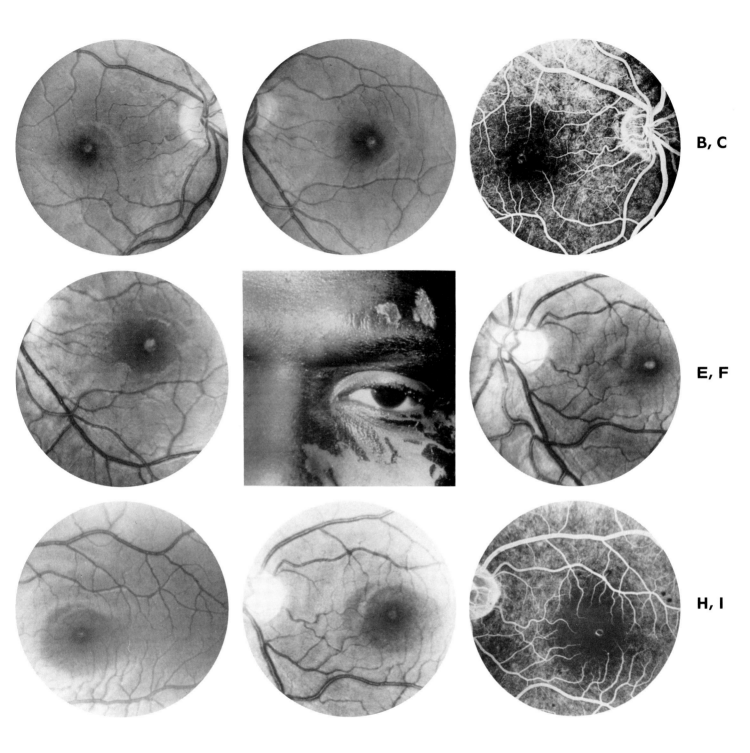

B, C

E, F

H, I

Lightning retinopathy

Acute visual loss associated with macular changes may occur in patients after being struck by lightning.[118,124,144,179] Macular "edema" simulating Berlin's edema seen early may be replaced by lesions described as a "cyst" (Fig. 8-15), "macular hole," or solar maculopathy. In spite of the appearance of the lesion and an initial loss of central vision, the prognosis for visual recovery is relative good.

Acute retinal damage caused by ophthalmic instruments

The toxic effects of light on the retina in experimental animals have been documented in the case of the indirect ophthalmoscope,[130,192,195,196] intraocular fiberoptic light,[131,202] and the operating microscope.* The visible and infrared wavelengths of light are probably most important in causing instrument-induced retinal damage.[175] Lesions similar to those produced experimentally in animals using the operating microscope and corneal contact lens have been observed in humans following extracapsular cataract extraction with and without intraocular lens implantation.† On the first and second postoperative days these patients may have a paracentral scotoma associated with an irregularly oval, yellow-white, deep retinal lesion that is most frequently located just above, below, or temporal to the center of the fovea (Fig. 8-16, A). Because of the frequent use of a bridle stay suture superiorly the lesion has been reported most often just below the center of the macula. The lesion stains intensely with fluorescein (Fig. 8-16, B). This is replaced over several days and weeks by a zone of fine mottling of the RPE (Fig. 8-16, C) that is most easily visualized as a focal area of hyperfluorescence angiographically. One case reported as an example of "pseudophakic serous maculopathy" was probably also caused by phototoxicity.[168] Although in most patients central visual acuity is unaffected, the scotoma may be permanent.[110,151] The retinal xanthophyll may play a role in ameliorating the effects of light damage to the center of the macula.[151,154] The reported incidence of photic maculopathy following extracapsular cataract extraction varies from 7 to 28%.[117,158] The most significant risk factor is the preoperative exposure time to the operating microscope light.[117] A variety of measures may prove effective in reducing chances of photic maculopathy in humans, including reduction of operating time, frequent covering of the cornea, oblique illumination, ultraviolet filters, utilization of an air bubble in the anterior chamber, and insertion of the intraocular lens with the plano surface forward.[127] Retinal burns, however, have occurred in spite of all of these precautions except the last mentioned.[113]

Retinal lesions identical to those produced experimentally with endoilluminators have occurred during the course of pars plana vitrectomy in humans.* Typically the burns are sharply defined, less than two disc diameters in size and they assume the shape of the light source used: oval if by filament and round if by fiber optic. Larger more pleomorphic burns, however, may occur. The greatest risk appears to occur during surgical removal of epiretinal membranes and cortical vitreous.[176,182] Reduction of time of exposure, use of low-power source, and avoidance of blue light and high temperature of infusion media are recommended to reduce the risk of a retinal burn.[176] Light damage to the retina may occur in the detached as well as the attached retina.[202]

FIG. 8-15   Lightning Maculopathy.

A to F, Lightning maculopathy occurred in this 25-year-old man who was struck by lightning along with four friends. One was killed; the others were made unconscious. The patient on awakening noted blurred vision and a glare sensation. Five weeks postinjury visual acuity in the right eye was 20/200 and 20/20, left eye. A full-thickness macular hole in the right eye and an impending hole in the left eye were described. Seven weeks after injury the visual acuity was 20/300 and 20/30. In the right eye there was a "cyst" surrounded by a cuff of subretinal fluid (**A**). A similar lesion with a halo of detachment was present in the left eye (**B**). Angiography revealed slight fluorescence in the right eye (**C**). One month later the acuity in the right eye was 20/100 and the cyst in the right eye was smaller (**D**). There was a yellow dot in the center of the left eye (**E**). A posterior subcapsular cataract was present in the right eye (**F**). Fourteen months after the injury the visual acuity was 20/20 in both eyes. Both eyes showed mild hyperpigmentation centrally and an irregular foveal reflex.

(From Handa and Jaffe.[144])

---

*References 116, 127, 148, 152, 154, 155, 159, 180.
†References 151, 153, 158, 160, 161, 168, 172, 177, 184, 186, 188.

*References 131, 162, 171, 173, 174, 176, 182.

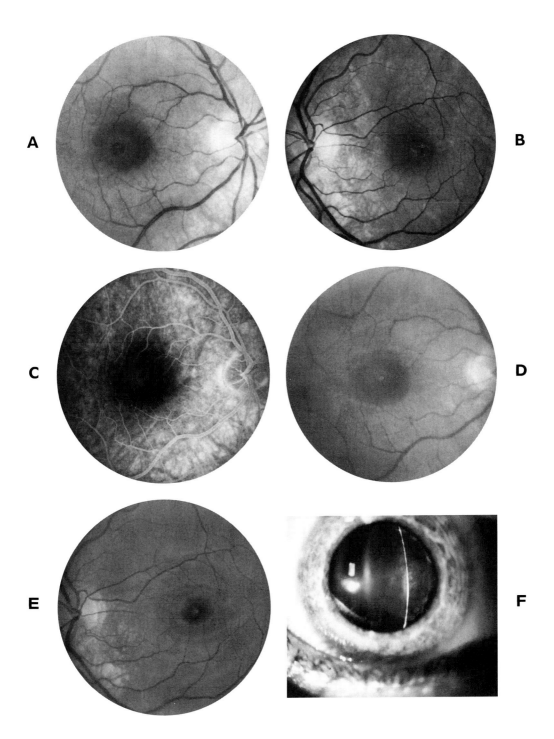

Histopathologic findings in animals and humans exposed to the operating microscope have shown evidence of photoreceptor and RPE damage in the area of the visible retinal burn.[136,161,180] Animal models have demonstrated that high oxygen tension in the blood is associated with worsening of light damage to the retina[153]; high levels of serum vitamin C, corticosteroids, and dimethylthiourea exert a protective effect.[163,185,193] Mitochondria are particularly susceptible to light damage, perhaps because they contain cytochromes that absorb the light.[164]

Although the operating microscope light has been suggested as a possible cause for clinically significant cystoid macular edema, there is little evidence to support this idea.*

Retinal injury from laser exposure

Accidental photocoagulation burns with ruby, argon, neodymium-YAG, and rhodamine dye lasers have been reported.† Fortunately, in most cases good visual function has been retained. Fig. 8-16, D to F, illustrates how a moderately intense solitary laser burn to the center of the fovea is compatible with return of good acuity in spite of destruction of the central photoreceptors.

Ophthalmologists who use operating microscopes or who do laser photocoagulation may have decreased color discrimination for colors in a tritan color-confusion axis.[110,112,138] There is a correlation between the years of laser use and the chronic reduction in color contrast sensitivity.

Wiebers et al. reported four patients with bilateral high-grade carotid artery stenosis who experienced episodic visual impairment related exclusively to light exposure.[199] They postulated that this may be related to delay in regeneration of visual pigments caused by ischemia.

*References 145, 147, 160, 166, 169, 192.
†References 107, 109, 113, 114, 128, 146, 167.

FIG. 8-16   Photic Maculopathy.

A to C, One day after exposure of the right macula of a phakic eye to the operating microscope for a period of 1 hour. The eye was blind because of a craniopharyngioma. Note the gray-white lesion located at the level of the RPE (**A**) and the intense fluorescein staining of the outer retina (**B**). Eight days after the exposure there was mottling of the RPE in the area of the lesion (**C**).

D to F, Acute ruby laser burn in the center of the fovea of a man with a ciliary body melanoma. Visual acuity before the burn was 20/20 and the fundus was normal (**D**). Five minutes after a moderately intense one-degree burn that generated a small steam bubble, there was a central gray foveal opacity (**E**). The visual acuity was 20/70. Two weeks later the acuity had returned to 20/25 at the time of enucleation. Photomicrograph (**F**) shows partial destruction of the central foveal area.

(**A** to **C** from Robertson DM, Feldman RB: *Am J Ophthalmol* 101:561, 1986; published with permission from The American Journal of Ophthalmology; copyright by The Ophthalmic Publishing Co.[184])

Retinal damage caused by chronic exposure to sunlight

The effect of long-term exposure to ambient light on the retina is the subject of considerable controversy. There is some evidence to suggest that age-related macular degeneration may be aggravated by the amount of exposure to the visible wavelengths of sunlight but not to ultraviolet light.[122,189,190,198]

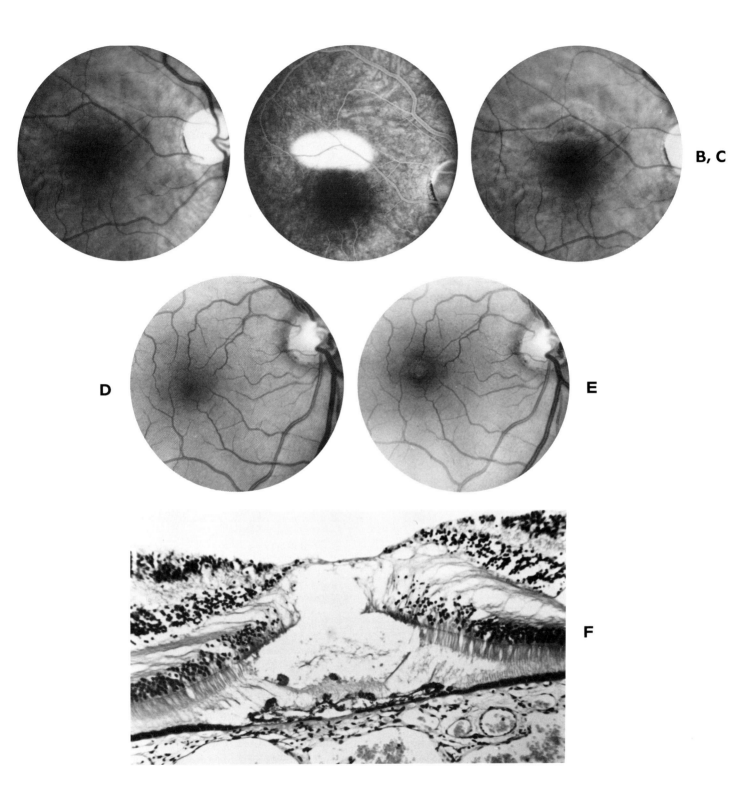

B, C

D

E

F

REFERENCES

Berlin's Edema (Commotio Retinae)

1. Bastek JV, Foos RY, Heckenlively J: Traumatic pigmentary retinopathy. *Am J Ophthalmol* 92:621-624, 1981.
2. Beckingsale AB, Rosenthal AR: Early fundus fluorescein angiographic findings and sequelae in traumatic retinopathy: case report. *Br J Ophthalmol* 67:119-123, 1983.
3. Berlin R: Zur sogenannten Commotio retinae. *Klin Monatsbl Augenheilkd* 11:42-78, 1873.
4. Blight R, Hart JCD: Structural changes in the outer retinal layers following blunt mechanical non-perforating trauma to the globe: an experimental study. *Br J Ophthalmol* 61:573-587, 1977.
5. Bunt-Milam AH, Black RA, Bensinger RE: Breakdown of the outer blood-retinal barrier in experimental *commotio retinae. Exp Eye Res* 43:397-412, 1986.
6. Cogan DG: Pseudoretinitis pigmentosa; report of two traumatic cases of recent origin. *Arch Ophthalmol* 81:45-53, 1969.
7. Gass JDM: *Stereoscopic atlas of macular diseases; diagnosis and treatment,* ed. 2, St. Louis, 1977, CV Mosby, p. 314.
8. Hart JCD, Frank HJ: Retinal opacification after blunt non-perforating concussional injuries to the globe; a clinical and retinal fluorescein angiographic study. *Trans Ophthalmol Soc UK* 95:94-100, 1975.
9. Kohno T, Ishibashi T, Inomata H, et al: Experimental macular edema of commotio retinae: preliminary report. *Jpn J Ophthalmol* 27:149-156, 1983.
10. Levin LA, Seddon JM, Topping T: Retinal pigment epithelial tears associated with trauma. *Am J Ophthalmol* 112:396-400, 1991.
11. Mansour AM, Green WR, Hogge C: Histopathology of commotio retinae. *Retina* 12:24-28, 1992.
12. Pulido JS, Blair NP: The blood-retinal barrier in Berlin's edema. *Retina* 7:233-236, 1987.
13. Sipperley JO, Quigley HA, Gass JDM: Traumatic retinopathy in primates; the explanation of commotio retinae. *Arch Ophthalmol* 96:2267-2273, 1978.
14. Williams DF, Mieler WF, Williams GA: Posterior segment manifestations of ocular trauma. *Retina* 10 (Suppl):S35-S44, 1990.

Macular Complications of Peripheral Chorioretinal Contusion and Rupture (Sclopetaria)

15. Goldzieher W: Beiträg zur Pathologie der orbitalen Schussverletzungen. *Z Augenheilkd* 6:277-285, 1901.
16. Martin DF, Awh CC, McCuen BW II, et al: Treatment and pathogenesis of traumatic chorioretinal rupture (sclopetaria). *Am J Ophthalmol* 117:190-200, 1994.
17. Perry HD, Rahn EK: Chorioretinitis sclopetaria; choroidal and retinal concussion injury from a bullet. *Arch Ophthalmol* 95:328-329, 1977.

Posttraumatic Macular Hole and Foveolar Pit

18. Burke JP, Orton HP, West J, et al: Whiplash and its effect on the visual system. *Graefes Arch Clin Exp Ophthalmol* 230:335-339, 1992.
19. Daily L: Further observations on foveolar splinter and macular wisps. *Arch Ophthalmol* 90:102-103, 1973.
20. Daily L: Macular and vitreal disturbances produced by traumatic vitreous rebound. *South Med J* 63:1197-1198, 1970.
21. Grey RHB: Foveo-macular retinitis, solar retinopathy, and trauma. *Br J Ophthalmol* 62:543-546, 1978.
22. Kelley JS, Hoover RE, George T: Whiplash maculopathy. *Arch Ophthalmol* 96:834-835, 1978.

Purtscher's Retinopathy

23. Beckingsale AB, Rosenthal AR: Early fundus fluorescein angiographic findings and sequelae in traumatic retinopathy: case report. *Br J Ophthalmol* 67:119-123, 1983.
24. Burton TC: Unilateral Purtscher's retinopathy. *Ophthalmology* 87:1096-1105, 1980.
25. Gass JDM: *Stereoscopic atlas of macular diseases; diagnosis and treatment,* ed. 2, St. Louis, 1977, CV Mosby, p. 185.
26. Jacob HS, Craddock PR, Hammerschmidt DE, Moldow CF: Complement-induced granulocyte aggregation; an unsuspected mechanism of disease. *N Engl J Med* 302:789-794, 1980.
27. Kelley JS: Purtscher's retinopathy related to chest compression by safety belts; fluorescein angiographic findings. *Am J Ophthalmol* 74:278-283, 1972.
28. Madsen PH: Traumatic retinal angiopathy (Purtscher). *Ophthalmologica* 165:453-458, 1972.
29. Marr WG, Marr EG: Some observations on Purtscher's disease: traumatic retinal angiopathy. *Am J Ophthalmol* 54:693-705, 1962.
30. Pratt MV, de Venecia G: Purtscher's retinopathy: a clinico-histopathological correlation. *Surv Ophthalmol* 14:417-423, 1970.
31. Purtscher O: Angiopathia retinae traumatica. Lymphorrhagien des Augengrundes. *Albrecht von Graefes Arch Ophthalmol* 82:347-371, 1912.
32. Urbanek J: Über Fettembolie des Auges. *Albrecht von Graefes Arch Ophthalmol* 131:147-173, 1934.

Retinal and Vitreous Hemorrhage Associated with Subarachnoid and Subdural Hemorrhage (Terson's Syndrome)

33. Castrén JA: Pathogeneses and treatment of Terson-syndrome. *Acta Ophthalmol* 41:430-434, 1963.
34. Clarkson JG, Flynn HW Jr, Daily MJ: Vitrectomy in Terson's syndrome. *Am J Ophthalmol* 90:549-552, 1980.
35. Garfinkle AM, Danys IR, Nicolle DA, et al: Terson's syndrome; a reversible cause of blindness following subarachnoid hemorrhage. *J Neurosurg* 76:766-771, 1992.
36. Keithahn MAZ, Bennett SR, Cameron D, Mieler WF: Retinal folds in Terson syndrome. *Ophthalmology* 100:1187-1190, 1993.
37. Khan SG, Frenkel M: Intravitreal hemorrhage associated with rapid increase in intracranial pressure (Terson's syndrome). *Am J Ophthalmol* 80:37-43, 1975.
38. Morris DA, Henkind P: Relationship of intracranial optic-nerve sheath and retinal hemorrhage. *Am J Ophthalmol* 64:853-859, 1967.
39. Schultz PN, Sobol WM, Weingeist TA: Long-term visual outcome in Terson syndrome. *Ophthalmology* 98:1814-1819, 1991.
40. Shaw HE Jr, Landers MB III: Vitreous hemorrhage after intracranial hemorrhage. *Am J Ophthalmol* 80:207-213, 1975.
41. Shaw HE Jr, Landers MB III, Sydnor CF: The significance of intraocular hemorrhages due to subarachnoid hemorrhage. *Ann Ophthalmol* 9:1403-1405, 1977.
42. Terson A: De l'hémorrhagie dans le corps vitré au cours de l'hémorrhagie cérébrale. *Clin Ophtalmol* 6:309, 1900.
43. Terson A: Le syndrome de l'hématome du corps vitré et de l'hémorrhagie intracranienne spontanés. *Ann Oculist* 163:666-673, 1926.
44. Velikay M, Datlinger P, Stolba U, et al: Retinal detachment with severe proliferative vitreoretinopathy in Terson syndrome. *Ophthalmology* 101:35-37, 1994.
45. Walsh FB, Hoyt WF: *Clinical neuro-ophthalmology,* ed. 3, Baltimore, 1969, Williams & Wilkins, p. 1786.

46. Weingeist TA, Goldman EJ, Folk JC, et al: Terson's syndrome; clinicopathologic correlations. *Ophthalmology* 93: 1435-1442, 1986.

Hemorrhagic Maculopathy Caused by Subarachnoid and Epidural Injections

47. Kushner FH, Olson JC: Retinal hemorrhage as a consequence of epidural steroid injection. *Arch Ophthalmol* 113:309-313, 1995.
48. Ling C, Atkinson PL, Munton CGF: Bilateral retinal haemorrhages following epidural injection. *Br J Ophthalmol* 77:316-317, 1993.
49. Oberman J, Cohn H, Grand MG: Retinal complications of gas myelography. *Arch Ophthalmol* 97:1905-1906, 1979.

Shaken Baby Syndrome

50. Budenz DL, Farber MG, Mirchandani HG, et al: Ocular and optic nerve hemorrhages in abused infants with intracranial injuries. *Ophthalmology* 101:559-565, 1994.
51. Buys YM, Levin AV, Enzenauer RW, et al: Retinal findings after head trauma in infants and young children. *Ophthalmology* 99:1718-1723, 1992.
52. Elner SG, Elner VM, Arnall M, Albert DM: Ocular and associated systemic findings in suspected child abuse; a necropsy study. *Arch Ophthalmol* 108:1094-1101, 1990.
53. Friendly DS: Ocular manifestations of physical child abuse. *Trans Am Acad Ophthalmol Otolaryngol* 75:318-332, 1971.
54. Gaynon MW, Koh K, Marmor MF, Frankel LR: Retinal folds in the shaken baby syndrome. *Am J Ophthalmol* 106:423-425, 1988.
55. Gilkes MJ, Mann TP: Fundi of battered babies. *Lancet* 2:468-469, 1967.
56. Greenwald MJ, Weiss A, Oesterle CS, Friendly DS: Traumatic retinoschisis in battered babies. *Ophthalmology* 93:618-625, 1986.
57. Han DP, Wilkinson WS: Late ophthalmic manifestations of the shaken baby syndrome. *J Pediatr Ophthalmol Strabismus* 27:299-303, 1990.
58. Harley RD: Ocular manifestations of child abuse. *J Pediatr Ophthalmol Strabismus* 17:5-13, 1980.
59. Jensen AD, Smith RE, Olson MI: Ocular clues to child abuse. *J Pediatr Ophthalmol* 8:270-272, 1971.
60. Lambert SR, Johnson TE, Hoyt CS: Optic nerve sheath and retinal hemorrhages associated with the shaken baby syndrome. *Arch Ophthalmol* 104:1509-1512, 1986.
61. Ludwig S, Warman M: Shaken baby syndrome: a review of 20 cases. *Ann Emerg Med* 13:104-107, 1984.
62. Massicotte SJ, Folberg R, Torczynski E, et al: Vitreoretinal traction and perimacular retinal folds in the eyes of deliberately traumatized children. *Ophthalmology* 98:1124-1127, 1991.
63. Ober RR: Hemorrhagic retinopathy in infancy: a clinicopathologic report. *J Pediatr Ophthalmol Strabismus* 17:17-20, 1980.
64. Riffenburgh RS, Sathyavagiswaran L: Ocular findings at autopsy of child abuse victims. *Ophthalmology* 98:1519-1524, 1991.
65. San Martin R, Steinkuller PG, Nisbet RM: Retinopathy in the sexually abused battered child. *Ann Ophthalmol* 13:89-91, 1981.
66. Spaide RF: Shaken baby syndrome; ocular and computed tomographic findings. *J Clin Neuro-Ophthalmol* 7:108-111, 1987.
67. Tongue AC: Editorial: The ophthalmologist's role in diagnosing child abuse. *Ophthalmology* 98:1009-1010, 1991.
68. Wilkinson WS, Han DP, Rappley MD, Owings CL: Retinal hemorrhage predicts neurologic injury in the shaken baby syndrome. *Arch Ophthalmol* 107:1472-1474, 1989.

Retinal Vessel Rupture Associated with Physical Extention (Valsalva Retinopathy)

69. Duane TD: Valsalva hemorrhagic retinopathy. *Am J Ophthalmol* 75:637-642, 1973.
70. Gabel V-P, Birngruber R, Gunther-Koszka H, Puliafito CA: Nd:YAG laser photodisruption of hemorrhagic detachment of the internal limiting membrane *Am J Ophthalmol* 107:33-37, 1989.
71. Gass JDM: Options in the treatment of macular diseases. *Trans Ophthalmol Soc UK* 92:449-468, 1972.
72. Gass JDM: *Stereoscopic atlas of macular diseases; diagnosis and treatment,* ed. 2, St. Louis, 1977, CV Mosby, p. 320.
73. Kalina RE, Kaiser M: Familial retinal hemorrhages. *Am J Ophthalmol* 74:252-255, 1972.
74. Kassoff A, Catalano RA, Mehu M: Vitreous hemorrhage and the Valsalva maneuver in proliferative diabetic retinopathy. *Retina* 8:174-176, 1988.
75. Linde R, Record R, Ferguson J: Resolution of preretinal hemorrhage. *Arch Ophthalmol* 95:1466-1467, 1977.
76. Pitta CG, Steinert RF, Gragoudas ES, Regan CDJ: Small unilateral foveal hemorrhages in young adults. *Am J Ophthalmol* 89:96-102, 1980.
77. Pruett RC, Carvalho ACA, Trempe CL: Microhemorrhagic maculopathy. *Arch Ophthalmol* 99:425-432, 1981.

Evulsion of the Optic Disc

78. Archer DB, Canavan YM: Contusional injuries of the distal optic nerve. *Trans Ophthalmol Soc NZ* 35:14-23, 1983.
79. Chang M, Eifrig DE: Optic nerve avulsion. *Arch Ophthalmol* 105:322-323, 1987.
80. Park JH, Frenkel M, Dobbie JG, Choromokos E: Evulsion of the optic nerve. *Am J Ophthalmol* 72:969-971, 1971.
81. Salzmann M: Die Ausreissung des Sehnerven (Evulsio nervi optici). *Z Augenheilkd* 9:489-505, 1903.
82. Williams DF, Williams GA, Abrams GW, et al: Evulsion of the retina associated with optic nerve evulsion. *Am J Ophthalmol* 104:5-9, 1987.

Ocular Decompression Retinopathy

83. Fechtner RD, Minckler D, Weinreb RN, et al: Complications of glaucoma surgery; ocular decompression retinopathy. *Arch Ophthalmol* 110:965-968, 1992.

Intraocular Foreign Bodies

84. Bego B, Turut P, Malthieu D, et al: Neo-vaisseaux sous-retiniens apres plaie chorio-retinienne pars corps etranger intra-oculaire (1 cas). *Bull Soc Ophtalmol Fr* 89:263-265, 1989.
85. Ferry AP: Lesions mistaken for malignant melanoma of the posterior uvea; a clinicopathologic analysis of 100 cases with ophthalmoscopically visible lesions. *Arch Ophthalmol* 72:463-469, 1964.
86. Lebowitz HA, Couch JM, Thompson JT, Shields JA: Occult foreign body simulating a choroidal melanoma with extrascleral extension. *Retina* 8:141-144, 1988.
87. Lipper S, Eifrig DE, Peiffer RL, Bagnell CR: Chorioretinal foreign body simulating malignant melanoma. *Am J Ophthalmol* 92:202-205, 1981.
88. Rones B, Zimmerman LE: An unusual choroidal hemorrhage simulating malignant melanoma. *Arch Ophthalmol* 70:30-32, 1963.

Chorioretinopathy and Optic Neuropathy Associated with Retrobulbar Injections.

89. Ahn JC, Stanley JA: Subarachnoid injection as a complication of retrobulbar anesthesia. *Am J Ophthalmol* 103:225-230, 1987.

90. Brookshire GL, Gleitsmann KY, Schenk EC: Life-threatening complication of retrobulbar block; a hypothesis. *Ophthalmology* 93:1476-1478, 1986.

91. Cohen SM, Sousa FJ, Kelly NE, Wendel RT: Respiratory arrest and new retinal hemorrhages after retrobulbar anesthesia. *Am J Ophthalmol* 113:209-211, 1992.

92. Duker JS, Belmont JB, Benson WE, et al: Inadvertent globe perforation during retrobulbar and peribulbar anesthesia; patient characteristics, surgical management, and visual outcome. *Ophthalmology* 98:519-526, 1991.

93. Friedberg HL, Kline OR Jr: Contralateral amaurosis after retrobulbar injection. *Am J Ophthalmol* 101:688-690, 1986.

94. Grizzard WS, Kirk NM, Pavan PR, et al: Perforating ocular injuries caused by anesthesia personnel. *Ophthalmology* 98:1011-1016, 1991.

95. Hay A, Flynn HW Jr, Hoffman JI, Rivera AH: Needle penetration of the globe during retrobulbar and peribulbar injections. *Ophthalmology* 98:1017-1024, 1991.

96. Hersch M, Baer G, Dieckert JP, et al: Optic nerve enlargement and central retinal-artery occlusion secondary to retrobulbar anesthesia. *Ann Ophthalmol* 21:195-197, 1989.

97. Javitt JC, Addiego R, Friedberg HL, et al: Brain stem anesthesia after retrobulbar block. *Ophthalmology* 94:718-724, 1987.

98. Katsev DA, Drews RC, Rose BT: An anatomic study of retrobulbar needle length. *Ophthalmology* 96:1221-1224, 1989.

99. Klein ML, Jampol LM, Condon PI, et al: Central retinal artery occlusion without retrobulbar hemorrhage after retrobulbar anesthesia. *Am J Ophthalmol* 93:573-577, 1982.

100. Lee DS, Kwon NJ: Shivering following retrobulbar block. *Can J Anaesth* 35:294-296, 1988.

101. Martin DF, Meredith TA, Topping TM, et al: Perforating (through-and-through) injuries of the globe; surgical results with vitrectomy. *Arch Ophthalmol* 109:951-956, 1991.

102. Mieler WF, Bennett SR, Platt LW, Koenig SB: Localized retinal detachment with combined central retinal artery and vein occlusion after retrobulbar anesthesia. *Retina* 10:278-283, 1990.

103. Morgan CM, Schatz H, Vine AK, et al: Ocular complications associated with retrobulbar injections. *Ophthalmology* 95:660-665, 1988.

104. Pautler SE, Grizzard WS, Thompson LN, Wing GL: Blindness from retrobulbar injection into the optic nerve. *Ophthalmic Surg* 17:334-337, 1986.

105. Schneider ME, Milstein DE, Oyakawa RT et al: Ocular perforation from a retrobulbar injection. *Am J Ophthalmol* 106:35-40, 1988.

Photic Maculopathy

106. Agarwal LP, Malik SRK: Solar retinitis. *Br J Ophthalmol* 43:366-370, 1959.

107. Alhalel A, Glovinsky Y, Treister G, et al: Long-term follow up of accidental parafoveal laser burns. *Retina* 13:152-154, 1993.

108. Anaclerio AM, Wicker HS: Self-induced solar retinopathy by patients in a psychiatric hospital. *Am J Ophthalmol* 69:731-736, 1970.

109. Anderson DR, Knighton RW, Feuer WJ: Evaluation of phototoxic retinal damage after argon laser iridotomy. *Am J Ophthalmol* 107:398-402, 1989.

110. Arden GB, Berninger T, Hogg CR, Perry S: A survey of color discrimination in German ophthalmologists; changes associated with the use of lasers and operating microscopes. *Ophthalmology* 98:567-575, 1991.

111. Beaumont P: Retinal burns from MIG-welding arcs. *Br J Ophthalmol* 73:852, 1989.

112. Berninger TA, Canning CR, Gündüz K, et al: Using argon laser blue light reduces ophthalmologists' color contrast sensitivity; argon blue and surgeons' vision. *Arch Ophthalmol* 107:1453-1458, 1989.

113. Boldrey EE, Ho BT, Griffith RD: Retinal burns occurring at cataract extraction. *Ophthalmology* 91:1297-1302, 1984.

114. Boldrey EE, Little HL, Flocks M, Vassiliadis A: Retinal injury due to industrial laser burns. *Ophthalmology* 88:101-107, 1981.

115. Brittain GPH: Retinal burns caused by exposure to MIG-welding arcs: report of two cases. *Br J Ophthalmol* 72:570-575, 1988.

116. Brod RD, Olsen KR, Ball SF, Packer AJ: The site of operating microscope light-induced injury on the human retina. *Am J Ophthalmol* 107:390-397, 1989.

117. Byrnes GA, Antoszyk AN, Mazur DO, et al: Photic maculopathy after extracapsular surgery; a prospective study. *Ophthalmology* 99:731-738, 1992.

118. Campo RV, Lewis RS: Lightning-induced macular hole. *Am J Ophthalmol* 97:792-794, 1984.

119. Cangelosi GC, Newsome DA: Solar retinopathy in persons on religious pilgrimage. *Am J Ophthalmol* 105:95-97, 1988.

120. Cialdini AP, Jalkh AE, Tolentino FI: Acute foveal outer retinopathy. *Arch Ophthalmol* 105:1490, 1987.

121. Cordes FC: Eclipse retinitis. *Am J Ophthalmol* 31:101-103, 1948.

122. Cruickshanks KJ, Klein R, Klein BEK: Sunlight and age-related macular degeneration; the Beaver Dam Eye Study. *Arch Ophthalmol* 111:514-518, 1993.

123. Dolphin K, Lincoff H: Bilateral radiant damage to the cornea and retina after exposure to a 700-V electric discharge. *Am J Ophthalmol* 114:775-776, 1992.

124. Duke-Elder S, MacFaul PA: *System of ophthalmology, vol. 14, part 2: Non-mechanical injuries,* St Louis, 1971, CV Mosby, pp. 813-835.

125. Ewald RA: Sun gazing associated with the use of LSD. *Ann Ophthalmol* 3:15-17, 1971.

126. Ewald RA, Ritchey CL: Sun gazing as the cause of foveomacular retinitis. *Am J Ophthalmol* 70:491-497, 1970.

127. Fechner PU, Barth R: Effect on the retina of an air cushion in the anterior chamber and coaxial illumination. *Am J Ophthalmol* 96:600-604, 1983.

128. Fowler BJ: Accidental industrial laser burn of macula. *Ann Ophthalmol* 15:481-483, 1983.

129. Freedman J, Gombos GM: Fluorescein fundus angiography in self-induced solar retinopathy; a case report. *Can J Ophthalmol* 6:124-127, 1971.

130. Friedman E, Kuwabara T: The retinal pigment epithelium. IV. The damaging effects of radiant energy. *Arch Ophthalmol* 80:265-279, 1968.

131. Fuller D, Machemer R, Knighton RW: Retinal damage produced by intraocular fiber optic light. *Am J Ophthalmol* 85:519-537, 1978.

132. Fuller DG: Severe solar maculopathy associated with the use of lysergic acid diethylamide (LSD). *Am J Ophthalmol* 81:413-416, 1976.

133. Gardner TW, Ai E, Chrobak M, Shoch DE: Photic maculopathy secondary to short-circuiting of a high-tension electric current. *Ophthalmology* 89:865-868, 1982.

134. Gass JDM: *Stereoscopic atlas of macular diseases; diagnosis and treatment,* ed. 2, St. Louis, 1977, CV Mosby, p. 322.

135. Gladstone GJ, Tasman W: Solar retinitis after minimal exposure. *Arch Ophthalmol* 96:1368-1369, 1978.

136. Green WR, Robertson DM: Pathologic findings of photic retinopathy in the human eye. *Am J Ophthalmol* 112:520-527, 1991.

137. Grey RHB: Foveo-macular retinitis, solar retinopathy, and trauma. *Br J Ophthalmol* 62:543-546, 1978.

138. Gündüz K, Arden GB: Changes in colour contrast sensitivity associated with operating argon lasers. *Br J Ophthalmol* 73:241-246, 1989.

139. Ham WT Jr, Mueller HA, Ruffolo JJ Jr, Guerry D III: Solar retinopathy as a function of wavelength: its significance for protective eyewear. *In:* Williams TP, Baker BN, editors: *The effects of constant light on visual processes,* New York, 1980, Plenum Press, pp. 319-346.

140. Ham WT Jr, Mueller HA, Ruffolo JJ Jr, et al: Action spectrum for retinal injury from near-ultraviolet radiation in the aphakic monkey. *Am J Ophthalmol* 93:299-306, 1982.

141. Ham WT Jr, Mueller HA, Sliney DH: Retinal sensitivity to damage from short wavelength light. *Nature* 260:153-154, 1976.

142. Ham WT Jr, Mueller HA, Williams RC, Geeraets WJ: Ocular hazard from viewing the sun unprotected and through various windows and filters. *Appl Optics* 12:2122-2129, 1973.

143. Ham WT Jr, Ruffolo JJ Jr, Mueller HA, et al: Histologic analysis of photochemical lesions produced in rhesus retina by short-wavelength light. *Invest Ophthalmol Vis Sci* 17:1029-1035, 1978.

144. Handa JT, Jaffe GJ: Lightning maculopathy; a case report. *Retina* 14:169-172, 1994.

145. Henry MM, Henry LM, Henry LM: A possible cause of chronic cystic maculopathy. *Ann Ophthalmol* 9:455-457, 1977.

146. Hirsch DR, Booth DG, Schocket S, Sliney DH: Recovery from pulsed-dye laser retinal injury. *Arch Ophthalmol* 110:1688-1689, 1992.

147. Hochheimer BF: A possible cause of chronic cystic maculopathy; the operating microscope. *Ann Ophthalmol* 13:153-155, 1981.

148. Hochheimer BF, D'Anna SA, Calkins JL: Retinal damage from light. *Am J Ophthalmol* 88:1039-1044, 1979.

149. Hope-Ross M, Travers S, Mooney D: Solar retinopathy following religious rituals. *Br J Ophthalmol* 72:931-934, 1988.

150. Hope-Ross MW, Mahon GJ, Gardiner TA, Archer DB: Ultrastructural findings in solar retinopathy. *Eye* 7:29-33, 1993.

151. Hupp SL: Delayed, incomplete recovery of macular function after photic retinal damage associated with extracapsular cataract extraction and posterior lens insertion. *Arch Ophthalmol* 105:1022-1023, 1987.

152. Irvine AR, Wood I, Morris BW: Retinal damage from the illumination of the operating microscope; an experimental study in pseudophakic monkeys. *Arch Ophthalmol* 102:1358-1365, 1984.

153. Jaffe GJ, Irvine AR, Wood IS, et al: Retinal phototoxicity from the operating microscope; the role of inspired oxygen. *Ophthalmology* 95:1130-1141, 1988.

154. Jaffe GJ, Wood IS: Retinal phototoxicity from the operating microscope: a protective effect by the fovea. *Arch Ophthalmol* 106:445-446, 1988.

155. Johnson RN, Schatz H, McDonald HR: Photic maculopathy: early angiographic and ophthalmoscopic findings and late development of choroidal folds. *Arch Ophthalmol* 105:1633-1634, 1987.

156. Kelly JS, Hoover RE, George T: Whiplash maculopathy. *Arch Ophthalmol* 96:834-835, 1978.

157. Kerr LM, Little HL: Foveomacular retinitis. *Arch Ophthalmol* 76:498-504, 1966.

158. Khwarg SG, Geoghegan M, Hanscom TA: Light-induced maculopathy from the operating microscope. *Am J Ophthalmol* 98:628-630, 1984.

159. Khwarg SG, Linstone FA, Daniels SA, et al: Incidence, risk factors, and morphology in operating microscope light retinopathy. *Am J Ophthalmol* 103:255-263, 1987.

160. Kraff MC, Sanders DR, Jampol LM, Lieberman HL: Effect of an ultraviolet-filtering intraocular lens on cystoid macular edema. *Ophthalmology* 92:366-369, 1985.

161. Kramer T, Brown R, Lynch M, et al: Molteno implants and operating microscope-induced retinal phototoxicity; a clinicopathologic report. *Arch Ophthalmol* 109:379-383, 1991.

162. Kuhn F, Morris R, Massey M: Photic retinal injury from endoillumination during vitrectomy. *Am J Ophthalmol* 111:42-46, 1991.

163. Lam S, Tso MOM, Gurne DH: Amelioration of retinal photic injury in albino rats by dimethylthiourea. *Arch Ophthalmol* 108:1751-1757, 1990.

164. Lawwill T: Effects of prolonged exposure of rabbit retina to low-intensity light. *Invest Ophthalmol* 12:45-51, 1973.

165. Lawwill T: Three major pathologic processes caused by light in the primate retina: a search for mechanisms. *Trans Am Ophthalmol Soc* 80:517-579, 1982.

166. Li Z-L, Tso MOM, Jampol LM, et al: Retinal injury induced by near-ultraviolet radiation in aphakic and pseudophakic monkey eyes; a preliminary report. *Retina* 10:301-314, 1990.

167. Liu HF, Gao GH, Wu DC, et al: Ocular injuries from accidental laser exposure. *Health Phys* 56:711-716, 1989.

168. Macy JI, Baerveldt G: Pseudophakic serous maculopathy. *Arch Ophthalmol* 101:228-231, 1983.

169. Mannis MJ, Becker B: Retinal light exposure and cystoid macular edema. *Arch Ophthalmol* 98:1133, 1980.

170. Marlor RL, Blais BR, Preston FR, Boyden DG: Foveomacular retinitis, an important problem in military medicine: Epidemiology. *Invest Ophthalmol* 12:5-16, 1973.

171. McDonald HR, Harris MJ: Operating microscope-induced retinal phototoxicity during pars plana vitrectomy. *Arch Ophthalmol* 106:521-523, 1988.

172. McDonald HR, Irvine AR: Light-induced maculopathy from the operating microscope in extracapsular cataract extraction and intraocular lens implantation. *Ophthalmology* 90:945-951, 1983.

173. McDonald HR, Verre WP, Aaberg TM: Surgical management of idiopathic epiretinal membranes. *Ophthalmology* 93:978-983, 1986.

174. Meyers SM, Bonner RF: Retinal irradiance from vitrectomy endoilluminators. *Am J Ophthalmol* 94:26-29, 1982.

175. Michaels M, Dawson WW, Feldman RB, Jarolem K: Infrared; an unseen and unnecessary hazard in ophthalmic devices. *Ophthalmology* 94:143-148, 1987.

176. Michels M, Lewis H, Abrams GW, et al: Macular phototoxicity caused by fiberoptic endoillumination during pars plana vitrectomy. *Am J Ophthalmol* 114:287-296, 1992.

177. Michels M, Sternberg P Jr: Operating microscope-induced retinal phototoxicity: pathophysiology, clinical manifestations and prevention. *Surv Ophthalmol* 34:237-252, 1990.

178. Naidoff MA, Sliney DH: Retinal injury from a welding arc. *Am J Ophthalmol* 77:663-668, 1974.

179. Noel L-P, Clarke WN, Addison D: Ocular complications of lightning. *J Pediatr Ophthalmol Strabismus* 17:245-246, 1980.

773

180. Parver LM, Auker CR, Fine BS: Observations on monkey eyes exposed to light from an operating microscope. *Ophthalmology* 90:964-972, 1983.

181. Penner R, McNair JN: Eclipse blindness; report of an epidemic in the military population of Hawaii. *Am J Ophthalmol* 61:1452-1457, 1966.

182. Poliner LS, Tornambe PE: Retinal pigment epitheliopathy after macular hole surgery. *Ophthalmology* 99:1671-1677, 1992.

183. Power WJ, Travers SP, Mooney DJ: Welding arc maculopathy and fluphenazine. *Br J Ophthalmol* 75:433-435, 1991.

184. Robertson DM, Feldman RB: Photic retinopathy from the operating room microscope. *Am J Ophthalmol* 101:561-569, 1986.

185. Rosner M, Lam TT, Fu J, Tso MOM: Methylprednisolone ameliorates retinal photic injury in rats. *Arch Ophthalmol* 110:857-861, 1992.

186. Ross WH: Light-induced maculopathy. *Am J Ophthalmol* 98:488-493, 1984.

187. Schatz H, Mendelblatt F: Solar retinopathy from sun-gazing under the influence of LSD. *Br J Ophthalmol* 57:270-273, 1973.

188. Stamler JF, Blodi CF, Verdier D, Krachmer JH: Microscope light-induced maculopathy in combined penetrating keratoplasty, extracapsular cataract extraction, and intraocular lens implantation. *Ophthalmology* 95:1142-1146, 1988.

189. Taylor HR, Muñoz B, West S, et al: Visible light and risk of age-related macular degeneration. *Trans Am Ophthalmol Soc* 88:163-173, 1990.

190. Taylor HR, West S, Muñoz B, et al: The long-term effects of visible light on the eye. *Arch Ophthalmol* 110:99-104, 1992.

191. Terrien F: Du pronostic des troubles visuels d'origine électrique. *Arch Ophthalmol (Paris)* 22:692-738, 1902.

192. Tso MOM: Photic maculopathy in rhesus monkey; a light and electron microscopic study. *Invest Ophthalmol* 12:17-34, 1973.

193. Tso MOM: Retinal photic injury in normal and scorbutic monkeys. *Trans Am Ophthalmol Soc* 85:498-556, 1987.

194. Tso MOM, LaPiana FG: The human fovea after sungazing. *Trans Am Acad Ophthalmol Otolaryngol* 79:OP788-OP795, 1975.

195. Tso MOM, Wallow IHL, Powell JO, Zimmerman LE: Recovery of the rod and cone cells after photic injury. *Trans Am Acad Ophthalmol Otolaryngol* 76:1247-1261, 1972.

196. Tso MOM, Woodford BJ: Effect of photic injury on the retinal tissues. *Ophthalmology* 90:952-963, 1983.

197. Uniat L, Olk RJ, Hanish SJ: Arc-welding maculopathy. *Am J Ophthalmol* 102:394-395, 1986.

198. West SK, Rosenthal FS, Bressler NM, et al: Exposure to sunlight and other risk factors for age-related macular degeneration. *Arch Ophthalmol* 107:875-879, 1989.

199. Wiebers DO, Swanson JW, Cascino TL, Whisnant JP: Bilateral loss of vision in bright light. *Stroke* 20:554-558, 1989.

200. Würdemann HV: The formation of a hole in the macula; light burn from exposure to electric welding. *Am J Ophthalmol* 19:457-460, 1936.

201. Yannuzzi LA, Fisher YL, Slakter JS, Krueger A: Solar retinopathy; a photobiologic and geophysical analysis. *Retina* 9:28-43, 1989.

202. Zilis JD, Machemer R: Light damage in detached retina. *Am J Ophthalmol* 111:47-50, 1991.

9

Toxic Diseases Affecting the Pigment Epithelium and Retina

Medications or other substances that find their way into the eye may cause visual dysfunction by virtue of a toxic effect on the sensory retina, the retinal pigment epithelium (RPE), and the optic nerve. In some instances (e.g., digitalis toxicity) visual symptoms may be unassociated with ophthalmoscopic changes in the fundus. In other instances the ophthalmoscopic changes may involve any one or a combination of the RPE, retina, and optic nerve head. Fluorescein angiography is particularly valuable in detecting mild toxic alterations of the RPE before they are apparent ophthalmoscopically.

▼ CHLOROQUINE (ARALEN) AND HYDROXYCHLOROQUINE (PLAQUENIL) RETINOPATHY

Chloroquine initially was used as antimalarial agent in World War II, but more recently it has been used in the treatment of amebiasis, rheumatoid arthritis, and systemic lupus erythematosus. Degeneration of the retinal pigment epithelium and sensory retina caused by prolonged use of chloroquine or hydroxychloroquine is one of the most important of the retinotoxic diseases.* Most patients who have developed retinopathy have received daily doses of chloroquine in excess of 250 mg or hydroxychloroquine in excess of 750 mg for at least a total dose of between 100 and 300 g.[28] There is evidence that the incidence of retinotoxic effects is lower following hydroxychloroquine than following chloroquine therapy.[17,21,24,28,29] Only four unequivocal cases of hydroxychloroquine retinopathy have been reported to date.[17,27,29] All had normal or reduced visual acuity, paracentral scotomata, and bull's-eye maculopathy. Two had evidence of peripheral retinopathy.[29] Although it has been suggested that patients receiving daily dosages of hydroxychloroquine up to 400 mg or 6.5 mg/kg of body weight per day may tolerate massive cumulative doses (for example 3923 g) without developing retinopathy,[17] such did occur in one patient who received 400 mg/day and a total dose of 2920 g.[29] I have recently seen another woman who after taking a total of 146 g (200 mg/day × 730 days) of hydroxychloroquine experienced rapid development of paracentral visual field loss and early bull's-eye maculopathy. The retinopathy caused by both drugs is probably a general toxic effect and not an idiosyncratic reaction. Vitreous fluorophotometry has demonstrated a breakdown in the blood–retinal barrier in patients receiving chloroquine but

*References 1, 3-5, 7, 9, 10, 12-16, 18-20, 22-26, 28, 31.

FIG. 9-1   Chloroquine Retinopathy.

A and B, After receiving chloroquine, 250 mg daily for 27 years for discoid disseminated lupus erythematosus, this 50-year-old woman noted blurring of vision in both eyes. Visual acuity was 20/30. She had a symmetric bull's-eye pattern of atrophy of the RPE in both eyes (**A**). Early arteriovenous-phase angiography revealed evidence of preservation of the choriocapillaris within the area of RPE atrophy centrally (**B**). Electroretinographic findings were normal.

C and D, This 53-year-old woman received a total dose of 454 g of hydroxychloroquine and chloroquine over a 36-month period. She showed progressive RPE and retinal degeneration for 16 years after stopping the medication.

E to I, This 50-year-old woman, who received chloroquine, 500 mg/day for 13 years for rheumatoid arthritis, began to notice a "halo" scotoma and nyctalopia in both eyes in February of 1977. Her visual acuity at that time was 20/30. She had a bull's-eye pattern of RPE atrophy bilaterally (**E**) that was most evident angiographically (**F**). Her electroretinographic findings were normal. The chloroquine was discontinued. Seven years later the bull's-eye pattern of atrophy had enlarged slightly and her visual acuity had decreased to 20/50 (**G and H**). Two years later she had experienced further loss of vision. The central island of RPE showed further evidence of atrophy angiographically (**I**). Visual acuity at that time was 20/200.

J to K, This 67-year-old woman developed bull's-eye maculopathy after receiving hydroxychloroquine 200 mg bid for 6 years. Her visual acuity was 20/50, right eye, and 20/70, left eye.

L, Histopathology of chloroquine maculopathy showing focal loss of the outer nuclear layer and the receptor elements, irregular depigmentation of the RPE, and preservation of the choriocapillaris.

(**C and D,** courtesy Dr. Ray T. Oyakawa, were made 6 years after photographs in a previous report by Brinkley et al.[3]; **K** from Wetterholm and Winter.[31])

not hydroxychloroquine.[21] The earliest sign of toxicity, which may occur before development of any other ophthalmoscopic or electrophysiologic abnormality, is a paracentral visual field loss. The patients's use of the Amsler grid may be helpful in detecting these early field defects.[7] The earliest ophthalmoscopic and angiographic alterations in the RPE occur in the parafoveal area (Fig. 9-1, *A* to *C,* and *E* to *K*). At this stage a paracentral scotoma and minimal or no loss of visual acuity are characteristic. An enlarging ring of atrophy of the RPE surrounding the fovea produces a bull's-eye–like lesion that is indistinguishable ophthalmoscopically from other causes of this lesion (see p. 336 in Chapter 5).

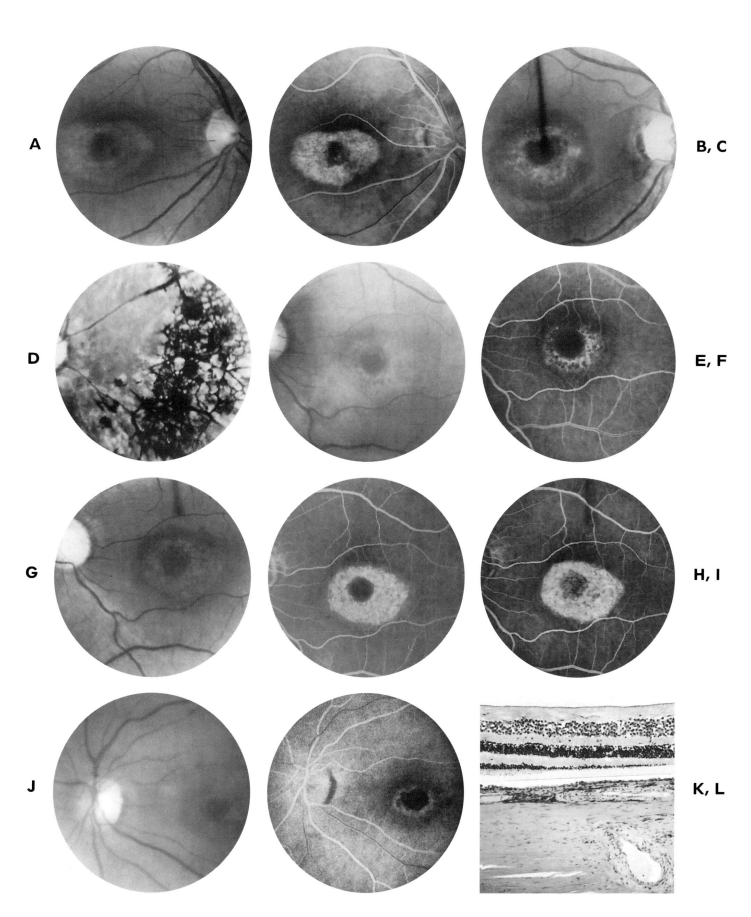

A

B, C

D

E, F

G

H, I

J

K, L

777

As the RPE alterations extend into the foveolar area, the patient loses central vision. Weiter has suggested that the retinal xanthophyll in the foveolar area may exert a photoprotective effect in the various causes of bull's-eye maculopathy.[30] In addition to changes in the posterior pole, continued use of the drug may cause extensive alterations in the RPE and retina peripherally (Fig. 9-1, D). These changes, together with narrowing of the retinal vessels and optic disc pallor, may resemble primary tapetoretinal dystrophies. Severe visual loss and blindness may eventually occur. Other ocular changes caused by chloroquine include whitening of the lashes, a whorl-like pattern of subepithelial corneal deposits, decreased corneal sensitivity, and extraocular muscle palsies.[10,16]

Fluorescein angiography is helpful in demonstrating the faint bull's-eye pattern of hyperfluorescence before its detection biomicroscopically, particularly in patients with blond fundi. In patients with darkly pigmented fundi, biomicroscopic evidence of RPE changes may precede angiographic changes.[6] The area of RPE depigmentation (Fig. 9-1, B, F, H, and I) in general corresponds with the area of field loss. There is minimal angiographic evidence of damage to the choriocapillaris in the areas of RPE depigmentation (Fig. 9-1, B) (see discussion in Chapter 2, p. 20). The detection of small paracentral scotomata to red light is one of the earliest findings in chloroquine toxicity. Use of static perimetry through the vertical meridian may be the most sensitive means of detecting the early visual field damage.[12] The electrooculogram and electroretinogram may be abnormal early. The electrooculogram may initially be supernormal (200% to 350%).[13]

Ideally patients requiring more than 200 mg chloroquine or 350 mg of hydroxychloroquine daily should have a complete eye examination, including visual acuity, visual fields, and fundus photography. If there is any biomicroscopic evidence of abnormality of the RPE or other signs of retinal degeneration or a family history of retinal degeneration, fluorescein angiography, EOG, and ERG should be considered as part of the baseline workup.

Histopathologically, depigmentation of the RPE, loss of the rod and cone receptor elements, and subretinal clumping of pigment occur in the macular area (Fig. 9-1, L).[2,31] Electron microscopic studies have revealed widespread changes in the retina, with the most severe occurring in the ganglion cells in spite of their relatively normal appearance by light microscopy.[22] There is experimental evidence that chloroquine is concentrated in the RPE and remains there long after cessation of treatment.[1,23] Although there is some evidence that the early electrophysiologic changes may be reversible, in most cases, once visual loss has occurred, it is irreversible and it may progress long after cessation of treatment (Fig. 9-1, E to I).[8,15,19,26] There may be an interval of 7 years or longer after cessation of chloroquine and the development of the first signs of retinopathy.[8] Some patients with disease attributed to late onset and progression of chloroquine retinopathy may in fact have had a genetically determined disease that can cause fundus changes identical to chloroquine retinopathy (e.g., cone dystrophy, rod–cone dystrophy, ceroid lipofuscinosis, and Stargardt's disease).

▼ THIORIDAZINE (MELLARIL) RETINOPATHY

Patients with acute thioridazine retinopathy typically experience blurred vision, dyschromatopsia (brownish coloration), or nyctalopia 3 to 8 weeks after receiving the drug in excess of 800 mg/day[11,32,34-41,43-47] and less frequently in lower doses.[32,39] Maximum daily dose seems more critical than cumulative dose. The fundus may be normal initially. Later a mild, fine, then coarse granular salt-and-pepper pigmentary retinopathy with a relatively uniform distribution involving the macula and sometimes the midperiphery as well may occur (Fig. 9-2, *A*). In some patients this may progress to include patchy or nummular areas of loss of the RPE and choriocapillaris (Fig. 9-2, *D* to *F*)[3,41,43,44] and may eventually progress to a severe diffuse tapetoretinal degeneration. Progression of the pigmentary changes but not necessarily functional changes may occur after the medication is discontinued.[35,42,43] Visual function may occasionally improve after cessation of toxic levels of the drug.[42] Other patients, however, may experience a late, slow progression of functional as well as anatomic changes. The progressive enlargement and confluence of patches of extrafoveal geographic atrophy of the RPE and choriocapillaris are similar to those seen in gyrate atrophy, Bietti's crystalline dystrophy, and choroideremia. Fluorescein angiography may be helpful in detecting mild RPE alterations (Fig. 9-2, *B* and *C*). The ERG responses may be normal early but become attenuated later in more severe cases.

Histopathologically, thioridazine retinopathy is associated with atrophy and disorganization of the photoreceptor outer segments followed by loss of the RPE and choriocapillaris.[44]

Retinotoxicity has been attributed to concentration of the drug within melanin granules in the uveal melanocytes and RPE.[44,46] Thioridazine has a structure similar to NP-207, an experimental drug that was never marketed because of severe retinotoxicity.[33] There is no specific treatment other than stopping the medication.

▼ CHLORPROMAZINE (THORAZINE) RETINOPATHY

Chlorpromazine rarely causes retinal toxicity. When taken in large doses in the range of 2400 mg/day over 12 months it may cause mild pigmentary changes in the retina (Fig. 9-2, *H* to *J*).[48-50] These rarely are associated with visual or functional deficits. Because patients receiving chlorpromazine have often received other medications that may have included potentially retinotoxic drugs, assignment of the exact cause of the retinopathy may be difficult. White and yellow-white granular deposits may occur in the axial part of the anterior subcapsular region of the lens, and in the posterior layers of the cornea in patients receiving 300 mg/day of chlorpromazine for 3 years or more.[49] The usual dosage of chlorpromazine is 40 to 75 mg per day, although dosages up to 800 mg daily are not uncommon.

▼ CLOFAZIMINE RETINOPATHY

Clofazimine is a red iminophenazine dye used concurrently with dapsone and rifampin as the treatment of choice for lepromatous leprosy, for treatment of dapsone-resistant leprosy, and for *Mycobacterium avium* complex infections in patients with AIDS. After several months of treatment, clofazimine crystals may accumulate in the ocular tissues. Reversible side effects include a superficial whorl pattern of anterior corneal pigmented lines, brownish discoloration of the conjunctiva and tears, and crystals in the iris and sclera. A large bull's-eye pattern of pigment epithelial atrophy (Fig. 9-2, *K* and *L*) has occurred in two patients following a 200 mg/day (total dose of approximately 48 g) and after 300 mg/day (total dose of approximately 40 g).[51,52] This was associated with reduced ERG b-waves and full-field photopic and scotopic as well as flicker amplitudes.

FIG. 9-2 **Thioridazine (Mellaril) Retinopathy.**

A to **C**, Mild visual loss occurred in a 21-year-old woman with schizophrenia who received thioridazine, 800 mg/day, for 3 years. The mild pigment epithelial alterations (**A**) were more apparent angiographically (**B** and **C**).

D to **G**, This 60-year-old woman received thioridazine daily for 11 years beginning at age 25 years. She was asymptomatic visually and had 20/20 visual acuity bilaterally until age 55, when she developed nyctalopia and paracentral scotomas. Her visual acuity was 20/25, right eye, and 20/50, left eye. She had widely scattered areas of geographic atrophy of the RPE that included the macular area (**D** to **F**). Angiography demonstrated evidence of generalized RPE depigmentation and choriocapillaris atrophy in the areas of geographic atrophy (**G**).

Chlorpromazine and Trifluoperazine Retinopathy.

H to **J**, This 41-year-old schizophrenic woman received chlorpromazine (Thorazine) and trifluoperazine (Stelazine) for many years. There was no definite history of treatment with thioridazine. Her visual acuity in both eyes was 20/30. She had diminished photopic and scotopic responses electroretinographically. The patchy and nummular areas of atrophy of the RPE were similar to those caused by thioridazine toxicity.

Clofazimine Retinopathy.

K and **L**, After 8 months of treatment with 48 grams of clofazimine for *Mycobacterium avium* complex associated with AIDS, this patient developed a bull's-eye pattern of RPE mottled depigmentation in the macula bilaterally. His visual acuity was 20/25. There was some generalized reduction of all components of his ERG responses. His color vision (AOHRR pseudoisochromatic plates) was normal.

(**K** and **L** from Cunningham et al.[52])

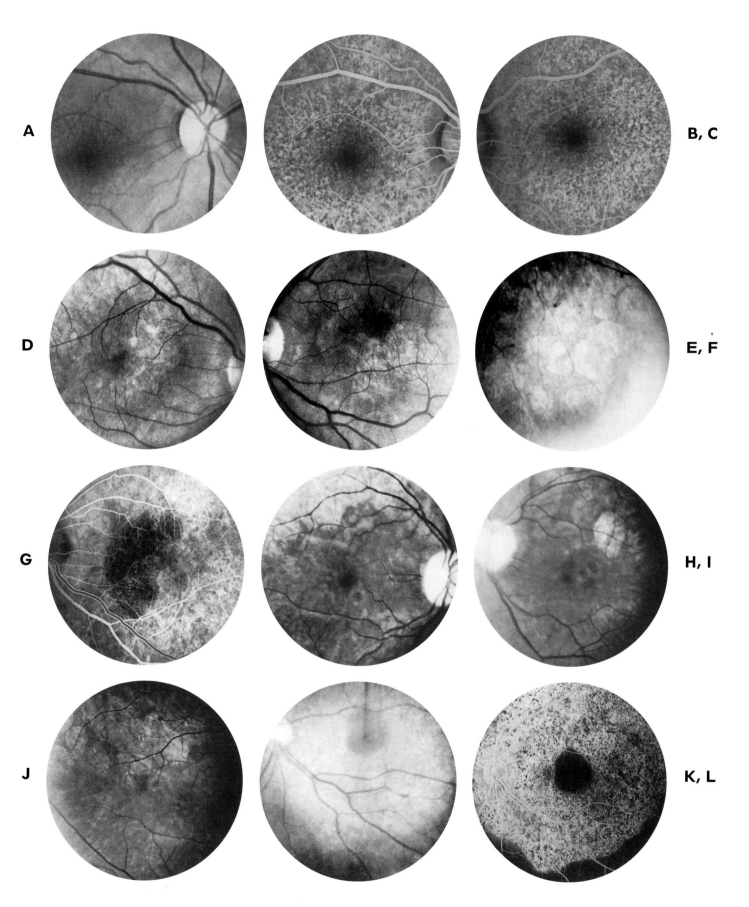

A

B, C

D

E, F

G

H, I

J

K, L

781

▼ DEFEROXAMINE MACULOPATHY

Intravenous administration of deferoxamine mesylate, 3 to 12 g/24 hours, for the treatment of transfusional hemosiderosis has produced rapid onset of visual loss; color vision abnormalities; nyctalopia; a ring scotoma; reduced electroretinographic, electrooculographic, dark-adaptation, and visual evoked responses; and mid- to high-frequency hearing loss of cochlear type.[53-56,58-61] The fundi may be normal initially or there may be a slight graying of the macula (Fig. 9-3, *A*). Both eyes are affected. Visual symptoms usually begin 7 to 10 days after the last treatment. Development of maculopathy may occur after chronic subcutaneous injection of deferoxamine.[57] Fluorescein angiography soon after the onset of visual symptoms in the presence of a normal-appearing fundus may show progressive staining at the level of the RPE in the macular areas, and in some cases leakage of dye from the optic disc vessels (Fig. 9-3, *B* and *C*). Pigmentary changes usually appear within several weeks (Fig. 9-3, *D*). After cessation of treatment, return of visual function occurs over 3 to 4 months and approximately 70% of patients recover normal acuity. The mechanism of retinal toxicity is unknown. Although chelation of iron is unlikely to be the explanation, removal of other metals, particularly copper, from the retinal pigment epithelium may be important.[55,59] Light microscopic and ultrastructural changes in the retinal pigment epithelium in an eye of a patient studied after recovery of visual function included patchy depigmentation and thinning, loss of microvilli from the apical surface, vacuolization of the cytoplasm, swelling and calcification of mitochondria, disorganization of the plasma membrane, and thickening of Bruch's membrane.[60]

FIG. 9-3 Deferoxamine Retinopathy.

A to **D,** This 64-year-old woman with chronic renal failure and renal dialysis developed severe osteoporosis that was thought to be related to excessive absorption of aluminum from the dialysate used to treat her renal insufficiency.[58] Following intravenous deferoxamine the patient noted dyschromatopsia, blurring of vision, and difficulty in reading. At the time of examination 15 days after her intravenous therapy her visual acuity was 20/30. She had 10-degree central relative scotomata. Funduscopic examination showed slight graying of the retina paracentrally **(A).** Fluorescein angiography showed a mottled pattern of hyperfluorescence throughout the macula and a central area of staining at the level of the RPE (**B** and **C**). She noted rapid improvement of her vision soon after her examination. When seen 8 months later, her only complaint was mild dyschromatopsia and her visual acuity was 20/20 in the right eye and 20/25 in the left eye. There was mottling of the RPE in the macular areas of both eyes **(D).**

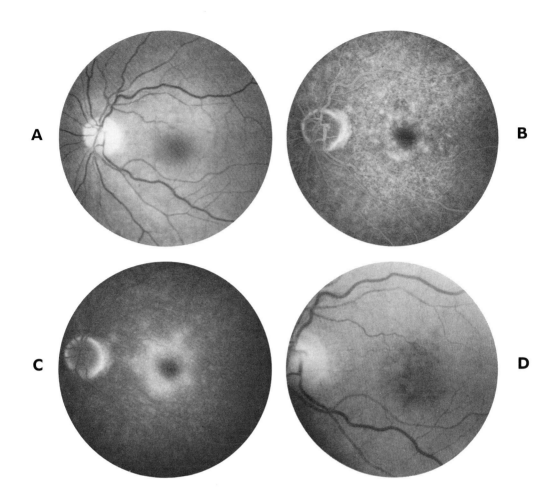

783

▼ SIDEROTIC RETINOPATHY

If iron-containing foreign bodies enter the eye, the iron may become oxidized and be bound to the ocular tissues, producing either localized siderosis or, particularly when the foreign body lodges in the vitreoretinal region, diffuse ocular siderosis (Fig. 9-4, *A* to *F*).[63,64,69] Evidence of ocular siderosis includes pupillary mydriasis, darkening of the iris, and orange deposits in the anterior subcapsular region of the lens. Posteriorly, hazy ocular media may preclude visualization of the fundus. Early optic disc hyperemia and fluorescein angiographic evidence of leakage may be present. Later a picture simulating pigmentary degeneration of the retina and progressive loss of peripheral visual fields may occur (Fig. 9-4, *A*). These changes may be associated with optic disc hyperemia. Abnormalities in the electroretinogram eventually occur and may be reversible following early removal of the intraocular iron foreign body.[66,67] Histopathologically, the iron is initially deposited primarily in the inner retina and RPE. Eventually, however, degeneration may affect all layers of the retina.

The natural course of a retained intraocular iron foreign body is variable. In some cases the foreign body may be absorbed or become encapsulated and the siderosis may stabilize or regress.[62] In some cases the hyperpigmentation of the encapsulated mass may simulate a choroidal melanoma (Figs. 9-4, *A*, and 8-10, *B* to *E*).[70] In general, intraocular iron foreign bodies should be removed, particularly from an eye showing evidence of siderosis.[71] Removal of foreign bodies deeply imbedded in the ocular wall or of largely oxidized foreign bodies may be difficult or impossible.

An acute pigment epitheliopathy, serous retinal detachment, and transient visual loss occurred in a patient with systemic hypertension and chronic glomerulonephritis after intravenous administration of iron dextran.[65]

Experimental injection of iron powder or iron-containing solutions into the vitreous may produce acute geographic areas of retinal whitening (Fig. 9-4, *G* to *L*), fluorescein angiographic evidence of

FIG. 9-4   Siderosis Bulbi.

A to **D**, This man was blind in the left eye because of siderosis following two unsuccessful attempts at removal of a retained intraocular foreign body 8 years previously. Note the dark brown mass (*arrow,* **A**) the severe atrophy of the retina and RPE and the delayed perfusion of the retina and choroidal blood vessels angiographically (**B** and **C**). Ultrasonography (**D**) confirmed the presence of the foreign body. The ERG was extinguished in the left eye.

E, Anterior subcapsular siderotic cataract.

F, Siderosis of the right iris in this patient with a retained intraocular foreign body.

Acute Siderotic Maculopathy in a Primate.

G to **L**, This squirrel monkey developed a circular white area in the macula 1 day after the intravitreal injection of 0.01 mg of iron as ferrous chloride (**G**). Fluorescein angiography revealed transmission of the choroidal fluorescence and later intense staining in the area of this whitening (**H**). Twenty-eight days later there was a circumscribed area of RPE depigmentation surrounded by a halo of hyperpigmentation in the macular area (**I**). A window defect in the RPE was evident angiographically (**J**). A phase-contrast micrograph made 1 day after intravitreal injection of iron powder showed pyknosis of the outer retinal cell nuclei and edema of the inner retina (**K**). A phase-contrast micrograph 28 days following intravitreal injection showed a sharp demarcation between the normal and the atrophic outer retinal layers in the macular region (**L**).

(**A** to **F** from Sneed[70]; **K** and **L** from Mascuili L, Anderson DR, Charles S: *Am J Ophthalmol* 74:638, 1972; published with permission from The American Journal of Ophthalmology; copyright by The Ophthalmic Publishing Co.[68])

severe disruption of the RPE (Fig. 9-4, *H*), and a diminished or nonrecordable electroretinogram within the first 24 hours after the injection.[68] A zone of focal atrophy of the RPE surrounded by a zone of pigment epithelial clumping develops within a few weeks (Fig. 9-4, *I* and *J*). Histologically, the primary damage is to the receptor cells and RPE (Fig. 9-4, *K* and *L*). Retinal damage is much more severe with ferrous than with ferric compounds.

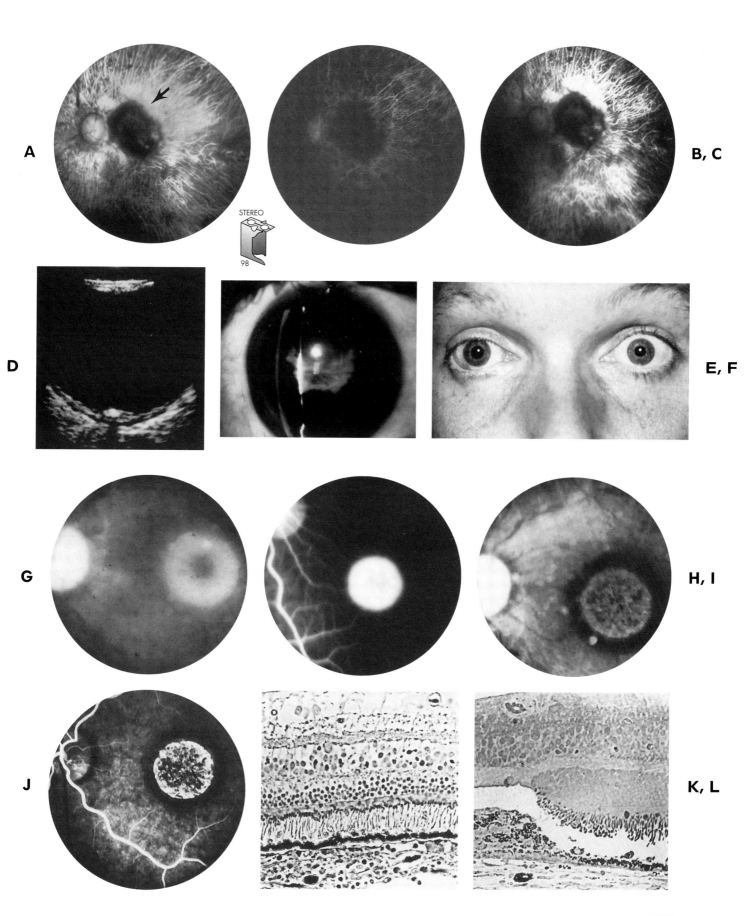

A

B, C

D

E, F

G

H, I

J

K, L

▼ CHALCOSIS MACULOPATHY

Patients with an intraocular copper foreign body may show a wide spectrum of reactions to its presence. In the case of a copper alloy, the inflammatory reaction may be minimal and a slow diffusion of copper occurs and impregnates limiting membranes of the eye to produce the picture of chalcosis that may include peripheral corneal ring, sunflower cataract (see Fig. 8-10, *I*), and heterochromia of the iris.[72-74] In addition, irregular yellowish-golden flakes may be deposited in the macular area away from the site of the foreign body (Fig. 9-5, *A* and *B*).[72,73] It is presumed that these apparently inert deposits are either copper carbonates or oxides. They apparently have little effect on visual acuity. Their location is uncertain, but they appear to be deep to the retinal vessels. These flakes disappear after removal of the foreign body (Fig. 9-5, *C*).[72,73] The electroretinogram is subnormal in approximately 50% of patients with chalcosis. Experimentally, copper has been found in the macrophages within the retina, in Müller cells, and in granular clumps scattered throughout the retina.[74,75]

▼ ARGYROSIS

Argyrosis may be associated with discoloration of the skin, mucous membranes, and many of the body organs. When this discoloration is confined to the eye following topical application of silver compounds to the eye, the blue-gray discoloration of the conjunctiva and cornea (Fig. 9-5, *D*) is referred to as argyria. The discoloration is caused by deposition of silver in the basement membrane of the conjunctiva and cornea, as well as in Descemet's membrane. Patients with argyrosis caused by chronic ingestion of silver-containing compounds may develop discoloration of the skin and body organs, as well as loss of the normal choroidal markings in the ocular fundus, a "dark" choroid fluorescein angiographically, and a leopard-spot mottling of the ocular fundus when viewed with red-free light (Fig. 9-5, *E* to *G*).[76] These fundus changes are probably caused by loss of transparency of Bruch's membrane as a result of deposition of silver in the membrane (Fig. 9-5, *H* and *I*).[76,77]

FIG. 9-5 Chalcosis.

A to **C,** Copper deposits in the macula of an 18-year-old patient with a posterior dislocated lens. He sustained an intraocular copper foreign body injury 5 years previously. These deposits disappeared 14 months after removal of the foreign body (**C**). His visual acuity was 20/20.

Argyrosis.

D, Bluish discoloration of the conjunctiva (argyrosis).

E to **G,** Dark choroid (**G**) associated with argyrosis of Bruch's membrane in a patient with systemic argyrosis caused by using a mouth wash containing silver (Collargent Acetarsol, Sarbach, Suresnes, France) 3 times a day for 3 years. Red light photograph shows no details of choroidal circulation and leopard-spot pattern of the fundus temporally (**E**) that is accentuated in the infrared light photograph (**F**).

H and **I,** Photomicrographs showing argyrosis of the RPE and Bruch's membrane (*arrows*). **H** is hematoxylin and eosin stain and **I** is Fontana stain.

(**A** to **C** from Delaney[72]; **E** and **G** from Cohen et al.[76]; **H** and **I** from Spencer et al.[77])

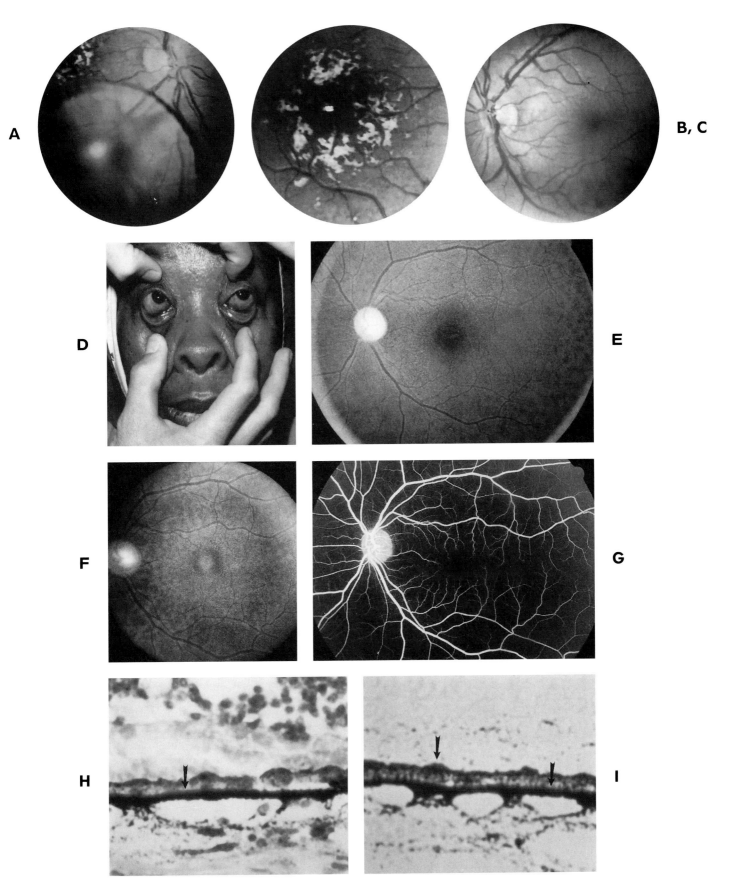

A

B, C

D

E

F

G

H

I

787

▼ CISPLATINUM AND BCNU (CARMUSTINE) RETINOPATHY

Intracarotid arterial chemotherapy with BCNU [1,3-*bis*-(9,2-chlorethyl)-1-nitrosourea], 300 to 400 mg, and cisplatinum [*cis*-diammine dichloroplatinum(II)], 200 mg, is used for treatment of recurrent malignant gliomas of the brain. This may cause precipitous ipsilateral visual loss and fundus changes of two different types. Patients receiving BCNU either alone or in combination with cisplatinum may develop visual loss associated with ophthalmoscopic signs of retinal infarction, retinal periarteritis and phlebitis, and papillitis.[78-81,83,85-87] Other findings may include cavernous sinus syndrome, partial sixth and third nerve palsies, severe conjunctival injection and chemosis, pain, and secondary glaucoma. Approximately 65% of patients treated develop these findings accompanied by visual loss about 6 weeks after the start of treatment. Once visual loss begins it is usually progressive and severe.

Intracarotid injection above the level of the ophthalmic artery does not protect from development of ocular complications.[83] Those treated with cisplatinum alone or in combination with BCNU may develop visual loss associated with a pigmentary retinopathy, with a central scotoma, and later diffuse constriction of the visual field.[78,81,82] The ERG may be nonrecordable in some patients.[82,85] The visual symptoms and pigmentary changes are usually mild following administration of cisplatinum alone and appear to be potentiated with the addition of BCNU.[82] Fig. 9-6 shows pigmentary retinopathy in two patients treated with cisplatinum and bleomycin. A similar pigmentary maculopathy has been reported after a combination of intracarotid injection of mannitol and methotrexate together with intravenous administration of cyclophosphamide.[84] Mannitol disruption of the blood–ocular barrier was thought to be instrumental in the macular changes, which typically do not occur with use of the two drugs alone.

▼ TAMOXIFEN RETINOPATHY

Tamoxifen citrate, a nonsteroidal antiestrogen, is used to treat patients with breast carcinoma. Patients who receive high doses of tamoxifen (total amount of drug in excess of 90 g) may develop loss of central vision, macular edema, and superficial white refractile deposits that are located primarily in the inner layers of the retina (Fig. 9-7, *A, B, D,* and *E*).[92-94,96] There may be punctate gray lesions

FIG. 9-6 Cisplatinum and Bleomycin Chorioretinal Toxicity.

A to E, This 46-year-old man had a right-sided intracarotid injection of cisplatinum and bleomycin for treatment of a glioblastoma of the brain. He noted the immediate sensation of heat behind the ipsilateral eye, and transient paralysis of the right arm. One day later he noted visual loss in the right eye. Eight days later visual acuity in the right eye was light perception only. The left eye was normal. Examination of the right fundus revealed swelling of the optic disc, narrowing of the retinal vessels, and subtle RPE mottling that was more apparent angiographically (**A** and **B**). Eight days later visual acuity was hand movements and there was prominent mottling of the RPE (**C** to **E**).

F, This 36-year-old man experienced rapid visual loss 2 weeks previously several days following a left-sided intracarotid injection of cisplatinum and bleomycin. His visual acuity was 20/20 right eye and 20/400 left eye. Note the mottling of the RPE in the left macula.

at the level of the outer retina and RPE that appear nonfluorescent (hypofluorescent) angiographically (Fig. 9-7, *F*). Refractile lesions are more numerous and larger in the paramacular area, are more heavily concentrated temporal to the macula, and show some tendency to clump. The number and size of the lesions do not change after cessation of tamoxifen. Light microscopy and electron microscopy show that the retractile lesions are located in the nerve fiber and inner plexiform layers.[92] They are intracellular and stain positively for glycosaminoglycans. The lesions appear to represent products of axonal degeneration. Histopathologically they are similar to corpora amylacea but are larger and more numerous in the paramacular area rather than the peripapillary area.

There is evidence that long-term low-dosage tamoxifen may cause retinopathy.[88-91,95] In a prospective study of 63 patients receiving a median dose of 20 mg/day of tamoxifen for a median duration of 25 months, four patients developed retinopathy and/or keratopathy 10, 27, 31, and 35 months after commencement of treatment.[95] The mean total dose in these four patients was 14.4 g. Decreased acuity, bilateral macular edema, and yellow-white dots in the paramacular and foveal areas occurred in all four patients and corneal opacities occurred in one patient. After withdrawal of drug, almost all ocular complications were reversible.[88,95] Heier and coworkers found mild deposition of intraretinal crystals in only two of 135 visually asymptomatic tamoxifen-treated patients (mean cumulative dose, 17.2 g).[91] The two patients with crystals had a cumulative dose of 10.9 and

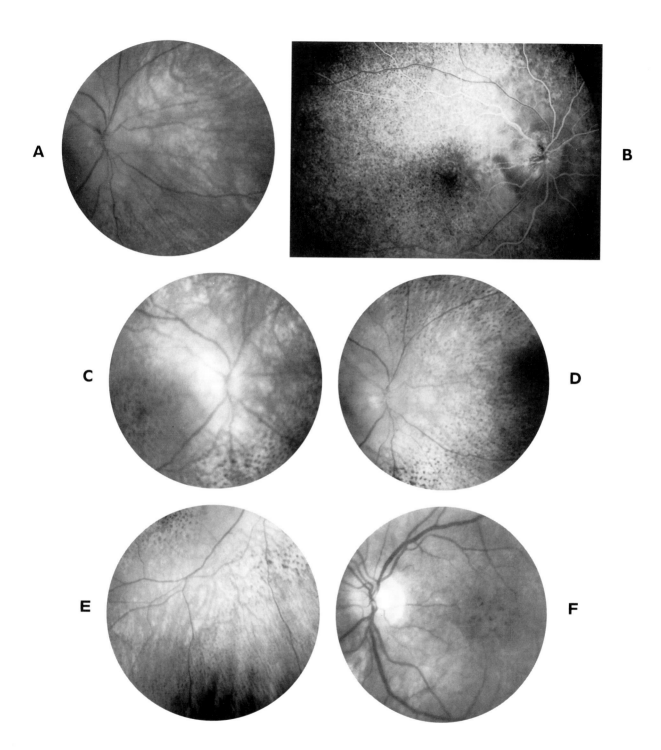

21.9 g, respectively. Transient bilateral optic disc edema, retinal hemorrhages, and macular edema may occasionally occur after starting low-dose tamoxifen daily.[88,90]

▼ OXALOSIS

Oxalosis is the deposition of calcium oxalate in various tissues of the body. The eye may be solely involved or may be involved as part of systemic oxalosis. Systemic oxalosis may be the result of (1) a primary hyperoxaluria secondary to an inborn error of metabolism (see Chapter 5), (2) a toxic reaction to ethylene glycol or methoxyflurane general anesthesia,[97-99] or (3) chronic renal failure and hemodialysis.[100] Ocular involvement in secondary systemic oxalosis has been observed after use of methoxyflurane, which is a nonflammable anesthetic. When administered to patients with renal dysfunction and particularly if administered over a prolonged period of time, it may cause irreversible renal failure secondary to the metabolic breakdown of the anesthetic to oxalic acid and fluoride ions (Fig. 9-7, *K*). These patients, as well as those with primary hyperoxaluria, may develop numerous yellow-white, punctate, crystalline lesions diffusely scattered throughout the posterior pole and midperiphery of the eyes (Figs. 5-39 and 9-7, *G* and *H*). In some the crystals appear to be most prominent in the pigment epithelium (Fig. 9-7, *H*),[97,98] and in others along the retinal arteries (Fig. 9-7, *G*).[99,100] In patients with methoxyflurane toxicity the retinal and pigment epithelial crystals may occur in the absence of changes in the optic disc, the macula, and the caliber of the retinal vessels seen in primary hyperoxaluria (see Fig. 5-39). Histopathologically, the flecks seen ophthalmoscopically are calcium oxalate crystals in the RPE, neurosensory retina, and ciliary epithelium (Fig. 9-7, *I* and *J*).[98]

The differential diagnosis includes the other forms of so-called flecked retina, including Bietti's crystalline dystrophy, nephropathic cystinosis, canthaxanthine retinopathy, Sjögren-Larsson's syndrome, talc retinopathy, fundus albi punctatus, retinitis punctata albescens, Stargardt's disease, Alport's syndrome, bilateral acquired juxtafoveolar telangiectasis, and vitamin A deficiency.

Calcium oxalate crystals may be found within the retina as an incidental finding in patients with long-standing retinal detachment and with morgagnian cataracts unassociated with evidence of systemic oxalosis.

FIG. 9-7 Tamoxifen Retinopathy.

A to C, Following a mastectomy for breast carcinoma this woman received a total dose of 67.5 g of tamoxifen over a period of 9 years. Her visual acuity was 20/200 in both eyes. Note the intraretinal crystals are more prominent in the left eye.

D to F, This 63-year-old woman who received a total dose of between 90 and 158 g of tamoxifen over a period of 29 months for treatment of metastatic breast carcinoma noted loss of central vision. Visual acuity was 20/50. There were superficial white refractile deposits that appeared to be in the inner layers of the retinas of both eyes (**A** and **B**). Note also the white spots in the periphery of the macula that angiographically appeared nonfluorescent (**C**). Later phase angiograms showed cystoid macular edema. Five months previously her visual acuity had been 20/30 in the right eye and 20/25 in the left eye and the fundi were normal.

Secondary Oxalosis.

G, Retinal oxalosis in a 34-year-old woman after 2 years of inhalation abuse of methoxyflurane. There were multiple, bright yellow-white crystals throughout the retina and pigment epithelium with a retinal arterial and periarterial predilection. She subsequently developed renal failure. Kidney biopsy revealed birefringent crystals in the renal tubule lumens.

H to K, Retinal oxalosis in a 63-year-old man who developed renal failure following methoxyflurane anesthesia (**H**). He subsequently died, and his eyes were obtained at autopsy. Note the birefringent oxalate crystals present in the retina (**I**), in the macular region, in the RPE (**J**), and in the kidney (**K**).

(**D** to **F** from McKeown et al.[94]; **G** from Novak et al.[99]; **H, J,** and **K** from Bullock JD, Albert DM: *Arch Ophthalmol* 93:26, 1975; copyright 1975, American Medical Association.[98])

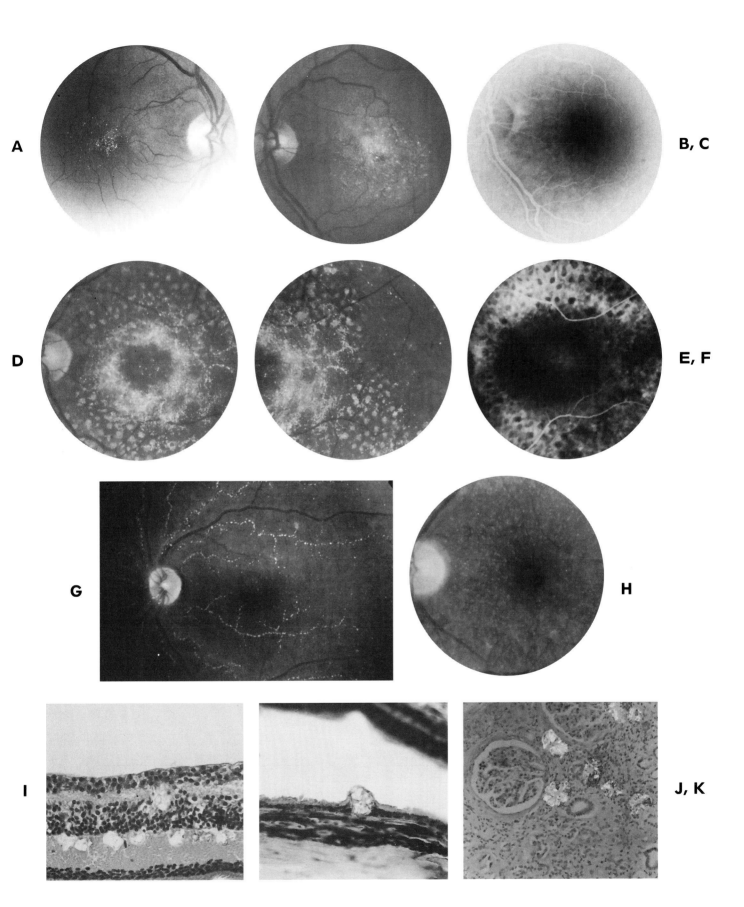

▼ CANTHAXANTHINE MACULOPATHY

Canthaxanthine is a carotinoid dye used in food and drug coloration. Some patients who use it orally (usually a total dose of 19 g or more within 24 months) as a tanning agent may develop a symmetric distribution of golden particles in a doughnut pattern in the superficial retina in the macular areas (Fig. 9-8).* The retinal crystals may be exaggerated in eyes with other diseases of the fundus (Fig. 9-8, *D* to *I*).[104] A few patients may develop similar crystals in the cornea at the level of Descemet's membrane.[119] Retrospective studies of pure canthaxanthine (Orobronze) consumers revealed an incidence of retinal deposits varying from 12% to 14%.[103,106] The occurrence of the deposits correlates with the total dose ingested. In two studies 37 g of canthaxanthine induced retinal deposits in 50% of the patients[103] and 60 g induced deposits in 100% of patients.[112] Predisposing factors that lead to onset of retinopathy at much lower dosage include focal disease of the RPE,[105,106] ocular hypertension,[105] and concurrent use of beta carotene (Fig. 9-8, *D* to *I*).[105] Hennekes reported the development of canthaxanthine retinopathy in a patient with retinitis pigmentosa after ingestion of 12 to 14 g over a period of 4 months.[111] The maculopathy is usually associated with normal visual acuity but reduced retinal sensitivity.[109] Some patients may demonstrate subnormal dark adaptation and electroretinographic responses.[102,115,116,120] The ERG changes in most patients are reversible after the ingestion of canthaxanthine is stopped.[101] EOG responses are normal.[110-112,116,121,123] Fluorescein angiography is typically normal but may show a bull's-eye pattern of faint hyperfluorescence (Fig. 9-8, *C*).

*References 103, 105-107, 110, 115, 117, 120.

FIG. 9-8 Canthaxanthine Retinopathy.

A to **C**, Note the glistening yellow crystals arranged in a doughnut shape in the superficial and deep retina in the macula of this patient who was a long-term user of skin-tanning agents. Note the perifoveolar ring of hyperfluorescence, which probably is caused by obstruction of the background fluorescence by the crystals rather than depigmentation of the RPE.

D to **F**, Unilateral deposition of canthaxanthine in the right eye of a patient with recurrent idiopathic central serous chorioretinopathy in the ipsilateral eye.

G, Asymmetric canthaxanthine retinopathy occurred in an asymptomatic 58-year-old woman with an old inferior temporal branch retinal vein obstruction in the left macula. She was complaining of blurred vision and "lemon-yellow pinwheel" photopsia in the left eye. Visual acuity was 20/20, right eye, and 20/40, left eye. There were more crystals in the left macula and there were intracorneal crystals in both eyes. She had taken oral canthaxanthine for many years.

H and **I**, Canthaxanthine retinopathy associated with chronic recurrent bilateral idiopathic central serous chorioretinopathy. He took canthaxanthine, one tablet per day for 4 months, 15 years before these photographs. Visual acuity was 20/300, right eye, and 20/25, left eye.

J and **K**, Crystalline retinopathy identical to that caused by canthaxanthine in a 48-year-old man with no history of supplemental canthaxanthine.

L, Mild unilateral crystalline retinopathy *(arrow)* of unknown cause in a middle-aged man.

(**A** and **B** from Cortin et al.[105])

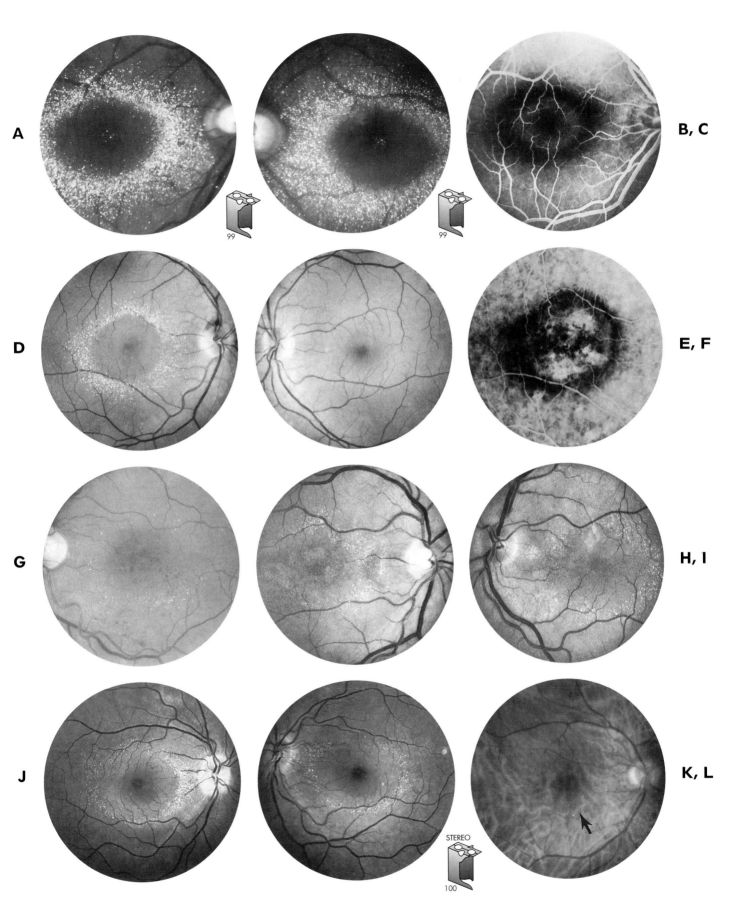

A

B, C

D

E, F

G

H, I

J

K, L

Morphologically these red, birefringent, and lipid-soluble carotenoid crystals are located in the inner layers of the entire retina and the ciliary body.[108] They are particularly large and numerous perifoveally, where they are clinically visible. They are located in a spongy degeneration of the inner neuropil and are associated with atrophy of the inner parts of Müller cells. They presumably represent a canthaxanthine–lipoprotein complex.[108]

The retinal crystals may gradually disappear a year or more after ingestion of canthaxanthine is discontinued, and some may remain for at least 7 years.[110,112,114] The delay in reversibility is in keeping with the observation that the plasma concentration of canthaxanthine takes at least 9 months to recover to normal levels in patients having received daily oral dosage of 100 mg for 3 months.[123] The return to normal values of static perimetry threshold in some patients suggests that the abnormality is not the result of an irreversible anatomic alteration, as suggested in experimental studies in rabbits.[124,125]

Retinopathy identical to that of canthaxanthine retinopathy may occur in some patients without a history of extradietary intake of canthaxanthine (Fig. 9-8, *J* and *K*).[118] Similar retinopathy has developed in one patient receiving long-term nitrofurantoin therapy.[113]

Administration of amounts of canthaxanthine comparable to those ingested by patients developing canthaxanthine retinopathy produced morphologic changes in the retina of rabbits and cats, but no retinal crystals.[122,124,125] The cats developed a progressive orange sheen to the ocular fundus that morphologically was associated with increased retinal pigment epithelial cell height and vacuolization caused by enlargement and disruption of phagosomes.[122]

▼ FLECKED RETINA ASSOCIATED WITH VITAMIN A DEFICIENCY

Patients with vitamin A deficiency secondary to inadequate dietary intake, malabsorption states resulting from celiac sprue, regional enteritis, jejunal bypass surgery, chronic liver disease, and hepatic transplantation may develop night blindness, corneal xerosis, and a peculiar peripheral retinal change characterized by the presence of multiple, yellow-white, somewhat granular spots at the level of the RPE (fundus xerophthalmicus; Uyemura's syndrome).[126-137] These flecks are of various sizes and shapes and simulate drusen. The retinal changes have been associated with marked constriction of the visual fields, abnormal dark adaptation, and electroretinographic changes, including disappearance of the a-wave followed by loss of the b-wave and greater reduction of the scotopic than the photopic responses. Following administration of vitamin A, there may be either complete or partial reversal of the fundus and electrophysiologic changes, depending on the chronicity of the deficiency.[134,136,137] The fundus changes are more likely to occur in those patients with vitamin A deficiency who develop evidence of corneal xerosis.

Fluorescein angiography in one case showed the fundus lesions to be hyperfluorescent, suggesting that they involve the RPE.[132,134]

Animals with vitamin A deficiency histopathologically develop disorganization of the rod outer segments and eventual loss of the visual cells.[128] It is probable that the transient yellow-white spots occurring in humans are related to the macrophagic response to loss of rod outer segments and RPE cell disruption similar to that which has been demonstrated histopathologically to account for the peculiar yellow-white spots that may be seen in patients with Leber's congenital amaurosis soon after birth (see p. 362).

One 50-year-old man with acquired night blindness associated with steatorrhea was noted to have the typical changes of fundus albipunctatus.[132] His abnormal dark adaptation curves improved after vitamin A administration, but the fundus remained unchanged. Although it was postulated that the albipunctate spots may have resulted from photoreceptor damage after chronic vitamin A deficiency, this seems unlikely since other investigators who have studied this disease have not noted persistence of the white spots following therapy.

▼ AMINOGLYCOSIDE MACULOPATHY

The inadvertent injection of large doses of gentamicin into either the anterior chamber after cataract extraction or the vitreous during a sub-Tenon's injection may produce a rapid and severe visual loss associated with a peculiar retinopathy that is most marked in the macular area (Fig. 9-9).[138,141,145-147,151] The patient is usually aware of profound loss of vision on the first postoperative day. Initially the fundus picture may simulate that seen in central retinal artery occlusion. There is marked whitening and swelling of the retina in the macular area associated with a cherry-red spot (Fig. 9-9, *D*, *F*, and *I*). Other surrounding areas of patchy retinal whitening may be evident. Retinal hemorrhages develop and become more numerous (Fig. 9-9, *A*, *F*, and *I*). Although intravitreal injection of levels of gentamicin up to 200 μg were previously considered safe for the treatment of endophthalmitis, macular infarction may occur in some patients after intravitreal injection of 0.1 or 0.2 mg of gentamicin sulfate.[140,150,154] Repetitive injections of nontoxic doses may produce retinal damage.[148] Fluorescein angiography typically shows a sharply defined zone of retinal vascular nonperfusion in the macular area associated with dye leakage from the neighboring retinal vessels (Fig. 9-9, *B*, *C*, *E*, *G*, *H*, *K*, and *L*).[147,151] The retinal whitening and hemorrhages may persist for many weeks or several months (Fig. 9-9, *J*). Optic atrophy and retinal pigmentary changes develop later and may be accompanied by rubeosis irides and hemorrhagic glaucoma. The visual prognosis is poor.

It is probable that the gentamicin and not the preservatives is the primary cause of the retinal infarction.[141,147] Although experimentally the presence or absence of the lens or vitreous does not change the toxic threshold to injected aminoglycosides, there is concern clinically that nontoxic doses of aminoglycosides may be toxic if injected intravitreally into vitrectomized eyes.[149,152] Although tobramycin and amikacin are less toxic than gentamicin, both have produced fundus findings similar to those caused by gentamicin.[140,143] The retinopathy has been observed most frequently following intravitreal injections of 0.4 mg of gentamicin after vitrectomy, but also in some cases after injection of 0.1 or 0.2 mg, doses that had previously been considered safe.[140] Prophylactic use of subconjunctival injection of gentamicin after routine surgery was the second most frequent cause of macular infarction. The retinopathy has been observed following the inadvertent intraocular injection of tobramycin after cataract extraction.[138,141,146] In one case this apparently resulted from diffusion of the subconjunctivally injected drug through the cataract wound.[146] The same maculopathy has occurred after intravitreal injections of amikacin.[141] Because of the frequency and severity of the complication Campochiaro and Lim recommended: (1) abandonment of prophylactic use of subconjunctival aminoglycosides after routine surgery, and (2) avoidance of intravitreal aminoglycosides in the prophylaxis of penetrating ocular trauma.

Experimentally, retinal toxicity to gentamicin may occur at levels as low as 100 μg injected into the vitreous.[144] In the rabbit model D'Amico et al. found lamellar storage material in the liposomes of retinal pigment epithelium and macrophages after injection of 100 μg into the vitreous; disruption of pigment epithelial cell organelles and loss of photoreceptors after 400 μg; and full-thickness retinal necrosis after 800 μg. These findings implicate the RPE as the primary site of toxicity.[144] Aminoglycoside maculopathy similar to that seen in humans has been produced in subhuman primates following intravitreal injection of 1000 to 10,000 μg of gentamicin.[139,142] Evidence suggests that the retinal whitening and the isoelectric electroretinographic findings that occur within minutes or hours after the injection are caused by direct damage to the inner retina by the drug before development of occlusion of the retinal vasculature. The latter is accompanied by retinal hemorrhages, damage to retinal pericytes and endothelial cells, and thrombosis. A possible mechanism to explain the retinal vascular occlusion was granulocytic plugging of the retinal capillary bed.[142]

In some patients aminoglycoside macular toxicity may be difficult to differentiate from that produced as a complication of intraneural injection during retrobulbar anesthesia or that resulting from spontaneous occlusion of the central retinal artery and vein. The vitreous inflammatory cell reaction, shallow retinal detachment, and delayed onset of retinal hemorrhages, as well as the characteristic angiographic pattern and prolonged retinal whitening associated with aminoglycoside toxicity are helpful in this regard.[145,146,153]

FIG. 9-9 Gentamicin Retinal Toxicity.

A to E, This 67-year-old man had accidental irrigation of the anterior chamber with 0.5 ml of gentamicin instead of acetylcholine after cataract extraction and placement of an intraocular lens. A posterior capsulotomy was done. Twenty minutes later the mistake was discovered, and the anterior chamber was irrigated. The next day the vision in the eye was light perception only. Two days postoperatively there was corneal edema and a semiopaque retina with peripheral retinal hemorrhages (A). Fluorescein angiography revealed extensive areas of nonperfusion of the retina in the posterior pole (B and C) and selective periarterial leakage (arrows, C). One month postoperatively the cornea was clear. There was a cherry-red spot surrounded by a milky white retina, dilated tortuous veins, many retinal hemorrhages, and pigmentary sheathing of the arteries (D). Angiography revealed persistence of the retinal vascular hypoperfusion (E). Visual acuity was hand movements. Six weeks later the patient developed evidence of neovascular glaucoma.

F to I, This 29-year-old man sustained an intraocular metallic foreign body injury. After removal of the foreign body transsclerally with a magnet, clindamycin, 250 μg, and gentamicin, 400 μg, were injected intravitreally. Ten hours postoperatively visual acuity was 20/200. Thirty-two hours postoperatively, the patient noted a dark central scotoma. Six days postoperatively there was whitening of the retina in the macular area associated with several blot hemorrhages (F). Angiography revealed nonperfusion of the retina in the macular area and leakage of dye from the surrounding vessels (G and H). Ten days postoperatively visual acuity was 5/200 and there was an increase in the area of retinal whitening and hemorrhages (I). Six months later the visual acuity was 10/200. There were atrophic retinal and RPE changes in the macula.

J to L, This woman had an extracapsular cataract extraction that was complicated by vitreous loss. Four days later she developed a hypopyon. A vitreous biopsy and intravitreal injection of gentamicin, vancomycin, and dexamethasone was done. Postoperatively she noted only bare light perception with the right eye. Four months postoperatively her visual acuity was 6/200. Funduscopic examination revealed some pigment cells in the vitreous, scattered retinal hemorrhages, whitening of the retina centrally (J), and several cotton-wool patches around the nasal aspect of the optic disc. Angiographically there was marked loss of the retinal blood vessels (K and L).

(A to I from McDonald et al.[147]; F to I, courtesy Dr. Matthew D. Davis.)

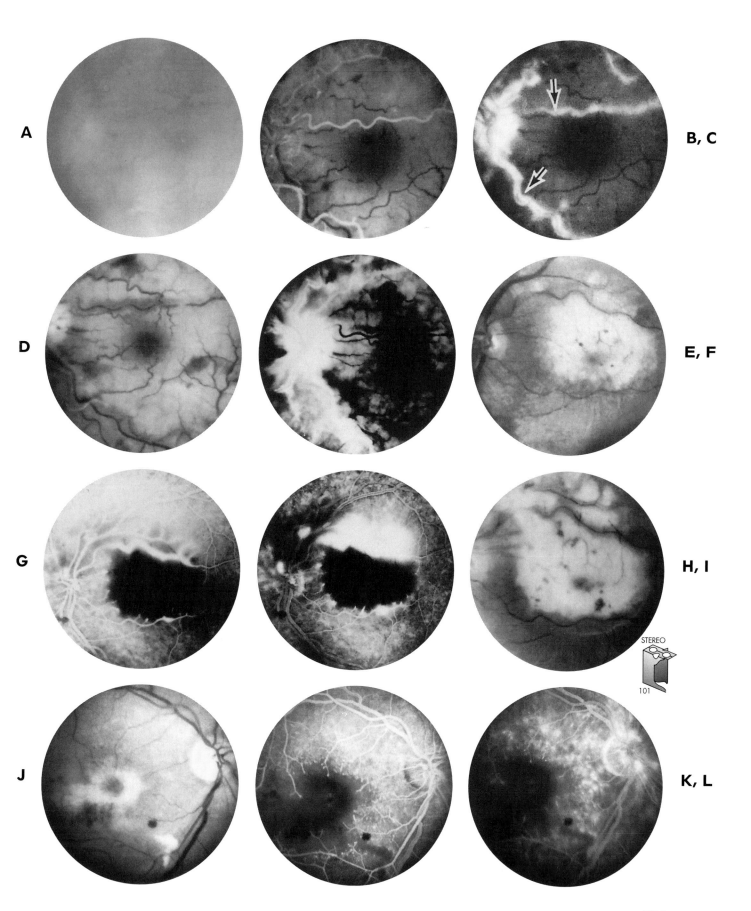

A

B, C

D

E, F

G

H, I

STEREO
101

J

K, L

797

▼ INTERFERON-ASSOCIATED RETINOPATHY

Patients receiving interferon-alfa 2a subcutaneously may develop multiple cotton-wool ischemic patches in the retina associated with retinal hemorrhages.[155] The pattern of the retinopathy may simulate Purtscher's retinopathy and be associated with decreased visual acuity (Fig. 9-10, A to C). The fundus changes are reversible after discontinuance of the therapy with interferon. Mild diabetes and systemic hypertension were present in 50% of the patients developing the retinopathy.[155] These observations suggest that patients with moderately severe diabetic, hypertensive, or other retinopathy associated with retinal capillary nonperfusion may be at greater risk of progression of the retinopathy and permanent visual loss following the administration of large amounts of interferon such as might be used in the treatment of patients with malignancies.

▼ METHAMPHETAMINE AND COCAINE RETINOPATHY

Inhalation of methamphetamine and cocaine may be followed by acute visual loss in one or both eyes. This may be associated with amaurosis fugax, retinal vasculitis with perivenous exudation and vitritis,[156] retinal and optic disc hemorrhages,[157] multiple cotton-wool patches, and central retinal artery occlusion (Fig. 9-10, D to H).[157,158] The adrenomimetic response and sudden increase in blood pressure after use of these drugs probably contribute to these retinal manifestations.

▼ LIDOCAINE–EPINEPHRINE TOXICITY

The inadvertent injection of lidocaine into the inner eye typically causes immediate corneal clouding, pupillary dilation, pupillary paralysis, and profound visual loss, all of which usually revert to normal within 24 hours.[159] In one patient there was persistence of a large central scotoma that was attributed to possible intraocular bleeding. Experimentally, intraocular lidocaine was unassociated with evidence of permanent retinal damage. Figure 9-10, I to L, illustrates the findings in a young man who apparently had an injection of 0.5 ml of lidocaine–epinephrine into the subretinal space in preparation for pterygium excision. Immediately after the injection his visual acuity was 1/200. When examined by a retinal specialist 2 hours later, the

FIG. 9-10 Interferon Retinopathy.

A to C, Bilateral Purtscher's-like retinopathy and visual loss occurred in this patient after receiving subcutaneous injections of interferon-alpha for 1 month for treatment of renal cell carcinoma. Note the angiographic evidence of retinal arteriolar occlusion (C).

Methamphetamine and Cocaine Retinopathy.

D and E, This 39-year-old man with a history of essential hypertension noted acute loss of vision in the left eye. He admitted snorting cocaine before his visual loss. Visual acuity was 20/20, right eye, and light perception only in the left eye. Note evidence of central retinal artery occlusion in the left eye and multiple cotton-wool patches in both eyes.

F to H, This man noted blurred vision in the left eye after snorting cocaine and an argument with his wife. He denied trauma. The right eye was normal. Note the multiple superficial retinal hemorrhages, one of which has a white center (arrow, G), boat-shaped preretinal hematomas, and intravitreal blood.

Lidocaine–Epinephrine Toxicity.

I to L, This 27-year-old man noted immediate pain and loss of vision during an anterior peribulbar injection of lidocaine and epinephrine in the upper nasal quadrant in preparation for pterygium removal. Fundus examination revealed a retinal detachment (presumably the anesthetic) that extended from the injection site into the posterior fundus. Laser photocoagulation was placed in the area of the subretinal blood and within 48 hours the subretinal fluid had resolved. Two weeks later the optic disc was pale and its margin was blurred (I). There were fine radiating lines in the macula. Angiography was unremarkable except for irregular hyperfluorescence in the area of laser treatment (J) and staining of the optic disc (K). Five weeks later his visual acuity was 20/80 and the optic disc was pale (L).

(A to C from Guyer et al.[155])

intraocular pressure was 16 mm Hg and the visual acuity was no light perception. There was mild whitening of the retina at the site of the injection and in the macular area. The retina was detached, presumably by lidocaine, nasally from the site of sclerochoroidal perforation near the equator to the posterior pole. The subretinal fluid was no longer evident when examined 2 days later. He experienced partial recovery of vision but was left with a large temporal and central scotoma corresponding with the area of retinal detachment and mild optic atrophy. The nature of the visual field defect suggests that the subretinal lidocaine–epinephrine rather than the transient rise in intraocular pressure was responsible for the permanent retinal visual loss.

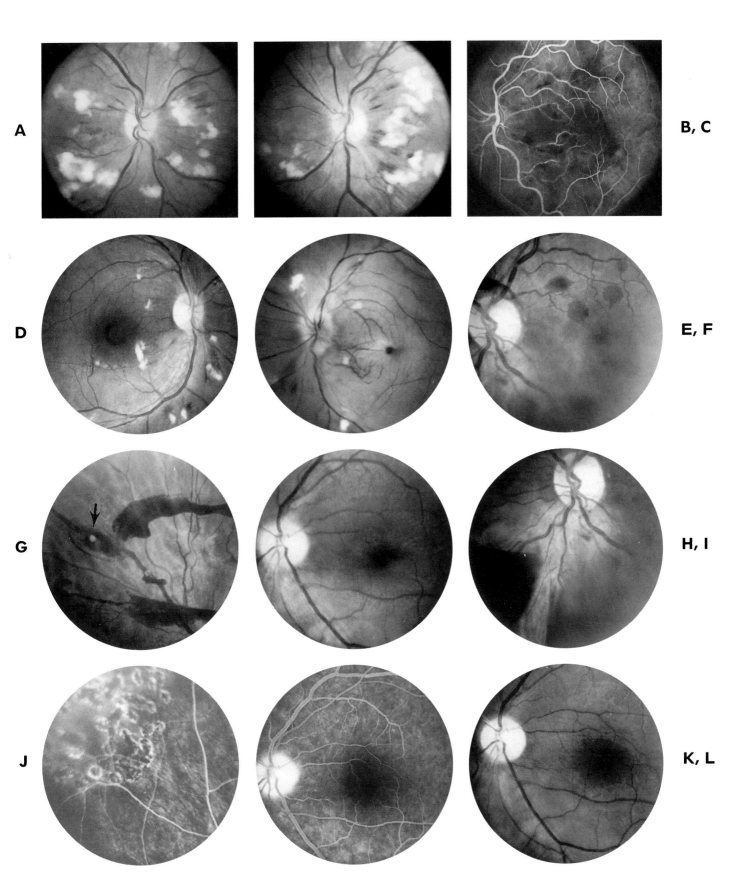

A

B, C

D

E, F

G

H, I

J

K, L

▼ QUININE TOXICITY

Following an overdose of quinine, whether by accidental ingestion or from attempts at abortion or suicide, patients develop nausea, vomiting, headache, tremor, tinnitus, and hypotension and may become obtunded or even comatose. When they awake within the first 24 hours, they may be totally blind. Examination of the fundus at that time reveals a slight loss of retinal transparency, mild dilation of the retinal veins, and normal caliber retinal arteries (Fig. 9-11, *A*).[160,161,163] Fluorescein angiography shows no abnormality other than slight obstruction of the background choroidal fluorescence (Fig. 9-11, *B*). Electroretinography may be normal or show slight changes such as slowing of the a-wave, transient increase in the depth of the a-wave, decrease in the b-wave, and loss of oscillatory potentials.[161] The electrooculogram usually shows no light rise.[165] Within several days the patient often recovers normal visual acuity but retains only a small island of central vision. The electrooculogram becomes progressively normal. The electroretinogram shows progressive loss of the b-wave. Recovery of retinal transparency, progressive narrowing of the retinal arteries, and pallor of the optic disc begin within several days after recovery of central vision (Fig. 9-11, *C* to *F*). Visual evoked potentials are abnormal. Dark adaptation usually shows delayed cone adaptation and little or no rod function. It is probable that the increase in background choroidal fluorescence that occurs soon after the acute visual loss is caused primarily by the return of normal retinal transparency, rather than loss of pigment from the RPE.

In animals with experimentally induced quinine retinal toxicity histopathologic examination of the early changes shows evidence of photoreceptor cell as well as ganglion cell alterations.[162,164] In later stages of the disease in humans, histopathologic examination shows loss of ganglion cells, nerve fiber layer, and receptor cells.

Pupillary abnormalities that may be permanent in these patients include poor reaction to light, tonic pupillary reaction, vermiform pupillary motion, and denervation supersensitivity.[163,165,167]

The normal caliber of the retinal arteries and the normal retinal and choroidal circulation time seen

FIG. 9-11 Quinine Retinal Toxicity.

This 25-year-old woman swallowed 12 to 15 tablets (3.7 to 4.7 g) of quinine as a suicidal gesture. This was followed by vomiting, buzzing in the ears, and blindness approximately 9 hours later. Examination 14½ hours after ingestion revealed no light perception in both eyes, mild loss of retinal transparency, and slight venous distention (**A**). Fluorescein angiography showed venous distention and slight loss of details of the choroidal fluorescence (**B**). Thirty-five hours after ingestion, she noted return of a small island of central vision. Her acuity was 20/20. The fundi were unchanged. Five days after ingestion there were optic disc pallor, narrowing of the retinal vessels, and partial clearing of the retinal haziness (**C**). Nine days after ingestion there was further clearing of the retina and pallor of the optic disc (**D** and **E**). Angiography was normal except for retinal vascular narrowing (**F**). After 6 months, visual acuity was 20/15 and 20 degrees of visual field remained in both eyes.

(**A** to **F** from Brinton et al.: *Am J Ophthalmol* 90:403 1980; published with permission from The American Journal of Ophthalmology; copyright by The Ophthalmic Publishing Co.[161])

during the acute stages of the disease suggest that vascular changes play little role in causing the retinal damage. The progressive narrowing of the retinal arterial tree that usually does not begin until after the patient has recovered central vision is probably caused by atrophy of the inner retinal layers as well as increased oxygen tension related to greater diffusion of oxygen from the choroid in the presence of loss of the visual cells. Thus, there is no rationale for retinal vascular dilators in the treatment of quinine toxicity. Lowering of the plasma level of quinine with repeated oral administration of activated charcoal theoretically may be beneficial.[166] There is, however, no treatment of proven value.

Quinine toxicity typically occurs with oral doses greater than 4 g, but there have been many case reports of toxicity with smaller doses. The recommended daily therapeutic dose is no more than 2 g, and the fatal oral dose for adults is approximately 8 g.

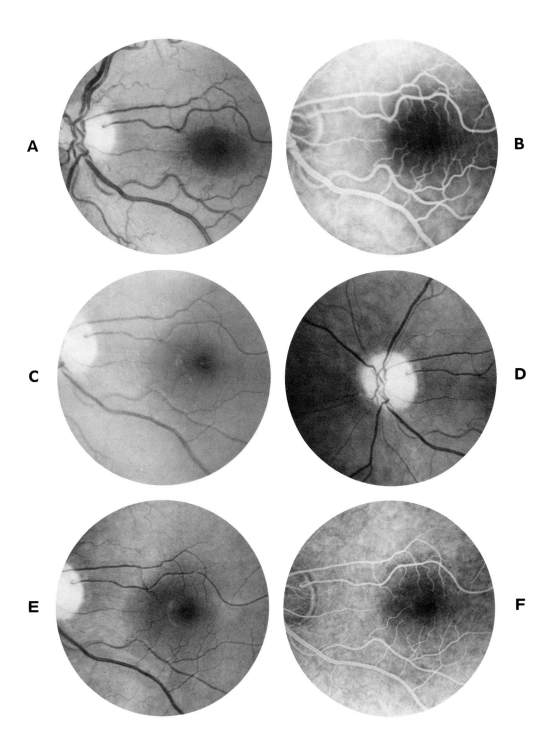

▼ METHYL ALCOHOL TOXICITY

Within 18 to 48 hours after the ingestion of methyl alcohol, which is metabolized to formaldehyde and formic acid, patients may experience symptoms ranging from spots before the eyes to complete blindness.[169] Diminution of pupillary reaction to light may occur in patients with impaired visual acuity as well as in some patients with normal acuity. The degree of pupillary light reflex impairment is of considerable prognostic significance. Patients with dilated, fixed pupils usually die or suffer severe visual damage. Funduscopic examination shows hyperemia of the optic disc, whitish striated edema of the disc margins and along the course of the major retinal vessels, and engorgement of the retinal veins (Fig. 9-12, A). Patients who survive and sustain severe visual damage develop optic atrophy in approximately 1 to 2 months (Fig. 9-12, C). A dense cecocentral scotoma, often sparing central fixation, is the most frequent field defect. Nerve fiber bundle defects and peripheral field constriction develop frequently and blindness may occur. Electroretinogram abnormalities involving the a- and b-waves occur.[175,176]

Experimental findings in rhesus monkeys suggest that the primary lesion in methyl alcohol poisoning is disruption of axoplasmic flow just at or behind the lamina cribrosa.[168,171,172] It is postulated that toxic metabolic breakdown products of methanol exert adverse effects on cytochrome oxidase and other oxidative enzymes, which causes swelling of the oligodendroglial cells in the retrolaminar optic nerve. This results in axonal compression, axoplasmic flow stasis, and optic disc edema.[168]

Recent reports of experimental methanol toxicity in rats and electrophysiologic and histopathologic studies in a human with methanol toxicity have demonstrated evidence that the retinal receptors and retinal pigment epithelium are affected.[170,173] The absorption, distribution, and metabolism of methanol and ethanol are similar. Since ethanol has a 100-fold greater affinity for alcohol dehydrogenase than methanol, treatment consists of early administration of ethanol and correction of metabolic acidosis.

▼ AMIODARONE OPTIC NEUROPATHY

Patients receiving amiodarone, an antiarrhythmic drug, may develop verticillate keratopathy, tremor, ataxia, pulmonary fibrosis, and occasionally visual loss associated with optic disc swelling and hemorrhages. These changes may be followed by optic

FIG. 9-12 Methyl Alcohol Ocular Toxicity.

A to **D**, This 53-year-old man experienced rapid loss of vision following the ingestion of methyl alcohol. Note the swelling and opacification of the optic nerve head and juxtapapillary retina (**A**). Angiography showed minimal staining of the optic nerve head (**B**). Eight weeks later the optic disc was pale and the visual loss persisted (**C**). Angiography showed hypofluorescence of the optic nerve head and evidence of juxtapapillary atrophy of the RPE (**D**) that was probably present at the time of the initial photographs (compare with **B**).

atrophy and narrowing of the retinal arteries in some patients.[177-179] It is uncertain whether or not this optic neuropathy is a peculiar complication of the drug or is a routine nonarteritic anterior ischemic optic neuropathy occurring in the group of patients who are predisposed to this complication.[180]

▼ CARBON MONOXIDE RETINOPATHY

Superficial retinal hemorrhages in a pattern very similar to that seen in Terson's syndrome (see Fig. 8-6) and in mountain climbers exposed to high altitudes (see next section) may occur in patients with acute or subacute exposure to carbon monoxide.[181-184] These may occur in association with papilledema and retinal venous engorgement and tortuosity. It is uncertain whether direct hypoxic damage to the vascular endothelium of the optic nerve and retina or compression of the retinal venous drainage associated with cerebral and optic nerve edema, or a combination of both, is responsible for the fundus changes.

▼ HIGH-ALTITUDE RETINOPATHY

Otherwise healthy individuals 6 to 96 hours after ascending to heights usually over 5000 m may develop retinal hemorrhages, papilledema, dilated retinal vessels, entopsias, and selective loss of color vision.[185-188] The retinal hemorrhages are superficial, are widely scattered, and frequently spare the macula. These patients may or may not have systemic symptoms of mountain sickness, including headache, insomnia, anorexia, and occasionally pulmonary edema, cerebral edema, and coma. Ocular and systemic blood pressures increase in patients with mountain sickness. Hypoxia causes decompensation of the vascular endothelium. In general the visual prognosis is good.

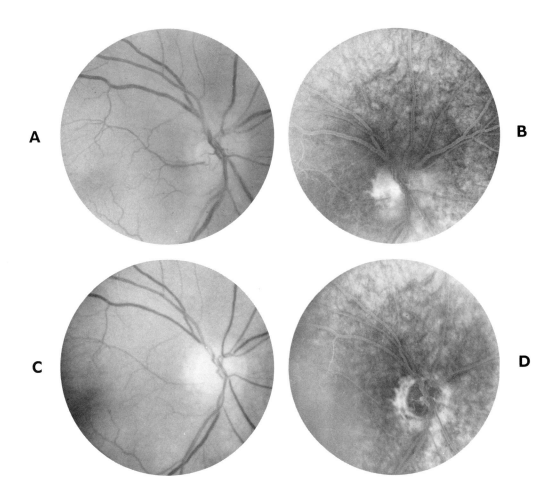

▼ INDOMETHACIN RETINOPATHY

There are a few reports of retinal changes attributed to indomethacin (Indocin); however, none present convincing evidence of a causal relationship between indomethacin therapy and the fundus changes.[189-191]

▼ DIGITALIS AND DIGOXIN RETINAL TOXICITY

Digitalis and digoxin may cause defective color vision, xanthopsia, and other aberrations of color vision, as well as abnormal dark adaptation and reduced photopic flicker ERG amplitudes.[192-194] The fundus appearance is unaffected. The patient may or may not complain of dyschromatopsia. Color vision testing is a useful measure in the diagnosis of toxicity of these drugs and may reveal both red–green and blue–yellow deficiencies.

▼ GLYCINE RETINAL TOXICITY ASSOCIATED WITH TRANSURETHRAL RESECTION

Glycine is the most commonly used irrigating substance during transurethral resection operations. Exposure of the prostate venous sinuses may allow excessive absorption of glycine, which when it reaches levels of approximately 4000 μmol/L (>30 mg/dl) may cause transient visual disturbances such as "darkening" of vision, or severe visual loss for up to several hours.[195] Funduscopic examination is normal. Visual loss is associated with ERG changes consisting of loss of oscillatory potentials and attenuation of 30-Hertz "flicker-following." This retinal dysfunction may be the result of glycine's role as an inhibitory neurotransmitter.

▼ NICOTINIC ACID MACULOPATHY

See Chapter 6, p. 492.

▼ EPINEPHRINE-INDUCED CYSTOID MACULOPATHY

See Chapter 6, p. 488.

▼ ACUTE MACULAR NEURORETINOPATHY AFTER INJECTION OF SYMPATHOMIMETICS

See Chapter 7, p. 694.

▼ CHLORTHALIDONE RETINOPATHY

See Chapter 4, p. 299.

REFERENCES

Chloroquine (Aralen) and Hydroxychloroquine (Plaquenil) Retinopathy

1. Bernstein H, Zvaifler N, Rubin M, Mansour AM: The ocular deposition of chloroquine. *Invest Ophthalmol* 2:384-392, 1963.
2. Bernstein HN, Ginsberg J: The pathology of chloroquine retinopathy. *Arch Ophthalmol* 71:238-245, 1964.
3. Brinkley JR Jr, Dubois EL, Ryan SJ: Long-term course of chloroquine retinopathy after cessation of medication. *Am J Ophthalmol* 88:1-11, 1979.
4. Carr RE, Gouras P, Gunkel RD: Chloroquine retinopathy; early detection by retinal threshold test. *Arch Ophthalmol* 75:171-178, 1966.
5. Carr RE, Henkind P, Rothfield N, Siegel IM: Ocular toxicity of antimalarial drugs; long-term follow-up. *Am J Ophthalmol* 66:738-744, 1968.
6. Cruess AF, Schachat AP, Nicholl J, Augsburger JJ: Chloroquine retinopathy; is fluorescein angiography necessary? *Ophthalmology* 92:1127-1129, 1985.
7. Easterbrook M: The use of Amsler grids in early chloroquine retinopathy. *Ophthalmology* 91:1368-1372, 1984.
8. Ehrenfeld M, Nesher R, Merin S: Delayed-onset chloroquine retinopathy. *Br J Ophthalmol* 70:281-283, 1986.
9. François J, de Rouck A, Cambie E, de Laey JJ: Rétinopathie chloroquinique. *Ophthalmologica* 165:81-99, 1972.
10. Grant WM: *Toxicology of the eye,* ed. 4, Springfield, IL, 1993, Charles C Thomas, pp. 371-382.
11. Gregory MH, Rutty DA, Wood RD: Differences in the retinotoxic action of chloroquine and phenothiazine derivatives. *J Pathol* 102:139-150, 1970.
12. Hart WM Jr, Burde RM, Johnston GP, Drews RC: Static perimetry in chloroquine retinopathy; perifoveal patterns of visual field depression. *Arch Ophthalmol* 102:377-380, 1984.
13. Heckenlively JR, Martin D, Levy J: Chloroquine retinopathy. *Am J Ophthalmol* 89:150, 1980.
14. Henkind P, Carr RE, Siegel IM: Early chloroquine retinopathy: clinical and functional findings. *Arch Ophthalmol* 71:157-165, 1964.
15. Henkind P, Gold DH: Ocular manifestations of rheumatic disorders; natural and iatrogenic. *Rheumatology* 4:13-59, 1973.
16. Henkind P, Rothfield NF: Ocular abnormalities in patients treated with synthetic antimalarial drugs. *N Engl J Med* 269:433-439, 1963.
17. Johnson MW, Vine AK: Hydroxychloroquine therapy in massive doses without retinal toxicity. *Am J Ophthalmol* 104:139-144, 1987.
18. Kearns TP, Hollenhorst RW: Chloroquine retinopathy; evaluation by fluorescein fundus angiography. *Arch Ophthalmol* 76:378-384, 1966.
19. Martin LJ, Bergen RL, Dobrow HR: Delayed onset chloroquine retinopathy: case report. *Ann Ophthalmol* 10:723-726, 1978.
20. Percival SPB, Behrman J: Ophthalmological safety of chloroquine. *Br J Ophthalmol* 53:101-109, 1969.
21. Raines MF, Bhargava SK, Rosen ES: The blood-retinal barrier in chloroquine retinopathy. *Invest Ophthalmol Vis Sci* 30:1726-1731, 1989.
22. Ramsey MS, Fine BS: Chloroquine toxicity in the human eye; histopathologic observations by electron microscopy. *Am J Ophthalmol* 73:229-235, 1972.
23. Rubin M, Bernstein HN, Zvaifler NJ: Studies on the pharmacology of chloroquine; recommendations for the treatment of chloroquine retinopathy. *Arch Ophthalmol* 70:474-481, 1963.
24. Rynes RI, Krohel G, Falbo A, et al: Ophthalmologic safety of long-term hydroxychloroquine treatment. *Arthritis Rheum* 22:832-836, 1979.
25. Sachs DD, Hogan MJ, Engleman EP: Chorioretinopathy induced by chronic administration of chloroquine phosphate (abstract). *Arthritis Rheum* 5:318-319, 1962.
26. Sassani JW, Brucker AJ, Cobbs W, Campbell C: Progressive chloroquine retinopathy. *Ann Ophthalmol* 15:19-22, 1983.
27. Shearer RV, Dubois EL: Ocular changes induced by long-term hydroxychloroquine (Plaquenil) therapy. *Am J Ophthalmol* 64:245-252, 1967.
28. Tobin DR, Krohel GB, Rynes RI: Hydroxychloroquine; seven-year experience. *Arch Ophthalmol* 100:81-83, 1982.
29. Weiner A, Sandberg MA, Gaudio AR, et al: Hydroxychloroquine retinopathy. *Am J Ophthalmol* 112:528-534, 1991.
30. Weiter JJ, Delori F, Dorey CK: Central sparing in annular macular degeneration. *Am J Ophthalmol* 106:286-292, 1988.
31. Wetterholm DH, Winter FC: Histopathology of chloroquine retinal toxicity. *Arch Ophthalmol* 71:82-87, 1964.

Thioridazine (Mellaril) Retinopathy

32. Applebaum A: An ophthalmoscopic study of patients under treatment with thioridazine. *Arch Ophthalmol* 69:578-580, 1963.
33. Burian HM, Fletcher MC: Visual functions in patients with retinal pigmentary degeneration following the use of NP 207. *Arch Ophthalmol* 60:612-629, 1958.
34. Connell MM, Poley BJ, McFarlane JR: Chorioretinopathy associated with thioridazine therapy. *Arch Ophthalmol* 71:816-821, 1964.
35. Davidorf FH: Thioridazine pigmentary retinopathy. *Arch Ophthalmol* 90:251-255, 1973.
36. de Margerie J: Ocular changes produced by a phenothiazine drug: thioridazine. *Trans Can Ophthalmol Soc* 25:160-175, 1962.
37. Fishman GA: Thioridazine hydrochloride (Mellaril) toxic pigmentary chorioretinopathy. *In:* Smith JL, editor: *Neuro-ophthalmology focus 1982,* New York, 1981, Masson, pp. 109-118.

38. Gregory MH, Rutty DA, Wood RD: Differences in the retinotoxic action of chloroquine and phenothiazine derivatives. *J Pathol* 102:139-150, 1970.

39. Heshe J, Engelstoft FH, Kirk L: Retinal injury developing under thioridazine therapy. *Nord Psykiatr T* 15:442-447, 1961.

40. Kimbrough BO, Campbell RJ: Thioridazine levels in the human eye. *Arch Ophthalmol* 99:2188-2189, 1981.

41. Kozy D, Doft BH, Lipkowitz J: Nummular thioridazine retinopathy. *Retina* 4:253-256, 1984.

42. Marmor MF: Is thioridazine retinopathy progressive? Relationship of pigmentary changes to visual function. *Br J Ophthalmol* 74:739-742, 1990.

43. Meredith TA, Aaberg TM, Willerson WD: Progressive chorioretinopathy after receiving thioridazine. *Arch Ophthalmol* 96:1172-1176, 1978.

44. Miller FS III, Bunt-Milam AH, Kalina RE: Clinical-ultrastructural study of thioridazine retinopathy. *Ophthalmology* 89:1478-1488, 1982.

45. Potts AM: The reaction of uveal pigment in vitro with polycyclic compounds. *Invest Ophthalmol* 3:405-416, 1964.

46. Potts AM: Uveal pigment and phenothiazine compounds. *Trans Am Ophthalmol Soc* 60:517-552, 1962.

47. Scott AW: Retinal pigmentation in a patient receiving thioridazine. *Arch Ophthalmol* 70:775-778, 1963.

Chlorpromazine (Thorazine) Retinopathy

48. DeLong SL, Poley BJ, McFarlane JR: Ocular changes associated with long-term chlorpromazine therapy. *Arch Ophthalmol* 73:611-617, 1965.

49. Mathalone MBR: Eye and skin changes in psychiatric patients treated with chlorpromazine. *Br J Ophthalmol* 51:86-93, 1967.

50. Weekley RD, Potts AM, Reboton J, May RH: Pigmentary retinopathy in patients receiving high doses of a new phenothiazine. *Arch Ophthalmol* 64:65-76, 1960.

Clofazimine Retinopathy

51. Craythorn JM, Swartz M, Creel DJ: Clofazimine-induced bull's-eye retinopathy. *Retina* 6:50-52, 1986.

52. Cunningham CA, Friedberg DM, Carr RE: Clofazimine-induced generalized retinal degeneration. *Retina* 10:131-134, 1990.

Deferoxamine Maculopathy

53. Blake DR, Winyard P, Lunec J, et al: Cerebral and ocular toxicity induced by desferrioxamine. *Q J Med* 56:345-355, 1985.

54. Cases A, Kelly J, Sabater F, et al: Ocular and auditory toxicity in hemodialyzed patients receiving desferrioxamine. *Nephron* 56:19-23, 1990.

55. Davies SC, Marcus RE, Hungerford JL, et al: Ocular toxicity of high-dose intravenous desferrioxamine. *Lancet* 2:181-184, 1983.

56. Lakhanpal V, Schocket SS, Jiji R: Deferoxamine (Desferal®)-induced toxic retinal pigmentary degeneration and presumed optic neuropathy. *Ophthalmology* 91:443-451, 1984.

57. Mehta AM, Engstrom RE Jr, Kreiger AE: Deferoxamine-associated retinopathy after subcutaneous injection. *Am J Ophthalmol* 118:260-262, 1994.

58. O'Hare JA, Murnaghan DJ: Evidence of increased parathyroid activity on discontinuation of high-aluminum dialysate in patients undergoing hemodialysis. *Am J Med* 77:229-232, 1984.

59. Pall H, Blake DR, Winyard P, et al: Ocular toxicity of desferrioxamine — an example of copper promoted auto-oxidative damage? *Br J Ophthalmol* 73:42-47, 1989.

60. Rahi AHS, Hungerford JL, Ahmed AI: Ocular toxicity of desferrioxamine: light microscopic histochemical and ultrastructural findings. *Br J Ophthalmol* 70:373-381, 1986.

61. Ravelli M, Scaroni P, Mombelloni S, et al: Acute visual disorders in patients on regular dialysis given desferrioxamine as a test. *Nephrol Dial Transplant* 5:945-949, 1990.

Siderotic Retinopathy

62. Broendstrup P: Two cases of temporary siderosis bulbi with spontaneous resorption and without impairment of function. *Acta Ophthalmol* 22:311-316, 1944.

63. Cibis PA, Brown EB, Hong SM: Ocular effects of systemic siderosis. *Am J Ophthalmol* 44(pt 2):158-172, 1957.

64. Cibis PA, Yamashita T, Rodrigues F: Clinical aspects of ocular siderosis and hemosiderosis. *Arch Ophthalmol* 62:180-187, 1959.

65. Hodgkins PR, Morrell AJ, Luff AJ, et al: Pigment epitheliopathy with serous detachment of the retina following intravenous iron dextran. *Eye* 6:414-415, 1992.

66. Knave B: Electroretinography in eyes with retained intraocular metallic foreign bodies; a clinical study. *Acta Ophthalmol Suppl* 100, 1969.

67. Kuhn F, Witherspoon CD, Skalka H, Morris R: Improvement of siderotic ERG. *Eur J Ophthalmol* 2:44-45, 1992.

68. Masciulli L, Anderson DR, Charles S: Experimental ocular siderosis in the squirrel monkey. *Am J Ophthalmol* 74:638-661, 1972.

69. Schocket SS, Lakhanpal V, Varma SD: Siderosis from a retained intraocular stone. *Retina* 1:201-207, 1981.

70. Sneed SR: Ocular siderosis. *Arch Ophthalmol* 106:997, 1988.

71. Sneed SR, Weingeist TA: Management of siderosis bulbi due to a retained iron-containing intraocular foreign body. *Ophthalmology* 97:375-379, 1990.

Chalcosis Maculopathy

72. Delaney WV Jr: Presumed ocular chalcosis: a reversible maculopathy. *Ann Ophthalmol* 7:378-380, 1975.

73. Felder KS, Gottlieb F: Reversible chalcosis. *Ann Ophthalmol* 16:638-641, 1984.

74. Rao NA, Tso MOM, Rosenthal AR: Chalcosis in the human eye; a clinicopathologic study. *Arch Ophthalmol* 94:1379-1384, 1976.

75. Rosenthal AR, Appleton B: Histochemical localization of intraocular copper foreign bodies. *Am J Ophthalmol* 79:613-625, 1975.

Argyrosis

76. Cohen SY, Quentel G, Egasse D, et al: The dark choroid in systemic argyrosis. *Retina* 13:312-316, 1993.

77. Spencer WH, Garron LK, Contreras F, et al: Endogenous and exogenous ocular and systemic silver deposition. *Trans Ophthalmol Soc UK* 100:171-178, 1980.

Cisplatinum and BCNU (Carmustine) Retinopathy

78. Caruso R, Wilding G, Ballintine E, Ozols R: Cisplatin retinopathy. ARVO Abstracts. *Invest Ophthalmol Vis Sci* 26(Suppl):34, 1985.

79. Greenberg HS, Ensminger WD, Chandler WF, et al: Intra-arterial BCNU chemotherapy for treatment of malignant gliomas of the central nervous system. *J Neurosurg* 61:423-429, 1984.

80. Grimson BS, Mahaley MS Jr, Dubey HD, Dudka L: Ophthalmic and central nervous system complications following intracarotid BCNU (Carmustine). *J Clin Neuro-Ophthalmol* 1:261-264, 1981.

81. Kupersmith MJ, Frohman LP, Choi IS, et al: Visual system toxicity following intra-arterial chemotherapy. *Neurology* 38: 284-289, 1988.

82. Kupersmith MJ, Seiple WH, Holopigian K, et al: Maculopathy caused by intra-arterially administered cisplatin and intravenously administered carmustine. *Am J Ophthalmol* 113:435-438, 1992.

83. Margo CE, Murtagh FR: Ocular and orbital toxicity after intracarotid cisplatin therapy. *Am J Ophthalmol* 116:508-509, 1993.

84. Millay RH, Klein ML, Shults WT, et al: Maculopathy associated with combination chemotherapy and osmotic opening of the blood-brain barrier. *Am J Ophthalmol* 102: 626-632, 1986.

85. Miller DF, Bay JW, Lederman RG, et al: Ocular and orbital toxicity of BCNU (Carmustine) and cisplatinum for malignant gliomas. *Ophthalmology* 92:402-406, 1985.

86. Ostrow S, Hahn P, Wiernik PH, Richards R: Ophthalmologic toxicity after cis-dichlorodiammine platinum(II) therapy. *Cancer Treat Rep* 62:1591-1594, 1978.

87. Shingleton BJ, Bienfang DC, Albert DM, et al: Ocular toxicity associated with high-dose carmustine. *Arch Ophthalmol* 100: 1766-1772, 1982.

Tamoxifen Retinopathy

88. Ashford AR, Donev I, Tiwari RP, Garrett TJ: Reversible ocular toxicity related to tamoxifen therapy. *Cancer* 61:33-35, 1988.

89. Chang T, Gonder JR, Ventresca MR: Low-dose tamoxifen retinopathy. *Can J Ophthalmol* 27:148-149, 1992.

90. Griffiths MFP: Tamoxifen retinopathy at low dosage. *Am J Ophthalmol* 104:185-186, 1987.

91. Heier JS, Dragoo RA, Enzenauer RW, Waterhouse WJ: Screening for ocular toxicity in asymptomatic patients treated with tamoxifen. *Am J Ophthalmol* 117:772-775, 1994.

92. Kaiser-Kupfer MI, Kupfer C, Rodrigues MM: Tamoxifen retinopathy; a clinicopathologic report. *Ophthalmology* 88:89-93, 1981.

93. Kaiser-Kupfer MI, Lippman ME: Tamoxifen retinopathy. *Cancer Treat Rep* 62:315-320, 1978.

94. McKeown CA, Swartz M, Blom J, Maggiano JM: Tamoxifen retinopathy. *Br J Ophthalmol* 65:177-179, 1981.

95. Pavlidis NA, Petris C, Briassoulis E, et al: Clear evidence that long-term low-dose tamoxifen treatment can induce ocular toxicity. A prospective study of 63 patients. *Cancer* 69:2961-2964, 1992.

96. Vinding T, Nielsen NV: Retinopathy caused by treatment with tamoxifen in low dosage. *Acta Ophthalmol* 61:45-50, 1983.

Oxalosis

97. Albert DM, Bullock JD, Lahav M, Caine R: Flecked retina secondary to oxalate crystals from methoxyflurane anesthesia: clinical and experimental studies. *Trans Am Acad Ophthalmol Otolaryngol* 79:OP817-OP826, 1975.

98. Bullock JD, Albert DM: Flecked retina; appearance secondary to oxalate crystals from methoxyflurane anesthesia. *Arch Ophthalmol* 93:26-30, 1975.

99. Novak MA, Roth AS, Levine MR: Calcium oxalate retinopathy associated with methoxyflurane anesthesia. *Retina* 8:230-236, 1988.

100. Wells CG, Johnson RJ, Qingli L, et al: Retinal oxylosis; a clinicopathologic report. *Arch Ophthalmol* 107:1638-1643, 1989.

Canthaxanthine Maculopathy

101. Arden GB, Oluwole JO, Polkinghorne P, et al: Monitoring of patients taking canthaxanthin and carotene: an electroretinographic and ophthalmological survey. *Hum Toxicol* 8:439-450, 1989.

102. Barker FM, Arden GB, Bird AC, et al: The ERG in canthaxanthin therapy. ARVO Abstracts. *Invest Ophthalmol Vis Sci* 28(Suppl):304, 1987.

103. Boudreault G, Cortin P, Corriveau L-A, et al: La rétinopathie à la canthaxanthine: 1. Étude clinique de 51 consommateurs. *Can J Ophthalmol* 18:325-328, 1983.

104. Chang TS, Aylward GW, Clarkson JG, Gass JDM: Asymmetric canthaxanthin retinopathy. *Am J Ophthalmol* 119:801-802, 1995.

105. Cortin P, Boudreault G, Rousseau AP, et al: La rétinopathie à la canthaxanthine: 2. Facteurs prédisposants. *Can J Ophthalmol* 19:215-219, 1984.

106. Cortin P, Corriveau LA, Rousseau A, et al: Canthaxanthine retinopathy. *J Ophthalmic Photogr* 6:68, 1983.

107. Cortin P, Corriveau LA, Rousseau AP, et al: Maculopathie en paillettes d'or. *Can J Ophthalmol* 17:103-106, 1982.

108. Daicker B, Schiedt K, Adnet JJ, Bermond P: Canthaxanthin retinopathy; an investigation by light and electron microscopy and physicochemical analysis. *Graefes Arch Clin Exp Ophthalmol* 225:189-197, 1987.

109. Harnois C, Cortin P, Samson J, et al: Static perimetry in canthaxanthin maculopathy. *Arch Ophthalmol* 106:58-60, 1988.

110. Harnois C, Samson J, Malenfant M, Rousseau A: Canthaxanthin retinopathy; anatomic and functional reversibility. *Arch Ophthalmol* 107:538-540, 1989.

111. Hennekes R: Periphere Netzhautdystrophie nach Canthaxanthin-Einnahme? *Fortschr Ophthalmol* 83:600-601, 1986.

112. Hennekes R, Weber U, Küchle HJ: Über canthaxanthinschäden der Netzhaut. *Z Prackt Augenheilkd* 6:7, 1985.

113. Ibanez HE, Williams DF, Bonuik I: Crystalline retinopathy associated with long-term nitrofurantoin therapy. *Arch Ophthalmol* 112:304-305, 1994.

114. Leyon H, Ros AM, Nyberg S, Algvere P: Reversibility of canthaxanthin deposits within the retina. *Acta Ophthalmol* 68:607-611, 1990.

115. Lonn LI: Canthaxanthin retinopathy. *Arch Ophthalmol* 105: 1590-1591, 1987.

116. McGuinness R, Beaumont P: Gold dust retinopathy after the ingestion of canthaxanthine to produce skin-bronzing. *Med J Aust* 143:622-623, 1985.

117. Metge P, Mandirac-Bonnefoy C, Bellaube P: Thésaurismose rétinienne à la canthaxanthine. *Bull Mem Soc Fr Ophtalmol* 95:547-549, 1983, publ 1984.

118. Oosterhuis JA, Remky H, Nijman NM, et al: Canthaxanthin-retinopathie ohne Canthaxanthin-Einnahme. *Klin Monatsbl Augenheilkd* 194:110-116, 1989.

119. Philip W: Carotinoid-Einlagerungen in der Netzhaut. *Klin Monatsbl Augenheilkd* 187:439-440, 1985.

120. Ros AM, Leyon H, Wennersten G: Crystalline retinopathy in patients taking an oral drug containing canthaxanthine. *Photodermatol* 2:183-185, 1985.

121. Saraux H, Laroche L: Maculopathie a paillettes d'or apres absorption de canthaxanthine. *Bull Soc Ophtalmol Fr* 83:1273-1275, 1983.

122. Scallon LJ, Burke JM, Mieler WF, et al: Canthaxanthine-induced retinal pigment epithelial changes in the cat. *Curr Eye Res* 7:687-693, 1988.

123. Weber U, Goerz G: Augenschadendurch Carotinoid-Einnahme. *Dtsch Arzteblatt* 25:181, 1985.

806

124. Weber U, Kern W, Novotny GEK, et al: Experimental carotenoid retinopathy. I. Functional and morphological alterations of the rabbit retina after 11 months dietary carotenoid application. *Graefes Arch Clin Exp Ophthalmol* 225:198-205, 1987.

125. Weber U, Michaelis L, Kern W, Goerz G: Experimental carotenoid retinopathy. II. Functional and morphological alterations of the rabbit retina after acute canthaxanthin application with small unilamellar phospholipid liposomes. *Graefes Arch Clin Exp Ophthalmol* 225:346-350, 1987.

Flecked Retina Associated with Vitamin A Deficiency

126. Bors F, Fells P: Reversal of the complications of self-induced vitamin A deficiency. *Br J Ophthalmol* 55:210-214, 1971.

127. Brown GC, Felton SM, Benson WE: Reversible night blindness associated with intestinal bypass surgery. *Am J Ophthalmol* 89:776-779, 1980.

128. Dowling JE: Night blindness, dark adaptation, and the electroretinogram. *Am J Ophthalmol* 50:875-889, 1960.

129. Fells P, Bors F: Ocular complications of self-induced vitamin A deficiency. *Trans Ophthalmol Soc UK* 89:221-228, 1969.

130. Fuchs A: White spots of the fundus combined with night blindness and xerosis (Uyemura's syndrome). *Am J Ophthalmol* 48:101-103, 1959.

131. Grey RHB: Visual field changes following hepatic transplantation in a patient with primary biliary cirrhosis. *Br J Ophthalmol* 75:377-380, 1991.

132. Levy NS, Toskes PP: Fundus albipunctatus and vitamin A deficiency. *Am J Ophthalmol* 78:926-929, 1974.

133. O'Donnell M, Talbot JF: Vitamin A deficiency in treated cystic fibrosis: case report. *Br J Ophthalmol* 71:787-790, 1987.

134. Sommer A, Tjakrasudjatma S, Djunaedi E, Green WR: Vitamin A-responsive panocular xerophthalmia in a healthy adult. *Arch Ophthalmol* 96:1630-1634, 1978.

135. Teng-Khoen-Hing: Fundus changes in hypovitaminosis A. *Ophthalmologica* 137:81-85, 1959.

136. Teng-Khoen-Hing: Further contributions to the fundus xerophthalmicus. *Ophthalmologica* 150:219-238, 1965.

137. Uyemura M: Ueber eine merkwürdige Augenhintergrundveränderung bei zwei Fällen von idiopathischer Hemeralopie. *Klin Monatsbl Augenheilkd* 81:471-473, 1928.

Aminoglycoside Maculopathy

138. Balian JV: Accidental intraocular tobramycin injection: a case report. *Ophthalmic Surg* 14:353-354, 1983.

139. Brown GC, Eagle RC, Shakin EP, et al: Retinal toxicity of intravitreal gentamicin. *Arch Ophthalmol* 108:1740-1744, 1990.

140. Campochiaro PA, Conway BP: Aminoglycoside toxicity—a survey of retinal specialists. *Arch Ophthalmol* 109:946-950, 1991.

141. Campochiaro PA, Lim JI, The Aminoglycoside Toxicity Study Group: Aminoglycoside toxicity in the treatment of endophthalmitis. *Arch Ophthalmol* 112:48-53, 1994.

142. Conway BP, Tabatabay CA, Campochiaro PA, et al: Gentamicin toxicity in the primate retina. *Arch Ophthalmol* 107:107-112, 1989.

143. D'Amico DJ, Caspers-Velu L, Libert J, et al: Comparative toxicity of intravitreal aminoglycoside antibiotics. *Am J Ophthalmol* 100:264-275, 1985.

144. D'Amico DJ, Libert J, Kenyon KR, et al: Retinal toxicity of intravitreal gentamicin; an electron microscopic study. *Invest Ophthalmol Vis Sci* 25:564-572, 1984.

145. Grizzard WS: Aminoglycoside macular toxicity after subconjunctival injection. *Arch Ophthalmol* 108:1206, 1990.

146. Judson PH: Aminoglycoside macular toxicity after subconjunctival injection. *Arch Ophthalmol* 107:1282-1283, 1989.

147. McDonald HR, Schatz H, Allen AW, et al: Retinal toxicity secondary to intraocular gentamicin injection. *Ophthalmology* 93:871-877, 1986.

148. Oum BS, D'Amico DJ, Kwak HW, Wong KW: Intravitreal antibiotic therapy with vancomycin and aminoglycoside: Examination of the retinal toxicity of repetitive injections after vitreous and lens surgery. *Graefes Arch Clin Exp Ophthalmol* 230:56-61, 1992.

149. Peyman GA: Aminoglycoside toxicity. *Arch Ophthalmol* 110: 446, 1992.

150. Pflugfelder SC, Hernández E, Fliesler SJ, et al: Intravitreal vancomycin; retinal toxicity, clearance, and interaction with gentamicin. *Arch Ophthalmol* 105:831-837, 1987.

151. Snider JD III, Cohen HB, Chenoweth RG: Acute ischemic retinopathy secondary to intraocular injection of gentamicin. In: Ryan SJ, Dawson AK, Little HL, editors: *Retinal diseases,* Orlando, FL, 1985, Grune & Stratton, pp. 227-232.

152. Talamo JH, D'Amico DJ, Hanninen LA, et al: The influence of aphakia and vitrectomy on experimental retinal toxicity of aminoglycoside antibiotics. *Am J Ophthalmol* 100:840-847, 1985.

153. Waltz K, Margo CE: Intraocular gentamicin toxicity. *Arch Ophthalmol* 109:911, 1991.

154. Zachary IG, Forster RK: Experimental intravitreal gentamicin. *Am J Ophthalmol* 82:604-611, 1976.

Interferon-Associated Retinopathy

155. Guyer DR, Tiedeman J, Yannuzzi LA, et al: Interferon-associated retinopathy. *Arch Ophthalmol* 111:350-356, 1993.

Methamphetamine and Cocaine Retinopathy

156. Shaw HE JR, Lawson JG, Stulting RD: Amaurosis fugax and retinal vasculitis associated with methamphetamine inhalation. *J Clin Neuro-Ophthalmol* 5:169-176, 1985.

157. Wallace RT, Brown GC, Benson W, Sivalingham A: Sudden retinal manifestations of intranasal cocaine and methamphetamine abuse. *Am J Ophthalmol* 114:158-160, 1992.

158. Zeiter JH, Corder DM, Madion MP, McHenry JG: Sudden retinal manifestations of intranasal cocaine and methamphetamine abuse. *Am J Ophthalmol* 114:780-781, 1992.

Lidocaine–Epinephrine Toxicity

159. Lincoff H, Zweifach P, Brodie S, et al: Intraocular injection of lidocaine. *Ophthalmology* 92:1587-1591, 1985.

Quinine Toxicity

160. Bacon P, Spalton DJ, Smith SE: Blindness from quinine toxicity, *Br J Ophthalmol* 72:219-224, 1988.

161. Brinton GS, Norton EWD, Zahn JR, Knighton RW: Ocular quinine toxicity. *Am J Ophthalmol* 90:403-410, 1980.

162. Caffi M, Rapizzi A: Sull'intossicazione sperimentale da chinino; ricerche sperimentali istologiche ed istochimiche sulla retina e sul nervo ottico di coniglio. *Minerva Oftalmol* 8:65-68, 1966.

163. Canning CR, Hague S: Ocular quinine toxicity. *Br J Ophthalmol* 72:23-26, 1988.

164. Casini F: Il metabolismo respiratorio della retina nell' intossicazione sperimentale da chinino. *Arch Ottalmol* 46:263-279, 1939.

165. Gangitano JL, Keltner JL: Abnormalities of the pupil and visual-evoked potential in quinine amblyopia. *Am J Ophthalmol* 89:425-430, 1980.

166. Guly U, Driscoll P: The management of quinine-induced blindness. *Arch Emerg Med* 9:317-322, 1992.
167. Knox DL, Palmer CAL, English F: Iris atrophy after quinine amblyopia. *Arch Ophthalmol* 76:359-362, 1966.

Methyl Alcohol Toxicity

168. Baumbach GL, Cancilla PA, Martin-Amat G, et al: Methyl alcohol poisoning. IV. Alterations of the morphological findings of the retina and optic nerve. *Arch Ophthalmol* 95:1859-1865, 1977.
169. Benton CD Jr, Calhoun FP Jr: The ocular effects of methyl alcohol poisoning: report of a catastrophe involving 320 persons. *Am J Ophthalmol* 36:1677-1685, 1953.
170. Fells JT, Murray TG, Lewandowski MF, et al: Methanol poisoning: clinical evidence of direct retinal dysfunction. ARVO Abstracts. *Invest Ophthalmol Vis Sci* 32:689, 1991.
171. Hayreh MS, Hayreh SS, Baumbach GL, et al: Methyl alcohol poisoning. III. Ocular toxicity. *Arch Ophthalmol* 95:1851-1858, 1977.
172. Martin-Amat G, Tephly TR, McMartin KE, et al: Methyl alcohol poisoning. II. Development of a model for ocular toxicity in methyl alcohol poisoning. II. Development of a model for ocular toxicity in methyl alcohol poisoning using the rhesus monkey. *Arch Ophthalmol* 95:1847-1850, 1977.
173. Murray TG, Burton TC, Rajani C, et al: Methanol poisoning; a rodent model with structural and functional evidence for retinal involvement. *Arch Ophthalmol* 109:1012-1016, 1991.
174. Pamies RJ, Sugar D, Rives LA, Herold AH: Methanol intoxication. How to help patients who have been exposed to toxic solvents. *Postgrad Med* 93:183-184,189-191,194, 1993.
175. Potts AM, Praglin J, Farkas I, et al: Studies on the visual toxicity of methanol. VIII. Additional observations on methanol poisoning in the primary test object. *Am J Ophthalmol* 40(pt 2):76-83, 1955.
176. Ruedemann AD Jr: The electroretinogram in chronic methyl alcohol poisoning in human beings. *Am J Ophthalmol* 54:34-53, 1962.

Amiodarone Optic Neuropathy

177. Garrett SN, Kearney JJ, Schiffman JS: Amiodarone optic neuropathy. *J Clin Neuro-Ophthalmol* 8:105-110, 1988.
178. Gittinger JW Jr, Asdourian GK: Papillopathy caused by amiodarone. *Arch Ophthalmol* 105:349-351, 1987.
179. Nazarian SM, Jay WM: Bilateral optic neuropathy associated with amiodarone therapy. *J Clin Neuro-Ophthalmol* 8:25-28, 1988.
180. Younge BR: Amiodarone optic neuropathy. *J Clin Neuro-Ophthalmol* 8:29, 1988.

Carbon Monoxide Retinopathy

181. Dempsey LC, O'Donnell JJ, Hoff JT: Carbon monoxide retinopathy. *Am J Ophthalmol* 82:692-693, 1976.
182. Ferguson LS, Burke MJ, Choromokos EA: Carbon monoxide retinopathy. *Arch Ophthalmol* 103:66-67, 1985.
183. Kelley JS, Sophocleus GJ: Retinal hemorrhages in subacute carbon monoxide poisoning; exposures in homes with blocked furnace flues. *JAMA* 239:1515-1517, 1978.
184. Murray WR: Amblyopia caused by inhalation of carbon monoxide gas. *Minn Med* 9:561-564, 1926.

High-Altitude Retinopathy

185. Lubin JR, Rennie D, Hackett P, Albert DM: High altitude retinal hemorrhage: a clinical and pathological case report. *Ann Ophthalmol* 14:1071-1076, 1982.
186. Rennie D, Morrissey J: Retinal changes in Himalayan climbers. *Arch Ophthalmol* 93:395-400, 1975.
187. Shults WT, Swan KC: High altitude retinopathy in mountain climbers. *Arch Ophthalmol* 93:404-408, 1975.
188. Wiedman M: High altitude retinal hemorrhage. *Arch Ophthalmol* 93:401-403, 1975.

Indomethacin Retinopathy

189. Burns CA: Indomethacin, reduced retinal sensitivity, and corneal deposits. *Am J Ophthalmol* 66:825-835, 1968.
190. Graham CM, Blach RK: Indomethacin retinopathy: case report and review. *Br J Ophthalmol* 72:434-438, 1988.
191. Henkes HE, van Lith GHM, Canta LR: Indomethacin retinopathy. *Am J Ophthalmol* 73:846-856, 1972.

Digitalis and Digoxin Retinal Toxicity

192. Chuman MA, LeSage J: Color vision deficiencies in two cases of digoxin toxicity. *Am J Ophthalmol* 100:682-685, 1985.
193. Robertson DM, Hollenhorst RW, Callahan JA: Receptor function in digitalis therapy. *Arch Ophthalmol* 76:852-857, 1966.
194. Weleber RG, Shults WT: Digoxin retinal toxicity; clinical and electrophysiologic evaluation of a cone dysfunction syndrome. *Arch Ophthalmol* 99:1568-1572, 1981.

Glycine Retinal Toxicity Associated with Transurethral Resection

195. Creel DJ, Wang JM, Wong KC: Transient blindness associated with transurethral resection of the prostate. *Arch Ophthalmol* 105:1537-1539, 1987.

10

Developmental Tumors of the Retinal Pigment Epithelium (RPE) and Retina

The terms "hamartoma," "choristoma," "phacoma (mother-spot)," and "nevus" are used to describe benign developmental tumors or placoid lesions. *Stedman's Medical Dictionary* defines a hamartoma as: "a focal malformation that resembles a neoplasm grossly and even microscopically, but results from faulty development in an organ; it is composed of an abnormal mixture of tissue elements, or an abnormal proportion of a single element, normally present at that site, which develops and grows at virtually the same rate as normal components, and is not likely to result in compression of the adjacent tissue (in contrast to neoplastic tissue)." A choristoma is defined as a "mass formed by maldevelopment of tissue of a type not normally found at that site." Phacoma is defined as, "a hamartoma found in phacomatosis," a group of hereditary diseases characterized by hamartomas of multiple tissues. A nevus is a "birthmark; a circumscribed malformation of the skin, especially if colored by hyperpigmentation or increased vascularity; it may be predominantly epidermal, adnexal, melanocytic, vascular, or mesodermal, or a localized overgrowth of melanin-forming cells arising in the skin early in life." Ophthalmologists have adopted the term "nevi" to refer to developmental melanocytic lesions of the uveal tract, and it has been recently suggested as an appropriate term to describe developmental placoid melanocytic lesions of the RPE.[13] Developmental uveal melanocytic nevi have been previously described in Chapter 3.

It is important to realize that reactive proliferation of RPE, retinal glial cells, and retinal vascular endothial cells can occasionally duplicate the clinical and histopathologic changes of all of the retinal hamartomatous lesions discussed in this chapter. Examples of these pseudohamartomas will be illustrated in this chapter.

▼ MELANOTIC NEVI OF THE UVEA AND OPTIC NERVE HEAD

See Chapter 3.

▼ MELANOTIC NEVI OF THE RETINAL PIGMENT EPITHELIUM

Solitary-type congenital hypertrophy of the retinal pigment epithelium (CHRPE)

Solitary-type CHRPEs are well-demarcated, very slightly elevated, gray-brown to black, oval, round, or occasionally geographic lesions with smooth or scalloped margins (Figs. 10-1 to 10-3).* They are usually solitary but may be multiple and grouped in a pattern suggesting animal tracks (Fig. 10-1, *A*). A CHRPE may occur anywhere in the fundus. There is often a halo of depigmentation just inside the outer edge of these lesions. Although most CHRPE are between one and two disc diameters, some may occupy an area equal to one quadrant of the fundus (Fig. 10-1, *B*). They have been observed in newborns.[7] Hypopigmented or depigmented lacunae within these lesions are frequently evident, particularly in older patients (Figs. 10-1, *B, D, E,* and *I,* and 10-2, *G* and *H*). These lacunae may show progressive enlargement, and eventually the entire lesion may become depigmented (Fig. 10-1, *G*). Although most of these lesions remain rather stationary, concentric enlargement has been demonstrated in up to 74% of cases (Fig. 10-1, *H* and *I*).[3,6,23] Occasionally, linear depigmented streaks and localized zones of mild hyperpigmentation occur at the anterior margin of these lesions.[6] Many CHRPE are associated with either a relative or an absolute scotoma corresponding to the site of the lesion.

Fluorescein angiography in patients with lightly pigmented fundi shows obstruction of the background choroidal fluorescence in the area of the lesion except in the fenestrated areas of hypopigmentation (Fig. 10-1, *C*). Angiographic evidence of alterations in the structure and permeability of the retinal vessels overlying these lesions may occasionally occur.[8,9,31] This includes capillary nonperfusion, capillary leakage, and chorioretinal anastomosis.

---

*References 2-4, 6, 14, 22, 26, 33.

FIG. 10-1   Congenital Hypertrophy of the RPE (CHRPE).

A, Multiple areas of CHRPE simulating large animal tracks.

B and **C,** Large area of CHRPE mistaken for a malignant melanoma in a 59-year-old woman who was asymptomatic. Note several areas of thinning of the RPE within the central portion of the lesion (*arrows,* **B**). There was an absolute field defect corresponding with the lesion. Angiography revealed obstruction of the background choroidal fluorescence except in the areas of thinning of the RPE (*arrow,* **C**).

D, A jet black CHRPE with small fenestrations (*arrow*) and absolute scotoma in the paramacular region of a young woman.

E, CHRPE associated with multiple fenestrations (*arrows*) and a peripheral nonpigmented ring.

F, CHRPE showing generalized hypopigmentation and a nonpigmented peripheral ring.

G, CHRPE showing generalized hypopigmentation that extends out to and includes a poorly defined, nonpigmented ring and a well-defined, pigmented ring.

H and **I,** Growth of CHRPE in a 47-year-old woman between January of 1978 (**H**) and June of 1985 (**I**).

J to **L,** Growth of CHRPE into the central macular area of the left eye.

(**E** and **F** from Buettner[4]; **A** to **D** from Gass[12]; **J** to **L** courtesy of Dr. Richard Dreyer.)

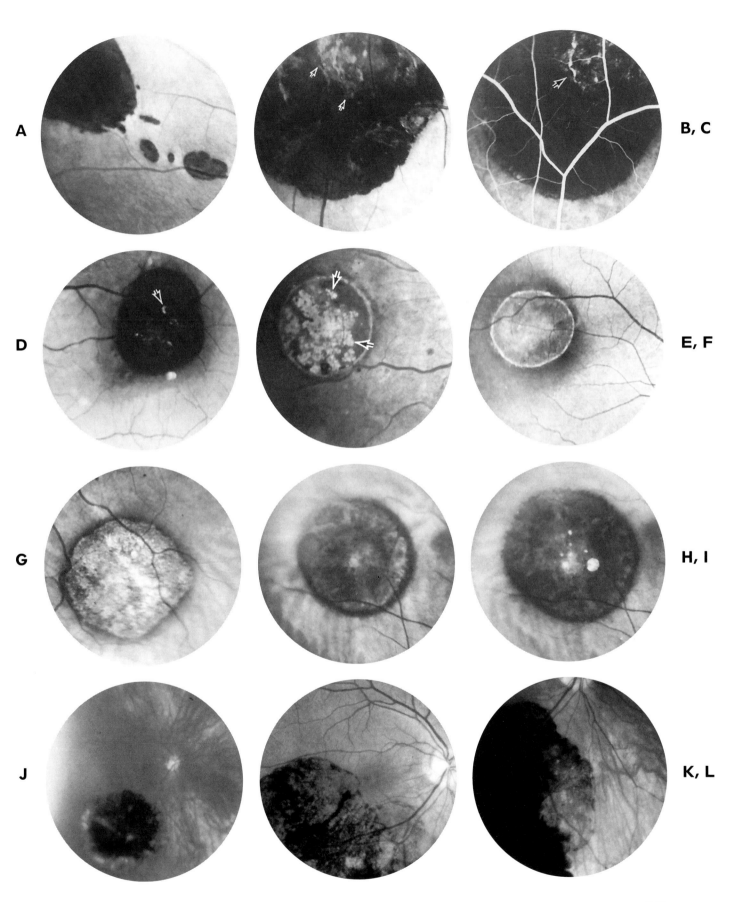

Histopathologically, CHRPE lesions are characterized by a single layer of enlarged retinal pigment epithelium (RPE) cells containing macromelanin granules that may be associated with varying degrees of degeneration of the overlying outer retinal layers (Fig. 10-2).[4,7,18,21] Some degree of RPE hyperplasia may also be evident.[38] Absence of lipofuscin in the hypertrophied RPE cells suggests that their incapacity to phagocytose and digest photoreceptor outer segments may be responsible for the receptor cell degeneration so often present overlying these lesions.[21] The structure of the macromelanosomes in CHRPE is similar to that described in X-linked ocular albinism.[21,35]

The differential diagnosis of CHRPE includes choroidal melanocytic nevi, secondary and primary hyperplasia of the RPE, and geographic dark fundus patches that are probably caused by subretinal bleeding and hemosiderin deposits, usually occurring in patients with sickle cell disease (see Figs. 6-44, C and D, and 6-45, I).[33] The large lesions, if not viewed binocularly, may be mistaken for malignant melanomas of the choroid (Fig. 10-1, B).

These lesions are similar histopathologically to lesions referred to as congenital grouped pigmentation of the RPE (see next subsection). Hypertrophy of the RPE has been identified histopathologically as being part of combined RPE and retinal hamartomas (see Figs. 10-8, K, and 10-10, E).

FIG. 10-2 Histopathologic Findings in Congenital Hypertrophy of the RPE (CHRPE).

A to **D,** Clinicopathologic correlation of a coin-shaped, flat, pigmented lesion noted on gross examination of an autopsy eye (**A**). Note the nonpigmented halo just inside the margins of the pigmented lesion. Histopathologic examination revealed a pigmented tumor to be composed of a single layer of large RPE cells (*right half of photomicrograph,* **B**). The main body of the lesion was separated from the normal surrounding RPE by a halo of partly depigmented RPE (*arrows,* **B**). There was extensive degeneration of the outer layers of retina overlying the entire lesion. A high-power view of the lesion revealed large RPE cells packed with large, round melanin granules (**C**). (Compare with the normal surrounding RPE in **D.**)

E, Histopathologic condition of another patient with CHRPE showing a sharp line of junction (*arrow*) separating the normal RPE on the left side of the photomicrograph and the hypertrophy of the RPE on the right side. Note that Bruch's membrane appears thickened and there is atrophy of the underlying choriocapillaris.

F, Electron microscopic view of the normal RPE (*left side*) and CHRPE RPE (*right side*) in the same case illustrated in **A** to **D**. Note thickening of the basement membrane (*bm*) of the RPE.

G and **H,** Clinicopathologic correlation of CHRPE associated with a large central fenestrated area noted on gross examination of an autopsy eye (**G**). Photomicrograph of the margin (*arrow,* **H**) of the hypertrophied RPE to the left of the arrow and the central fenestrated area showed loss of RPE in the fenestrated area and proliferation of glial cells along the inner surface of Bruch's membrane (**H**).

(**A** to **C** and **F** to **H** from Buettner.[4])

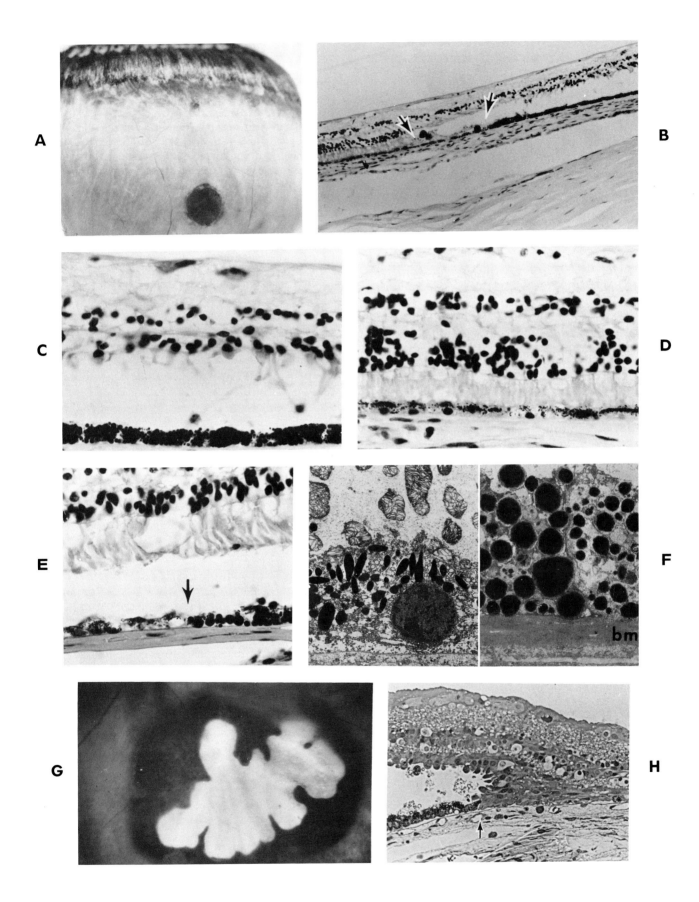

A

B

C

D

E

F

bm

G

H

813

Multiple CHRPE associated with familial adenomatous polyposis and Gardner's syndrome

Multiple isolated CHRPE lesions occur usually in both eyes of a high percentage of patients with this dominantly inherited familial cancer syndrome that includes intestinal polyposis, osteomas of the skull, and various soft tissue tumors, including fibromas, lipomas, and epidermal and sebaceous cysts.* The risk for intestinal malignancy during adult life is virtually 100%. The soft tissue tumors tend to occur during the first two decades, the bony tumors in the second decade, and the polyps in adulthood (mean age 30 years). Osteomas of the orbit may occur.[37] Approximately 50% of patients will develop adenocarcinoma of the colon by 35 years of age. There is a disproportionate risk of other cancers (carcinoma of ampulla of Vater, adrenal gland, thyroid gland, and bladder), a variety of sarcomas, and neuroepithelial tumors (Turcot syndrome) (Fig. 10-3, *G* to *I*).[22] Multiple CHRPE affecting both eyes is a reliable marker for Gardner's syndrome. Multiple CHRPE appears to be specific for Gardner's syndrome and is not found in the other familial intestinal polyposis syndromes (familial polyposis without extraintestinal manifestations, Peutz-Jeghers syndrome) or in patients with familial nonpolyposis colorectal cancers.[35] The CHRPE lesions in Gardner's syndrome often show a peculiar oval shape with a fishtail-like change at one or both poles (Fig. 10-3, *C, E,* and *F*).[14] In some cases the lesions appear to be located in close approximation to the major retinal vessels and may be associated with abnormalities in the overlying retinal vessels.[30] Histopathologically, some of the lesions appear similar to solitary CHRPE. Others show in addition hamartomatous malformations of the RPE featuring cellular hypertrophy, hyperplasia and retinal invasion, and formation of a mushroom-shaped tumor (Fig. 10-3, *K* and *L*).[17,36]

*References 1, 10, 11, 13, 15-17, 19, 20, 22, 27-32, 35-37.

FIG. 10-3   Familial Multifocal Congenital Hypertrophy of the RPE (CHRPE).

A to F, Multiple, oval areas of flat CHRPE were present bilaterally in the 30-year-old mother (**A**), the 8-year-old son (**B** and **D**), and the 10-year-old daughter (**E** and **F**). Note the depigmented halo near the margin of the lesions, their radial orientation in respect to the posterior pole, and the fishtail-shaped hypopigmented area at one or both ends of the lesions *(arrows)*. The lesions showed varying degrees of pigmentation. The eye examinations were otherwise normal in these patients. Medical evaluation failed to find evidence of intestinal polyposis or other disease.

G to I, Turcot's syndrome with multiple CHRPE (**G**); adenomatous polyps of the stomach, duodenum, and colon (**I**); and a cerebellar medulloblastoma *(arrow,* **H**) occurred in this 20-year-old man, who presented with nausea, headaches, and vomiting after head trauma.

J and K, Histopathology of CHRPE lesions found in the eyes of a patient with Gardner's syndrome. **J,** Hypertrophy of RPE. **K,** Hyperplasia and hypertrophy of RPE. **L,** Hypertrophy and hyperplasia RPE with extension through the full thickness of the retina.

(**G** to **I** from Munden et al.[22]; **J** and **K** from Traboulsi et al.[36])

Patients with multiple CHRPE lesions in one eye or bilateral lesions, or with a solitary lesion and a family history of intestinal polyposis should be evaluated for evidence of Gardner's syndrome. There is no evidence that typical solitary or grouped CHRPE lesions represent a marker for Gardner's syndrome.[31] Multifocal CHRPE lesions have occurred in a family with microcephaly and hyperreflexia[24] and in one family in Miami without any other abnormalities (Fig. 10-3).[14]

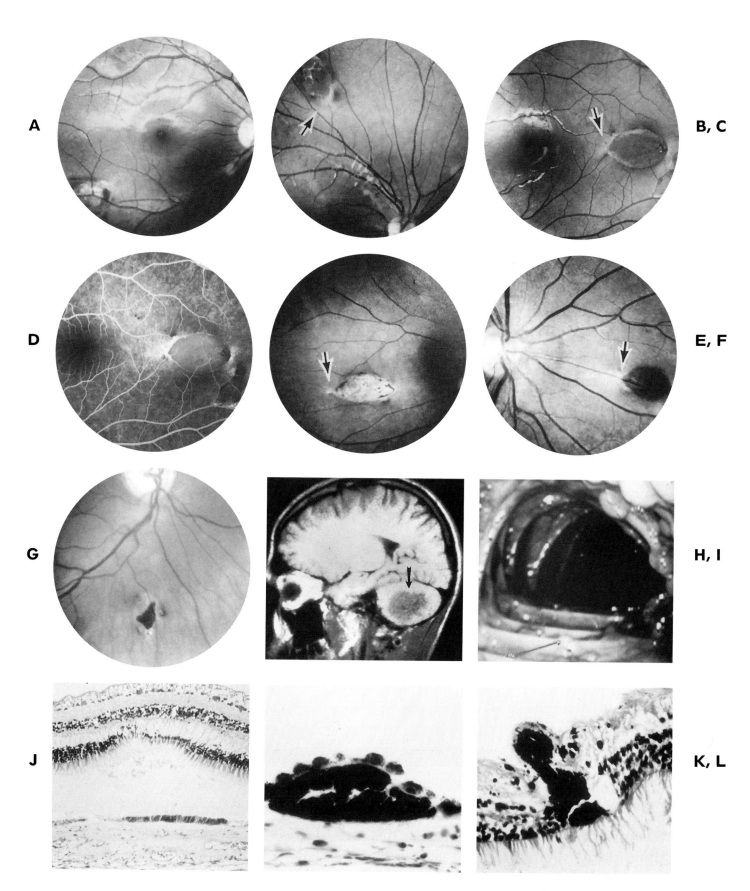

A

B, C

D

E, F

G

H, I

J

K, L

Grouped-type congenital pigmented nevi of the retinal pigment epithelium, "bear tracks"

This is a rare congenital anomaly characterized by sharply circumscribed, small, variably sized, pigment spots that are often arranged in groups to resemble the footprints of animals (Fig. 10-4).[42,44,46,50,51] They are usually grouped in one sector of the fundus with the smaller spots located at the apex directed toward the optic disc. They infrequently are present in the macular area. Extensive areas of the fundus may be affected and be associated with bilateral involvement (Fig. 10-4, D and E).[43,45,49,52] Familial cases involving two successive generations are reported.[40,41,48] The retina overlying "bear tracks" appears normal biomicroscopically and angiographically.[46] Electrooculographic findings are normal. These lesions are believed to be stationary, but long-term followup studies have not been done. Grouped nevi have infrequently occurred in association with other anomalies or disorders.[39,49]

These lesions histopathologically are similar to congenital hypertrophy of the RPE (CHRPE).[47,50] Unlike CHRPE most of the melanin granules retain their ellipsoidal shape and hypertrophy and hyperplasia of the RPE are less prominent.[47] Clinically, some patients may show lesions typical of both grouped nevi and CHRPE (Figs. 10-1, A, and 10-4, G).

FIG. 10-4 **Congenital Grouped Pigmentation of the RPE.**

A to **C,** Uniocular involvement in three patients. Each showed lesions in one quadrant or less. None had macular involvement. All had normal visual function.

D to **F,** Marked peripheral involvement in both eyes of this patient with normal visual function. **F,** Higher power view of the upper nasal quadrant of the right fundus.

G, Several large peripheral zones of hypertrophy of the RPE accompanied grouped pigmentation in this patient.

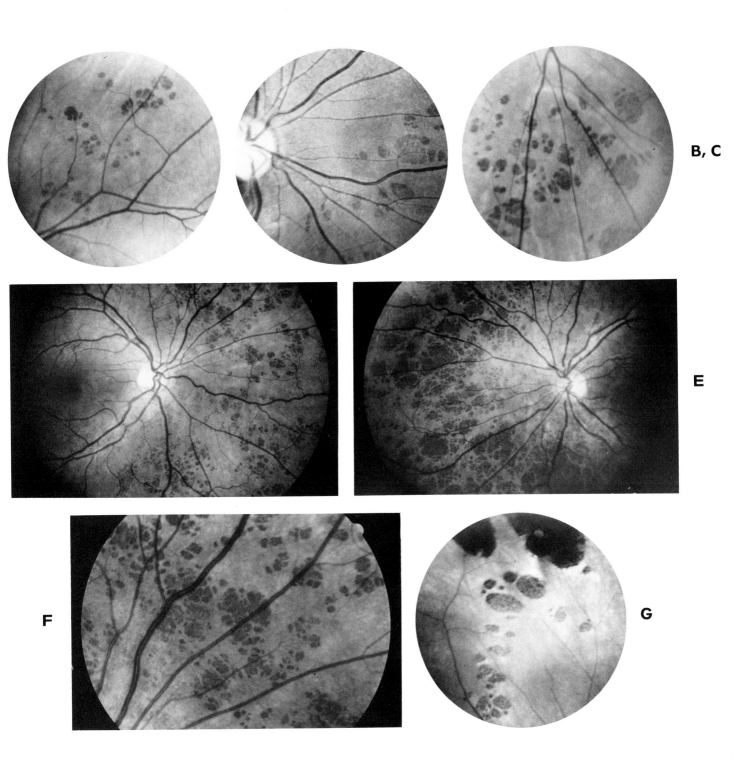

B, C

E

F

G

817

▼ ALBINOTIC AND NONPIGMENTED NEVI OF THE RETINAL PIGMENT EPITHELIUM

Grouped-type congenital albinotic and hypomelanotic nevi of the retinal pigment epithelium, "polar bear tracks"

Congenital grouped albinotic nevi are multiple, white, variably sized spots involving the RPE in a pattern similar to that in congenital grouped pigmentation of the RPE (Fig. 10-5).[13,14,24,53] They may occur in one or both eyes and may be mistaken for other flecked retina diseases (e.g., drusen, fundus flavimaculatus, pattern dystrophy, fundus albipunctatus, and Gaucher's disease). Like pigmented bear tracks, these albinotic spots occur rarely and tend to be more numerous and larger in the peripheral fundus, and they usually do not involve the macular area. They appear to represent focal thickening of the RPE that is filled with a white material. This white material may be diffusely distributed or may be more concentrated in the periphery of the lesion (Fig. 10-5, A and C). In some cases the spots appear to be devoid of white material, and the underlying choroidal vessels are visible. In other cases, some of the spots may appear to contain dark gray pigment. The overlying retina appears normal, except that larger retinal vessels may appear to be locally narrowed (Fig. 10-5, C and D). The lesions are probably relatively stable, but further long-term followup studies are required to document this. Although considered to be functionally of no significance, one patient with macular as well as peripheral lesions developed neovascularization (Fig. 10-5, G and H).

Fluorescein angiography shows variable degrees of transmission of the choroidal fluorescence through these lesions (Fig. 10-5, B).

Although longer followup of these rarely encountered patients is required, it is probable that the albinotic spots represent a congenital anomaly of the RPE closely akin to congenital grouped hyperpigmentation of the RPE. In the case of the albinotic spots, the RPE cells appear to be stuffed

FIG. 10-5 Congenital Grouped RPE Albinotic Nevi.

A to **C,** Except for the albinotic spots the results of an eye examination that included color vision testing, electroretinography, electrooculography, and dark-adaptation studies were normal in this healthy 15-year-old girl. Note the peripheral distribution of white material in some of the larger spots (*arrows,* **A**) and slight narrowing of a retinal artery overlying one spot (*arrow,* **C**). Angiography showed variable transmission of the choroidal fluorescence through the spots (**B**).

D and **E,** Albinotic spots in one eye of a 40-year-old asymptomatic woman. Note narrowing of retinal vein *(arrow)* overlying a large spot.

F, Albinotic spots in one eye of an asymptomatic young man.

G and **H,** This healthy 14-year-old girl was observed for 3 years with grouped albinotic spots in both eyes before she was seen because of loss of central vision in the left eye associated with choroidal neovascularization (*arrow,* **H**). Her electroretinographic and electrooculographic findings were normal.

(**D** and **E,** courtesy Dr. Alvaro Rodriguez; **G** and **H,** courtesy Dr. Harry W. Flynn.)

with a white material, possibly an abnormal precursor of melanin rather than enlarged melanin granules as in grouped hyperpigmentation of the RPE.

I believe that these albinotic RPE spots are identical to those reported by Kandori and associates[54-56] in association with stationary night blindness that was manifest primarily by abnormal dark adaptation. None of the four patients seen at the Bascom Palmer Eye Institute had nyctalopia. Studies, including dark adaptation, electroretinography, and electrooculography, were normal in the two patients illustrated in Fig. 10-5, A to C, and G to H. Park et al.[57] reported similar white spots in one of two siblings with pigmented RPE lesions, microcephaly, mental retardation, and autosomal dominant hyperreflexia.

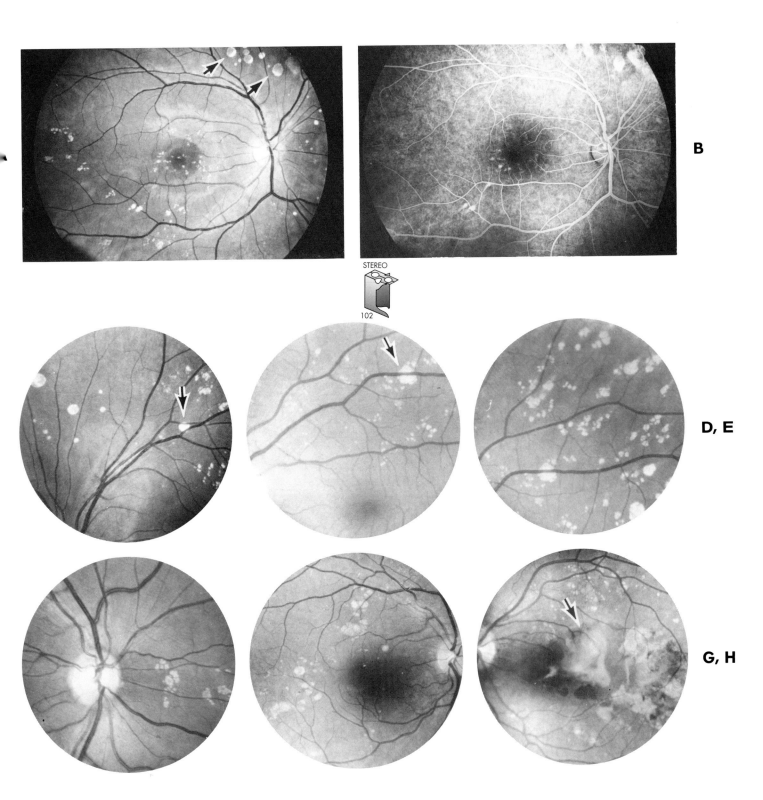

B

STEREO
102

D, E

G, H

Solitary-type hypomelanotic and albinotic nevi

These solitary, sharply circumscribed, hypopigmented reddish-orange or white lesions of the RPE, which have been previously referred to as "congenital hypomelanotic freckle" or "retinal albinotic spots," are most frequently observed in the peripheral fundus and in the temporal half of the macula.[12,13,58-60] These latter lesions often have an oval or fish-shaped appearance similar to that seen in the CHRPE lesions associated with Gardner's syndrome (Fig. 10-6, *A* and *D* to *F*).[59] They are often discovered on routine eye examination in children. They may be unassociated with a demonstrable visual field defect. Although they may show a slight milky white color, they are rarely as densely white as the grouped albinotic RPE nevi. Unlike most acquired atrophic lesions of the RPE, hypopigmented RPE nevi typically have no margin or irregular hyperpigmentation. Angiographically the choriocapillaris underlying these lesions appears to be normal (Fig. 10-6, *B* and *C*). Microscopically, hypopigmented RPE nevi show a sharp transition from normal RPE to flat nonpigmented epithelium (Fig. 10-6, *G* and *H*).[12,23,60] Unlike the presentation in most cases of congenital hypertrophy of the RPE, the overlying retina is normal. The underlying choroid is also unaffected. So far there are no histopathologic studies of solitary nevi that have clinically appeared to show evidence of white pigment production.

FIG. 10-6 **Large Solitary Amelanotic Spot or Nevus of the RPE.**

A to C, Amelanotic RPE nevus first noted on a routine eye examination 6 years previously in an asymptomatic 51-year-old Black woman with 20/15 visual acuity bilaterally. She had only a faint relative scotoma to 3/1000 color test objects. Note the relatively intact choriocapillaris (**B** and **C**).

D, Amelanotic nevus in a 12-year-old boy with normal acuity, Amsler grid, and Goldmann visual field examinations.

E, Paired amelanotic nevi in an asymptomatic patient.

F, Hypopigmented RPE nevus with focus of RPE hyperplasia and atrophy.

G to J, Amelanotic nevus or freckle noted on gross examination of a fresh eye removed at autopsy (**G**). Histopathologic examination revealed a focal area of depigmentation of the artifactitiously detached RPE (*arrows,* **H**). A high-power view showed a sharp transition (*arrows*) between the nonpigmented, flattened RPE cells and the relatively normal, surrounding RPE cells (*arrows,* **I** and **J**).

(**D** from Roseman and Gass[59]; **E** and **F**, courtesy Dr. Mark J. Daily; **G** to **J** from Gass.[12])

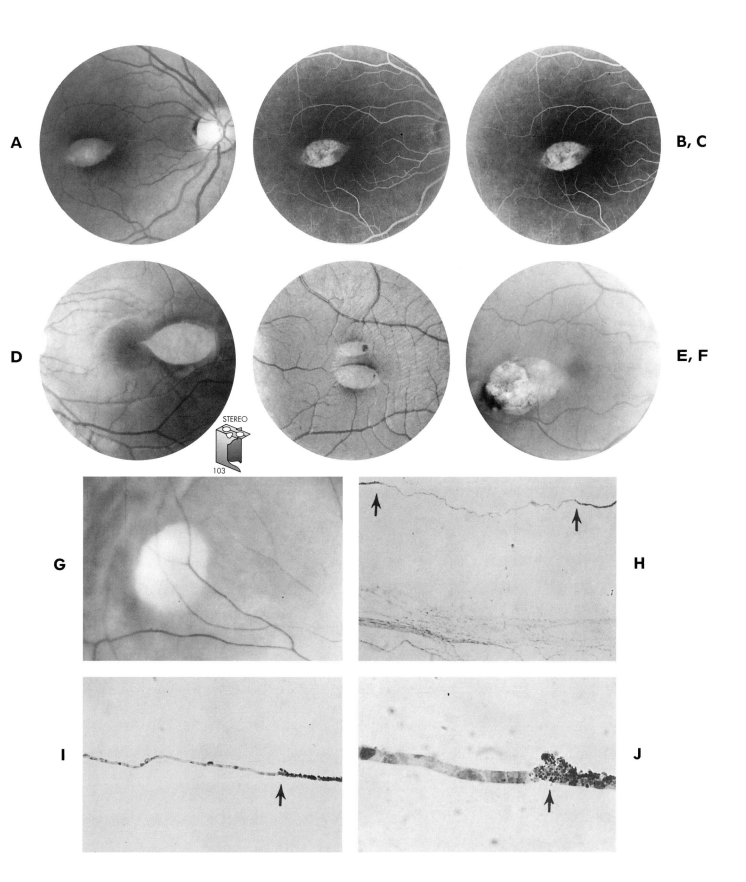

A

B, C

D

STEREO
103

E, F

G

H

I

J

▼ RETINAL PIGMENT EPITHELIAL HAMARTOMA (CONGENITAL HYPERPLASIA OF THE RETINAL PIGMENT EPITHELIUM, PIGMENT EPITHELIAL ADENOMA)

I have seen children as well as adults with focal, solitary, nodular, black subretinal lesions that extend anteriorly into and usually through the entire thickness of the retina and that probably are hamartomas composed of hyperplastic RPE (Fig. 10-7).[13,14] The hamartomas are unassociated with any changes in the surrounding RPE or retina but may occur in association with other fundus anomalies (Fig. 10-7, *A*). Like solitary hypomelanotic RPE nevi, these lesions are frequently discovered in the temporal macular area of normal children or young adults on routine eye examination. Fluorescein angiography reveals that these lesions are nonfluorescent early but may show evidence of some staining late (Fig. 10-7, *B* and *C*).

To date no change in the size of these lesions has been documented. Some of the large pigment epithelial adenomas in eyes enucleated because of suspected choroidal melanomas probably are also of developmental origin.[61-66]

FIG. 10-7   Congenital Hyperplasia of the RPE.

A to **C,** On a routine eye examination a focal elevated pigmented lesion that extended through the full thickness of the retina was noted in the right macula of an asymptomatic 12-year-old girl (**A**). Note the edge of the anomalous optic disc (**A** and **C**). Fluorescein angiography showed that the lesion extended through and covered the surface of the retina and that it stained in the late photographs (**B** and **C**). **Color plate 104** shows stereoscopic photographs made 16 years after **A.**

D and **E,** An elevated pigmented lesion extending through the full thickness of the retina was noted in an asymptomatic 57-year-old man. His visual acuity in the right eye was 20/25 and in the left eye was 20/20. He had a past history of having watched an eclipse as a child. The left fundus was normal. Angiography revealed that the lesion extended through the full thickness of the retina, obscured the retinal vessels, and stained centrally in the late photographs (**E**).

F, This pigmented lesion involving the full thickness of the retina was discovered in an 11-year-old girl whose visual acuity in the right eye was 20/15 and in the left eye was 20/20. The left fundus was normal.

G, Diagram of intraretinal congenital RPE hyperplasia. **1,** Superficial. **2,** Preretinal extension. **3,** Preretinal extension with superficial vascularization.

(**F,** courtesy Dr. R. Kennon Guerry; **G** from Gass.[13])

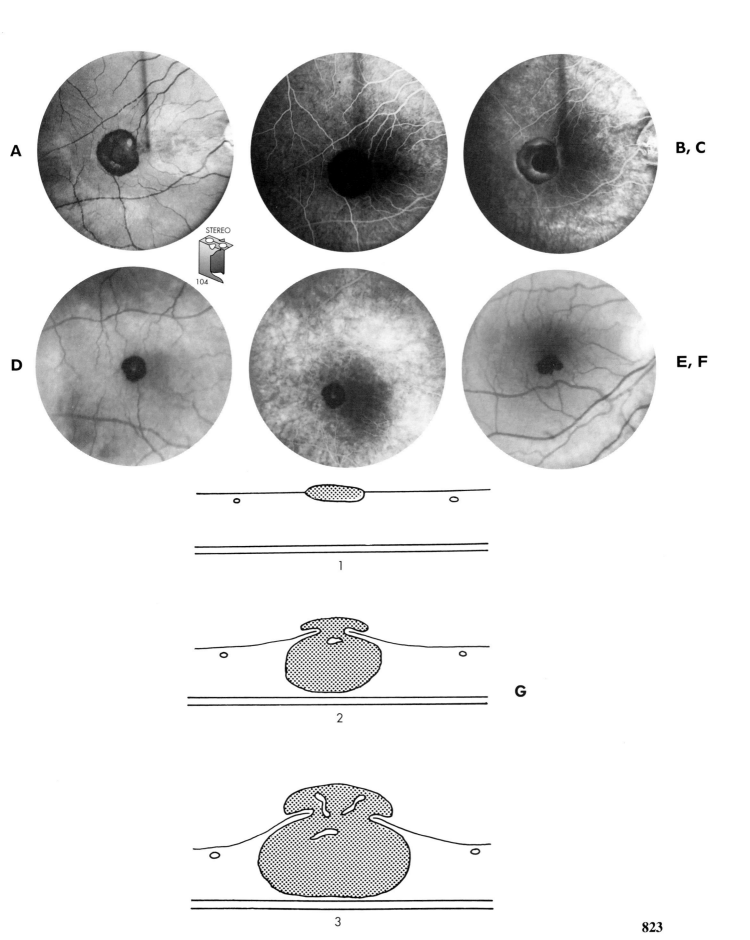

A

B, C

D

E, F

STEREO

104

G

1

2

3

▼ COMBINED PIGMENT EPITHELIAL AND RETINAL HAMARTOMA

Combined pigment epithelial and retinal hamartomas are peculiar, slightly elevated, partly pigmented lesions, which may be mistaken for a postinflammatory scar or a malignant melanoma, and which may be present anywhere in the fundus.* The clinical history, appearance of the tumor, and its structure vary with its location.

Combined pigment epithelial and retinal hamartoma involving the optic disc

Patients with tumors that involve the optic nerve head and juxtapapillary retina typically are seen in young adults because of blurred and distorted vision in one eye. The visual acuity is usually 20/100 or better. Biomicroscopic examination reveals an ill-defined, slightly elevated, partly pigmented tumor involving part of the optic nerve head and adjacent retina (Fig. 10-8). The tumor is composed of a fine granular distribution of pigment, giving it a charcoal-gray filigree appearance.† The presence of many fine capillaries within the tumor may be partly obscured from view by a semitranslucent gray membrane that is always present on the inner retinal surface. Patients become symptomatic either because of metamorphopsia caused by contraction of this membrane that produces traction folds in the retina that extend into the central macular area (Fig. 10-8, *A*), or less frequently because of subretinal and intraretinal exudation derived from the capillary component of the tumor (Fig. 10-8, *D*). This exudation may reabsorb spontaneously and leave atrophic changes in the RPE surrounding the tumor. Other complications that may occur infrequently include choroidal neovascularization, retinal hemorrhages, and vitreous hemorrhages.[85,104] The early phases of angiography demonstrate dilated, multiple, fine blood vessels within the tumor, and later phases show evidence of leakage of dye from these vessels (Fig. 10-8, *B, C, E, F, H,* and *I*).[78,81,103] Histopathologically, the optic disc tumors show evidence of a hamartomatous malformation involving hyperplasia of the RPE, glial cells, and blood vessels (Fig. 10-8, *J* and *K*).‡ Many of these lesions remain stable. Some may develop exudative changes and show an increase in opacification of the glial component of the tumor. The surface glial mem-

*References 70, 76, 77, 78, 81, 92, 95, 98, 99, 101-103.
†References 63, 70-72, 75-79, 81, 84, 89, 92, 103.
‡References 70, 76, 78, 81, 89, 101, 103.

FIG. 10-8 Combined RPE and Retinal Hamartoma (CRPE-RH) of the Juxtapapillary Retina and Optic Disc Head.

A to C, A circumscribed, slightly elevated, finely mottled, pigmented lesion was noted in a 21-year-old man with a 1-year history of progressive distortion of the vision in his left eye. Two years previously his visual acuity had been 20/20. He had multiple flat pigmented lesions on the buttocks and arms. His past medical history was otherwise negative. Visual acuity in the left eye was 20/50. Flecks of pigmented tissue extended anteriorly into the thickened retina and optic nerve tissue and partly covered the major retinal vessels as they entered the optic nerve head (**A**). This was associated with an epiretinal glial membrane. Prominent retinal traction folds extended from this membrane into the macula. There were many fine, dilated, tortuous capillaries within the tumor. These were best seen angiographically (**B**). There was slight leakage of dye from vessels in the later angiograms (**C**).

D to F, Serous detachment of the macula and circinate retinopathy caused by a juxtapapillary retinal and RPE hamartoma in a 55-year-old woman (**D**). Angiography revealed a capillary angiomatous component of this lesion (**E** and **F**, *stereo*).

G to I, Small hypopigmented combined RPE and retinal hamartoma in a 66-year-old asymptomatic man who was suspected of having ischemic optic neuropathy (**G**). An epiretinal membrane on the surface of the lesion partly obscured the retinal vessels and the mottled pigmentation within the tumor (**G**). Angiography revealed evidence of the capillary angiomatous nature of this lesion as well as some dilation of the retinal capillaries in the papillomacular bundle (**H** and **I**).

J and K, Clinicopathologic correlation of a juxtapapillary CRPE-RH in a 29-year-old man with an 8-week history of blurred vision in his left eye (**J**). Melanoma was suspected, and the eye was enucleated. Histopathologic examination revealed disorganization of the normal architecture of the optic nerve head and retina associated with hyperplasia of the retinal blood vessels, RPE, and glial tissue (**K**). Cords and sheets of RPE proliferation extended throughout the tumor and surrounded blood vessels (*arrows,* **K**). Note the proliferation of fibrous tissue near the surface of the retina.

(A to C from Vogel et al.[103]; J and K from Machemer.[89])

brane causing the retinal folding is an integral part of the tumor and accounts for the fact that surgical stripping of the membrane is difficult and has little chance of restoring central vision.[90,97]

These tumors, particularly if lightly pigmented, when discovered in infants or young children may be mistaken for retinoblastoma and *Toxocara canis.* In patients with more heavily pigmented tumors, the differential diagnosis includes melanocytoma,

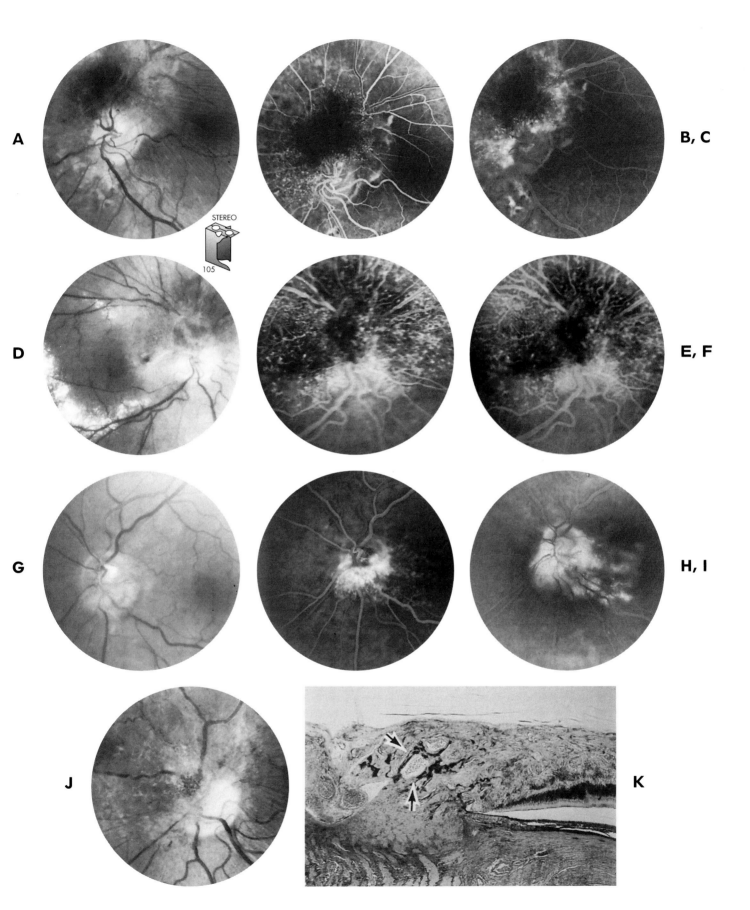

A

B, C

D

E, F

G

H, I

J

K

STEREO
105

malignant melanoma, and reactive hyperplasia of the RPE. The optic disc tumors with minimal pigmentation may be difficult or impossible to differentiate from capillary angiomas or from epipapillary and juxtapapillary epiretinal membranes associated with other causes.[96] One patient's hypopigmented tumor was misdiagnosed as ischemic optic neuropathy (Fig. 10-8, *G* to *I*). Reactive proliferation of retinal endothelial, glial, and RPE cells may duplicate any of the retinal and RPE hamartomas. The author has seen the spontaneous development of lesions indistinguishable from a juxtapapillary and a peripheral combined pigment epithelial and retinal hamartoma in two adult patients where previously there was no lesion (Fig. 10-12, *G* and *H*).[83]

FIG. 10-9 Combined RPE and Retinal Hamartomas (CRPE-RH) Without Intrinsic Involvement of the Optic Disc Head.

A, CRPE-RH in the macula of the left eye of an otherwise healthy 7-year-old girl with amblyopia in the left eye.

B to D, CRPE-RH in the macular region of an 8-year-old boy (**A**). His right fundus was normal. Fluorescein angiography demonstrated tortuosity, dilation, and abnormal permeability of the retinal vessels in the region of the tumor (**B to D**). *Arrows* indicate the temporal border of the flat pigmented portion of the tumor (**C**).

E and F, Peripheral CRPE-RH simulating a retinoblastoma and malignant melanoma of the choroid in a 19-month-old girl who was the product of an uncomplicated full-term pregnancy and delivery. Her birth weight was 8 pounds. At age 5 months intermittent exotropia was noted. There was dragging of the retinal vessels and displacement of the macula (*arrow,* **F**) in a superotemporal direction by a slightly elevated, partly pigmented tumor that was located near the equator superotemporally (**E**). Much of the central portion of the pigmented lesion was obscured by gray-white, semitranslucent, thickened retinal tissue and an epiretinal membrane (**E**). Note the dilation and tortuosity of the retinal vessels and the feathery appearance of the flat pigmented portion of the tumor (*arrows,* **E**) where it blended imperceptibly into the normal RPE. By the age of 40 months the child's visual acuity in the affected eye was counting fingers only and the lesion was unchanged.

G to J, Midperipheral CRPE-RH (**H**) associated with heterotopia of the macula and congenital optic disc pit (**I**). Note the dilated capillaries and leakage of fluorescein (**I** and **J**).

K and L, Healthy 4-year-old boy referred for possible retinoblastoma discovered during evaluation of poor vision in the right eye. He had anisometropic amblyopia with 20/60 vision, right eye, and 20/30 vision, left eye. There was a slightly elevated pigmented lesion covered by gray-white retinal tissue and tortuous retinal vessels near the superotemporal border of the left macula (**L**).

(**A** to **F** from Gass.[12])

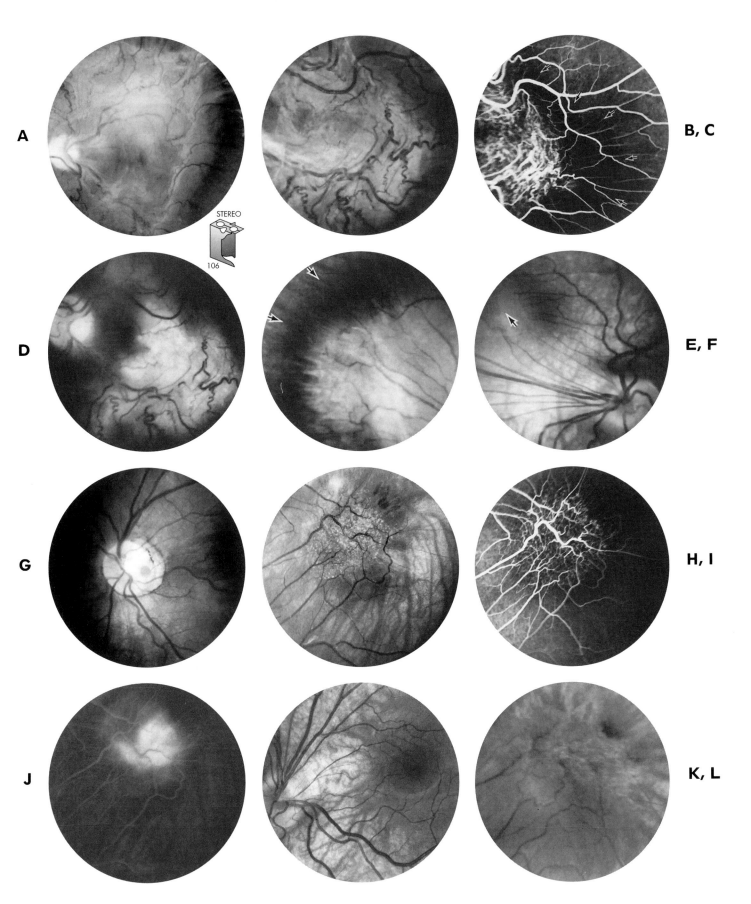

A

B, C

D

E, F

G

H, I

J

K, L

STEREO
106

827

Combined pigment epithelial and retinal hamartoma without optic disc involvement

These tumors, which are often only slightly elevated, are usually discovered in one eye of an infant or child with strabismus and subnormal visual acuity.[75,78,81,88,91] They are associated with increased number, dilation, and tortuosity of the retinal vessels, evidence of gray epiretinal fibrous tissue, and hyperpigmentation confined to the level of the RPE. This pigmentation is greatest at the border of the lesion, where its feathery edges blend imperceptibly into the surrounding normal RPE. Unlike tumors involving the optic disc, these show no evidence of RPE cells or capillary angiomatous tissue near their inner surface. These tumors may involve the peripapillary area (Fig. 10-10), the macula (Figs. 10-9 and 10-11), or the peripheral fundus (Fig. 10-9, *H* to *L*). Those in the temporal half of the eye peripherally are often associated with displacement of the macula toward the lesion (Fig. 10-9, *G* to *L*). Fluorescein angiography usually shows marked tortuosity and leakage of dye from the retinal vessels within these macular and peripheral tumors (Figs. 10-9, *A* to *D*, and 10-11, *D* to *G*). These patients, most of whom are children, have no history of prematurity and have none of the changes in the far periphery of the fundus typical of retinopathy of prematurity. Subretinal exudation may occasionally occur from the tumor vessels. I have seen one patient in whom this exudation resulted in progressive detachment of the retina, rubeotic glaucoma, and loss of the eye (Fig. 10-11, *A* to *C*). The histopathologic findings in the peripheral lesions differ from those involving the optic disc in that they show less disorganization of the retina, no RPE migration and less evidence of capillary proliferation within the retina, and evidence of hypertrophy of the RPE (Fig. 10-10, *D* and *E*).[88]

FIG. 10-10   Peripapillary Combined RPE and Retinal Hamartoma (CRPE-RH).

A to **C,** CRPE-RH surrounding the right optic disc (*arrows,* **A** and **B**) in an infant. Within several years there was further condensation of the fibrous tissue on the tumor surface (**C**).

D, Large peripapillary RPE and retinal hamartoma in a 16-year-old boy. Melanoma was suspected, and the eye was enucleated. Histopathologic examination revealed hypertrophy of the RPE (*arrows,* **E**), mild dysplasia of the retina, and epiretinal fibrous tissue.

(**A** to **C** courtesy Dr. John P. Shock, Jr; **D** and **E** from Laqua H, Wessing A: *Am J Ophthalmol* 87:34, 1979; published with permission from The American Journal of Ophthalmology, copyright by The Ophthalmic Publishing Co.[88])

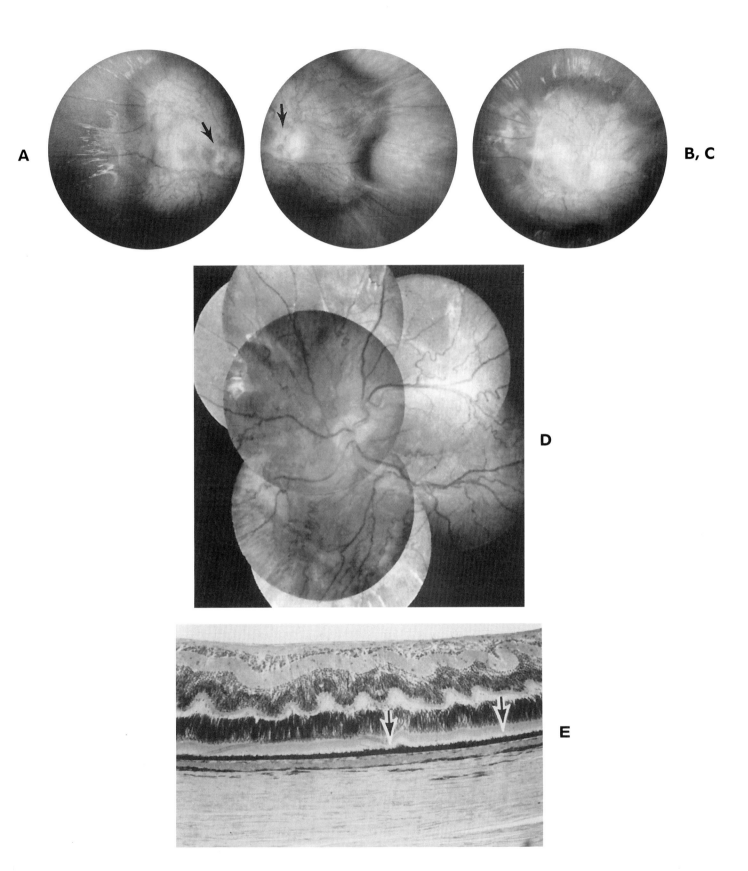

I have seen these hamartomas, or lesions simulating them, occur in patients with cutaneous hemangiomas, sex-linked juvenile retinoschisis, a congenital pit of the optic disc in the opposite eye and in patients with neurofibromatosis (Figs. 10-9, G to J, and 10-11).[80] The association of these hamartomas with neurofibromatosis is now well established.* Neurofibromatosis has been subdivided into at least two major disorders, NF-1 and NF-2, with gene defects on two different chromosomes.[67,93] The combined pigment epithelial and retinal hamartomas in these patients with neurofibromatosis usually involve the macula (Fig. 10-11), may be bilateral, and have occurred most commonly in neurofibromatosis type 2.[69,82,87]

---

*References 13, 14, 67-69, 73, 74, 79, 80, 82, 86, 87, 93, 100.

FIG. 10-11   Combined Retinal and RPE Hamartomas Occurring in Patients with Neurofibromatosis.

A to **C,** A combined RPE and retinal hamartoma of the macular region in a 30-month-old girl with suspected retinoblastoma or malignant melanoma (**A** and **B**). Left exotropia was noted at 2 months of age. There was inferotemporal displacement of the optic nerve head and retinal vessels by a large (eight disc diameters), elevated, partly pigmented mass in the macular and paramacular areas. The central portion of the pigmented lesion was obscured by thickened translucent retinal tissue and a gray preretinal membrane. The patient had several prominent *café-au-lait* spots on the abdomen (**C**). Several years later she developed an exudative retinal detachment and rubeotic glaucoma, and the eye was enucleated.

D to **G,** Bilateral hypopigmented combined retinal and RPE hamartomas in an infant with neurofibromatosis.

H to **J,** Bilateral hypopigmented combined and RPE hamartomas in a child with neurofibromatosis.

(**A** and **B** from Gass[81]; **D** to **G** from Palmer et al.[94]; **H** to **J,** courtesy Dr. Lanning B. Kline.)

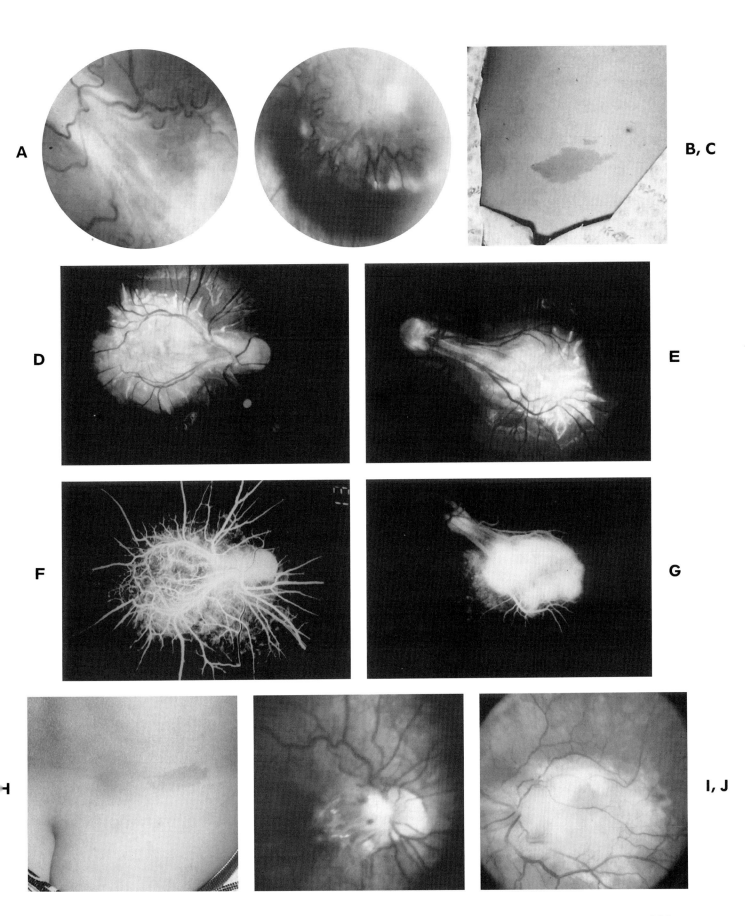

▼ REACTIVE HYPERPLASIAS OF THE RETINAL PIGMENT EPITHELIUM SIMULATING HAMARTOMAS AND NEOPLASIAS

A variety of stimuli are capable of exciting the highly reactive RPE to proliferate to form mass lesions that may simulate RPE and uveal hamartomatous and neoplastic lesions (Figs. 10-12 and 10-13).[105-112] One of these stimuli is recurrent and chronic focal choroiditis occurring at the site of chorioretinal scars in patients with the presumed ocular histoplasmosis syndrome (Fig. 10-13, *F* to *L*). The lesions may be pigmented or nonpigmented and they may be difficult to distinguish from choroidal melanomas biomicroscopically, angiographically, or ultrasonographically. Histopathologically, some of the lesions may demonstrate cytologic features suggestive of a RPE neoplasia (Fig. 10-13, *H* to *L*). These highly reactive lesions may be locally destructive but are apparently incapable of metastasis. Histopathologically, the index of suspicion of reactive hyperplasia should be high if the lesion arises within or adjacent to a chorioretinal scar, particularly in the juxtapapillary area. Figure 10-13, *A* to *E*, demonstrates the unusual development of mass lesions presumed to be reactive RPE hyperplasia arising within congenital familial macular colobomata.

FIG. 10-12   Vitreoretinal Traction Causing Lesions Simulating Combined RPE and Retinal Hamartoma (CRPE-RH).

A to **F,** Vitreoretinal traction was associated with an elevated gray retinal lesion with dilated retinal vessels surrounded by a zone of RPE darkening in the inferior fundus of this boy with bilateral X-linked foveomacular schisis (**A** and **B**). Angiography showed dilated, distorted, and partly occluded retinal vessels (**C**). One year later lipid exudate extended into the macular area (**D** to **E**) and there was increased vitreous condensation and band formation (**F**).

G and **H,** This patient developed loss of vision associated with vitreomacular traction in the left eye. Note the tenting of the retina by a vitreous band (*arrow,* **G**). Four months later the juxtapapillary retina was tented anteriorly by further vitreous condensation and traction. Note the darkening of the RPE (*arrow,* **H**) that surrounds the mass and caused it to simulate CRPE-RH.

I and **J,** Focal vitreoretinal traction caused an elevated pigmented lesion associated with distortion of the retinal vessels and a gray epiretinal membrane simulating CRPE-RH (**I**). Four years later the vitreous and part of the epiretinal membrane (*arrow,* **J**) spontaneously detached from the retina.

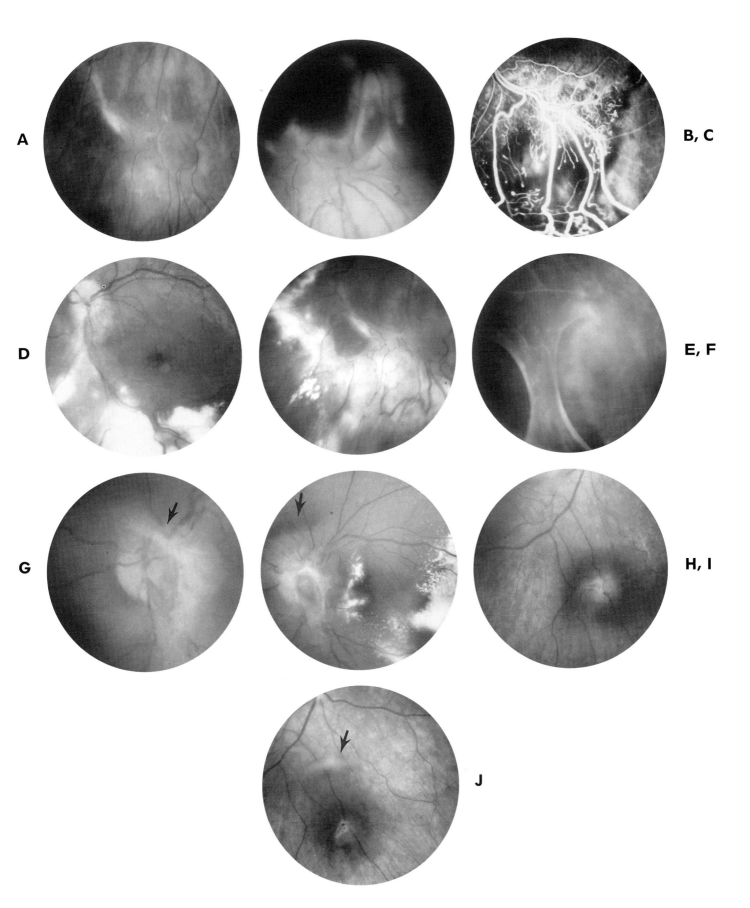

A

B, C

D

E, F

G

H, I

J

FIG. 10-13   Reactive Hyperplasia of the RPE Simulating RPE Hamartomas and Choroidal Melanomas.

A to **E,** A nodule of RPE hyperplasia (*arrows,* **A** and **B**) developed within congenital macular staphylomas of this 25-year-old woman. Visual acuity was 20/400 bilaterally. Over a period of several years the RPE nodule in the left eye enlarged and a melanoma was suspected (**C**). Angiography revealed the presence of blood vessels within the nodule (*arrow,* **D**) and late staining (**E**). Bilateral macular scars noted in early childhood in her and her brother were attributed to toxoplasmosis. Her grandfather had macular degeneration.

F and **G,** A small pigmented nodule (*arrow,* **F**) developed on the right optic disc of this patient with multifocal chorioretinal and juxtapapillary scars typical of the presumed ocular histoplasmosis syndrome (POHS). Angiography showed dilation of the capillaries in the surface of the nodule (**G**) and late staining.

H to **L,** This 64-year-old woman with bilateral POHS developed a slowly enlarging mass on the left optic disc (**H**) that for a period of 8 years was unassociated with loss of visual acuity, before development of an extension of lipid exudate into the macula (**J**). Because of concern of a melanoma a needle biopsy was done. The results were equivocal and the eye was enucleated. Histopathologically the tumor was composed of large hypopigmented RPE cells showing minimal mitotic activity (**K** and **L**). The tumor was interpreted as a low-grade adenocarcinoma of the RPE by Shields et al.[109] but in the author's opinion represents reactive RPE hyperplasia.

(**H** to **L** from Shields et al.[109])

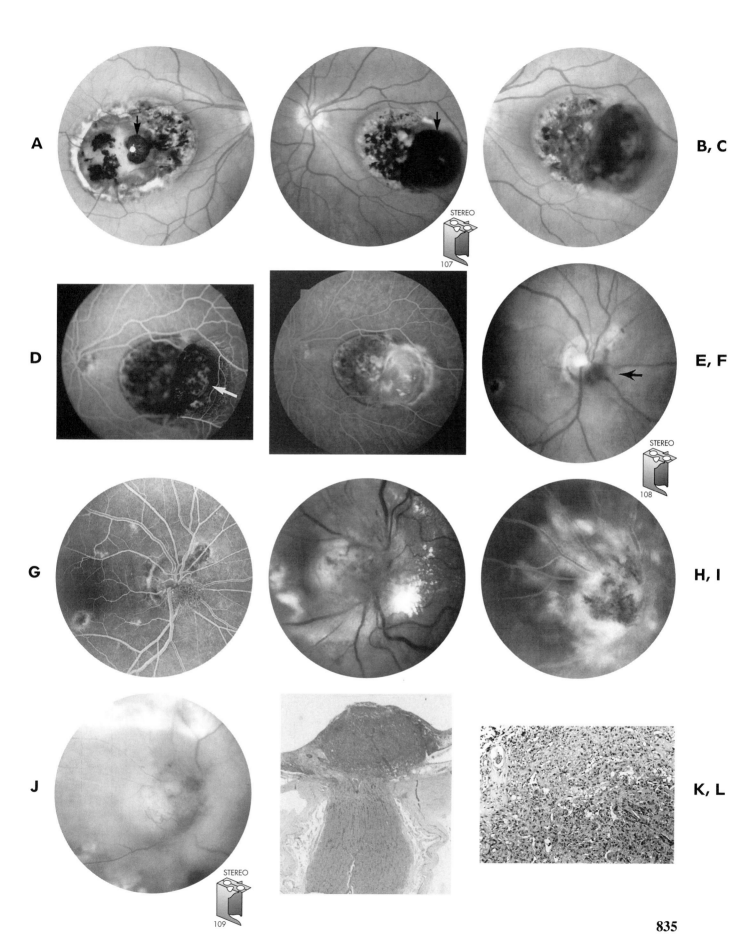

▼ RETINAL AND OPTIC DISC ASTROCYTIC HAMARTOMAS

Retinal and optic disc astrocytic hamartomas may occur as a solitary finding in normal patients, in patients with dominantly inherited tuberous sclerosis (Bourneville's disease), or rarely in patients with neurofibromatosis (von Recklinghausen's disease).* The intraocular tumors are typically globular, white, well-circumscribed, elevated lesions arising from the inner surface of the retina or optic nerve head (Figs. 10-14 to 10-16). Multiple lesions are common in patients with tuberous sclerosis (Fig. 10-14, A to F). Early in life the tumors may be semitranslucent, be free of calcification, and be mistaken for retinoblastoma (Figs. 10-14, A and D, and 10-15, F).† In infants and children they may occasionally arise where earlier no lesion was present. Later in life they assume a more densely white color and may develop multiple nodular areas of calcification, giving it a mulberry appearance (Figs. 10-14, A and D; 10-15, E; and 10-16, A). Clear cystic spaces may be present within the tumor (Fig. 10-14, D). The tumors may show varying degrees of vascularization that are more evident angiographically than ophthalmoscopically (Figs. 10-14, B and C, and 10-16, E and F). The tumor's blood vessels are usually permeable to fluorescein. In addition to nodular retinal tumors, flat or slightly elevated, white, circular or oval astrocytic hamartomas of the inner retinal layers are common (Fig. 10-14, D). These sessile tumors show less tendency to undergo calcific degeneration. In general, retinal astrocytic hamartomas show minimal evidence of growth and no treatment is indicated. Occasionally, however, particularly in younger individuals, progressive enlargement and calcification of these tumors may be demonstrated (Fig. 10-16, J to L).[138] Visual loss may be caused by tumor growth, vitreous hemorrhage, or intraretinal and subretinal exudation (Fig. 10-17, D to F).‡ This exudation may spontaneously resolve[139] or in some patients may do so only after photocoagulation of the tumor (Fig. 10-17, D to F).[115] In some, the rapid growth and necrosis may be mistaken for a nonpigmented melanoma (Fig. 10-16, J to L).§ In other patients the highly vascular component of the tumor may

*References 113-115, 118-122, 124-132, 134, 138, 146-149.
†References 117, 127, 131, 137, 146, 149.
‡References 113, 115, 125, 135, 141, 142, 147.
§References 116, 132, 136, 141, 142, 144.

FIG. 10-14   Astrocytic Hamartoma of the Retina in Patients with Tuberous Sclerosis.

A to C, Multiple astrocytic hamartomas of the optic nerve head and retina in a 35-year-old woman with tuberous sclerosis (**A**). She had a lifelong history of generalized seizures. She had five mentally retarded children. Examination revealed sebaceous adenoma and subungual fibromas of the fingers and toes (Fig. 10-15, B). Multiple endophytic astrocytic hamartomas of the retina were present in the left fundus. The lesions were elevated, globular, and semitranslucent. Retinal vessels could be seen within some of these tumors. Several of the tumefactions showed evidence of early calcification (*arrow,* A). Angiography revealed a capillary network within the hamartomas (**B** and **C**). These capillaries were permeable to fluorescein dye, and there was evidence of diffusion of the dye into the vitreous (**C**).

D to F, A partly calcified cystic astrocytic hamartoma in a 9-year-old girl with tuberous sclerosis. She had a history of seizures but was not mentally retarded. Note the mulberry-like areas of calcification within the large cystic lesions. Two smaller hamartomas were present within the optic nerve head (*arrow*) and inferior to the papillomacular bundle. Fluorescein angiography demonstrated dilation of the capillary network and staining within these tumors (**E** and **F**).

G to I, Large astrocytic hamartoma of the left macula of an 8-year-old boy with tuberous sclerosis. He had sebaceous adenoma and a large fibroma of the left lower lid (**G**).

simulate a retinal angioma (Figs. 10-16, G to I, and 10-17, A to C).[145] In the case of spontaneous necrosis astrocytomas may simulate necrotizing retinochoroiditis.[117] The fossilized mulberry tumors involving the optic nerve head should be distinguished from hyaline bodies of the optic nerve head. These latter are calcified masses of extracellular material unrelated to astrocytic hamartomas. When calcified astrocytic hamartomas of the optic disc are small, they may be difficult or impossible to distinguish from hyaline bodies.[119] Demonstration of growth of these small lesions in patients with retinitis pigmentosa has suggested that these lesions in patients with retinitis pigmentosa are astrocytic hamartomas.[120,140,143] Retinal telangiectasis, retinitis proliferans, and retinal exudation developed in one eye of a patient with familial tuberous sclerosis but no evidence of a retinal astrocytoma.[133]

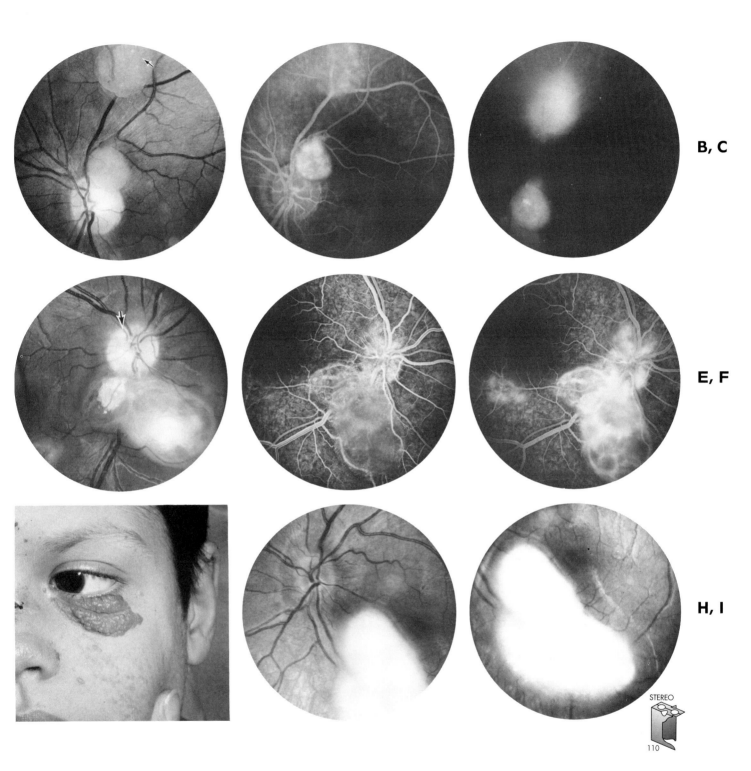

B, C

E, F

H, I

Histopathologically, these tumors are typically composed of spindle-shaped fibrous astrocytes, some of which are elongated and contain small oval nucleoli (Figs. 10-15, *F,* and 10-16, *L*). Other tumors are composed of large, bizarre, pleomorphic astrocytic cells, that in at least one case showed ultrastructural and histochemical similarities to Müller cells.[131] Cystic areas containing serous exudate and blood, as well as areas of calcified degeneration, may be present. Some of these tumors may be of Müller cell origin.[131]

FIG. 10-15   Astrocytic Hamartoma of the Retina in Patients with Tuberous Sclerosis.

A, Sebaceous adenoma of the nose and cheeks and a solitary hamartoma of the forehead.

B, Subungual fibroma *(arrow).*

C, Skull X-ray film of patient shown in **A** showed multiple calcified astrocytic hamartomas *(arrows)* characteristic of tuberous sclerosis.

D, Enhanced computed tomography scan showed multiple astrocytic hamartomas in the paraventricular system of a patient with tuberous sclerosis.

E, Photomicrograph of calcified astrocytic hamartoma of the optic disc and adjacent retina of a 17-year-old boy with sebaceous adenoma. The calcified central portion of the tumor was lost in sectioning.

F, Endophytic noncalcified astrocytic hamartoma of the peripheral retina of the same patient in **E.**

(**E** and **F** from Zimmerman and Walsh.[149])

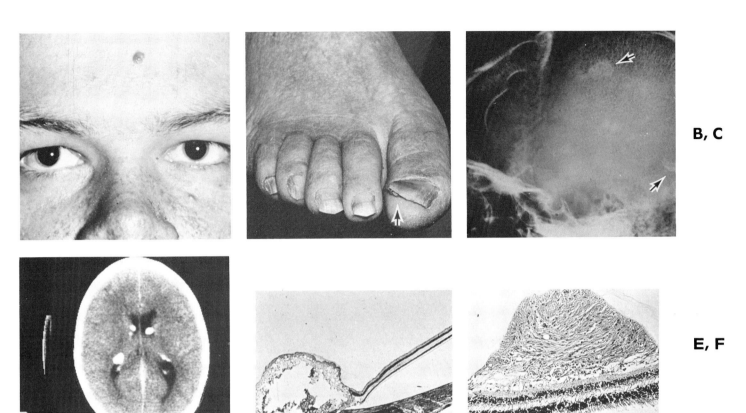

B, C

E, F

A careful search should be made for the various manifestations of tuberous sclerosis in any patient with a white retinal tumor. These include the classic triad of seizures, mental deficiency, and sebaceous adenoma (fibroangiomas) as well as other manifestations including white ash-leaf spots on the skin and iris, soft yellow-brown cutaneous fibromas (Figs. 10-14, *G,* and 10-15, *A*), subungual fibromas (Fig. 10-15, *B*), renal hamartomas, cardiac rhabdomyomas, calcified cerebral astrocytic hamartomas (Fig. 10-15, *C* and *D*), cystic lung disease, and bony changes, including cystic changes of the phalanges and cortical thickening of the metatarsal and metacarpal bones.[134] Computed tomography and roentgenographic techniques are useful in the detection of the intraocular tumors.[119] In infants and children these tumors can appear identical to retinoblastoma or may mimic necrotizing retinochoroiditis.[118] In older patients they may be confused with regressed retinoblastoma or retinoma (Fig. 10-16, *G* to *I*), capillary hemangiomas of the retina, or a localized retinal scar secondary to previous hemorrhage or inflammation.

FIG. 10-16 Astrocytic Hamartomas of the Retina and Optic Nerve Head in Patients Without Tuberous Sclerosis.

A to **C,** Large calcified exophytic astrocytic hamartoma of the retina in a 15-year-old boy without other evidence of tuberous sclerosis (**A**). He gave an 8-year history of defective vision in the right eye first noted while firing a gun. The family history and past medical history were negative. Visual acuity in the affected eye was 20/300. Angiography (**B** and **C**) revealed an extensive capillary network that extended down into the tumor. There was leakage of dye from this network and pooling of dye within the cystic areas of the tumor (*arrow,* **C**).

D to **F,** Cystic astrocytic hamartoma of the retina in a 10-year-old girl without other evidence of tuberous sclerosis (**D**). This was an incidental finding, and her eye examination was otherwise normal. Note the white, finely polycystic tumor arising from the inner retinal layers just superior to the left macular region (**D**). Note that most of the retinal vessels are hidden within this cottony tumor. Fluorescein angiography revealed a network of retinal vessels within the tumor and late leakage of the dye (**E** and **F**).

G to **I,** Elevated, vascularized, partly calcified retinal mass in a healthy 17-year-old boy with no family history of tuberous sclerosis or retinoblastoma.

J to **L,** Nonpigmented, pedunculated, vascularized astrocytic hamartoma in the juxtapapillary region of a 41-year-old man with a 3-week history of blurred vision in the right eye (**J** and **K**). This was misinterpreted as a melanoma because of an increased phosphorus-32 uptake test (100%). Histopathologic examination of the enucleated eye revealed a retinal astrocytic hamartoma (**L**).

(**J** to **L** from Ramsey RC et al.: *Am J Ophthalmol* 88:32, 1979; published with permission from The American Journal of Ophthalmology; copyright by The Ophthalmic Publishing Co.)[141]

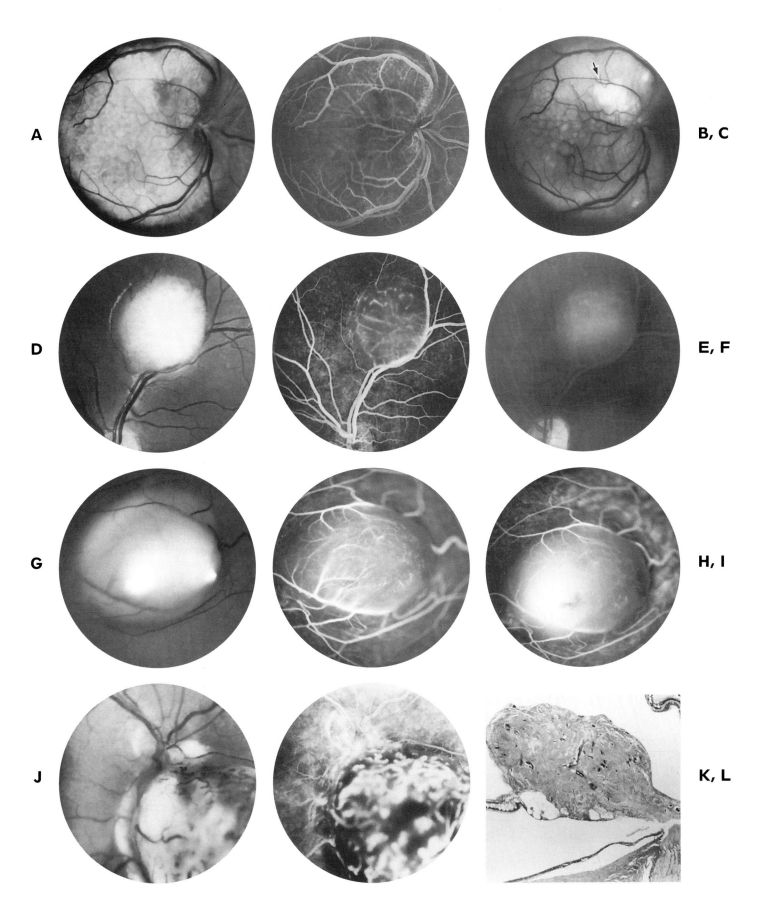

A

B, C

D

E, F

G

H, I

J

K, L

▼ REACTIVE ASTROCYTIC HYPERPLASIA SIMULATING AN ASTROCYTIC HAMARTOMA

I have seen four healthy adult patients with focal vascularized retinal masses that appeared similar to astrocytic hamartomas. In two cases the lesions subsequently disappeared spontaneously (Fig. 10-17, *A* to *C*).[127] In one boy with bilateral pars planitis an exophytic vascularized white retinal mass developed during observation (Fig. 10-17, *J* to *K*). It is probable that most of these lesions and some of those reported in the literature as sporadic astrocytomas are products of reactive proliferation of the retinal glial cells caused by focal retinitis, focal retinal vascular leakage, chorioretinitis, vitreoretinal traction, and, less often, subretinal neovascularization. (See discussion in Chapter 7, p. 604 and Fig. 7-2, *I* to *L*).

FIG. 10-17 Lesions of Uncertain Etiology Simulating Retinal Astrocytic Hamartomas.

A to **C,** Endophytic retinal tumor in a 38-year-old woman with a 3-month history of blurred vision in her left eye (**A**). Her past history revealed convulsions unassociated with fever at 1 year of age. It was otherwise unremarkable. There were many dilated blood vessels present within the tumor, which was located in the retina inferior to the left macula (**A**). Angiography demonstrated an extensive vascular network within the tumor and late leakage of dye (**B** and **C**). Medical evaluation failed to reveal other evidence of tuberous sclerosis. The patient was reexamined 10 months later, and there was no change in the appearance of the lesion. Examination 3 years after her initial visit revealed that the lesion had disappeared, leaving only a minor disturbance in the retina in the area of the tumor. Because of its spontaneous disappearance, it is doubtful that it was an astrocytic hamartoma.

D to **F,** Sessile presumed astrocytic hamartoma in a healthy 42-year-old man with a recent history of blurred vision in the left eye. He had a small angioma and a pigmented nevus of the conjunctiva in the same eye. His visual acuity was 20/25, left eye, and 20/20, right eye. Note the ill-defined gray-whitening of the retina in the inferonasal macular area (*arrowheads,* **D**) and the cystoid macular edema (*arrow,* **D**). Angiography revealed evidence of a capillary network within the lesion and evidence of intraretinal edema (**E** and **F**). Two months following laser photocoagulation the vision had improved to 20/20. He had no other findings of tuberous sclerosis.

G to **I,** This 28-year-old woman complained of blurred vision in the left eye. Examination of the right eye was normal. In the left eye she had a gray, slightly elevated retinal tumor that straddled the major retinal vascular arcades in the superior macular area (**G**). Angiography showed evidence of the vascular nature of this lesion (**H** and **I**). There were no other stigmata of tuberous sclerosis. Several months later she had developed extensive exudative maculopathy. She was lost to followup.

J to **L,** An elevated, vascularized, and partly calcified tumor developed in this 17-year-old boy who when he was first examined at 10 years of age had the typical findings of bilateral pars planitis and no evidence of an intraocular mass. Stereoangiograms (**H** and **I**) revealed the highly vascular nature of this exophytic mass, which probably was the result of a reactive proliferation of the retinal vasculature and glial cells in response to the intraocular inflammatory disease.

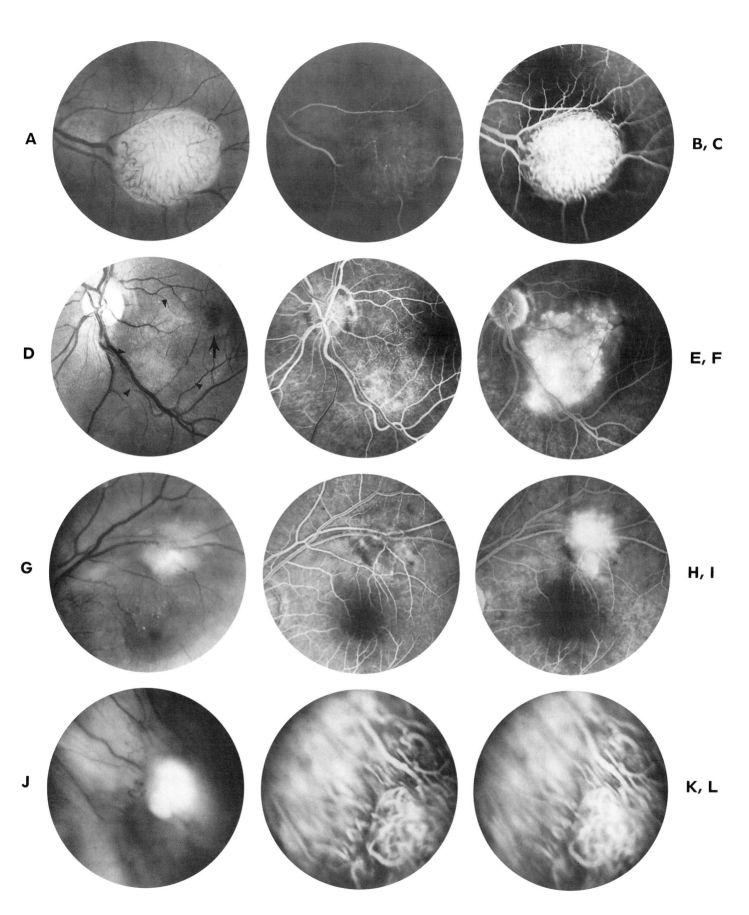

A

B, C

D

E, F

G

H, I

J

K, L

▼ RETINAL VASCULAR HAMARTOMAS

There are two distinct retinal vascular hamartomas, both of which may be associated with similar hamartomas elsewhere in the body.

Retinal and optic disc cavernous hemangiomas

Retinal and optic disc cavernous hemangiomas are sessile tumors composed of clusters of thin-walled saccular aneurysms filled with dark venous blood that give the appearance of a cluster of grapes projecting from the inner retinal surface (Figs. 10-15, *A, B, E, G*, and *J*, and 10-19, *A*). They can be clearly differentiated from other retinal vascular malformations, including retinal telangiectasis, retinal capillary angioma (angiomatosis retinae), and arteriovenous malformations.* Small isolated clumps of aneurysms are often present around the tumor mass. Varying amounts of a gray fibrous membrane may partly cover the anterior tumor surface. Plasma–erythrocytic separation within the aneurysms is common. The caliber of the major retinal vessels is unaffected by the tumor. Exudation is rare. A small hemorrhage may occasionally be present on its surface (Fig. 10-19, *A*). Evidence of bleeding into the vitreous has been reported in approximately 10% of cases but is usually minimal and unassociated with any visual loss.[177] These lesions may be seen initially at any age, but the average age is 23 years. They are more common in females (female to male ratio of 3:2). Most patients have only a solitary lesion affecting one eye; however, multiple lesions may occur in one eye or occasionally in both eyes. The visual acuity is usually normal unless the macula is directly involved with the malformation (Fig. 10-18, *A* and *E*). Visual loss associated with macular pucker,[177] macular traction,[160] and amblyopia[80] occurs infrequently (Fig. 10-18, *G* to *I*). The tumor is associated with a relative or an absolute scotoma that corresponds to the tumor size. Fluorescein angiography demonstrates that the vascular tumor is relatively isolated from the retinal circulation (Figs. 10-18, *C, D, F, H, I, K,* and *L,* and 10-19, *B* and *C*). Perfusion of the hamartoma occurs but is delayed and appears incomplete. The plasma–erythrocytic layering within the saccular aneurysms is conspicuous in the later phases of fluorescein angiography (Fig. 10-18, *I* and *L*). Extravascular leakage of dye from the tumor vessels does not occur in most instances.

*References 150, 151, 153, 156, 158, 160-162, 164, 166, 169-172, 174, 179, 180, 182, 185, 188, 189.

FIG. 10-18 Cavernous Hemangioma of the Retina.

A to **D,** Large macular cavernous hemangioma of the retina was first observed in this 17-year-old girl who presented at age 5 years because of left esotropia. Her visual acuity in the left eye was 20/30. Note the fluid level in some of the incompletely perfused aneurysms in **C** and **D**. Minimal change occurred in its appearance during this period of followup, but the visual acuity decreased to counting fingers only. She had no evidence of angiomas elsewhere.

E and **F,** Cavernous hemangioma in the left macula of a healthy 7-year-old boy (**E**). Note the delay in dye perfusion of this tumor (**F**). Five years later the tumor was unchanged.

G to **I,** Cavernous hemangioma of the retina in a 30-month-old girl who developed right esotropia at 6 months of age. Her general health and physical examination were normal except for the presence of a few spider angiomas on her hands and wrists. An identical twin sister was normal except for similar spider angiomas on the hands. There was an irregularly elevated vascular mass in the supertemporal quadrant of the right eye (**G**) that was composed of dilated, oval or rounded, thin-walled, saccular blood vessels that gave the appearance of a mass of grapes lying on the inner retinal surface and protruding into the vitreous. The tumor extended from the ora serrata almost into the macular area of the right eye. Fluorescein angiography showed slow and incomplete filling of the aneurysms making up the tumor (**H** and **I**). Note delay in venous drainage (*arrow,* **H**) from the area of the tumor. Approximately 30 minutes after dye injection there was still incomplete perfusion of the tumor. Note the level of dye in the large tumor cyst (*arrow,* **I**). The patient was lying on her left side in the operating room during the angiographic study.

J to **L,** Cavernous hemangioma of the optic nerve head in an asymptomatic 51-year-old woman. Visual acuity was 20/15. Angiography revealed slow perfusion, plasma–erythrocytic separation, and minimal staining (**K** and **L**).

(**G** to **L** from Gass.[160])

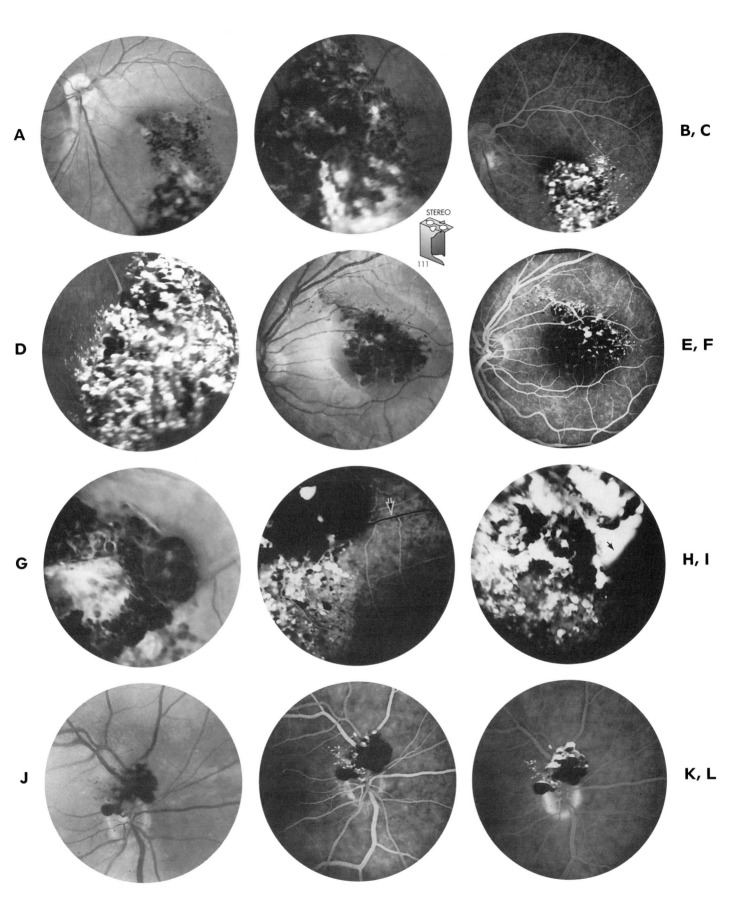

Whereas most retinal and optic nerve cavernous hemangiomas occur sporadically, there is evidence that some patients may have a dominantly inherited neurocutaneous syndrome that includes cavernous hemangiomas of the optic nerves, chiasm, optic tracts, the pre-Rolandic area of the cerebral cortex, the midbrain, brainstem, and cerebellum (Fig. 10-20, F), as well as the skin (Fig. 10-20, E).* The angiomas of the brain may cause seizures or subarachnoid hemorrhages. Twin retinal vessels, defined as a pair of vessels, separated by less than one venule width, that run a parallel course for more than one disc diameter, located at least two disc areas distant from the optic disc, have been described in the carriers as well as affected members of families with cavernous hemangiomas of the eye and brain, as well as in family members of patients with von Hippel-Lindau disease.[152] Cavernous hemangiomas do not increase in size. The amount of fibrous tissue on the anterior surface increases over a period of time and is associated with partial obliteration of the tumor.

Histopathologically, the tumor is composed of multiple thin-walled interconnecting aneurysms of variable size, occupying the inner half of the retina and in some patients the optic nerve (Fig. 10-20, A to D).[156,160,169,176,184] The endothelial lining of the large vascular channels ultrastructurally appears normal.[176] The gray membrane that overlies part of the angiomas in some cases is of glial origin.[176]

---

*References 154, 157, 160, 161, 165, 166, 168, 173, 175, 178, 180-182, 184, 186-189.

FIG. 10-19   Cavernous Hemangioma of the Retina.

A to C, Cavernous hemangioma discovered in a 27-year-old woman who was hospitalized because of a generalized seizure. An electroencephalogram revealed low voltage in the left cerebral hemisphere. A skull roentgenogram and a carotid arteriogram were normal. Her father died at 49 years of age with status epilepticus. Autopsy of the father revealed a focal cavernous hemangioma in the midbrain, pons, and cerebellum (Fig. 10-20, F). The woman's eye examination was normal except for the presence of a slightly elevated sessile cavernous hemangioma involving the inferonasal quadrant of the right eye (**A**). A small subretinal and deep retinal hemorrhage was present (*arrow,* **A**). Angiography revealed delayed and incomplete perfusion of the cavernous hemangioma (**B** and **C**). Note evidence of plasma layering *(arrows)* and minimal evidence of extravascular escape of dye. A general physical examination revealed a stellate angiomatous hamartoma of the right chin and several cherry angiomas of the thigh.

D, Diagram showing structural differences of (**1**) normal retinal vessels, (**2**) diffuse and focal vascular dilation and permeability alteration in retinal telangiectasis, and (**3**) localized vascular malformation (hamartoma) arising from the capillary bed in cavernous hemangioma.

(From Gass.[160])

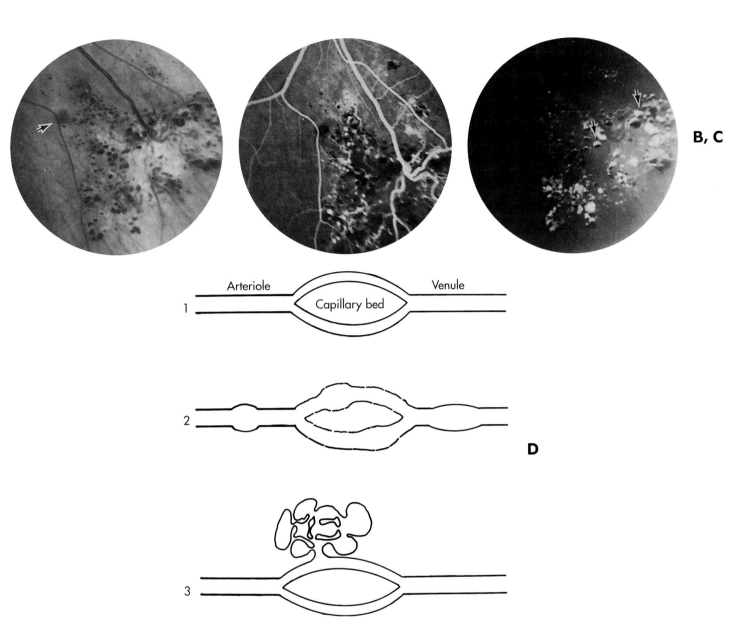

B, C

D

Arteriole   Venule

1   Capillary bed

2

3

Photocoagulation has been used to obliterate these lesions but is unnecessary as long as the patient shows no signs of developing vitreous hemorrhage.[162,169,170] In one case of severe vitreous hemorrhage, the tumor was partly excised during a pars plana vitrectomy.[167] Some of the cerebral cortical angiomas causing seizures or subarachnoid hemorrhage may be resectable.[183]

Before 1971, retinal cavernous hemangioma was not recognized as a distinct retinal vascular hamartoma. The more sessile and smaller lesions (Fig. 10-19, *A*) were often misdiagnosed as congenital retinal telangiectasis.[159] Figure 10-1, *C*, diagrammatically indicates the basic structural difference between retinal telangiectasis, which is a congenital anomaly affecting the structure and integrity of the intrinsic retinal vasculature, and a retinal cavernous hemangioma, which is a localized vascular tumefaction composed of cavernous vascular channels that are partly isolated from normal retinal circulation. Some of the more globular retinal cavernous hemangiomas have been reported in the older literature as angiomatosis retinae.[179]

It is uncertain whether the retinal vascular lesion reported in one patient with central nervous system symptoms and the dermatologic disorder angioma serpiginosum is related to retinal cavernous hemangioma.[163] A lesion that angiographically was similar to a retinal cavernous hemangioma was observed in an infant with blue rubber bleb nevus syndrome.[155] The fact that the lesion spontaneously disappeared over a 4-month period suggests that it may not have been a cavernous hemangioma.

FIG. 10-20   **Cavernous Hemangioma of the Retina.**

A and **B,** Histopathologic condition of cavernous hemangioma of the retina in a 2-year-old girl whose eye was enucleated with the mistaken diagnosis of retinoblastoma. The sessile retinal tumor was composed of multiple, thin-walled, dilated blood vessels that replaced the inner half of the retina (**A**). The arrow indicates pigment-laden macrophages in the subretinal space. The retinal detachment was artifactitious. A high-power view of the lesion revealed dilated, endothelium-lined aneurysms interconnected by narrow channels (*arrows,* **B**). These relatively isolated vascular saccules account for the sluggish circulation and plasma–erythrocytic separation demonstrated angiographically in these lesions.

C, Histologic condition of cavernous hemangioma of the optic nerve and adjacent retina.

D, Histopathologic condition of a retrobulbar cavernous hemangioma of the optic nerve head. This was an incidental finding in the optic nerve of a 3-month-old White girl who was born prematurely with a birth weight of 2 pounds, 14 ounces.

E, A slightly raised cutaneous cavernous hemangioma on the arm of a patient with a retinal cavernous hemangioma. This patient had generalized seizures. One son, who had multiple cutaneous angiomas on the face, leg, and foot, died soon after surgical excision of a cavernous hemangioma of the brain.

F, Cavernous hemangioma of the midbrain in the father of the patient illustrated in Fig. 10-19, *A* to *C.*

(**A** from Hogan and Zimmerman[169]; **B** from Gass[160]; **C** from Davies and Thumin[156]; **D** from Spencer[184]; **E** courtesy Dr. L.L. Calkins; **F** from Gass[160] from AFIP negative no. 70-6110, hematoxylin and eosin, × 7.)

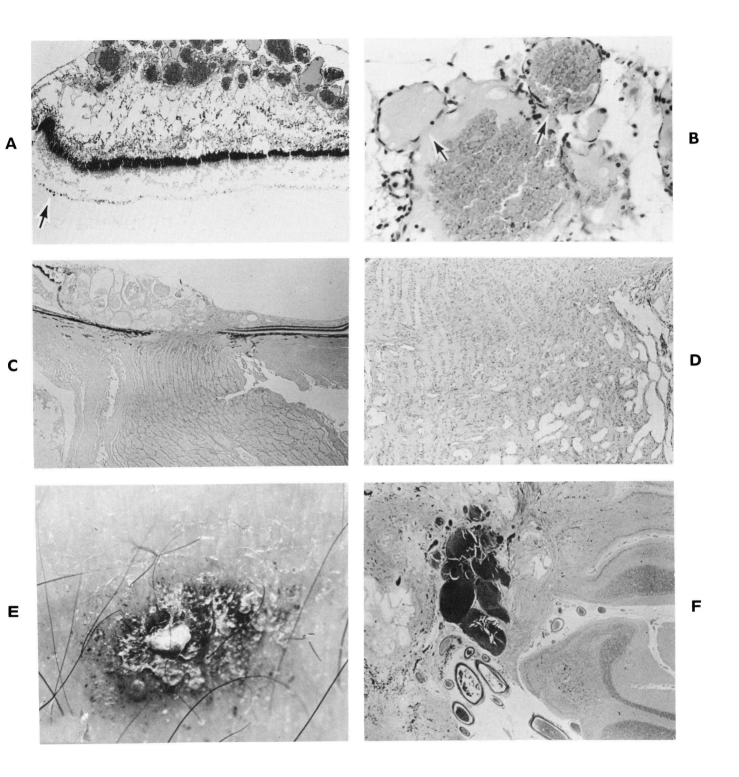

Retinal and optic disc capillary hemangiomas

The terms "retinal and optic disc capillary hemangiomas," "angiomatosis retinae," and "von Hippel's disease"[213] are used synonymously to refer to congenital hereditary capillary angiomatous hamartomas of the retina and optic nerve head.* When associated with central nervous system and other organ involvement the condition is referred to as von Hippel-Lindau disease.[219,220] Von Hippel-Lindau (VH-L) disease is a dominantly inherited systemic hamartia that includes not only capillary angiomas of the retina, cerebellum, brainstem, and spinal cord, but also angiomas, adenomas, and cysts affecting the kidney, liver, pancreas, epididymis, and mesosalpinx. The diagnosis of VH-L is justified when either a retinal angioma or a CNS angioma occurs together with one or more visceral cysts or tumors in one patient or when a single lesion of the VH-L complex is found in a relative at risk. Ocular manifestations of VH-L are often the first to appear. Retinal angiomas and CNS angioma each eventually occur in approximately 50% of patients with VH-L. Pheochromocytomas occur in approximately 10% of patients with VH-L.[210,212,221] Approximately 25% of patients with VH-L develop clear cell renal carcinomas typically during the late stages of the disease.[193,201,221] Polycythemia occurs in approximately 15% of patients. Twin retinal vessels, a retinal sign of dominantly inherited retinal cavernous hemangioma (see previous discussion of retinal cavernous hemangioma), occur in approximately 70% of patients with familial VH-L disease and in 50% of at-risk family members without ocular angiomas.[199] Since most patients who present with a solitary retinal angioma and a negative family history suggesting VH-L fail to show other evidence of the disease, the medical evaluation of these patients with sporadic tumors probably does not need to be as comprehensive as in patients with multiple ocular tumors or other evidence of familial involvement. The gene mutation responsible for VH-L maps to the region of chromosome 3 associated with renal cell carcinoma.[239]

*References 191, 193, 205, 206, 210-213, 219-221, 223, 225, 227, 230, 232, 234-236, 241, 242, 248.

FIG. 10-21 Capillary Hemangiomas of the Retina.

A, Diagram showing sites of origin of retinal capillary angiomas.

I, Endophytic angioma of the optic nerve head. II, Endophytic peripheral retinal angioma. III, Exophytic juxtapapillary angioma. IV, Exophytic peripheral retinal angioma. V, Intraneural angioma.

B to D, This 36-year-old woman noted blurred vision in the left eye caused by a juxtapapillary capillary hemangioma (arrow, A). She had no other stigmata of von Hippel-Lindau disease. Stereoscopic angiography revealed the sessile capillary angiomatous nature of the lesion (C and D).

E to J, Juxtapapillary (E) and peripheral capillary hemangioma (F) in a 10-year-old girl with no evidence of extraocular involvement with angiomatosis. Angiography revealed the capillary nature of the tumors (G and H), shunting of blood from the arterial to the venous side of the circulation in the region of the peripheral tumor (H), and late staining (I and J).

(A from Gass.[202])

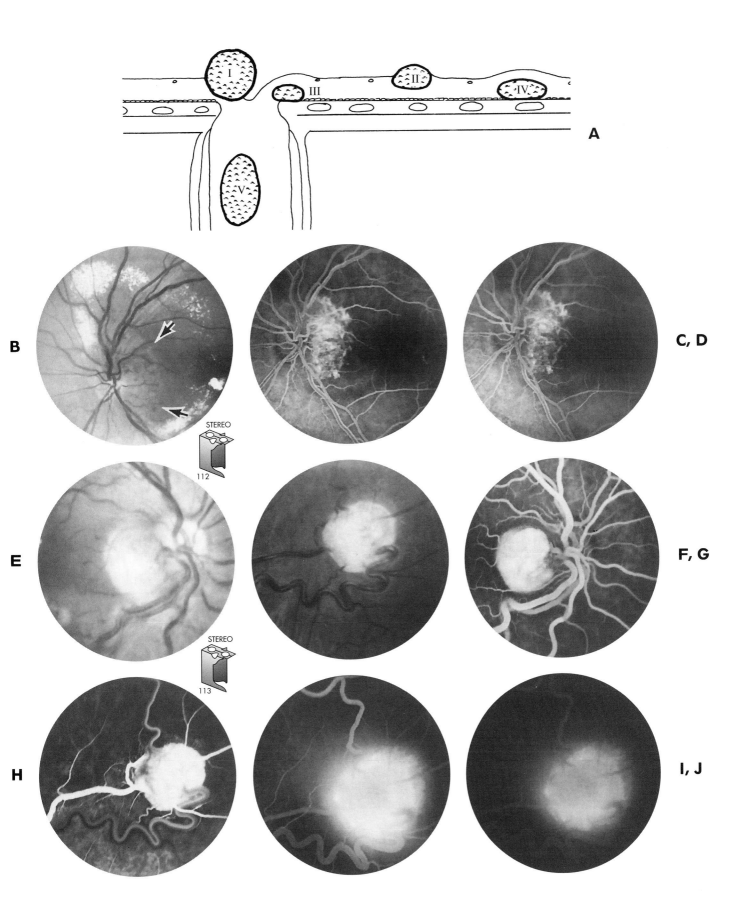

A

B

C, D

E

F, G

H

I, J

851

Capillary hemangiomas are typically red or pink tumors that may arise from the superficial retina or optic nerve head and protrude inward (endophytic angiomas) (Figs. 10-21, *A-I, A-II;* 10-21, *E;* 10-22, *H;* and 10-24, *G* to *I*). When located peripheral to the optic disc, these endophytic tumors are usually associated with arteriovenous shunting between a dilated tortuous feeding artery and a draining vein (Fig. 10-22, *H* and *I*). Capillary hemangiomas may also arise from the outer retinal layers (exophytic capillary hemangiomas) (Figs. 10-21, *A-III, A-IV;* 10-21, *B;* 10-22, *A;* 10-23, *A, F,* and *G;* and 10-24, *A* and *D* to *F*). These tumors are usually not associated with evidence of arteriovenous shunting, and there is a predilection for them to develop in the juxtapapillary area. When they arise in this area they are frequently sessile and may be misdiagnosed as papilledema or juxtapapillary choroidal neovascularization because of their predilection for causing juxtapapillary serous detachment of the retina and circinate exudation extending into the macular region (Figs. 10-21, *B;* 10-23, *A, F,* and *G;* and 10-24, *A* and *E*).[205,241] Loss of central vision may occur secondary to the accumulation of yellow, lipid-rich exudate in the macula derived from peripheral retinal angiomas. The mechanism for this accumulation is similar to that in patients with peripheral retinal telangiectasia (see p. 495). Loss of vision may also be caused by an epiretinal membrane distorting the macula remote from the site of the angioma (Fig. 10-22, *A* to *C*). There is a striking predilection for these epiretinal membranes to spontaneously peel and for vision to return to nearly normal after treatment of the peripheral angioma (Fig. 10-22, *A* to *F*).[202,203,218,237,238] For this reason, vitrectomy for excision of the epiretinal membrane should be considered only after a 4- to 6-month period of observation. Floaters and visual loss may also be caused by development of a retinal tear adjacent to an angioma and subsequent rheg-

matogenous retinal detachment.[202,228] Vitreous traction developing at the anterior surface of the retinal angioma and adjacent retina is responsible for the retinal tear. Vitreous traction may also be a factor in the development on the tumor surface of proliferative retinopathy, vitreous hemorrhage either spontaneously or following treatment of the tumor, and tractional retinal detachment. A retrobulbar capillary angioma (Fig. 10-21, *A-E*) should be considered in patients with angiomatosis and unexplained visual loss.

FIG. 10-22   Capillary Angiomas of the Retina and Optic Nerve.

A to **F,** Peripheral retinal capillary angiomas (**A** and **B**) and macular pucker (**C**) in a 23-year-old woman complaining of recent loss of central vision in the right eye. Her past medical history and family history were unremarkable. Visual acuity in the right eye was 20/70 and in the left eye was 20/15. In addition to the solitary angioma in the superotemporal fundus (**A**), there was a small angioma nasally (*arrow*, **B**). Fluorescein angiography demonstrated both lesions (**D** and **E**). The retinal tumors were treated with cryopexy and photocoagulation. Soon afterward the preretinal membrane spontaneously detached from the inner surface of the macula and remained attached to the optic nerve head (*arrow*, **F**). Her visual acuity improved to 20/25 + 3.

G to **K,** Exudative maculopathy (**G**) caused by an endophytic angioma nasal to the right optic disc (**H** and **I**) in this 23-year-old woman who presented with a 2-month history of blurred vision in the right eye. Her family history and past medical history were negative. A CT scan of the brain was negative. Visual acuity was 20/70, right eye, and 20/20, left eye. Laser photocoagulation of the feeder artery and tumor resulted in a vitreous hemorrhage (**J**). Six years later her visual acuity was 20/40. Note the vitreoretinal traction, nasal displacement of the optic disc and foveal center (*arrow*, **K**), and resolution of the macular exudation.

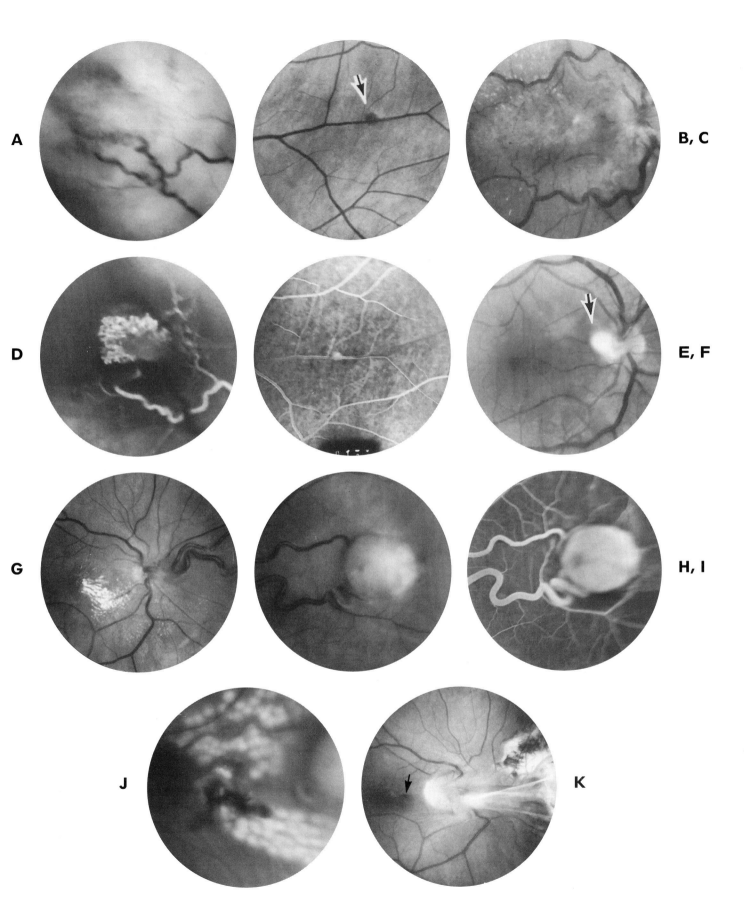

A

B, C

D

E, F

G

H, I

J

K

Stereoscopic fluorescein angiography is invaluable in detecting exophytic sessile juxtapapillary capillary hemangiomas (Figs. 10-21, *B,* and 10-23).[205] Because these tumors protrude into the subretinal space adjacent to the optic disc and because they frequently arise in the papillomacular bundle area in symptomatic patients, they are difficult to treat with photocoagulation (Fig. 10-23, *A* to *F* and *G* to *L*). Fluorescein angiography in peripheral endophytic lesions shows evidence of arteriovenous shunting (Figs. 10-21, *J,* and 10-22, *I*). Angiography usually shows no evidence of fluorescein staining in the macular region in those patients with lipid-rich accumulations secondary to peripheral angiomas. Angiography is particularly useful in the detection of very small lesions that may be barely visible biomicroscopically (Fig. 10-22, *B* and *E*).*

Light and electron microscopy reveal that these tumors are composed of a mass of retinal capillaries, many of which have a normal endothelium, basement membrane, and pericytes (Fig. 10-25).† In some cases, capillaries making up these tumors may show abnormal fenestrations.[215,226] Stromal cells, which some have attributed to astrocytes, separate the vascular channels and frequently contain large lipid-filled vacuoles. New vessels may develop on the anterior surface of these tumors and extend into the vitreous (Fig. 10-25, *D*). Exophytic tumors may have vascular communication with the choroid in some cases.

---

*References 202, 214, 216, 222, 233, 241, 245.
†References 206, 209, 215, 226, 229, 240, 246.

FIG. 10-23   Retinal Capillary Angioma.

A to **E,** Sessile juxtapapillary retinal angioma (**A**) misdiagnosed as papilledema in a 31-year-old woman with a 5-month history of intermittent headaches. She had recently been hospitalized for a thorough neurologic evaluation, which was negative. Her visual acuity in both eyes was 20/20. Angiography revealed a capillary angioma, largely confined to the outer two-thirds of the retina (**B** and **C**). She developed chronic serous detachment of the macula, and her visual acuity decreased to 20/50 in the right eye. She had two courses of argon laser grid pattern treatment (**D**) to the tumor that resulted in resolution of the intraretinal and subretinal exudate (**E**). At the time of her last photograph, made 9 years after her initial treatment, her visual acuity was 20/30.

F to **L,** This 19-year-old woman had a history of blurred vision and optic disc lesions first noted at age 15 years. She was asymptomatic in the right eye. Visual acuity was 20/30, right eye, and 20/400, left eye. There was exudative maculopathy associated with a juxtapapillary capillary angioma bilaterally (*arrows,* **F** and **G**). The angioma in the left eye was treated with argon green laser (**H**) and was retreated 4 months later. At that time the acuity in the right eye had decreased to 20/50 and the angioma (**J**) was treated with laser. One month later the angioma in the right eye (**K**) was retreated. Forty-two months later her visual acuity in the right eye was 20/40 and the left eye was 20/60. There was improvement in the exudation in both eyes (**I** and **L**). At the time of her initial examination an MRI of the brain revealed a left cerebellar hemangioblastoma that was successfully removed. There was no family history of angiomatosis.

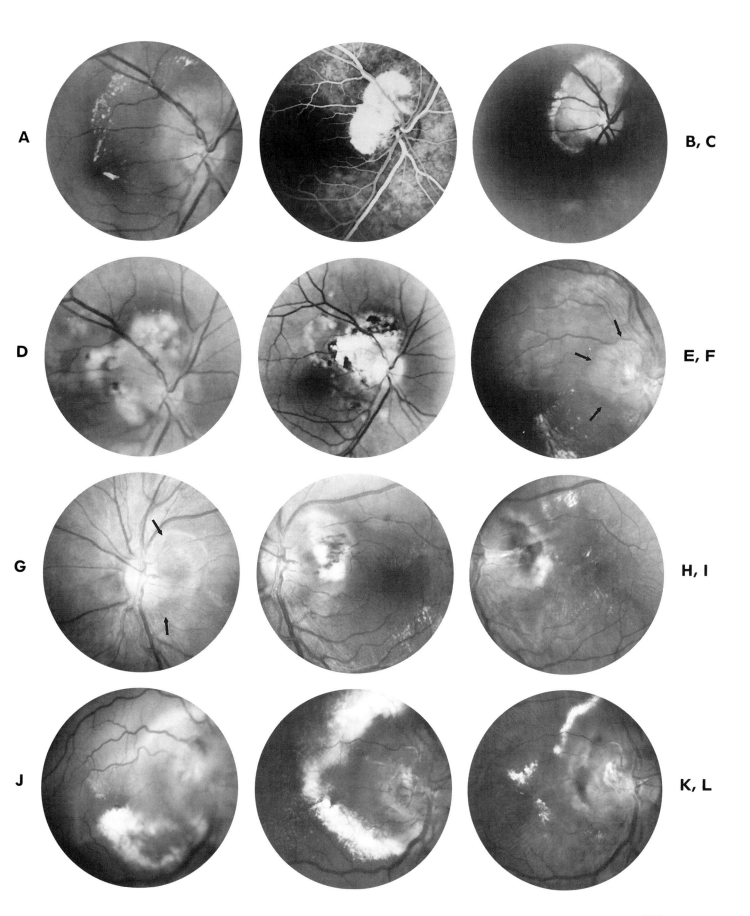

Because of their capillary nature and predilection for the development of arteriovenous fistulas and exudation, these tumors are capable of reactive proliferation and continued growth even into adulthood. Progressive intraretinal and subretinal exudation and detachment are part of the natural course of the disease. Spontaneous fibrotic involution of angiomas, however, occasionally occurs.[235,246] Identification of capillary angiomas ophthalmoscopically and by fluorescein angiography during the early stages is important because treatment with photocoagulation[192,194,204,207,216] or cryotherapy[190,204,243-245] at this stage of the disease is easier. The sessile exophytic juxtapapillary hemangiomas associated with loss of macular vision are difficult to treat because of the frequency with which they are located in the papillomacular bundle and because laser treatment is ineffective in stopping the exudation derived from the outer portion of the tumor that protrudes into the subretinal space. The use of photocoagulation to create a barrier between juxtapapillary angiomas and the center of the macula before their causing macular detachment and exudation may prove to be of value (Fig. 10-24, *D to I*). Treatment of the peripheral angiomas with photocoagulation or cryotherapy or both is generally effective in lesions whose diameter does exceed one disc diameter. Treatment of larger lesions is complicated by excessive subretinal exudation and a predilection for the development of retinitis proliferans on the surface of these tumors. Techniques for treating large retinal angiomas include repeated applications of laser to the feeding artery to reduce the tumor perfusion before treating the tumor directly, use of transscleral penetrating diathermy, and pars plana vitrectomy and direct diathermy to the tumor.[196,217] The use of a transvitreal arterial clip together with diathermy and removal of the posterior vitreous may prove to be useful in the treatment of large angiomas.[204] Surgical excision of these lesions has been reported.[231]

FIG. 10-24   Natural Course of Retinal and Optic Disc Capillary Angiomas.

A to F, Exophytic capillary angioma in a 17-year-old boy complaining of blurred vision in the left eye (*arrows,* **A** and **B**). At that time there were no other lesions in either eye. Medical evaluation for extraocular evidence of angiomatosis was negative. Over the subsequent 10 years he had gradual enlargement of the angiomatous mass that grew through the center of his macula despite laser photocoagulation. During this time he developed a small angioma in the inferior fundus of the same eye and a small angioma on the right optic disc (*arrow,* **C**). This remained unchanged from 1979 until 1992, when he returned because he had noticed a paracentral scotoma in the right eye (**D**). Meanwhile he had developed total retinal detachment and had no light perception in the left eye. Laser treatment along the temporal margin of the tumor was advised and was refused. He returned in 1995 complaining of difficulty reading. His acuity was 20/15 but he had a large cecocentral scotoma associated with exudative retinal detachment and further enlargement of the angioma (**E**). In an effort to isolate the tumor from the center of the macula a row of krypton red laser burns was placed near the temporal margin of the tumor (*arrow,* **F**). Nine months later the exudate was gone and he was asymptomatic.

G to I, Gradual enlargement of juxtapapillary angioma occurred in this patient. **G,** March 1983. **H,** March 1985. **I,** September 1996. Several years later the patient had severe loss of central vision because of exudative retinal detachment. Use of a barrier-type laser treatment and direct treatment of the angioma early (**G** and **H**) may have prevented or delayed the loss of central vision.

J to L, A juxtapapillary angioma (*arrows,* **K**) developed 5 years later at the site of a choroidal rupture (*arrow,* **J**) in this 19-year-old woman with Stargardt's disease. Her sister had Stargardt's disease, but her family history was negative otherwise. This tumor may be a secondary angioma resulting from reactive glial-vascular proliferation at the site of chorioretinal scarring.

(**G to I,** courtesy Dr. Arnold Patz; **J to L,** from Retsas et al.[231a])

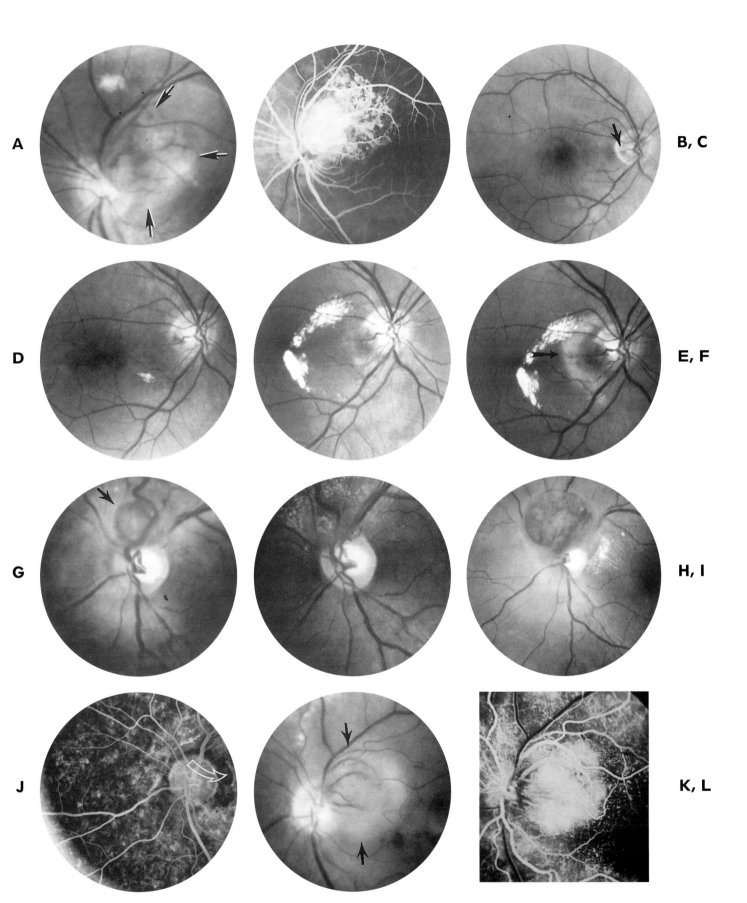

A

B, C

D

E, F

G

H, I

J

K, L

The differential diagnosis for juxtapapillary capillary angiomas includes juxtapapillary choroidal neovascularization, hypopigmented combined retinal and RPE hamartoma, papilledema,[197,198] juxtapapillary choroidal hemangiomas and osteomas, and reactive retinal glial and vascular proliferation (see discussion in the next section). Stereoscopic fluorescein angiography is the most important study in the differential diagnosis. The differential diagnosis of peripheral capillary hemangiomas is not difficult in the presence of a dilated, tortuous retinal artery and vein extending from the optic disc to the tumor.

▼ REACTIVE RETINAL VASCULAR PROLIFERATION SIMULATING RETINAL CAPILLARY HAMARTOMAS

There may be some difficulty in differentiating peripheral exophytic angiomas from retinal telangiectasis or pseudoangiomatous masses caused by reactive vascular proliferation in patients with retinopathy of prematurity, branch vein occlusion, diabetic retinopathy, familial exudative vitreoretinopathy, X-linked juvenile retinoschisis, chronic rhegmatogenous retinal detachment, and retinitis proliferans (Fig. 10-24, *J* to *L*).[195,200,208,218,224,231a]

▼ RETINAL TELANGIECTASIS AND ARTERIOVENOUS ANEURYSM

Retinal telangiectasias and arteriovenous aneurysms are not truly tumors and are discussed in Chapter 6.

FIG. 10-25 **Histopathology of Capillary Hemangioma of the Retina and Optic Nerve Head.**

A to **D,** Histopathologic condition of preexudative phase of retinal angioma in a 48-year-old man who complained of paresthesias of the arms and legs. His mother had died of a brain tumor at 40 years of age. His neurologic examination was normal. His cerebrospinal fluid protein was 300 mg/dl. A myelogram revealed a block at the first cervical vertebra, and a right brachial arteriogram revealed a large vascular tumor at the level of the brainstem. A cerebellar hemangioblastoma was found at the time of craniotomy. The patient died soon afterward. An autopsy revealed multiple cysts of the right kidney and pancreas. Gross examination of the right eye revealed two nodular retinal angiomas. The larger one (*arrow,* **A**) measured 1.5 mm. The retinal vessels leading to both angiomas were dilated. Histopathologic examination revealed dilated feeder vessels (*arrow,* **B**) supplying the capillary tumor, which replaced the normal retinal architecture and protruded into the vitreous cavity. A high-power view of the tumor showed that it was composed of capillary-sized blood vessels lined by flattened endothelial cells (**C**). Strands of fibroglial tissue and capillaries were present on the surface of the tumor and extended into the vitreous (*arrow,* **D**).

E and **F,** Clinicopathologic correlation of an exophytic capillary angioma of the optic nerve head and peripapillary retina simulating chronic papilledema in a 29-year-old man who first noted blurred vision in his right eye in 1959. He had similar swelling of both optic discs associated with exudative detachment of the surrounding retina (**E**). Over the subsequent 3 years he had progressive loss of vision in both eyes, and because of the uncertainty of the diagnosis the left eye was enucleated. His family history was positive for an angioblastic meningioma in his mother, a pheochromocytoma in a niece and a nephew, and bilateral optic nerve lesions similar to those in the patient in a nephew. Histopathologic examination revealed an exophytic capillary hemangioma involving the juxtapapillary retina and optic nerve head (*arrows,* **F**).

(**A** to **D** from Nicholson et al.[229]; **E** and **F** from Darr et al.[198])

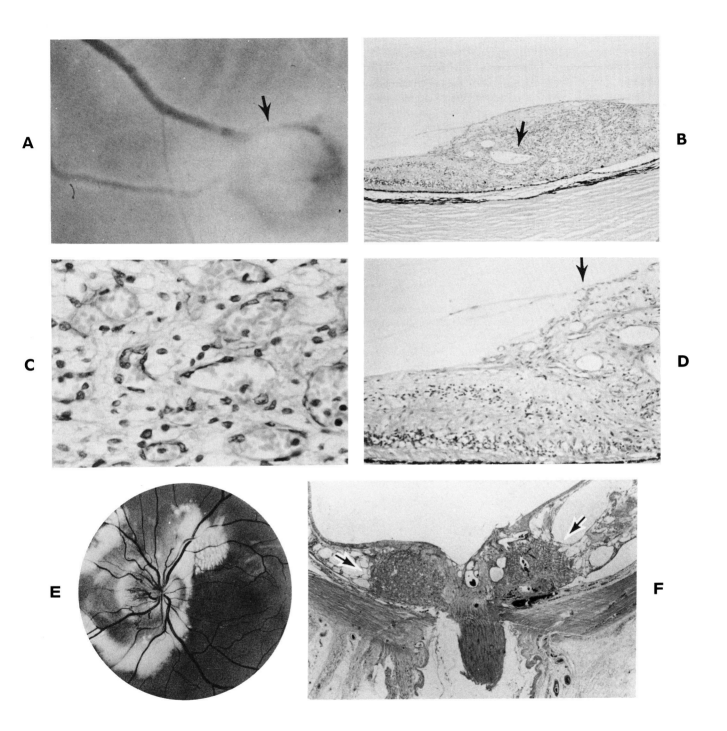

REFERENCES

Solitary-Type and Multiple Congenital Hypertrophy of the Retinal Pigment Epithelium (CHRPE)

1. Aiello LP, Traboulsi EI: Pigmented fundus lesions in a preterm infant with familial adenomatous polyposis. *Arch Ophthalmol* 111:302-303, 1993.

2. Blair NP, Trempe CL: Hypertrophy of the retinal pigment epithelium associated with Gardner's syndrome. *Am J Ophthalmol* 90:661-667, 1980.

3. Boldrey EE, Schwartz A: Enlargement of congenital hypertrophy of the retinal pigment epithelium. *Am J Ophthalmol* 94:64-66, 1982.

4. Buettner H: Congenital hypertrophy of the retinal pigment epithelium. *Am J Ophthalmol* 79:177-189, 1975.

5. Buettner H: Kongenitale Hypertrophie des Pigmentepithels der Netzhaut und Gardner-Syndrom. *Fortschr Ophthalmol* 83:597-599, 1986.

6. Chamot L, Zografos L, Klainguti G: Fundus changes associated with congenital hypertrophy of the retinal pigment epithelium. *Am J Ophthalmol* 115:154-161, 1993.

7. Champion R, Daicker BC: Congenital hypertrophy of the pigment epithelium: light microscopic and ultrastructural findings in young children. *Retina* 9:44-48, 1989.

8. Cleary PE, Gregor Z, Bird AC: Retinal vascular changes in congenital hypertrophy of the retinal pigment epithelium. *Br J Ophthalmol* 60:499-503, 1976.

9. Cohen SY, Quentel G, Guiberteau B, Coscas GJ: Retinal vascular changes in congenital hypertrophy of the retinal pigment epithelium. *Ophthalmology* 100:471-474, 1993.

10. Diaz-Llopis M, Menezo JL: Congenital hypertrophy of the retinal pigment epithelium in familial adenomatous polyposis. *Arch Ophthalmol* 106:412-413, 1988.

11. Gardner EJ, Richards RC: Multiple cutaneous and subcutaneous lesions occurring simultaneously with hereditary polyposis and osteomatosis. *Am J Hum Genet* 5:139-147, 1953.

12. Gass JDM: *Differential diagnosis of intraocular tumors; a stereoscopic presentation,* St. Louis, 1974, CV Mosby, pp. 221-246.

13. Gass JDM: Focal congenital anomalies of the retinal pigment epithelium. *Eye* 3:1-18, 1989.

14. Gass JDM: *Stereoscopic atlas of macular diseases; diagnosis and treatment,* ed. 3, St. Louis, 1987, CV Mosby, pp. 606-611.

15. Giardiello FM, Offerhaus GJ, Traboulsi EI, et al: Value of combined phenotypic markers in identifying inheritance of familial adenomatous polyposis. *Gut* 32:1170-1174, 1991.

16. Heinemann M-H, Baker RH, Miller HH, DeCross JJ: Familial polyposis coli: the spectrum of ocular and other extracolonic manifestations. *Graefes Arch Clin Exp Ophthalmol* 229:213-218, 1991.

17. Kasner L, Traboulsi EI, Delacruz Z, Green WR: A histopathologic study of the pigmented fundus lesions in familial adenomatous polyposis. *Retina* 12:35-42, 1992.

18. Kurz GH, Zimmerman LE: Vagaries of the retinal pigment epithelium. *Int Ophthalmol Clin* 2(2):441-464, 1962.

19. Lewis RA, Crowder WE, Eierman LA, et al: The Gardner syndrome; significance of ocular features. *Ophthalmology* 91:916-925, 1984.

20. Llopis MD, Menezo JL: Congenital hypertrophy of the retinal pigment epithelium and familial polyposis of the colon. *Am J Ophthalmol* 103:235-236, 1987.

21. Lloyd WC 3d, Eagle RC JR, Shields JA, et al: Congenital hypertrophy of the retinal pigment epithelium; electron microscopic and morphometric observations. *Ophthalmology* 97:1052-1060, 1990.

22. Munden PM, Sobol WM, Weingeist TA: Ocular findings in Turcot syndrome (glioma-polyposis). *Ophthalmology* 98:111-114, 1991.

23. Norris JL, Cleasby GW: An unusual case of congenital hypertrophy of the retinal pigment epithelium. *Arch Ophthalmol* 94:1910-1911, 1976.

24. Parke JT, Riccardi VM, Lewis RA, Ferrell RE: A syndrome of microcephaly and retinal pigmentary abnormalities without mental retardation in a family with coincidental autosomal dominant hyperreflexia. *Am J Med Genet* 17:585-594, 1984.

25. Purcell JJ Jr, Shields JA: Hypertrophy with hyperpigmentation of the retinal pigment epithelium. *Arch Ophthalmol* 93:1122-1126, 1975.

26. Reese AB, Jones IS: Benign melanomas of the retinal pigment epithelium. *Am J Ophthalmol* 42:207-212, 1956.

27. Romania A, Zakov ZN, Church JM, Jagelman DG: Retinal pigment epithelium lesions as a biomarker of disease in patients with familial adenomatous polyposis; a follow-up report. *Ophthalmology* 99:911-913, 1992.

28. Romania A, Zakov ZN, McGannon E, et al: Congenital hypertrophy of the retinal pigment epithelium in familial adenomatous polyposis. *Ophthalmology* 96:879-884, 1989.

29. Santos A, Morales L, Hernandez-Quintela E, et al: Congenital hypertrophy of the retinal pigment epithelium associated with familial adenomatous polyposis. *Retina* 14:6-9, 1994.

30. Schmidt D, Jung CE, Wolff G: Changes in the retinal pigment epithelium close to retinal vessels in familial adenomatous polyposis. *Graefes Arch Clin Exp Ophthalmol* 232:96-102, 1994.

31. Shields JA, Shields CL, Shah PG, et al: Lack of association among typical congenital hypertrophy of the retinal pigment epithelium, adenomatous polyposis, and Gardner syndrome. *Ophthalmology* 99:1709-1713, 1992.

32. Stein EA, Brady KD: Ophthalmologic and electro-oculographic findings in Gardner's syndrome. *Am J Ophthalmol* 106:326-331, 1988.

33. Sugar HS, Wolff L: Geographic dark posterior fundus patches. *Am J Ophthalmol* 83:847-852, 1977.

34. Traboulsi EI, Maumenee IH, Krush AJ, et al: Congenital hypertrophy of the retinal pigment epithelium predicts colorectal polyposis in Gardner's syndrome. *Arch Ophthalmol* 108:525-526, 1990.

35. Traboulsi EI, Maumenee IH, Krush AJ, et al: Pigmented ocular fundus lesions in the inherited gastrointestinal polyposis syndromes and in hereditary nonpolyposis colorectal cancer. *Ophthalmology* 95:964-969, 1988.

36. Traboulsi EI, Murphy SF, de la Cruz ZC, et al: A clinico-pathologic study of the eyes in familial adenomatous polyposis with extracolonic manifestations (Gardner's syndrome). *Am J Ophthalmol* 110:550-561, 1990.

37. Whitson WE, Orcutt JC, Walkinshaw MD: Orbital osteoma in Gardner's syndrome. *Am J Ophthalmol* 101:236-241, 1986.

38. Wirz K, Lee WR, Coaker T: Progressive changes in congenital hypertrophy of the retinal pigment epithelium; an electron microscopic study. *Graefes Arch Clin Exp Ophthalmol* 219:214-221, 1982.

Grouped-Type Congenital Pigmented Nevi of the Retinal Pigment Epithelium, "Bear Tracks"

39. Collier M: Les manifestations oculaires associées à la dyschondroplasie d'Ollier (a propos d'un cas comportant une pigmentation congénitale de la rétine. *Bull Soc Ophtalmol Fr* no. 4:161-169, 1961.

40. De Jong PTVM, Delleman JW: Familial grouped pigmentation of the retinal pigment epithelium. *Br J Ophthalmol* 72:439, 1988.

41. Gašparová D, Szedélyová L: Familial occurrence of grouped pigmentation of the ocular fundus. *Cesk Oftalmol* 36:406-408, 1980.

42. Höeg N: Die gruppierte Pigmentation des Augengrundes. *Klin Monatsbl Augenheilkd* 49(1):49-77, 1911.

43. Loewenstein A, Steel J: Special case of melanosis fundi: bilateral congenital group pigmentation of the central area. *Br J Ophthalmol* 25:417-423, 1941.

44. Mauthner L: *Lehrbuch der Ophthalmoscopie,* Vienna, 1868, Tendler, p. 388.

45. McGregor IS: Macular coloboma with bilateral grouped pigmentation of the retina. *Br J Ophthalmol* 29:132-136, 1945.

46. Morse PH: Fluorescein angiography of grouped pigmentation of the retina. *Ann Ophthalmol* 5:27-30, 1973.

47. Regillo CD, Eagle RC Jr, Shields JA, et al: Histopathologic findings in congenital grouped pigmentation of the retina. *Ophthalmology* 100:400-405, 1993.

48. Renardel de Lavalette VW, Cruysberg JRM, Deutman AF: Familial congenital grouped pigmentation of the retina. *Am J Ophthalmol* 112:406-409, 1991.

49. Schwarz GT: Case report of congenital grouped pigmentation of the retina with maculocerebral degeneration. *Am J Ophthalmol* 26:72-74, 1943.

50. Shields JA, Tso MOM: Congenital grouped pigmentation of the retina; histopathologic description and report of a case. *Arch Ophthalmol* 93:1153-1155, 1975.

51. Silvan Lopez F: Pigmentación agrupada retiniana. *Arch Soc Oftalmol Hisp-Am* 8:448-456, 1948.

52. Welter SL: "Naevus pigmentosus des Augenhintergrundes." *Klin Monatsbl Augenheilkd* 78:682-687, 1927.

Grouped-Type Congenital Albinotic and Hypomelanotic Nevi of the Retinal Pigment Epithelium, "Polar Bear Tracks"

53. Fuhrmann C, Bopp S, Laqua H: Congenital grouped albinotic spots: a rare anomaly of the retinal pigment epithelium. *Ger J Ophthalmol* 1:103-104, 1992.

54. Kandori F: Very rare case of congenital nonprogressive night blindness with fleck retina. *J Clin Ophthalmol* 13:384-386, 1959.

55. Kandori F, Setogawa T, Tamai A: Electroretinographical studies on "fleck retina with congenital nonprogressive night blindness." *Acta Soc Ophthalmol Jpn* 70:1311-1325, 1966.

56. Kandori F, Tamai A, Kurimoto S, Fukunaga K: Fleck retina. *Am J Ophthalmol* 73:673-685, 1972.

57. Parke JT, Riccardi VM, Lewis RA, Ferrell RE: A syndrome of microcephaly and retinal pigmentary abnormalities without mental retardation in a family with coincidental autosomal dominant hyperreflexia. *Am J Med Genet* 17:585-594, 1984.

Solitary-Type Hypomelanotic and Albinotic Nevi

58. Kraupa E: Beiträge zur Morphologie des Augenhintergrundes III. *Klin Monatsbl Augenheilkd* 67:15-26, 1921.

59. Roseman RL, Gass JDM: Solitary hypopigmented nevus of the retinal pigment epithelium in the macula. *Arch Ophthalmol* 110:1358-1359, 1992; correction p. 1762.

60. Schlernitzauer DA, Green WR: Peripheral retinal albinotic spots. *Am J Ophthalmol* 72:729-732, 1971.

Retinal Pigment Epithelial Hamartoma (Congenital Hyperplasia of the Retinal Pigment Epithelium, Pigment Epithelial Adenoma)

61. Blodi FC, Reuling FH, Sornson ET: Pseudomelanocytoma at the optic nerve head; an adenoma of the retinal pigment epithelium. *Arch Ophthalmol* 73:353-355, 1965.

62. Duke JR, Maumenee AE: An unusual tumor of the retinal pigment epithelium in an eye with early open-angle glaucoma. *Am J Ophthalmol* 47:311-317, 1959.

63. Font RL, Zimmerman LE, Fine BS: Adenoma of the retinal pigment epithelium; histochemical and electron microscopic observations. *Am J Ophthalmol* 73:544-554, 1972.

64. Garner A: Tumours of the retinal pigment epithelium. *Br J Ophthalmol* 54:715-723, 1970.

65. Jampel HD, Schachat AP, Conway B, et al: Retinal pigment epithelial hyperplasia assuming tumor-like proportions; report of two cases. *Retina* 6:105-112, 1986.

66. Tso MOM, Albert DM: Pathological condition of the retinal pigment epithelium; neoplasms and nodular non-neoplastic lesions. *Arch Ophthalmol* 88:27-38, 1972.

Combined Pigment Epithelial and Retinal Hamartoma

67. Aoki S, Barkovich AJ, Nishimura K, et al: Neurofibromatosis types 1 and 2; cranial MR findings. *Radiology* 172:527-534, 1989.

68. Bouzas EA, Parry DM, Eldridge R, Kaiser-Kupfer MI: Familial occurrence of combined pigment epithelial and retinal hamartomas associated with neurofibromatosis 2. *Retina* 12:103-107, 1992.

69. Bouzas EA, Parry DM, Eldridge R, Kaiser-Kupfer MI: Visual impairment in patients with neurofibromatosis 2. *Neurology* 43:622-623, 1993.

70. Cardell BS, Starbuck MJ: Juxtapapillary hamartoma of retina. *Br J Ophthalmol* 45:672-677, 1961.

71. Corcostegui B, Mendez M, Corcostegui G, Gil Gibernau JJ: Éléments diagnostiques des hamartomes de la rétine et de l'épithélium pigmentaire. *Bull Mem Soc Fr Ophtalmol* 96:152, 1985.

72. Cosgrove JM, Sharp DM, Bird AC: Combined hamartoma of the retina and retinal pigment epithelium: the clinical spectrum. *Trans Ophthalmol Soc UK* 105:106-113, 1986.

73. Cotlier E: Cafe-au-lait spots of the fundus in neurofibromatosis. *Arch Ophthalmol* 95:1990-1992, 1977.

74. Destro M, D'Amico DJ, Gragoudas ES, et al: Retinal manifestations of neurofibromatosis; diagnosis and management. *Arch Ophthalmol* 109:662-666, 1991.

75. Flood TP, Orth DH, Aaberg TM, Marcus DF: Macular hamartomas of the retinal pigment epithelium and retina. *Retina* 3:164-170, 1983.

76. Font RL, Moura RA, Shetlar DJ, et al: Combined hamartoma of sensory retina and retinal pigment epithelium. *Retina* 9:302-311, 1989.

77. Friberg TR, Gulledge SL: Hamartomas of the retina and pigment epithelium. *Can J Ophthalmol* 17:56-60, 1982.

78. Gass JDM: *Differential diagnosis of intraocular tumors; a stereoscopic presentation,* St. Louis, 1974, CV Mosby, p. 221.

79. Gass JDM: Discussion of paper by Schachat AP, Shields JA, Fine SL, et al: Combined hamartomas of the retinal and retinal pigment epithelium. *Ophthalmology* 91:1615, 1984.

80. Gass JDM: *Stereoscopic atlas of macular diseases; diagnosis and treatment,* ed. 3, St. Louis, 1987, CV Mosby, p. 624.

81. Gass JDM: An unusual hamartoma of the pigment epithelium and retina simulating choroidal melanoma and retinoblastoma. *Trans Am Ophthalmol Soc* 71:171-185, 1973.

82. Good WV, Brodsky MC, Edwards MS, Hoyt WF: Bilateral retinal hamartomas in neurofibromatosis type 2. *Br J Ophthalmol* 75:190, 1991.

83. Hrisomalos NF, Mansour AM, Jampol LM, et al: "Pseudo"-combined hamartoma following papilledema. *Arch Ophthalmol* 105:1634-1635, 1987.

84. Jabbour O, Payeur G: Malformation congénitale de l'épithélium pigmentaire et de la rétine. *J Fr Ophtalmol* 6:149-154, 1983.

85. Kahn D, Goldberg MF, Jednock N: Combined retinal-retina pigment epithelial hamartoma presenting as a vitreous hemorrhage. *Retina* 4:40-43, 1984.

86. Kaye LD, Rothner AD, Beauchamp GR, et al: Ocular findings associated with neurofibromatosis type II. *Ophthalmology* 99:1424-1429, 1992.

87. Landau K, Dossetor FM, Hoyt WF, Muci-Mendosa R: Retinal hamartoma in neurofibromatosis 2. *Arch Ophthalmol* 108:328-329, 1990.

88. Laqua H, Wessing A: Congenital retino-pigment epithelial malformation, previously described as hamartoma. *Am J Ophthalmol* 87:34-42, 1979.

89. Machemer R: Die Primäre retinale Pigmentepithelhyperplasie. *Albrecht von Graefes Arch Ophthalmol* 167:284-295, 1964.

90. McDonald HR, Abrams GW, Burke JM, Neuwirth J: Clinicopathologic results of vitreous surgery for epiretinal membranes in patients with combined retinal and retinal pigment epithelial hamartomas. *Am J Ophthalmol* 100:806-813, 1985.

91. McLean EB: Hamartoma of the retinal pigment epithelium. *Am J Ophthalmol* 82:227-231, 1976.

92. Mele A, Cennamo G, Sorrentino V, Capobianco S: Fluoroangiographic and echographic study on a juxtapapillary hamartoma of the retinal pigment epithelium. *Ophthalmologica* 189:180-185, 1984.

93. Mulvihill JJ, Parry DM, Sherman JL, et al: NIH Conference. Neurofibromatosis 1 (Recklinghausen disease) and neurofibromatosis 2 (bilateral acoustic neurofibromatosis); an update. *Ann Intern Med* 113:39-52, 1990.

94. Palmer ML, Carney MD, Combs JL: Combined hamartomas of the retinal pigment epithelium and retina. *Retina* 10:33-36, 1990.

95. Reynolds WD, Goldstein BG: Retinal pigment epithelial hamartoma. *Ophthalmology* 90:117-119, 1983.

96. Rosenberg PR, Walsh JB: Retinal pigment epithelial hamartoma—unusual manifestations. *Br J Ophthalmol* 68:439-442, 1984.

97. Sappenfield DL, Gitter KA: Surgical intervention for combined retinal-retinal pigment epithelial hamartoma. *Retina* 10:119-124, 1990.

98. Schachat AP, Glaser BM: Retinal hamartoma, acquired retinoschisis, and retinal hole. *Am J Ophthalmol* 99:604-605, 1985.

99. Schachat AP, Shields JA, Fine SL, et al: Combined hamartomas of the retina and retinal pigment epithelium. *Ophthalmology* 91:1609-1614, 1984.

100. Sivalingam A, Augsburger J, Perilongo G, et al: Combined hamartoma of the retina and retinal pigment epithelium in a patient with neurofibromatosis type 2. *J Pediatr Ophthalmol Strabismus* 28:320-322, 1991.

101. Theobald GD, Floyd G, Kirk HQ: Hyperplasia of the retinal pigment epithelium simulating a neoplasm: report of two cases. *Am J Ophthalmol* 45(Pt 2):235-240, 1958.

102. Vogel MH, Wessing A: Die Proliferation des juxtapapillären retinalen Pigmentepithels. *Klin Monatsbl Augenheilkd* 162:736-743, 1973.

103. Vogel MH, Zimmerman LE, Gass JDM: Proliferation of the juxtapapillary retinal pigment epithelium simulating malignant melanoma. *Doc Ophthalmol* 26:461-481, 1969.

104. Wang C-L, Brucker AJ: Vitreous hemorrhage secondary to juxtapapillary vascular hamartoma of the retina. *Retina* 4:44-47, 1984.

Reactive Hyperplasias of the Retinal Pigment Epithelium Simulating Hamartomas and Neoplasias

105. Garner A: Tumours of the retinal pigment epithelium. *Br J Ophthalmol* 54:715-723, 1970.

106. Laqua H: Tumors and tumor-like lesions of the retinal pigment epithelium. *Ophthalmologica* 183:34-38, 1981.

107. Minckler D, Allen AW Jr: Adenocarcinoma of the retinal pigment epithelium. *Arch Ophthalmol* 96:2252-2254, 1978.

108. Ramahefasolo S, Coscas G, Regenbogen L, Godel V: Adenocarcinoma of retinal pigment epithelium. *Br J Ophthalmol* 71:516-520, 1987.

109. Shields JA, Eagle RC Jr, Barr CC, et al: Adenocarcinoma of retinal pigment epithelium arising from a juxtapapillary histoplasmosis scar. *Arch Ophthalmol* 112:650-653, 1994.

110. Shields JA, Eagle RC Jr, Shields CL, De Potter P: Pigmented adenoma of the optic nerve head simulating a melanocytoma. *Ophthalmology* 99:1705-1708, 1992.

111. Tso MOM, Albert DM: Pathological condition of the retinal pigment epithelium; neoplasms and nodular non-neoplastic lesions. *Arch Ophthalmol* 88:27-38, 1972.

112. Vogel MH, Wölz U: Malignes Epitheliom des retinalen Pigmentepithels. *Klin Monatsbl Augenheilkd* 175:592-596, 1979.

Retinal and Optic Disc Astrocytic Hamartomas

113. Atkinson A, Sanders MD, Wong V: Vitreous haemorrhage in tuberous sclerosis; report of two cases. *Br J Ophthalmol* 57:773-779, 1973.

114. Barksy D, Wolter JR: The retinal lesion of tuberous sclerosis: An angiogliomatous hamartoma? *J Pediatr Ophthalmol* 8:261-265, 1971.

115. Bloom SM, Mahl CF: Photocoagulation for serous detachment of the macula secondary to retinal astrocytoma. *Retina* 11:416-422, 1991.

116. Bornfeld N, Messmer EP, Theodossiadis G, et al: Giant cell astrocytoma of the retina; clinicopathologic report of a case not associated with Bourneville's disease. *Retina* 7:183-189, 1987.

117. Cleasby GW, Fung WE, Shekter WB: Astrocytoma of the retina; report of two cases. *Am J Ophthalmol* 64:633-637, 1967.

118. Coppeto JR, Lubin JR, Albert DM: Astrocytic hamartoma in tuberous sclerosis mimicking necrotizing retinochoroiditis. *J Pediatr Ophthalmol Strabismus* 19:306-313, 1982.

119. Daily MJ, Smith JL, Dickens W: Giant drusen (astrocytic hamartoma) of the optic nerve seen with computerized axial tomography. *Am J Ophthalmol* 81:100-101, 1976.

120. De Bustros S, Miller NR, Finkelstein D, Massof R: Bilateral astrocytic hamartomas of the optic nerve heads in retinitis pigmentosa. *Retina* 3:21-23, 1983.

121. Destro M, D'Amico DJ, Gragoudas ES, et al: Retinal manifestations of neurofibromatosis; diagnosis and management. *Arch Ophthalmol* 109:662-666, 1991.

122. Eng LF, Rubinstein LJ: Contribution of immunohistochemistry to diagnostic problems of human cerebral tumors. *J Histochem Cytochem* 26:513-522, 1978.

123. Farber MG, Smith ME, Gans LA: Astrocytoma of the ciliary body. *Arch Ophthalmol* 105:536-537, 1987.

124. Font RL, Ferry AP: The phakomatoses. *Int Ophthalmol Clin* 12(1):1-50, 1972.

125. Foos RY, Straatsma BR, Allen RA: Astrocytoma of the optic nerve head. *Arch Ophthalmol* 74:319-326, 1965.

126. Garron LK, Spencer WH: Retinal glioneuroma associated with tuberous sclerosis. *Trans Am Acad Ophthalmol Otolaryngol* 68:1018-1021, 1964.

127. Gass JDM: *Differential diagnosis of intraocular tumors; a stereoscopic presentation,* St. Louis, 1974, CV Mosby, p. 312.

128. Gass JDM: The phakomatoses. *In:* Smith JL, editor: *Neuro-ophthalmology; symposium of the University of Miami and the Bascom Palmer Eye Institute,* vol. 2, St. Louis, 1965, CV Mosby, pp. 223-268.

129. Gutman I, Dunn D, Behrens M, et al: Hypopigmented iris spot: an early sign of tuberous sclerosis. *Ophthalmology* 89:1155-1159, 1982.

130. Harley RD, Grover WD: Tuberous sclerosis; description and report of 12 cases. *Ann Ophthalmol* 1:477-481, 1970.

131. Jakobiec FA, Brodie SE, Haik B, Iwamoto T: Giant cell astrocytoma of the retina; a tumor of possible Mueller cell origin. *Ophthalmology* 90:1565-1576, 1983.

132. Jordano J, Galera H, Toro M, Carreras B: Astrocytoma of the retina: Report of a case. *Br J Ophthalmol* 58:555-559, 1974.

133. Jost BF, Olk RJ: Atypical retinitis proliferans, retinal telangiectasis, and vitreous hemorrhage in a patient with tuberous sclerosis. *Retina* 6:53-56, 1986.

134. Jozwiak S: Diagnostic value of clinical features and supplementary investigations in tuberous sclerosis in children. *Acta Paediatr Hung* 32:71-88, 1992.

135. Kroll AJ, Ricker DP, Robb RM, Albert DM: Vitreous hemorrhage complicating retinal astrocytic hamartoma. *Surv Ophthalmol* 26:31-38, 1981.

136. Margo CE, Barletta JP, Staman JA: Giant cell astrocytoma of the retina in tuberous sclerosis. *Retina* 13:155-159, 1993.

137. McLean JM: Glial tumors of the retina in relation to tuberous sclerosis. *Am J Ophthalmol* 41:428-432, 1956.

138. Nyboer JH, Robertson DM, Gomez MR: Retinal lesions in tuberous sclerosis. *Arch Ophthalmol* 94:1277-1280, 1976.

139. Panzo GJ, Meyers SM, Gutman FA, et al: Spontaneous regression of parafoveal exudates and serous retinal detachment in a patient with tuberous sclerosis and retinal astrocytomas. *Retina* 4:242-245, 1984.

140. Pillai S, Limaye SR, Saimovici L-B: Optic disc hamartoma associated with retinitis pigmentosa. *Retina* 3:24-26, 1983.

141. Ramsay RC, Kinyoun JL, Hill CW, et al: Retinal astrocytoma. *Am J Ophthalmol* 88:32-36, 1979.

142. Reeser FH, Aaberg TM, Van Horn DL: Astrocytic hamartoma of the retina not associated with tuberous sclerosis. *Am J Ophthalmol* 86:688-698, 1978.

143. Robertson DM: Hamartomas of the optic disk with retinitis pigmentosa. *Am J Ophthalmol* 74:526-531, 1972.

144. Sahel JA, Frederick AR Jr, Pesavento R, Albert DM: Idiopathic retinal gliosis mimicking a choroidal melanoma. *Retina* 8:282-287, 1988.

145. Schwartz PL, Beards JA, Maris PJG: Tuberous sclerosis associated with a retinal angioma. *Am J Ophthalmol* 90:485-488, 1980.

146. Shami MJ, Benedict WL, Myers M: Early manifestation of retinal hamartomas in tuberous sclerosis. *Am J Ophthalmol* 115:539-540, 1993.

147. Wang C-L, Brucker AJ: Vitreous hemorrhage secondary to juxtapapillary vascular hamartoma of the retina. *Retina* 4:44-47, 1984.

148. Wolter JR, Mertus JM: Exophytic retinal astrocytoma in tuberous sclerosis; report of a case. *J Pediatr Ophthalmol* 6:186-191, 1969.

149. Zimmerman LE, Walsh FB: Clinical pathologic conference. *Am J Ophthalmol* 42:737-747, 1956.

Retinal and Optic Disc Cavernous Hemangiomas

150. Amalric P, Biau C: L'angiographie fluorescéinique chez l'enfant. *Arch Ophtalmol (Paris)* 28:55-60, 1968.

151. Augsburger JJ, Shields JA, Goldberg RE: Classification and management of hereditary retinal angiomas. *Int Ophthalmol* 4:93-106, 1981.

152. Bottoni F, Canevini MP, Canger R, Orzalesi N: Twin vessels in familial retinal cavernous hemangioma. *Am J Ophthalmol* 109:285-289, 1990.

153. Colvard DM, Robertson DM, Trautmann JC: Cavernous hemangioma of the retina. *Arch Ophthalmol* 96:2042-2044, 1978.

154. Corboy JR, Galetta SL: Familial cavernous angiomas manifesting with an acute chiasmal syndrome. *Am J Ophthalmol* 108:245-250, 1989.

155. Crompton JL, Taylor D: Ocular lesions in the blue rubber bleb naevus syndrome. *Br J Ophthalmol* 65:133-137, 1981.

156. Davies WS, Thumim M: Cavernous hemangioma of the optic disc and retina. *Trans Am Acad Ophthalmol Otolaryngol* 60:217-218, 1956.

157. Dobyns WB, Michels VV, Groover RV, et al: Familial cavernous malformations of the central nervous system and retina. *Ann Neurol* 21:578-583, 1987.

158. Drummond JW, Hall DL, Steen WH Jr, Lusk JE: Cavernous hemangioma of the optic disc. *Ann Ophthalmol* 12:1017-1018, 1980.

159. Frenkel M, Russe HP: Retinal telangiectasia associated with hypogammaglobulinemia. *Am J Ophthalmol* 63:215-220, 1967.

160. Gass JDM: Cavernous hemangioma of the retina; a neuro-oculo-cutaneous syndrome. *Am J Ophthalmol* 71:799-814, 1971.

161. Gass JDM: *Differential diagnosis of intraocular tumors; a stereoscopic presentation,* St. Louis, 1974, CV Mosby, p. 294.

162. Gass JDM: Treatment of retinal vascular anomalies. *Trans Am Acad Ophthalmol Otolaryngol* 83:OP432-OP442, 1977.

163. Gautier-Smith PC, Sanders MD, Sanderson KV: Ocular and nervous system involvement in angioma serpiginosum. *Br J Ophthalmol* 55:433-443, 1971.

164. Gislason I, Stenkula S, Alm A, et al: Cavernous haemangioma of the retina. *Acta Ophthalmol* 57:709-717, 1979.

165. Giuffrè G: Cavernous hemangioma of the retina and retinal telangiectasis; distinct or related vascular malformations? *Retina* 5:221-224, 1985.

166. Goldberg RE, Pheasant TR, Shields JA: Cavernous hemangioma of the retina; a four-generation pedigree with neuro-cutaneous manifestations and an example of bilateral retinal involvement. *Arch Ophthalmol* 97:2321-2324, 1979.

167. Haller JA, Knox DL: Vitrectomy for persistent vitreous hemorrhage from a cavernous hemangioma of the optic disk. *Am J Ophthalmol* 116:106-107, 1993.

168. Hassler W, Zentner J, Wilhelm H: Cavernous angiomas of the anterior visual pathways. *J Clin Neuro-Ophthalmol* 9:160-164, 1989.

169. Hogan MJ, Zimmerman LE: *Ophthalmic pathology; an atlas and textbook,* ed. 2, Philadelphia, 1962, WB Saunders, p. 533.

170. Klein M, Goldberg MF, Cotlier E: Cavernous hemangioma of the retina: report of four cases. *Ann Ophthalmol* 7:1213-1221, 1975.

171. Krause U: A case of cavernous haemangioma of the retina. *Acta Ophthalmol* 49:221-231, 1971.

172. Lewis RA, Cohen MH, Wise GN: Cavernous haemangioma of the retina and optic disc; a report of three cases and a review of the literature. *Br J Ophthalmol* 59:422-434, 1975.

173. Malik S, Cohen BH, Robinson J, et al: Progressive vision loss; a rare manifestation of familial cavernous angiomas. *Arch Neurol* 49:170-173, 1992.

174. Mansour AM, Jampol LM, Hrisomalos NF, Greenwald M: Cavernous hemangioma of the optic disc. *Arch Ophthalmol* 106:22, 1988.

175. McCormick WF, Hardman JM, Boulter TR: Vascular malformations ("angiomas") of the brain, with special reference to those occurring in the posterior fossa. *J Neurosurg* 28:241-251, 1968.

176. Messmer E, Font RL, Laqua H, et al: Cavernous hemangioma of the retina; immunohistochemical and ultrastructural observations. *Arch Ophthalmol* 102:413-418, 1984.

177. Messmer E, Laqua H, Wessing A, et al: Nine cases of cavernous hemangioma of the retina. *Am J Ophthalmol* 95:383-390, 1983.

178. Neame H: Angiomatosis retinae, with report of pathological examination. *Br J Ophthalmol* 32:677-689, 1948.

179. Niccol W, Moore RF: A case of angiomatosis retinae. *Br J Ophthalmol* 18:454-457, 1934.

180. Pancurak J, Goldberg MF, Frenkel M, Crowell RM: Cavernous hemangioma of the retina; genetic and central nervous system involvement. *Retina* 5:215-220, 1985.

181. Roberson GH, Kase CS, Wolpow ER: Telangiectases and cavernous angiomas of the brainstem: "Cryptic" vascular malformations; a report of a case. *Neuroradiology* 8:83-89, 1974.

182. Schwartz AC, Weaver RG Jr, Bloomfield R, Tyler ME: Cavernous hemangioma of the retina, cutaneous angiomas, and intracranial vascular lesion by computed tomography and nuclear magnetic resonance imaging. *Am J Ophthalmol* 98:483-487, 1984.

183. Simard JM, Garcia-Bengochea F, Ballinger WE Jr, et al: Cavernous angioma: A review of 126 collected and 12 new cases. *Neurosurgery* 18:162-172, 1986.

184. Spencer WH: Primary neoplasms of the optic nerve and its sheaths: clinical features and current concepts of pathogenetic mechanisms. *Trans Am Ophthalmol Soc* 70:490-528, 1972.

185. Turut P, François P: Hémangiome caverneux de la rétine. *J Fr Ophtalmol* 2:393-404, 1979.

186. Voigt K, Yasargil MG: Cerebral cavernous haemangiomas or cavernomas; incidence, pathology, localization, diagnosis, clinical features and treatment; review of the literature and report of an unusual case. *Neurochirurgia* 19:59-68, 1976.

187. Wallner EF Jr, Moorman LT: Hemangioma of the optic disc. *Arch Ophthalmol* 53:115-117, 1955.

188. Weskamp C, Cotlier I: Angioma del cerebro y de la retina con malformaciones capilares de la piel. *Arch Oftalmol Buenos Aires* 15:1-10. 1940.

189. Yen M-Y, Wu C-C: Cavernous hemangioma of the retina and agenesis of internal carotid artery with bilateral oculomotor palsies. *J Clin Neuro-Ophthalmol* 5:258-262, 1985.

Retina and Optic Disc Capillary Hemangiomas

190. Amoils SP, Smith TR: Cryotherapy of angiomatosis retinae. *Arch Ophthalmol* 81:689-691, 1969.

191. Annesley WH Jr, Leonard BC, Shields JA, Tasman WS: Fifteen year review of treated cases of retinal angiomatosis. *Trans Am Acad Ophthalmol Otolaryngol* 83:OP446-OP453, 1977.

192. Apple DJ, Goldberg MF, Wyhinny GJ: Argon laser treatment of von Hippel-Lindau retinal angiomas. II. Histopathology of treated lesions. *Arch Ophthalmol* 92:126-130, 1974.

193. Benson M, Mody C, Rennie I, Talbot J: Haemangioma of the optic disc. *Graefes Arch Clin Exp Ophthalmol* 228:332-334, 1990.

194. Blodi CF, Russell SR, Pulido JS, Folk JC: Direct and feeder vessel photocoagulation of retinal angiomas with dye yellow laser. *Ophthalmology* 97:791-795, 1990.

195. Campochiaro PA, Conway BP: Hemangiomalike masses of the retina. *Arch Ophthalmol* 106:1409-1413, 1988.

196. Cardosa RD, Brockhurst RJ: Perforating diathermy coagulation for retinal angiomas. *Arch Ophthalmol* 94:1702-1715, 1976.

197. Dabezies OH, Walsh FB, Hayes GJ: Papilledema with hamartoma of hypothalmus. *Arch Ophthalmol* 65:174-180, 1961.

198. Darr JL, Hughes RP Jr, McNair JN: Bilateral peripapillary retinal hemangiomas; a case report. *Arch Ophthalmol* 75:77-81, 1966.

199. de Jong PTVM, Verkaart RJF, van de Vooren MJ, et al: Twin vessels in von Hippel-Lindau disease. *Am J Ophthalmol* 105:165-169, 1988.

200. De Laey JJ, Heintz B, Pollet L: Retinal angioma and juvenile sex-linked retinoschisis. *Ophthalmic Paediatr Genet* 13:73-76, 1992.

201. Fritch CD: Multiple carcinomatosis and von Hippel-Lindau disease requiring bilateral nephrectomy. *Ann Ophthalmol* 12:1307-1309, 1980.

202. Gass JDM: *Differential diagnosis of intraocular tumors; a stereoscopic presentation,* St. Louis, 1974, CV Mosby, p. 265.

203. Gass JDM: Photocoagulation of macular lesions. *Trans Am Acad Ophthalmol Otolaryngol* 75:580-608, 1971.

204. Gass JDM: Treatment of retinal vascular anomalies. *Trans Am Acad Ophthalmol Otolaryngol* 83:OP432-OP442, 1977.

205. Gass JDM, Braunstein R: Sessile and exophytic capillary angiomas of the juxtapapillary retina and optic nerve head. *Arch Ophthalmol* 98:1790-1797, 1980.

206. Goldberg MF, Duke JR: von Hippel-Lindau disease; histopathologic findings in a treated and an untreated eye. *Am J Ophthalmol* 66:693-705, 1968.

207. Goldberg MF, Koenig S: Argon laser treatment of von Hippel-Lindau retinal angiomas. I. Clinical and angiographic findings. *Arch Ophthalmol* 92:121-125, 1974.

208. Gottlieb F, Fammartino JJ, Stratford TP, Brockhurst RJ: Retinal angiomatous mass; a complication of retinal detachment surgery. *Retina* 4:152-157, 1984.

209. Grossniklaus HE, Thomas JW, Vigneswaran N, Jarrett WH III: Retinal hemangioblastoma; a histologic, immunohistochemical, and ultrastructural evaluation. *Ophthalmology* 99:140-145, 1992.

210. Hagler WS, Hyman BN, Waters WC III: von Hippel's angiomatosis retinae and pheochromocytoma. *Trans Am Acad Ophthalmol Otolaryngol* 75:1022-1034, 1971.

211. Haining WM, Zweifach PH: Fluorescein angiography in von Hippel-Lindau disease. *Arch Ophthalmol* 78:475-479, 1967.

212. Hardwig T, Robertson DM: von Hippel-Lindau disease: A familial, often lethal, multi-system phakomatosis. *Ophthalmology* 91:263-270, 1984.

213. Hippel E von: Über eine sehr seltene Erkrankung der Natzhaut; Klinische Beobachtungen. *Albrecht von Graefes Arch Ophthalmol* 59:83-106, 1904.

214. Imes RK, Monteiro MLR, Hoyt WF: Incipient hemangioblastoma of the optic disk. *Am J Ophthalmol* 98:116, 1984.

215. Jakobiec FA, Font RL, Johnson FB: Angiomatosis retinae: an ultrastructural study and lipid analysis. *Cancer* 38:2042-2056, 1976.

216. Jesberg DO, Spencer WH, Hoyt WF: Incipient lesions of von Hippel-Lindau disease. *Arch Ophthalmol* 80:632-640, 1968.

217. Johnson MW, Flynn HW Jr, Gass JDM: Pars plana vitrectomy and direct diathermy for complications of multiple retinal angiomas. *Ophthalmic Surg* 23:47-50, 1992.

218. Laatikainen L, Immonen I, Summanen P: Peripheral retinal angiomalike lesion and macular pucker. *Am J Ophthalmol* 108:563-566, 1989.

219. Lindau A: Studien über Kleinhirncysten; Bau, Pathogenese und Beziehungen zur Angiomatosis Retinae. *Acta Pathol Microbiol Scand Suppl* 1, 1926, p. 77.

220. Lindau A: Zur Frage der Angiomatosis retinae und ihrer Hirnkomplikationen. *Acta Ophthalmol* 4:193-226, 1926.

221. Machemer R, Williams JM Sr: Pathogenesis and therapy of traction detachment in various retinal vascular diseases. *Am J Ophthalmol* 105:170-181, 1988.

222. Magnússon L, Törnquist R: Incipient lesions in angiomatosis retinae. *Acta Ophthalmol* 51:152-158, 1973.

223. Maher ER, Moore AT: von Hippel-Lindau disease. *Br J Ophthalmol* 76:743-745, 1992.

224. Medlock RD, Shields JA, Shields CL, et al: Retinal hemangioma-like lesions in eyes with retinitis pigmentosa. *Retina* 10:274-277, 1990.

225. Melmon KL, Rosen SW: Lindau's disease; review of the literature and study of a large kindred. *Am J Med* 36:595-617, 1964.

226. Mottow-Lippa L, Tso MOM, Peyman GA, Chejfec G: von Hippel angiomatosis; a light, electron microscopic, and immunoperoxidase characterization. *Ophthalmology* 90:848-855, 1983.

227. Nerad JA, Kersten RC, Anderson RL: Hemangioblastoma of the optic nerve; report of a case and review of literature. *Ophthalmology* 95:398-402, 1988.

228. Nicholson DH, Anderson LS, Blodi C: Rhegmatogenous retinal detachment in angiomatosis retinae. *Am J Ophthalmol* 101:187-189, 1986.

229. Nicholson DH, Green WR, Kenyon KR: Light and electron microscopic study of early lesions in angiomatosis retinae. *Am J Ophthalmol* 82:193-204, 1976.

230. Oosterhuis JA, Rubinstein K: Haemangioma at the optic disc. *Ophthalmologica* 164:362-374, 1972.

231. Peyman GA, Rednam KRV, Mottow-Lippa L, Flood T: Treatment of large von Hippel tumors by eye wall resection. *Ophthalmology* 90:840-847, 1983.

231a. Retsas C, Sarks J, Shanahan J: Angiomatose rétinienne associée á une maladie de Stargardt. A pros d'un cas clique. *J Fr Ophtalmol* 12:857-862, 1989.

232. Ridley M, Green J, Johnson G: Retinal angiomatosis: the ocular manifestations of von Hippel-Lindau disease. *Can J Ophthalmol* 21:276-283, 1986.

233. Salazar FG, Lamiell JM: Early identification of retinal angiomas in a large kindred with von Hippel-Lindau disease. *Am J Ophthalmol* 89:540-545, 1980.

234. Schindler RF, Sarin LK, MacDonald PR: Hemangiomas of the optic disc. *Can J Ophthalmol* 10:305-318, 1975.

235. Schmidt D, Neumann HPH: Atypische retinale Veränderungen bei v. Hippel-Lindau-Syndrom. *Fortschr Ophthalmol* 84:187-189, 1987.

236. Schmidt D, Neumann HPH, Witschel H: Mikroläsionen der Retina bei Patienten mit v. Hippel-Lindau-Syndrom. *Fortschr Ophthalmol* 83:233-235, 1986.

237. Schwartz PL, Fastenberg DM, Shakin JL: Management of macular puckers associated with retinal angiomas. *Ophthalmic Surg* 21:550-556, 1990.

238. Schwartz PL, Trubowitsch G, Fastenberg DM, Stein M: Macular pucker and retinal angioma. *Ophthalmic Surg* 18:677-679, 1987.

239. Seizinger BR, Rouleau GA, Ozelius LJ, et al: von Hippel-Lindau disease maps to the region of chromosome 3 associated with renal cell carcinoma. *Nature* 332:268-269, 1988.

240. Souders BF: Juxtapapillary hemangioendothelioma of the retina; report of a case. *Arch Ophthalmol* 41:178-182, 1949.

241. Takahashi T, Wada H, Tani E, et al: Capillary hemangioma of the optic disc. *J Clin Neuro-Ophthalmol* 4:159-162, 1984.

242. Thomas JV, Schwartz PL, Gragoudas ES: Von Hippel's disease in association with von Recklinghausen's neurofibromatosis. *Br J Ophthalmol* 62:604-608, 1978.

243. Watzke RC: Cryotherapy for retinal angiomatosis; a clinicopathologic report. *Arch Ophthalmol* 92:399-401, 1974.

244. Watzke RC, Weingeist TA, Constantine JB: Diagnosis and management of von Hippel-Lindau disease. *In:* Peyman GA, Apple DJ, Sanders DR, editors: *Intraocular tumors,* New York, 1977, Appleton-Century-Crofts, pp. 199-217.

245. Welch RB: von Hippel-Lindau disease: The recognition and treatment of early angiomatosis retinae and the use of cryosurgery as an adjunct to therapy. *Trans Am Ophthalmol Soc* 68:367-424, 1970.

246. Whitson JT, Welch RB, Green WR: Von Hippel-Lindau disease: case report of a patient with spontaneous regression of a retinal angioma. *Retina* 6:253-259, 1986.

247. Wing GL, Weiter JJ, Kelly PJ, et al: von Hippel-Lindau disease; angiomatosis of the retina and central nervous system. *Ophthalmology* 88:1311-1314, 1981.

248. Yimoyines DJ, Topilow HW, Abedin S, McMeel JW: Bilateral peripapillary exophytic retinal hemangioblastomas. *Ophthalmology* 89:1388-1392, 1982.

11

Neoplastic Diseases of the Retina and Optic Disc

▼ RETINOBLASTOMA

Infants and young children with strabismus, leukocoria, and occasionally heterochromia irides may present with visual loss caused by one or more retinoblastomas (Fig. 11-1, *A*).* The diagnosis of retinoblastoma is made in 90% of patients before 5 years of age.[37] Approximately 200 cases occur each year in the United States.[14] Bilateral involvement occurs in 20% to 35% of cases. Second-eye involvement is delayed in approximately 20% to 25% of cases. The mean age of diagnosis is 13 months for those with bilateral retinoblastoma versus a mean age of 24 months in those with unilateral retinoblastoma.[41] Retinoblastomas are typically globular, white, usually well-circumscribed tumors that may arise anywhere in the fundus (Fig. 11-1, *B* and *C*). They may grow inward toward the vitreous (endophytic) or outward (exophytic) into the subretinal space and may or may not be associated with ophthalmoscopic evidence of focal areas of calcification (Fig. 11-1, *J*). Varying degrees of vascularization of the tumor occur, and this is usually seen best with fluorescein angiography (Fig. 11-1, *D, E, K,* and *L*).[20,35,51] Telangiectasis of the retinal vessels on the surface of exophytic tumors may occur. Biomicroscopic and angiographic evidence of communication of these dilated vessels with blood vessels extending into the depth of the tumor serves to differentiate retinoblastomas from primary retinal telangiectasis associated with underlying exudative detachment (Coats' syndrome) (Fig. 11-1, *A* to *E*).[20] Seeding of the tumor along the inner retinal surface and into the vitreous occurs frequently in advanced cases (Fig. 11-1, *G* to *I*). Extension of retinoblastoma into the anterior chamber may occur.[22] As many as 80% of eyes containing retinoblastoma have calcification demonstrable by ultrasound, roentgenography, or scans. Computerized tomography (CT) is superior to magnetic resonance imaging (MRI) in detecting calcification.[30] However, MRI is superior to CT scan in defining anatomic differences in pseudoglioma and in detecting extraocular extension of the tumor.[30]

Diffuse infiltrating retinoblastoma is an unusual type of retinoblastoma (1.5% of cases). It may simulate uveitis, is unassociated with formation of a discrete mass, and may be accompanied by

---

*References 1, 3, 4, 6, 9-12, 14, 16-21, 23, 24, 35, 37, 38, 40, 42, 47, 49, 51, 59, 60.

FIG. 11-1 Retinoblastoma.

A, Heterochromia irides, the presenting manifestation of retinoblastoma, in the right eye of this infant.

B to F, Large exophytic retinoblastoma. Note dilated tortuous retinal vessels that extend down into the substance of the tumor (**B** and **C**) and angiographic evidence of staining (**D** and **E**). Large blood vessels (*arrows*) were evident histopathologically near the surface of the tumor (**F**).

G to I, Multiple white tumor seeds were evident on the retinal surface posteriorly in this child with a peripherally located retinoblastoma. They showed no angiographic evidence of blood vessels (*arrows,* **H**). Note the necrotic center of the tumor seeds (*arrow*) evident histopathologically (**I**).

J to L, Small retinoblastoma or retinoma showing calcification (*arrow,* **J**) in a 4-year-old Indian child who had enucleation of his left eye 1 month before examination. Histopathologic examination of that eye revealed retinoblastoma with invasion of the optic nerve. He was referred for treatment of this solitary lesion noted in the right eye. He had a 6-year-old brother who had an enucleation of one eye at 6 months of age. His mother (Fig. 11-2, **A** to **E**) had a retinoma. Fluorescein angiography revealed a fine capillary network within and immediately surrounding the tumor (**K** and **L**). There was extensive leakage of dye from these vessels. This patient died of widespread metastasis several months later. The clinical and angiographic appearance of this solitary nodule is quite similar to that of retinal astrocytic hamartomas (see Fig. 10-14) and retinoma (Fig. 11-2, *F* and *G*).

---

a pseudohypopyon.[8,52] Computerized tomography and ultrasonography are of limited value in diagnosis of diffuse retinoblastoma. Other features of this form of retinoblastoma are older average age of presentation (6 years, compared to 13 to 24 months); slight male predominance (64%); all reported cases have been unilateral and none has been familial; and anterior chamber paracentesis is helpful in making the diagnosis. A few patients with extensive involvement of the retina may develop orbital cellulitis that is not necessarily associated with extraocular extension of the tumor.[57]

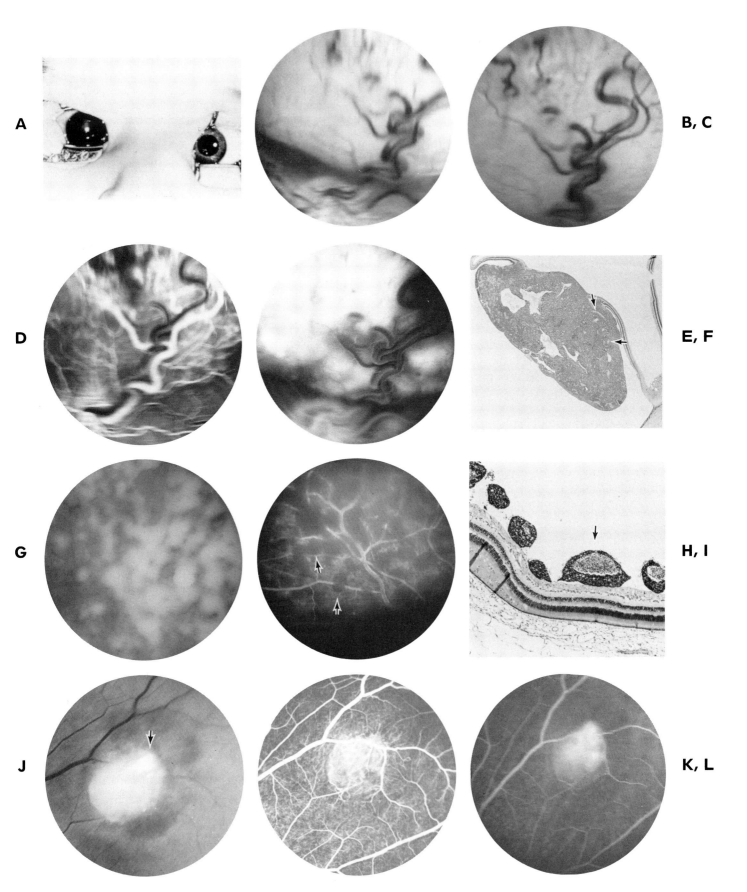

A

B, C

D

E, F

G

H, I

J

K, L

869

Although most patients with retinoblastoma present as young children, retinoblastoma has been reported in patients as old as 60 years.[59] Maximum survival rates for both unilateral and bilateral retinoblastoma occur when the diagnosis is made after 7 years of age (96% survival).[2,46] Survival is poorest when diagnosis occurs between years 2 and 7 (81% survival) and intermediate when diagnosis occurs between birth and 2 years of age.[2] Retinoblastoma, when it kills, almost always does so within 5 years of enucleation. Risk factors include invasion of optic nerve and orbit, histologic evidence of cataract, delay in the diagnosis of retinoblastoma, and bilaterality.[25]

The differential diagnosis in patients with localized white retinal tumors includes retinomas (Fig. 11-2), astrocytic hamartomas (see Fig. 10-16), *Toxocara canis* granuloma (see Fig. 3-49), and combined pigment epithelial and retinal hamartomas (see Fig. 10-11).[54] In patients with large tumors and leukocoria, the differential diagnosis includes retinal telangiectasis (Coats' syndrome), *Toxocara canis,* retinopathy of prematurity, familial exudative vitreoretinopathy, persistent hyperplastic primary vitreous, retinal dysplasia, traumatic chorioretinopathy, calcified intraocular abscess, and incontinentia pigmenti.[23,40,53,54] Detection of abnormal levels of lactate dehydrogenase and enolase in the aqueous humor of patients with retinoblastoma may be of some help in the differential diagnosis of unusual or atypical cases.[1,5,8,53]

FIG. 11-2   Retinomas.

A to **E,** This asymptomatic 23-year-old mother of the patient illustrated in Figure 11-1, *J* to *L,* had three retinomas (**A** to **C**). The one in the right macula had club-shaped calcified opacities (*arrow,* **A**) within the zone of atrophic retina. Angiography showed perfusion of a network of retinal vessels and underlying large choroidal vessels in the area of the lesion (**D**). There was some staining of the periphery of the lesion (**E**).

F, Probable retinoma or astrocytic hamartoma in an asymptomatic 4-year-old child with no other ocular abnormalities and a negative family history.

G to **I,** Retinoma with calcification (*arrow,* **G**) in a 21-year-old asymptomatic mother who had a child with bilateral retinoblastomas. Note the "fish-flesh" tumor (**G**) and the rich vascular network and localized staining evident angiographically (**H** and **I**).

(**F** courtesy Dr. Bernard H. Doft.)

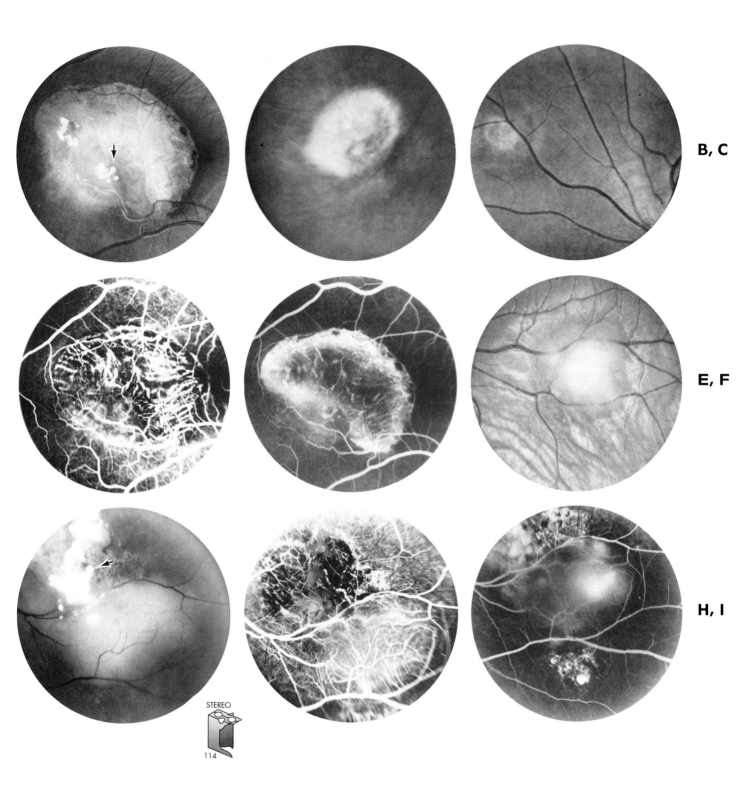

B, C

E, F

STEREO
114

H, I

Previously, enucleation was the treatment of choice in patients with uniocular involvement. In patients with bilateral retinoblastoma, the eye with greatest involvement was usually enucleated and the less involved eye was treated with irradiation (external beam and episcleral plaques), cryopexy, or photocoagulation. These latter forms of therapy are now being used in selected patients with uniocular involvement and small to medium-sized tumors.* The visual results following external beam irradiation treatment of retinoblastomas involving the macular have been favorable but are dependent upon the tumor size and proximity to the center of the fovea.[26,63] Although the overall mortality of patients with retinoblastoma is 15% to 16%, nearly all of these deaths occur in patients with advanced type IV or V involvement.[24] Direct spread of the tumor via the optic nerve is the most important cause of death. Experimental evidence suggests that vitamin D may prove to be an effective chemotherapeutic agent against retinoblastoma.[13]

---

*References 3, 6, 9, 43-45, 48, 50, 55, 56, 63.

In approximately one-third of cases, retinoblastoma is heritable with an autosomal dominant pattern.[10,17,19] Forty percent to 50% of the offspring of these patients with retinoblastoma will develop retinoblastoma (Fig. 11-1, *J* to *L*). Only 20% of the heritable cases will have a positive family history. Most heritable cases arise as a mutation. The retinoblastoma gene can be identified if the patient has bilateral retinoblastoma or if he or she has other affected family members. In 1% to 2% of retinoblastoma patients, the retinoblastoma gene is associated with the deletion of chromosome 13q14. A retinoma ("spontaneously regressed retinoblastoma") or phthisis bulbi occurring in a patient with other evidence of retinoblastoma are clinical signs that suggest the presence of a retinoblastoma gene (Fig. 11-2).[18,19] Hereditary cases usually have bilateral retinoblastomas. The presence of multiple retinomas in a single individual or a single retinoma in a patient with relatives with retinoblastoma implies gene carrier status for those individuals and puts their children at approximately 50% risk of tumor development. The gene for RB predisposition (RB 1) has been mapped to chromosome region 13q14.[36] Genetic linkage analysis has confirmed that the hereditary nondeletion form of the disease results from mutations on the same locus. Linkage analysis in retinoblastoma families is important in detecting the hereditary nature of RB in families with low penetrance.[36,64]

Retinomas, formerly called spontaneously regressed retinoblastomas, are semitranslucent, "fish-flesh" retinal tumors associated with "cottage cheese" calcification and RPE disturbances (Fig. 11-2).[4,22,59] Retinoma was suggested as the name for these benign tumors resulting from an incomplete mutation.[18,19] Approximately two-thirds of patients with a retinoma will have retinoblastoma in the fellow eye or have a family history of retinoblastoma. Approximately 50% of their offspring will develop retinoblastoma. Malignant transformation of a retinoma has occurred.[15] Fluorescein angiography reveals evidence of a vascular network within retinomas and some evidence of dye leakage (Fig. 11-2, *D, E, H,* and *I*).[19,20,35] There is often evidence of RPE and choriocapillaris atrophy in the area of the retinoma (Fig. 11-2, *D*). Anastomosis between the retinal and choroidal vessels may occur.[19] Histopathologically, retinomas are composed of differentiated neural elements and not the classic retinoblastoma cell.[59] Ophthalmoscopically retinomas appear identical to so-called regressed retinoblastoma following irradiation treatment. It has been suggested that this portion of the tumor remaining after treatment may be the result of a coexistent retinoma.[18,19] The overall cumulative 5-year survival rate for patients with retinoblastoma is approximately 90%.[43,61] The chance of survival after treatment of retinoblastoma is directly related to the degree of invasion of the optic nerve as determined by histopathologic examination of the affected eye.[31,32] Approximately 30% of eyes enucleated for retinoblastoma have evidence of optic nerve invasion that is graded as follows: grade I, superficial invasion; grade II, extension to cribriform plate; grade III, beyond the cribriform plate; grade IV, up to and including the surgical margin. The respective mortality rates for each of the grades are 10%, 29%, 42%, and 78%.[31] Grade of involvement of the optic nerve and age at time of diagnosis have been shown by multivariate analysis to be factors significantly associated with survival. Choroidal invasion may also be a risk factor.[31,32]

The rate of recurrence and development of new tumors after treatment may be as high as 40% in patients with hereditary retinoblastoma.[33] Nearly all recurrences occur within the first 2 years after treatment.

Some patients with heritable retinoblastoma may develop an associated pinealoma (RB-P).[27,29,34] Ninety-five percent of RB-P patients have bilateral retinoblastomas and in most cases the disease is fatal. Most of the patients present with symptoms of increased intracranial pressure caused by obstructive hydrocephalus.

Patients with the retinoblastoma gene have a high incidence of development of other cancers with a mean latent period of 10 years.[28,39,62] The reported incidence of these second tumors has varied: 4% to 20% in 10 years, 14% to 50% in 20 years, and 14% to 90% in 30 years. In one study, the 30-year cumulative incidence was 35.1% for patients who received irradiation therapy compared to an incidence rate of 5.8% for those who did not receive irradiation.[39] The 30-year incidence rate of second tumors was 29.3% within the field of irradiation and 8.1% outside the field. The rate outside the field was the same as nonirradiated patients (5.8%). These findings indicate that carriers of the RB gene have an increased incidence of second tumors, and that the incidence rate is further increased in patients who receive irradiation therapy. Attempts are now in progress to identify and characterize the oncogene for retinoblastoma.[7]

▼ LEUKEMIC CHORIORETINOPATHY AND OPTIC NEUROPATHY

Loss of central vision in patients with either acute or chronic leukemia may be caused either by direct leukemic invasion of the uveal tract, retina, vitreous, or optic nerve or by other associated hematologic abnormalities, including anemia and hyperviscosity or a combination of both.

Leukemic choroidopathy

Postmortem eyes of patients with leukemia demonstrate histopathologically a mild leukemic infiltration of the uveal tract, but most do not show ophthalmoscopic evidence of choroidal involvement during life. In some patients, however, the infiltrate becomes sufficiently intense to cause damage to the overlying RPE and serous retinal detachment.[65-68,70-72,74,86,114] Detachment of the retinal pigment epithelium may also occur.[73] The clinical picture may be mistaken for central serous chorioretinopathy (Fig. 11-3, *A*), or in the case of more widespread retinal detachment, Harada's disease (Fig. 11-3, *D* and *E*). Fluorescein angiography is useful in detecting the areas of RPE damage underlying the serous detachment (Fig. 11-3, *B*, *C*, and *F*). The sites of leakage of dye from the underlying choroid are usually multiple pinpoint areas similar to those seen in Harada's disease and other infiltrative diseases of the choroid. The choroidal infiltrate may occasionally produce a localized or diffuse choroidal tumor. Leukemic tumefactions of the choroid are more frequently associated with acute lymphatic leukemia.

Occasionally, striking leopard-spot changes may occur in the RPE in patients with extensive choroidal involvement with leukemia (Fig. 11-3, *G* to *J*).[67,69,73] It is unclear whether the extensive RPE necrosis and clumping of pigment that occurs in these cases is caused by the leukemic infiltration of the choriocapillaris, chemotherapy, or a combination of both.

FIG. 11-3 Macular Detachment Caused by Leukemic Infiltration of Choroid.

A to **C,** Choroidal tumor and serous detachment of the macula secondary to leukemia in a 59-year-old White woman who developed blurred vision and metamorphopsia in the left eye. Near the temporal margin of the left optic disc there was a moundlike elevation of the choroid and a shallow serous retinal detachment that extended into the macular region (*black and white arrows,* **A**). A small amount of subretinal blood (*black arrow*) was present. Angiography revealed multiple, small, pinpoint areas of diffusion of dye from the surface of the tumor as well as evidence of leakage of dye from the optic nerve capillaries into the subretinal exudate (**B** and **C**). The patient was admitted to the hospital, and bone marrow examination revealed acute myelomonocytic leukemia. The patient died soon afterward.

D to **F,** Bilateral bullous retinal detachment simulating Harada's disease in a 25-year-old patient with acute leukemia (**D** and **E**). His initial medical evaluation revealed leukopenia but no evidence of leukemia. Angiography revealed multiple focal areas of dye leakage from the choroid and later a flagstone pattern of staining beneath the retina (**F**). Although the cause of the peculiar placoid pattern of late fluorescein staining is unknown, its appearance suggests that there were multiple relatively flat areas of detachment of the RPE, which in this patient may have been caused by leukemic infiltration from the choroid into the sub-RPE space. The retinal detachment disappeared after corticosteroid treatment. He died, however, about 6 weeks later, and autopsy revealed myelogenous leukemia.

G to **J,** Peculiar clumping of the pigment epithelium in a 6-year-old patient treated for acute lymphocytic leukemia. He had been treated with vincristine, prednisone, methotrexate, and cyclophosphamide. He developed alopecia and severe visual loss. The visual loss was more noticeable at night than during the day. He died 3 months later and histopathologic examination revealed multiple clumps of RPE cells (*arrow,* **J**) and mild leukemic infiltration of the choroid. It is unknown whether the changes in the RPE were primarily attributable to anoxia secondary to the anemia or leukemic infiltration of the choriocapillaris or to the toxic effects of drugs used in therapy.

(**G** to **J** from Clayman HM et al: *Am J Ophthalmol* 74:416, 1972; published with permission from The American Journal of Ophthalmology; copyright by The Ophthalmic Publishing Co.[67])

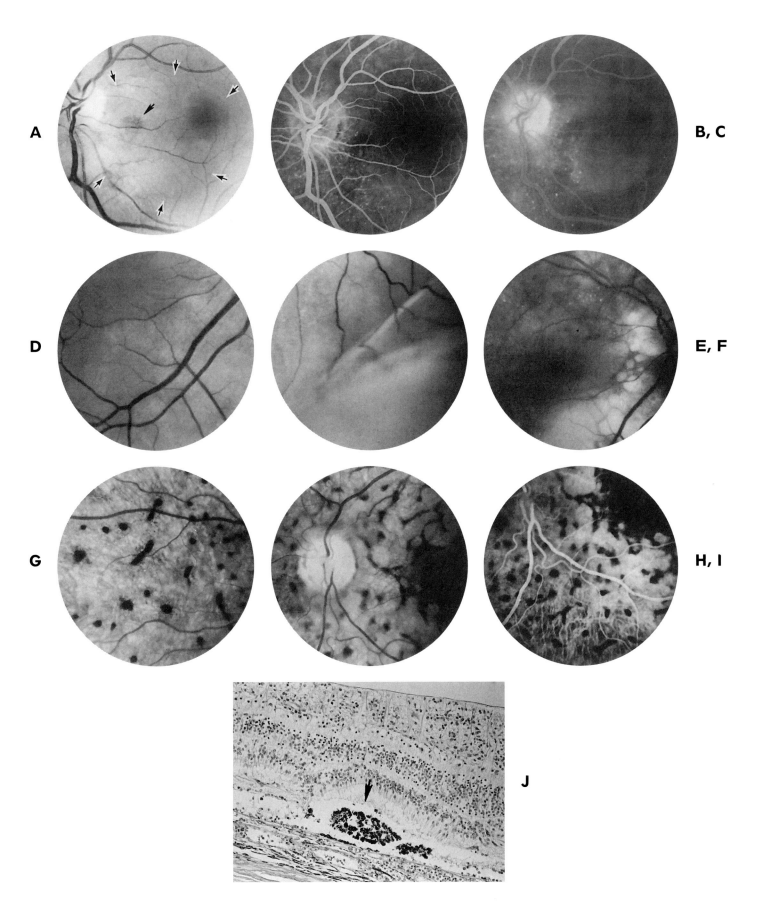

Leukemic retinopathy

The most striking fundus pictures associated with leukemia involve the retina and they typically occur in patients with acute leukemia, frequently during a period of relapse and frequently associated with severe and coexisting anemia (Fig. 11-4).* These patients may develop dilation, tortuosity, and beading of the retinal veins; retinal vascular sheathing; cotton-wool patches; superficial flame-shaped hemorrhages; deep, round hemorrhages; white-centered hemorrhages; and subhyaloid and subinternal limiting membrane hemorrhages (Fig. 11-4). These changes are similar to those seen in patients with severe anemia from any cause as well as dysproteinemias (see Fig. 6-61, *A* to *F*).[88,95,105] Some patients may develop grayish-white nodular leukemic retinal infiltrations and perivascular retinal infiltration (Fig. 11-5).[96,106] Patients, particularly with chronic myelogenous leukemia, may develop peripheral retinal microaneurysms,[83,93] retinal vascular closure,[82,102,112] and retinal and optic disc neovascularization.† Increased blood viscosity and reduced blood flow associated with prolonged and marked leukocytosis[85,99,103] and thrombocytosis[98] are probably the cause of these latter changes. Fluorescein angiography is helpful in detecting these alterations. Leopard-spot retinal pigment epithelial alterations seen in these patients, often during the stage of remission, are probably caused by choroidal infiltration (Fig. 11-3, *G* to *I*).[89,92,97,111] Pigment epithelial and retinal degeneration may occur in one or both eyes and occasionally be accompanied by development of a macular hole.[92,111]

*References 75, 78, 79, 81, 83, 86, 90, 100, 101, 108-110, 113.
†References 82, 85, 98, 99, 103, 109.

FIG. 11-4   Hemorrhagic Retinopathy Associated with Acute Leukemia.

A to **E,** This man with acute myelogenous leukemia developed bilateral loss of vision. Five months later after chemotherapy his vision had improved and there was marked improvement in the retinopathy.

F to **H,** This man with acute lymphatic leukemia experienced bilateral loss of vision. Note the white-centered hemorrhages and superficial retinal hematoma (*arrow,* **G**).

I and **J,** Before death this patient with chronic granulocytic leukemia had extensive perivascular infiltration and nodular white and hemorrhagic masses in the retina. Histopathologic examination of the eyes revealed massive perivascular leukemic infiltration and hemorrhagic nodular leukemic tumefactions lying beneath the internal limiting membrane (*arrow*).

(From Kuwabara T, Aiello L: *Arch Ophthalmol* 72:494, 1964; copyright 1964, American Medical Association.[96])

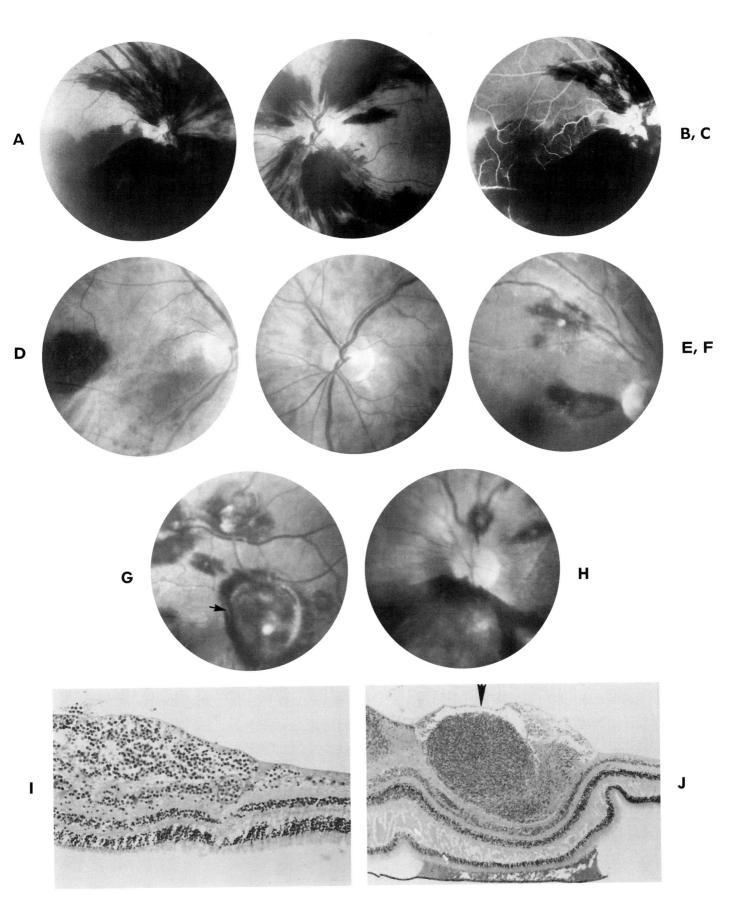

Leukemic optic neuropathy

Acute visual loss may be caused by leukemic invasion of the optic nerve, usually in children with acute lymphocytic leukemia (Fig. 11-5, *A* to *F, K,* and *L*). In some patients the infiltration may be confined to the retrobulbar area or may involve the optic nerve head.[77,84,91,104,108,114] Visual loss in these latter patients may be minimal, and the swollen optic nerve may be mistaken for papilledema associated with increased intracranial pressure (Fig. 11-5, *K*). These patients show a dramatic response to antimetabolite, corticosteroid, or orbital irradiation therapy, which should be instituted promptly after a CT study and lumbar puncture to exclude papilledema.[107] Infiltration of the optic nerve may be associated with occlusion of the central retinal artery and vein.[76,109] Progressive visual loss and optic atrophy may occasionally occur coincident with a worsening of chronic lymphocytic leukemia.[80]

Leukemic infiltration of the vitreous

An occasional patient with acute leukemia may lose vision caused by vitreous cellular infiltration, and vitrectomy may be of value in making the diagnosis as well as improving the vision.[110]

Other unusual causes for visual loss in patients with leukemia include iris infiltration,[94] anterior segment ischemia,[79] open angle glaucoma,[87] and corneal ring ulcer.[113]

FIG. 11-5 Leukemic Infiltration of the Retina and Optic Nerve.

A to **F,** This 6-year-old girl developed lymphocytic leukemia in December of 1966. She was treated with vincristine, prednisone, and methotrexate. Because of visual loss she was seen at the Bascom Palmer Eye Institute on November 8, 1967. Visual acuity in the right eye was finger counting and in the left eye was hand movements. The optic nerve head in both eyes was obscured by a massive cellular infiltration that extended into the retina in the peripapillary region (**A** and **B**). There was pronounced perivenous infiltration. By December 3, 1967, the degree of infiltration in the right eye had improved (**C**). There was further improvement by March 13, 1968 (**D**). On June 11, 1968, her visual acuity had returned to 20/20 in this eye. By November 14, 1968, the patient was quite well and was attending school. Her vision in the right eye was 20/20. Most of the perivascular infiltration had disappeared (**E**). The optic nerve head was pale, and its margins were blurred. The visual acuity in the left eye was 20/200, and there was still evidence of perivascular infiltration (**F**).

G to **J,** Leukemic infiltration of the retina. This 8-year-old girl with acute leukemia developed loss of central vision in the left eye. The optic nerve head was blurred, and there were scattered retinal hemorrhages in the macula and elsewhere in the fundus (**G**). In the periphery there was pronounced perivascular sheathing presumed to be secondary to leukemic infiltration (**H**). Fluorescein angiography revealed dilation and microaneurysmal formation in the retinal capillary bed and widespread leakage of dye from the capillaries and veins (**I** and **J**).

K and **L,** This 6-year-old girl developed leukemic transformation of a lymphosarcoma of the mediastinum. In June of 1970 she was treated with a regimen of vincristine, methotrexate, and prednisone. Remission was achieved, but by September the child developed signs and symptoms of central nervous system involvement. Intrathecal methotrexate was given on September 1, 1970. On September 10, 1970, her vision in the right eye was light perception with projection and the left eye was 20/20. The right optic nerve head and peripapillary retina (**K**) were swollen and white in color. This was presumed to be related to leukemic infiltration. The optic disc in the left eye was normal. A subconjunctival injection of triamcinolone was given, and a course of oral prednisone, 20 mg three times per day, was begun. On October 15, 1970 visual acuity was 20/20 in each eye. The swelling of the right optic disc had largely disappeared (**L**). There was loss of pigment from the RPE associated with multiple black clumps of pigment surrounding the optic disc. Her general condition deteriorated, and she died on December 27, 1970.

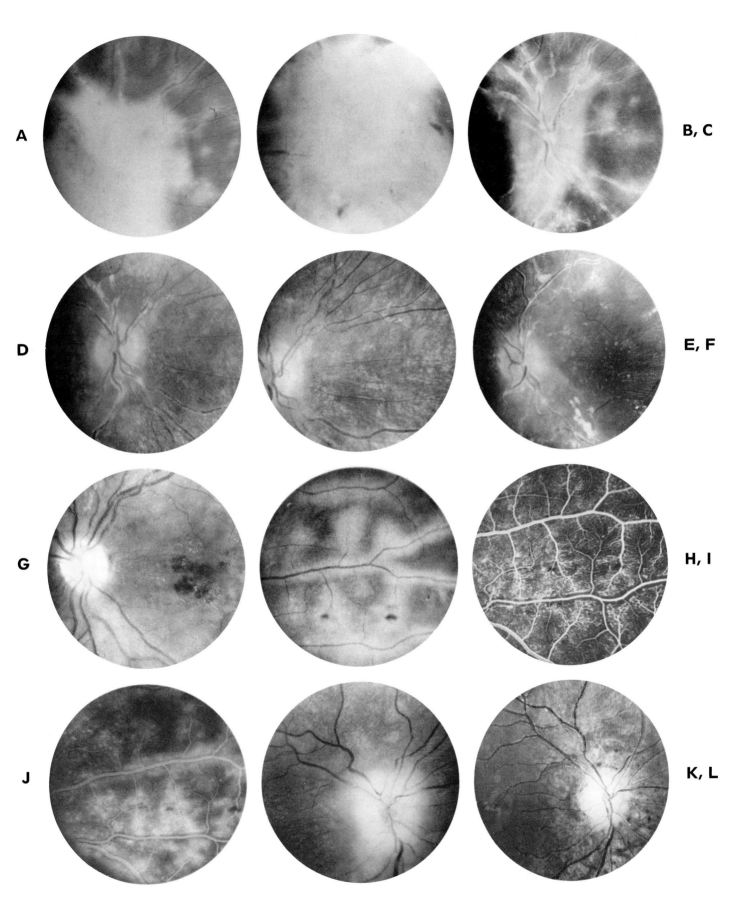

A

B, C

D

E, F

G

H, I

J

K, L

▼ RETINAL AND UVEAL TRACT INVOLVEMENT WITH THE LYMPHOMAS

The classification of lymphomas is in a constant state of flux. For purposes of this presentation, lymphomas will be subdivided as follows: (1) Hodgkin's lymphoma, (2) large-cell non-Hodgkin's lymphoma, (3) neoplastic angioendotheliomatosis, (4) lymphocytic lymphoma, (5) Burkitt's lymphoma, (6) mycosis fungoides, (7) multiple myeloma, and (8) lymphoid granulomatosis. Benign reactive lymphoid hyperplasia of the uveal tract, considered by some to be a low-grade lymphoma, is discussed in Chapter 3, p. 184.

Hodgkin's disease

Hodgkin's disease is a lymphoma that involves lymph nodes and lymphatics early and other organ systems later. Ocular involvement is infrequent and only rarely has been confirmed histopathologically.[115-117]

Large-cell non-Hodgkin's lymphoma (reticulum cell sarcoma, histiocytic lymphoma)

Large-cell non-Hodgkin's lymphoma was previously considered a relatively rare cause for ocular morbidity. There is abundant evidence, however, that the incidence of this tumor is increasing.[131] Only part of this increase can be explained on the basis of the increase in the number of immunosuppressed patients with organ transplants and with acquired immune deficiency syndrome.* There are two major subgroups of large-cell non-Hodgkin's lymphoma. The most common is the ocular–CNS type, in which the lymphoma is confined to the eye and central nervous system.† The other systemic type occurs less commonly, and the eye and central nervous system are infrequently affected.[130]

The ocular–central nervous system form of large-cell non-Hodgkin's lymphoma

The lymphoma cells in the ocular–central nervous system form of the disease appear to arise primarily in the vitreous and in the sub-RPE space and only secondarily extend into the retina and choroid.[134,135] Patients are usually in the sixth to seventh decade of life when they present to the ophthalmologist with a wide variety of clinical pictures that may simulate many ocular disorders (Figs. 11-6, 11-7, and 11-8). Young adults and chil-

---

*References 89, 118, 136, 143, 145, 155, 163, 166, 175.
†References 119, 120, 122, 124, 125, 128, 131, 134, 148, 149, 159, 161, 164, 169-171, 173, 175.

FIG. 11-6 Diagram Illustrating the Pathologic Anatomy Underlying the Variety of Clinical Pictures Caused by the Ocular–CNS Form of Large-Cell Non-Hodgkin's Lymphoma.

Lymphoma cells infiltrate the vitreous (*small arrow,* **A**) and the sub-RPE space and produce initially small placoid lesions simulating multiple evanescent white dot syndrome, slightly elevated lesions (**B**) simulating multifocal choroiditis, or larger sub-RPE masses (**C**) that are pathognomonic for non-Hodgkin's lymphoma. Invasion of the overlying retina (**E**) produces white lesions simulating acute retinitis, and ischemic retina infarction. As these retinal lesions expand they may invade and occlude retinal vessels and produce a clinical picture of acute retinal necrosis. Spontaneous necrosis and resolution of the lymphoma may occur early (**D**), and produce multifocal chorioretinal scars simulating the presumed ocular histoplasmosis syndrome, or later (**F**), and cause large geographic areas or diffuse areas of RPE atrophy simulating degenerative and postinflammatory scarring.

dren are occasionally affected.[172] The ocular–CNS form of large-cell lymphoma most frequently masquerades as posterior uveitis in patients complaining of floaters caused by the vitreous infiltration with lymphomatous and inflammatory cells. Most of the patients with vitreous infiltration will soon afterward develop multiple fundus lesions, which initially may be nonelevated and appear similar to multifocal choroiditis (Fig. 11-8, *G*) or multiple evanescent white dot syndrome (Fig. 11-8, *A*), but which typically enlarge to form solitary, sharply defined, blisterlike, yellowish-white sub-RPE tumors that are usually sufficiently characteristic to permit an accurate diagnosis (Figs. 11-6, *C*; 11-7; and 11-8, *B*).[134,135,138,139] The fine speckling of pigment on the surface of these amelanotic subretinal mounds is the biomicroscopic clue to the sub-RPE location of the tumors, which may be confluent and massive in size. The tumor may extend through the RPE into the overlying sensory retina and vitreous, where it produces a localized white lesion that may simulate that of acute retinitis (Figs. 11-6, *E*; 11-7, *I;* and 11-8, *G* and *H*). Infiltration of the major retinal vessels may cause a fundus picture of branch arterial occlusion (Fig. 11-8, *G* to *L*), and hemorrhagic infarction of the retina simulating that seen in acute retinal necrosis caused by the herpetic viruses.[136,161] An occasional patient presents with visual loss caused by lymphomatous infiltration of the retrobulbar portion of the optic nerve simulating retrobulbar neuritis or infiltration of the optic nerve head simulating papillitis.[141,142,147] One or

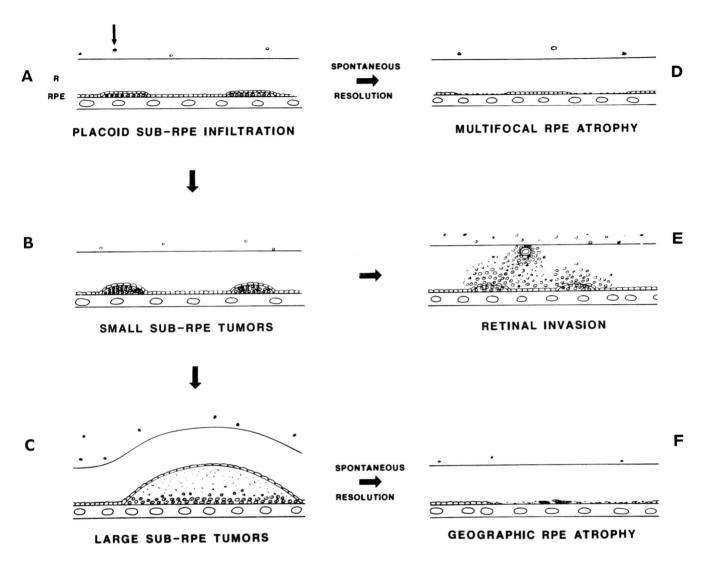

A

R

RPE

PLACOID SUB-RPE INFILTRATION

SPONTANEOUS

RESOLUTION

D

MULTIFOCAL RPE ATROPHY

B

SMALL SUB-RPE TUMORS

E

RETINAL INVASION

C

LARGE SUB-RPE TUMORS

SPONTANEOUS

RESOLUTION

F

GEOGRAPHIC RPE ATROPHY

both eyes may be affected. The disease becomes bilateral in 80% of the cases. There may be a delay of months or several years until involvement of the second eye. Iridocyclitis and secondary glaucoma may occur later in the course of the disease. In some patients there is a remarkable tendency for the subpigment epithelial lesions to resolve spontaneously. When this occurs early multifocal small scars simulating that in the presumed ocular histoplasmosis syndrome occur (Figs. 11-6, *D*, and 11-8, *G*).[153] When large lesions resolve, large foci of geographic atrophy of the pigment epithelium may simulate that seen in degenerative or postinflam-

matory disorders (Figs. 11-6, *F* and 11-7, *E*). When present, the multiple solid RPE masses are virtually pathognomonic for large-cell lymphoma.[135] Ocular signs and symptoms usually antedate those caused by central nervous system involvement.[154] If large-cell lymphoma is suspected the patient should have a general medical evaluation, including neurologic examination, CT or MRI scan, and lumbar puncture. In most cases this evaluation will be negative. Examination of the cerebrospinal fluid in some patients may demonstrate a lymphocytosis but infrequently demonstrates the presence of malignant cells. Vitreous biopsy may be necessary to confirm the diagnosis.* This should be done only when an experienced team for cytologic evaluation of vitreous aspirates is available. Even under the best of circumstances, after obtaining the specimen via a syringe and large-bore needle, proper concentrating and staining of the vitreous cells, and examination by a skilled cytologist, a definitive diagnosis may not be possible. In some patients cytologic examination of the vitreous aspirant may reveal only inflammatory cells.[148] Direct biopsy of the choroid–RPE complex in the area of a visible lesion offers the best chance for a definitive diagnosis but the procedure has a higher morbidity.[150] Cytologic examination is more important than lymphocyte surface markers in arriving at the correct diagnosis of large-cell lymphoma.[123,174] Irregular nuclear contours, lobation of nuclei, coarse irregular chromatin, and the presence of nucleoli are cytologic features of large-cell lymphoma (Fig. 11-7, *J*). Most large-cell lymphomas are of B-cell derivation.[133] Many are polyclonal rather than monoclonal. If the evaluation of the patient reveals evidence of a CNS lesion, biopsy via CT-guided stereotactic needle biopsy is an effective means at arriving at a diagnosis.[128,159] Treatment of CNS lymphoma involves chemotherapy followed by radiation therapy.[128]

---

*References 121, 123, 146, 148, 156-158, 160, 173.

FIG. 11-7   Large-Cell Non-Hodgkin's Lymphoma, Ocular–CNS Type (Reticulum Cell Sarcoma).

A to **H,** This 60-year-old woman was seen in December of 1968 with widespread areas of solid yellow-white detachments of the RPE in her left eye (**A, B,** and **D**). Angiographically these lesions were largely nonfluorescent (**C**). Medical evaluation was negative. These lesions disappeared spontaneously and the patient had 20/20 vision (**E**). When she returned 4 years later there were widespread RPE atrophic changes in the left eye. In the right eye she had the same picture illustrated in the left eye in **D.** Ten weeks later she died after experiencing Jacksonian seizures. Gross examination of the right eye revealed multiple necrotic white tumors beneath the detached RPE (*arrows,* **F**). Note detachment of the thinned and clumped RPE (*upper arrow,* **G**) and liquefactive necrosis of tumor between the RPE and viable tumor lying along the inner surface of Bruch's membrane (*lower arrow,* **G**). Viable reticulum cell sarcoma (*arrow*) was lying along the inner surface of Bruch's membrane (**H**). Note chronic inflammatory cells in the choroid.

I to **K,** Subpigment epithelial reticulum cell sarcoma in a 62-year-old man after vitrectomy. Note tumor (*arrow,* **I**) breaking through the RPE. Vitreous aspirate showed cells with enlarged hyperchromatic indented nuclei and minimal cytoplasm (*arrow,* **J**) characteristic of reticulum cell sarcoma. Resolution of tumor occurred 5 months after external beam irradiation (**K**).

(**A** to **K** from Gass et al.[135])

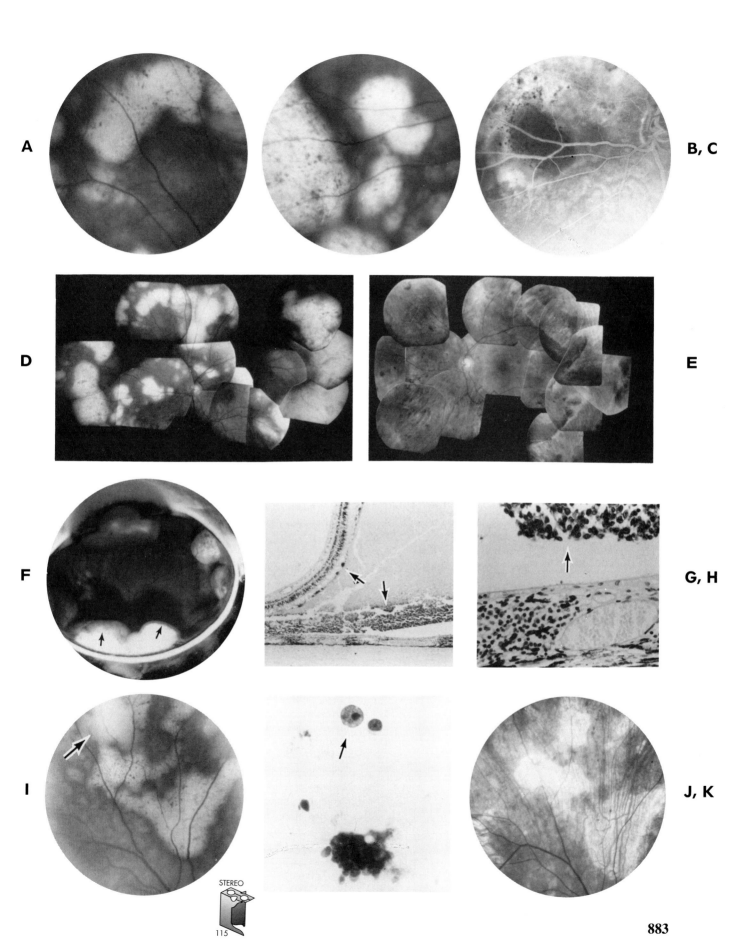

A

B, C

D

E

F

G, H

I

STEREO
115

J, K

883

Histopathologically patients with ocular–CNS large-cell lymphoma typically show multiple areas of lymphomatous infiltration of the sub-RPE space (Fig. 11-7, *F* to *H*).* The large sub-RPE lesions are composed primarily of necrotic tumor that is separated from Bruch's membrane by a thin layer of viable hyperchromatic tumor cells (Fig. 11-7, *F* to *H*). In most patients the uveal tract is free of tumor but is infiltrated with lymphocytes, mostly reactive T lymphocytes, and plasma cells (Fig. 11-7, *H*). In some cases the tumor may extend into the underlying choroid or the overlying retina and vitreous (Fig. 11-8, *G* to *L*). Histopathologic examination of eyes after spontaneous resolution of the lymphoma shows multiple geographic areas of RPE atrophy or placoid disciform scars that may simulate either postinflammatory scars or a diffuse chorioretinal dystrophy.[134,135]

The course of this disease is variable, but some patients may survive 5 years or longer. The ocular lesions in large-cell lymphoma do not respond well to systemic corticosteroids or immunosuppressive therapy. Irradiation, however, usually causes rapid resolution of the sub-RPE infiltration. Prophylactic irradiation of the central nervous system may prolong survival, although nearly all patients eventually die from central nervous system involvement.[125,129,154] The vitreous cellular reaction that is partly inflammatory in nature responds poorly to irradiation, and vitrectomy may be necessary for visual as well as diagnostic purposes before institution of irradiation therapy.

---

*References 120, 134, 135, 139, 158, 168.

FIG. 11-8 Large-Cell Non-Hodgkin's Lymphoma, Ocular–CNS Type (Reticulum Cell Sarcoma).

A to F, This 56-year-old woman note blurred vision and floaters in the right eye. Vitritis and multiple, small, white or gray-white subretinal lesions confined to the right eye were interpreted as multiple evanescent white dot syndrome (*arrows,* **A**). When examined 1 month later her visual acuity was 5/200, right eye, and 20/20, left eye. She had developed a sub-RPE mass (*arrow,* **B**) and a Swiss cheese–like subretinal infiltration in the right eye. Angiography showed evidence of RPE changes centrally as well as staining in the area of the infiltrate. The right eye was normal. The diagnosis was large-cell lymphoma with probable involvement of the retrobulbar optic nerve. Medical evaluation was negative. Four months later the tumor had resolved temporally but had extended nasally (**C**). Repeated evaluations for evidence of lymphoma were negative. She refused vitreous biopsy. The lesions in the right eye resolved spontaneously and over the subsequent 40 months she developed similar lesions in the left eye. Vitreous biopsy was positive for lymphoma. Three years after her onset of symptoms she developed evidence of lymphoma in the brain. She received irradiation treatment to the eyes and brain. When last examined her visual acuity was 20/200, right eye, and 20/400, left eye. There was widespread evidence of degeneration of the RPE but no evidence of tumor in either eye (**E and F**). Five years after her initial visit she was alive and tumor free. Forgetfulness and depression were attributed to postirradiation changes.

G to L, This apparently healthy 71-year-old woman developed a superotemporal branch retinal artery occlusion caused by intraretinal invasion of a sub-RPE lymphoma in the right eye (**G**). At the time of initial presentation she had vitreous cellular infiltration and multiple atrophic chorioretinal scars in the right eye. The left eye was normal except for a single focal scar and lesions in the macula interpreted as drusen. Six weeks later the retinal whitening extended into other quadrants (**H**) and multiple yellow plaques (*arrows*) had developed in the formally occluded retinal artery. Angiographically there was evidence of narrowing of the artery caliber in the area of these plaques (*arrows,* **I**). She subsequently developed the clinical picture of acute retinal necrosis and rubeotic glaucoma in the right eye that was enucleated. Histopathologic examination revealed large mounds of necrotic lymphoma beneath the RPE, extensive retinal necrosis, tumor invasion of the retinal arteries, and occlusion of the artery (*arrow,* **K**) on the optic disc and narrowing of the retinal artery (*arrows,* **L**) by tumor and atheromatous deposits. Medical evaluation for other evidence of lymphoma was negative. She developed multiple focal lesions simulating choroiditis in the left eye (**J**). Note that some were hypofluorescent (*arrows,* **J**). Fourteen months after her initial presentation she developed hemiparesis and brain scan evidence of a lymphoma.

(**G** to **L** from Gass and Trattler.[136])

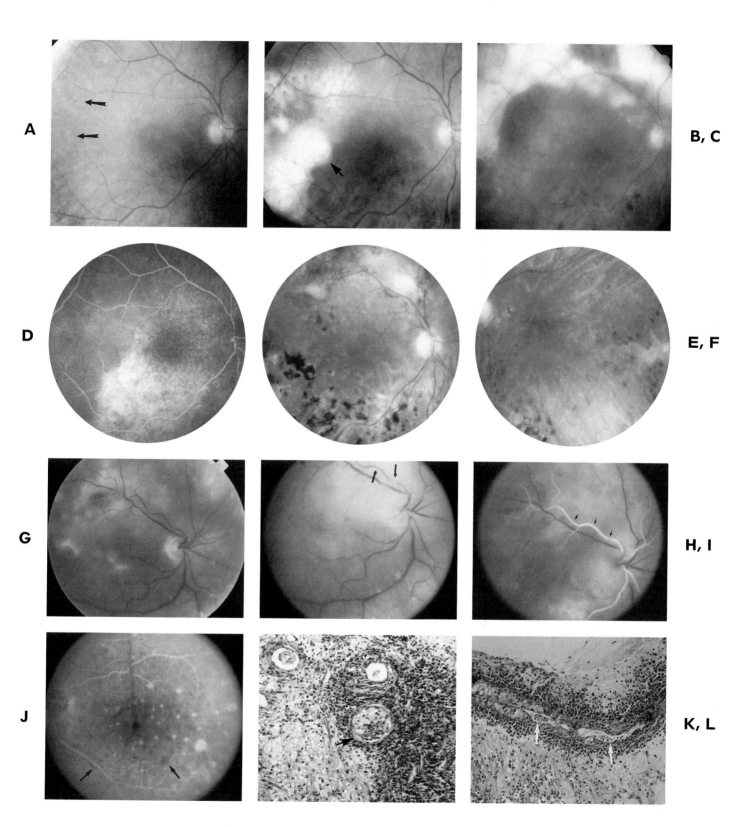

Systemic form of large-cell non-Hodgkin's lymphoma

Approximately 25% of the patients with large-cell non-Hodgkin's lymphoma have the systemic form of the disorder. The eye and brain are infrequently affected. When the eye is involved, the lymphomatous infiltration occurs primarily in the ciliary body and choroid.* Some of these lymphomas are T-cell lymphomas.[140,144,162] A few patients may develop diffuse infiltration of the posterior choroid. Choroidal and/or sub-RPE infiltration may produce a peculiar fundus picture composed of a reticular pattern of yellowish flecks simulating fundus flavimaculatus and serous detachment of the retina in the macular area (Fig. 11-9).[137] This may be confined to only one eye and may be the presenting manifestation of the systemic lymphoma. Fluorescein angiography reveals multifocal areas of hypofluorescence corresponding with the retinal flecks and an increase in the background choroidal fluorescence between the flecks in the early arteriovenous-phase angiograms (Fig. 11-9, C and E). Usually within several months these patients develop evidence of lymph node and other organ involvement with sparing the central nervous system. The biomicroscopic and angiographic findings in the macular areas simulate that of fundus flavimaculatus, as well as the fundus changes in patients with benign diffuse uveal melanocytic proliferation in association with a systemic carcinoma (see Fig. 3-86), with organ transplant retinopathy (see Fig. 3-68), and idiopathic uveal effusion syndrome (see Fig. 3-70). The author has observed one patient having a systemic lymphoma with this peculiar fundus picture in one eye and with multiple large sub-RPE tumors in his opposite eye, typical of that in the ocular–CNS form of large-cell non-Hodgkin's lymphoma. The findings in this case demonstrate what others have previously observed: that there is some overlap in the two forms of large-cell non-Hodgkin's lymphoma.[139] The findings in these patients suggest the possibility that the peculiar fundus flavimaculatus–like picture may be caused by diffuse damage to the RPE caused by sub-RPE infiltration by lymphoma cells that rapidly undergo spontaneous necrosis before forming tumefactions.

---

*References 122, 126, 127, 144, 165, 167.

FIG. 11-9 Retinal Involvement Simulating Fundus Flavimaculatus in Systemic Large-Cell Non-Hodgkin's Lymphoma.

A to C, This healthy 53-year-old woman noted recent blurring of vision in the right eye. Her visual acuity was 20/25 in the right eye and 20/15 in the left eye. Amsler grid testing revealed paracentral scotomata in the right eye. In the right eye there were 2+ vitreous cells and the fundus showed a reticular pattern of yellowish clumping of pigment simulating fundus flavimaculatus at the level of the RPE throughout the macula and juxtapapillary area (**A**). There were several areas of subretinal white infiltration superonasally (**B**). The left eye was normal. Early angiograms revealed the pigment clumps to be hypofluorescent on a background of greater than normal choroidal fluorescence (**C**). There was late staining in the area of the white infiltrate. Angiograms of the left eye were normal. Medical evaluation for inflammatory and neoplastic disease was negative. Her visual blurring gradually improved, and 7 weeks later her visual acuity was 20/20. She still noted slight loss of light and color sensitivity. Six months after the onset of visual symptoms she noted axillary lymphadenopathy. Tumors were discovered in the left supraclavicular area, retroperitoneal area, and left breast. Biopsy revealed a histiocytic, non-Hodgkin's lymphoma (reticulum cell sarcoma). She received systemic corticosteroid and antimetabolite therapy, and 14 months after the onset of visual symptoms she was apparently in remission. She has not returned for eye examination but can read the newspaper with the right eye and is still asymptomatic in the left eye.

D to I, This apparently healthy 67-year-old man developed blurred vision in the left eye in association with a fundus picture simulating fundus flavimaculatus (**D**). Angiography (**E** and **F**) was similar to that in C. His visual acuity was 20/20. Medical evaluation was negative. Six weeks later his acuity had declined to 20/80. There was an increase in the damage to the RPE (**G** to **I**). Several months later he developed lymphadenopathy. Biopsy revealed a large-cell lymphoma.

Retinal Involvement in Lymphocytic Lymphoma.

J to L, Rapid visual loss occurred in both eyes of a 48-year-old woman caused by well-differentiated lymphocytic lymphoma. There was marked retinal perivascular and optic disc infiltration in both eyes. This infiltration cleared within a month after cobalt irradiation treatment, and visual acuity improved from counting fingers to 20/60 in both eyes.

(**A** to **I** from Gass et al.[137]; **J** to **L** from Lewis RA, Clark RB: *Am J Ophthalmol* 79:48, 1975; published with permission from The American Journal of Ophthalmology; copyright by The Ophthalmic Publishing Co.[179])

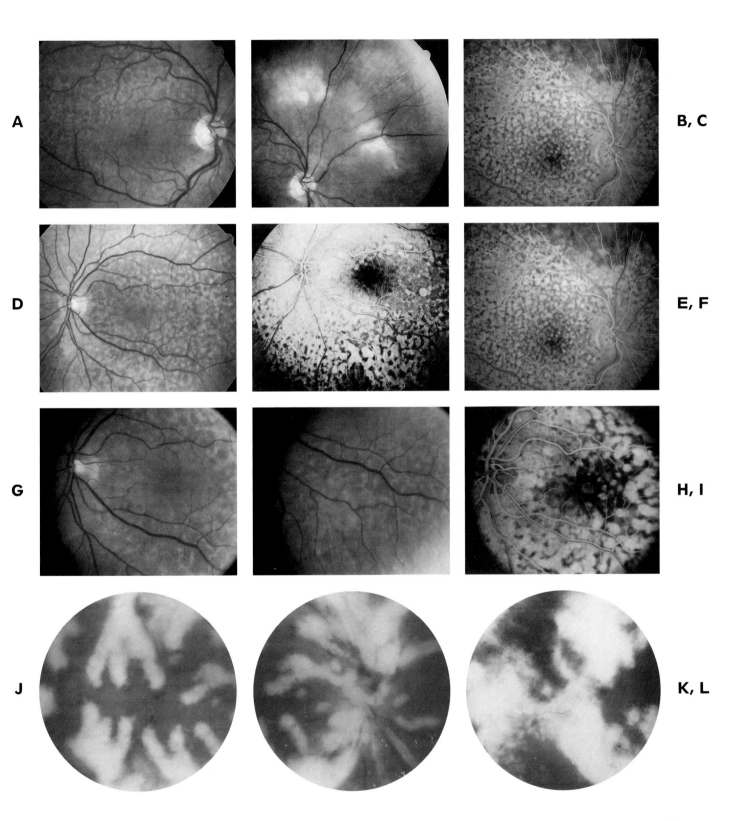

There are other examples of patients with an overlap of the ocular findings in the lymphomas. Patients with mycosis fungoides, which is a cutaneous T-cell lymphoma, may develop systemic lymphoma late in the course of the disease. This may rarely include diffuse infiltration of the choroid and retina, as well as sub-RPE infiltration similar to that in large-cell lymphoma.[128,132,153] Adult T-cell leukemia/lymphoma is a recently described clinicopathologic entity characterized by an extremely aggressive course, a leukemic or lymphomatous proliferation of hyperlobated peripheral T-cells, and an association with infection by a retrovirus, human T-lymphotrophic virus type 1 (HTLV-1).[151,152] These patients develop infiltration of multiple organ systems, which may include a pattern of intraocular involvement similar to that in patients with ocular–CNS non-Hodgkin's lymphoma and acute retinal necrosis.

Angioendotheliomatosis

Neoplastic angioendotheliomatosis is a rare form of extranodal large-cell lymphoma characterized by multifocal proliferation of neoplastic mononuclear cells within the lumen of blood vessels. It is a rare, fatal disease characterized by widespread intravascular proliferations of malignant cells of putative endothelial origin. Clinically, fever of unknown origin and dermatologic and bizarre neurologic manifestations predominate. Ocular changes include iridocyclitis, keratic precipitates, vitritis, papilledema, and retinal vascular alterations, including hemorrhages and retinal artery occlusion.[118,176,177] Infiltration of the choroid producing a clinical picture simulating Harada's disease may occur occasionally. Histologically, there is panuveal involvement with granulomatous iridocyclitis in addition to vascular and secondary pigmentary changes resembling somewhat hypertensive choroidopathy. The vascular endothelial cells show signs of malignant transformation.

▼ LYMPHOCYTIC LYMPHOMA

Lymphocytic lymphoma only rarely involves the eye (Fig. 11-9, *J* to *L*).[178,179] Lewis and Clark[179] reported a peculiar pattern of widespread retinal infiltration in a 48-year-old woman with a well-differentiated lymphocytic lymphoma involving the abdominal, cervical, and submandibular areas. Retinal infiltration cleared within 1 month following treatment with cyclophosphamide, vincristine, and oral prednisone. Kattah and associates[178]

FIG. 11-10   Hemorrhagic Optic Neuropathy and Visual Loss Caused by Multiple Myeloma.

This 67-year-old woman reported blurred vision in the left eye of 1 week's duration. Visual acuity was 20/30 in the right eye and counting fingers at 8 feet in the left eye. The right fundus was normal. There were some cells in the vitreous of the left eye. Note cotton-wool patches and opacification (*arrows*, **A**) of the optic nerve head posterior to the hemorrhages. Angiography showed minimal capillary dilation and staining of the optic disc (**B** and **C**). The clinical impression was myeloma infiltration of the optic nerve. She had a total dose of 2000 R of cobalt-60 to the posterior pole over a 2-week period. Three months later her visual acuity was 20/70 and the optic disc was slightly pale (**D**).

reported leptomeningeal and optic nerve involvement in a 26-year-old patient.

Burkitt's lymphoma

Burkitt's lymphoma is a poorly differentiated lymphocytic lymphoma with peculiar epidemiologic, clinical, and histopathologic features. The tumor frequently infiltrates the orbit, occasionally extends into the eye[181] but rarely arises within the eye.[180-182] In this latter instance, the infiltration of the optic disc and retina simulates that in leukemia.

Mycosis fungoides

Mycosis fungoides, a malignant lymphomatous disease derived from T lymphocytes, arises in the skin and may be confused with psoriasis. Later it may involve other body organs. It infrequently affects the central nervous system and eye.[185,186,188] Infiltration of the vitreous,[183,186,187] choroid,[184] sub-RPE space,[183] optic nerve, and retina[185,186,187] has been reported.

Multiple myeloma

Multiple myeloma is a neoplastic disease of plasma cells that in its advanced stages produces osteoporosis, punched-out bony lesions, multiple fractures, and bone tumors. Proptosis caused by bony involvement may be the first sign of the disease.[189] Rarely, the optic nerve may be infiltrated and cause a picture of optic neuritis and, in some cases, central retinal artery occlusion.[190,191] One patient seen at Bascom Palmer Eye Institute with optic nerve involvement responded promptly to external beam irradiation (Fig. 11-10).[134]

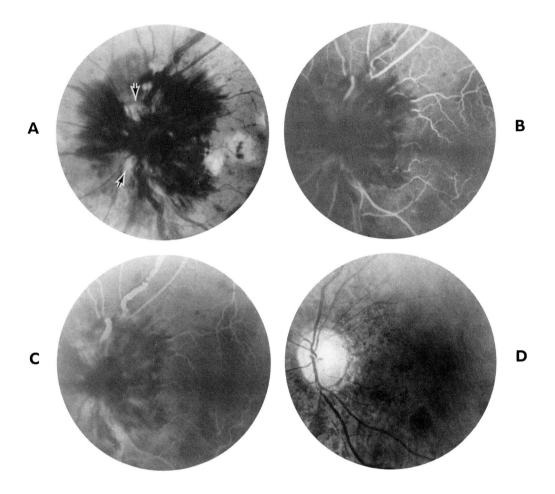

Lymphomatoid granulomatosis

Lymphomatoid granulomatosis is an angiocentric and angiodestructive lymphoproliferative disorder that has some features in common with Wegener's granulomatosis and malignant lymphoma.[192-194] Patients usually present with bilateral pulmonary infiltrates and cutaneous, central nervous system, and renal involvement. Atypical lymphoreticular cells invade blood vessels. Most ophthalmic manifestations of the disease are the result of cranial nerve involvement. Intraocular involvement, however, may occur and be associated with peripheral retinal vasculitis, involving both veins and arteries, and posterior uveitis.[194] In some instances the vasculitis in the eye may be largely confined to the choroid and produce a fundus picture simulating acute posterior multifocal placoid pigment epitheliopathy.[192] The mortality rate in patients with lymphomatoid granulomatosis is high and treatment is ineffective.[194]

▼ METASTATIC CARCINOMA AND CUTANEOUS MALIGNANT MELANOMA TO THE RETINA

Metastatic carcinoma to the retina occurs infrequently.* It usually occurs in one eye but may affect both eyes.[198] Initially the retinal metastasis may be indistinguishable from an ischemic infarct of the retina (Fig. 11-11, *A*). As the tumor enlarges, it produces a more dense, whitish opacification of the retina that may simulate necrotizing retinitis caused by toxoplasmosis, cytomegalovirus, or other infections (Fig. 11-11, *E*). Overlying vitreous cells may or may not be present.[196,197,216] Cytologic examination of the vitreous in such cases may establish the diagnosis.[203,207,216] The borders of metastatic lesions in the retina are more irregular than in choroidal metastasis. In approximately one-half of the reported cases, choroidal involvement was also present. Multiple perivascular white infiltrates may accompany the main tumor mass.[216]

---

*References 196, 197, 200-202, 204, 205, 211-216.

FIG. 11-11   Metastatic Carcinoma to the Retina and Vitreous.

A to **D,** This 42-year-old woman who had received treatment for metastatic breast carcinoma complained of floaters. Examination revealed coarse vitreous opacities near the surface of the retina (**A** and **B**). Fluorescein angiography revealed patchy areas of leaking retinal vessels (**C** and **D**). Vitreous biopsy revealed metastatic breast carcinoma.

E to **I,** This 49-year-old man complained of dizziness, headaches, dysarthria, and right hemiparesis. Examination revealed a solitary white retinal lesion in the left eye (**E**). Computerized tomography and magnetic resonance imaging of the brain revealed multiple nodular lesions (**F**). Chest roentgenogram revealed enlarged mediastinal nodes and a nodular density in the right middle lobe (**G**). Postmortem examination of the eyes revealed a solitary metastatic oat cell carcinoma lesion in the retina (**H** and **I**). Note that the choroid (*arrow,* **H**) is unaffected.

(**A** to **I** from Leys et al.[205])

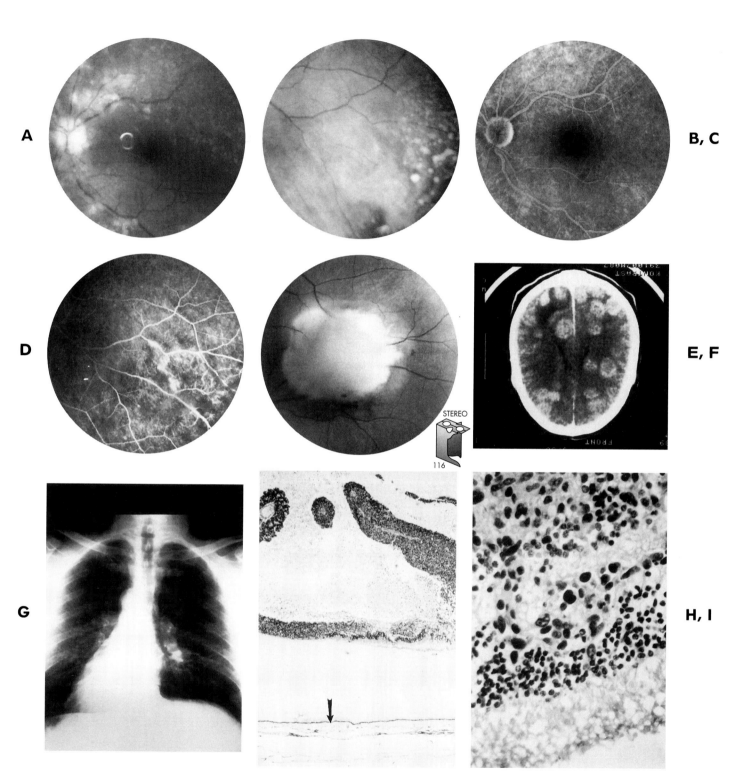

A

B, C

D

E, F

STEREO
116

G

H, I

891

Cutaneous melanoma may occasionally metastasize to the eye, and in approximately 20% of such cases it does so to the retina rather than to the uveal tract (Fig. 11-12).* In some cases it may metastasize to the vitreous and cause the patient to complain of vitreous floaters that are the result of brown, cellular, spherical clumps of melanoma cells suspended in the vitreous cavity (Fig. 11-12, *A*). These cell clumps are sufficiently characteristic and different from the irregular clumps of proliferating RPE cells (tobacco dust) that the diagnosis of metastatic melanoma should be suspected. The vitreous infiltration may be accompanied by superficial gray-brown infiltrates arranged in a dendritic pattern with feathery edges infiltrating the nerve fiber layer of the retina surrounding the optic nerve head (Fig. 11-12, *B*). Large, beige-colored plaques or clusters of the tumor cells in the vitreous may partly obscure the fundus from view. In other cases there may be localized irregular plaques of melanoma cells within the retina (Fig. 11-12, *C* and *D*). In spite of subconjunctival injection and systemic treatment with antimetabolites, the tumor in the eye may proliferate and cause rubeosis and secondary glaucoma.[210]

The reasons for the rarity of metastatic cancer to the retina compared to the uveal tract are uncertain. Differences in blood flow (turbulent flow in the choroid versus laminar flow in the retina), absence of fenestrations in the retinal vascular endothelium, and inhibitory factors present in the vitreous are possibly important.[199]

---

*References 195, 198, 203, 206, 208-210, 215.

FIG. 11-12   Metastatic Cutaneous Melanoma to the Retina and Vitreous.

A and B, A 43-year-old woman noted floaters in the left eye. Three years previously she had a cutaneous melanoma excised. Cobalt treatment was given because of a positive lymph node biopsy. Visual acuity was 20/20. Slit-lamp examination of the left eye revealed golden brown spherules in the anterior vitreous cavity **(A)** and pigmented cells emanating from the region of the optic disc **(B).** Angiography revealed some staining of the optic disc. The patient died 4 months later in spite of antimetabolite therapy.

C and D, Retinal metastasis in a 44-year-old man 3 years after excision of a cutaneous melanoma.

(**A** and **B** from Robertson DM et al: Metastatic tumor to the retina and vitreous cavity from primary melanoma of the skin; treatment with systemic and subconjunctival chemotherapy, *Ophthalmology* 88:1296, 1981[210]; **C** and **D** from Letson AD, Davidorf FH: *Arch Ophthalmol* 100:605, 1982; copyright 1982, American Medical Association.[203])

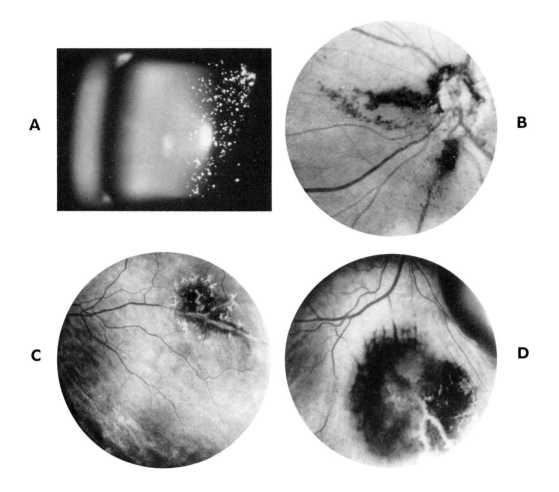

893

▼ PARANEOPLASTIC RETINOPATHY ASSOCIATED WITH CARCINOMA (CANCER-ASSOCIATED RETINOPATHY OR CAR SYNDROME)

The rapid development of visual loss associated with bizarre visual sensations, nyctalopia, ring scotoma, flat electroretinographic response, progressive retinal arterial narrowing, and no or minimal changes in the RPE and optic disc may occur as a remote effect of a systemic carcinoma, most frequently a small-cell carcinoma of the lung (Fig. 11-13, A).[218-227,229-236] A few vitreous cells were noted in one case,[223] and aqueous cells in another.[225] Fluorescein angiography in two cases showed evidence of mottled hyperfluorescence in both eyes.[223,225] Blindness may occur within 4 months. The visual symptoms may antedate the discovery of the carcinoma. Histopathologic examination shows severe degeneration and loss of the receptor cells and unlike retinitis pigmentosa, minimal damage to the RPE and normal choriocapillaris.[218,219,223,230,231] In one case there was loss of ganglion cells.[221] Electron microscopy in one patient revealed immature melanin granules with melanolysosomes, suggesting abnormal melanin synthesis and resorption.[218] This suggested to the authors that increased melanin synthesis and melanin content within the RPE in response to a hormonelike substance produced by the cancer may compromise its ability to phagocytose and maintain normal turnover of receptor outer segments. This in turn may cause photoreceptor cell degeneration.

Cogan et al. reported a unique case of paraneoplastic retinopathy simulating a cone dystrophy in a patient with recurrent blindness on exposure to bright light, total achromatopsia, bilateral central scotomas, narrowing of the retinal arteries, and decreased ERG amplitudes affecting predominantly cone function.[219] Medical evaluation disclosed a pelvic pleomorphic carcinoma of presumed uterine origin. She died because of metastatic disease 9 months after ocular symptoms developed. Histopathologic examination of eyes revealed loss of the retinal receptors and prominent atrophic and proliferative changes in the pigment epithelium that were most marked in the macular areas (Fig. 11-13, B and C).

Keltner and associates[223] found antibodies to normal fresh retina in the serum of one patient with the CAR syndrome and postulated an autoimmune mechanism for retinal degeneration. Thurkill et al. identified serum antibodies to a specific antigen (CAR antigen) with a molecular weight of 23,000

FIG. 11-13   Cancer-Associated Retinopathy.

A, Cancer-associated retinopathy in an elderly man who noted the rapid progression of loss of peripheral vision and nyctalopia. Note the narrowed retinal vessels and absence of evidence of RPE changes other than the juxtapapillary atrophy that was present in both eyes.

B and **C,** A 72-year-old-woman developed total achromatopsia, bilateral central scotomas, predominant suppression of cone response by ERG, and narrowing of the retinal arteries. She died 9 months later from metastatic carcinoma. Histopathologic examination revealed loss of photoreceptors most marked in the macular areas (**B** and **C**) and selective loss of cones elsewhere.

Acute Vogt-Koyanagi-Harada-like Syndrome in a Patient with Metastatic Cutaneous Melanoma.

D to **I,** This 71-year-old woman had had a melanoma of the dorsum of her foot removed 3 years previously. Two weeks before admission she had noted headache, progressive vitiligo of the skin of the face and arms (**D** and **E**), deafness, floaters, and progressive loss of vision in both eyes. Her visual acuity was light perception with poor projection in both eyes. She had 2 + aqueous cells and flare and keratic precipitates, 3 + vitreous cells, and large areas of depigmentation of the choroid and posterior fundus (**F** and **G**). Her general physical examination revealed inguinal lymphadenopathy but no other evidence of metastatic disease. The nodes were positive for melanoma. Computed tomography of the brain and abdomen were negative, and electroretinographic responses were extinguished in both eyes. Lumbar puncture revealed 130 lymphocytes and spinal fluid protein of 90 mg/dl. Treatment with systemic corticosteroids resulted in rapid return of visual function to 20/50 in the right eye and 20/70 in the left eye. Ten months after the onset of visual symptoms, the vitreous inflammation was minimal and there were scattered focal areas of depigmentation of the choroid in both eyes (**H** and **I**). The patient led an active life and was able to read until the time of her death, caused by metastatic melanoma 15 months later.

(**B** and **C** from Cogan et al[219]; **D** to **I** from Gass.[241])

daltons in these patients.[232,234] They postulated that the demonstration of hypersensitivity to specific antigens in CNS tissue is characteristic of paraneoplasia and is a potentially useful indication of occult neoplasia. Paraneoplastic disorders have been identified in association with different types of neoplasia: melanoma, cervical, colon, prostate, and breast cancer. The most common associated cancer is small-cell carcinoma of the lung. The retinal specific immunologic reactions, suggestive of autoimmunity, manifesting as high-titered antibody reactions with the 23 kd retinal CAR antigen, are now known to be located

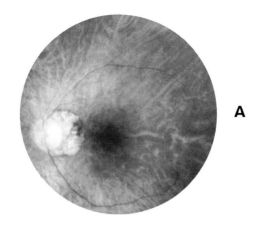

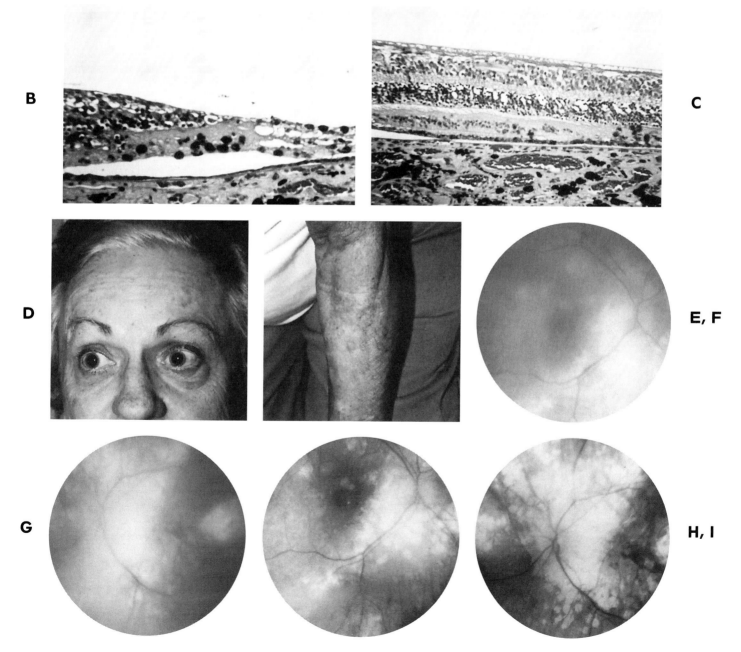

within the retinal receptors.[223,232,233] Thurkill et al. hypothesize that a carcinoma–retina immunologic cross-reaction is responsible for the induction of the unique antibody response encountered in patients with CAR, with vision loss developing as a cancer-evoked autoimmune retinopathy.[235]

There is some evidence that the visual deficit in some of these patients may show improvement following corticosteroid and chemotherapy.[219,222,224,225] In general, however, the visual prognosis is poor.

Neurologic disease, including optic neuropathy, occurring as a remote effect of cancer (e.g., cerebellar degeneration, brainstem encephalitis, motor neuron degeneration, peripheral neuropathy, polymyositis, and myasthenia) has been known for many years, but its pathogenesis is likewise uncertain.[217,225,228]

Patients with bilateral diffuse uveal melanocytic proliferation associated with occult carcinoma may also develop severe loss of retinal receptor function that cannot be fully explained on the basis of either the choroidal infiltrate that typically spares the choriocapillaris, or exudative retinal detachment (see Chapter 3, p. 236). The pathogenesis of the receptor cell dysfunction is probably similar to that in other carcinoma-associated retinopathies.

▼ PARANEOPLASTIC CHORIORETINOPATHY ASSOCIATED WITH MELANOMA-ASSOCIATED RETINOPATHY OR MAR SYNDROME

Acute paraneoplastic night blindness may occur occasionally in patients with metastatic cutaneous melanoma.[237,238,241,243-245] This may be associated with acute anterior and posterior uveitis, patchy depigmentation of the choroid, vitiligo, dysacousis, and severe visual loss (Fig. 11-13, *D* to *I*).[237,239,241] This syndrome occurred in one patient receiving bacillus Calmette-Guerin (BCG) treatment for cutaneous melanoma.[239] The visual symptoms are associated with an electroretinogram that may simulate that occurring in patients with congenital stationary night blindness[244] or that may be extinguished.[239] It is probable that the acute changes in the eye, skin, and ear are an unusual immunologic response to the melanoma, although this could not be verified in the patient seen at Bascom Palmer Eye Institute (Fig. 11-13, *D* to *I*). Sera of patients with melanoma-associated paraneoplastic retinopathy (MAR) may demonstrate high titers of immunoglobulins reactive to retinal bipolar cells.

Patients with MAR, unlike those with CAR, experience primarily central visual loss rather than ring scotomas and, early, their ERG does not show the severely depressed or absent a-wave indicative of photoreceptor dysfunction.[245] Vitiligo has been reported in association with cutaneous melanomas in as many as 20% of cases. In a few patients it may be accompanied by intraocular inflammation.[230,240] Other diseases linking vitiligo and intraocular inflammation, particularly chorioretinitis and patchy depigmentation of the fundus, include sympathetic uveitis[240] and vitiliginous chorioretinitis (bird-shot chorioretinitis).[242] The frequent association of nyctalopia in vitiliginous chorioretinitis, its occasional occurrence in association with sympathetic uveitis, and its occurrence in the patient illustrated in Fig. 7-39 indicates that the receptor cells as well as the melanocytes may also be the target of the immunologic reaction.

REFERENCES

Retinoblastoma

1. Abramson DH: Lactate dehydrogenase and retinoblastoma. *In:* Jakobiec FA, editor: *Ocular and adnexal tumors,* Birmingham, AL, 1978, Aesculapius Publishing, pp. 454-459.
2. Abramson DH: Retinoblastoma. *Pediatr Emerg Casebook* 3(5), 1985.
3. Abramson DH, Ellsworth RM, Haik B: Cobalt plaques in advanced retinoblastoma. *Retina* 3:12-15, 1983.
4. Abramson DH, Ellsworth RM, Kitchin FD, Tung G: Second nonocular tumors in retinoblastoma survivors; are they radiation-induced? *Ophthalmology* 91:1351-1355, 1984.
5. Abramson DH, Greenfield DS, Ellsworth RM, et al: Neuron-specific enolase and retinoblastoma; clinicopathologic correlations. *Retina* 9:148-152, 1989.
6. Abramson DH, Marks RF, Ellsworth RM, et al: The management of unilateral retinoblastoma without primary enucleation. *Arch Ophthalmol* 100:1249-1256, 1982.
7. Albert DM: Historic review of retinoblastoma. *Ophthalmology* 94:654-662, 1987.
8. Bhatnagar R, Vine AK: Diffuse infiltrating retinoblastoma. *Ophthalmology* 98:1657-1661, 1991.
9. Buys RJ, Abramson DH, Ellsworth RM, Haik B: Radiation regression patterns after cobalt plaque insertion for retinoblastoma. *Arch Ophthalmol* 101:1206-1208, 1983.
10. Carlson EA, Letson RD, Ramsay NKC, Desnick RJ: Factors for improved genetic counseling for retinoblastoma based on a survey of 55 families. *Am J Ophthalmol* 87:449-459, 1979.
11. Char DH: Current concepts in retinoblastoma. *Ann Ophthalmol* 12:792-804, 1980.
12. Char DH, Hedges TR III, Norman D: Retinoblastoma; CT diagnosis. *Ophthalmology* 91:1347-1350, 1984.
13. Cohen SM, Saulenas AM, Sullivan CR, Albert DM: Further studies of the effect of vitamin D on retinoblastoma; inhibition with 1,25-dihydroxycholecalciferol. *Arch Ophthalmol* 106:541-543, 1988.
14. Devesa SS: The incidence of retinoblastoma. *Am J Ophthalmol* 80:263-265, 1975.
15. Eagle CR Jr, Shields JA, Donoso L, Milner RS: Malignant transformation of spontaneously regressed retinoblastoma,

retinoma/retinocytoma variant. *Ophthalmology* 96:1389-1395, 1989.

16. Ellsworth RM: The practical management of retinoblastoma. *Trans Am Ophthalmol Soc* 67:462-534, 1969.

17. François J, DeBie S, Matton-Van Leuven MT: Genesis and genetics of retinoblastoma. *J Pediatr Ophthalmol Strabismus* 16:85-100, 1979.

18. Gallie BL, Ellsworth RM, Abramson DH, Phillips RA: Retinoma: spontaneous regression of retinoblastoma or benign manifestation of the mutation? *Br J Cancer* 45:513-521, 1982.

19. Gallie BL, Phillips RA, Ellsworth RM, Abramson DH: Significance of retinoma and phthisis bulbi for retinoblastoma. *Ophthalmology* 89:1393-1399, 1982.

20. Gass JDM: *Differential diagnosis of intraocular tumors; a stereoscopic presentation,* St. Louis, 1974, CV Mosby, p. 331.

21. Goldberg L, Danziger A: Computed tomographic scanning in the management of retinoblastoma. *Am J Ophthalmol* 84:380-382, 1977.

22. Haik BG, Dunleavy SA, Cooke C, et al: Retinoblastoma with anterior chamber extension. *Ophthalmology* 94:367-370, 1987.

23. Howard GM: Erroneous clinical diagnoses of retinoblastoma and uveal melanoma. *Trans Am Acad Ophthalmol Otolaryngol* 73:199-202, 1969.

24. Jensen RD, Miller RW: Retinoblastoma: epidemiologic characteristics. *N Engl J Med* 285:307-311, 1971.

25. Kopelman JE, McLean IW, Rosenberg SH: Multivariate analysis of risk factors for metastasis in retinoblastoma treated by enucleation. *Ophthalmology* 94:371-377, 1987.

26. Lam BL, Judisch GF, Sobol WM, Blodi CF: Visual prognosis in macular retinoblastomas. *Am J Ophthalmol* 110:229-232, 1990.

27. Lueder GT: Successful therapy for trilateral retinoblastoma. *Am J Ophthalmol* 114:646-647, 1992.

28. Lueder GT, Judisch GF, O'Gorman TW: Second nonocular tumors in survivors of heritable retinoblastoma. *Arch Ophthalmol* 104:372-373, 1986.

29. Lueder GT, Judisch GF, Wen B: Heritable retinoblastoma and pinealoma. *Arch Ophthalmol* 109:1707-1709, 1991.

30. Mafee MF, Goldberg MF, Cohen SB, et al: Magnetic resonance imaging versus computed tomography of leukocoric eyes and use of in vitro proton magnetic resonance spectroscopy of retinoblastoma. *Ophthalmology* 96:965-976, 1989.

31. Magramm I, Abramson DH, Ellsworth RM: Optic nerve involvement in retinoblastoma. *Ophthalmology* 96:217-222, 1989.

32. Messmer EP, Heinrich T, Höpping W, et al: Risk factors for metastases in patients with retinoblastoma. *Ophthalmology* 98:136-141, 1991.

33. Messmer EP, Sauerwein W, Heinrich T, et al: New and recurrent tumor foci following local treatment as well as external beam radiation in eyes of patients with hereditary retinoblastoma. *Graefes Arch Clin Exp Ophthalmol* 228:426-431, 1990.

34. Nelson SC, Friedman HS, Oakes WJ, et al: Successful therapy for trilateral retinoblastoma. *Am J Ophthalmol* 114:23-29, 1992.

35. Ohnishi Y, Yamana Y, Minei M, Ibayashi H: Application of fluorescein angiography in retinoblastoma. *Am J Ophthalmol* 93:578-588, 1982.

36. Onadim Z, Hykin PG, Hungerford JL, Cowell JK: Genetic counselling in retinoblastoma: importance of ocular fundus examination of first degree relatives and linkage analysis. *Br J Ophthalmol* 75:147-150, 1991.

37. Pendergrass TW, Davis S: Incidence of retinoblastoma in the United States. *Arch Ophthalmol* 98:1204-1210, 1980.

38. Reese AB: *Tumors of the eye,* ed. 3, Hagerstown MD, 1976, Harper & Row, pp. 90-124.

39. Roarty JD, McLean IW, Zimmerman LE: Incidence of second neoplasms in patients with bilateral retinoblastoma. *Ophthalmology* 95:1583-1587, 1988.

40. Robertson DM, Campbell RJ: Analysis of misdiagnosed retinoblastoma in a series of 726 enucleated eyes. *Mod Probl Ophthalmol* 18:156-159, 1977.

41. Rubenfeld M, Abramson DH, Ellsworth RM, Kitchin FD: Unilateral vs. bilateral retinoblastoma; correlations between age at diagnosis and stage of ocular disease. *Ophthalmology* 93:1016-1019, 1986.

42. Rubin ML, Kaufman HE: Spontaneously regressed probable retinoblastoma; report of a case. *Arch Ophthalmol* 81:442-445, 1969.

43. Sanders BM, Draper GJ, Kingston JE: Retinoblastoma in Great Britain 1969-80: incidence, treatment, and survival. *Br J Ophthalmol* 72:576-583, 1988.

44. Shields CL, Shields JA, De Potter P, et al: Plaque radiotherapy in the management of retinoblastoma. *Ophthalmology* 100:216-224, 1993.

45. Shields CL, Shields JA, Minelli S, et al: Regression of retinoblastoma after plaque radiotherapy. *Am J Ophthalmol* 115:181-187, 1993.

46. Shields CL, Shields JA, Shah P: Retinoblastoma in older children. *Ophthalmology* 98:395-399, 1991.

47. Shields JA, Augsburger JJ: Current approaches to the diagnosis and management of retinoblastoma. *Surv Ophthalmol* 25:347-372, 1981.

48. Shields JA, Giblin ME, Shields CL, et al: Episcleral plaque radiotherapy for retinoblastoma. *Ophthalmology* 96:530-537, 1989.

49. Shields JA, Leonard BC, Michelson JB, Sarin LK: B-scan ultrasonography in the diagnosis of atypical retinoblastomas. *Can J Ophthalmol* 11:42-51, 1976.

50. Shields JA, Parsons H, Shields CL, Giblin ME: The role of cryotherapy in the management of retinoblastoma. *Am J Ophthalmol* 108:260-264, 1989.

51. Shields JA, Sanborn GE, Augsburger JJ, et al: Fluorescein angiography of retinoblastoma. *Retina* 2:206-214, 1982.

52. Shields JA, Shields CL, Eagle RC, Blair CJ: Spontaneous pseudohypopyon secondary to diffuse infiltrating retinoblastoma. *Arch Ophthalmol* 106:1301, 1988.

53. Shields JA, Shields CL, Eagle RC, et al: Calcified intraocular abscess simulating retinoblastoma. *Am J Ophthalmol* 114:227-229, 1992.

54. Shields JA, Shields CL, Parsons HM: Differential diagnosis of retinoblastoma. *Retina* 11:232-243, 1991.

55. Shields JA, Shields CL, Parsons H, Giblin ME: The role of photocoagulation in the management of retinoblastoma. *Arch Ophthalmol* 108:205-208, 1990.

56. Shields JA, Shields CL, Sivalingam V: Decreasing frequency of enucleation in patients with retinoblastoma. *Am J Ophthalmol* 108:185-188, 1989.

57. Shields JA, Shields CL, Suvarnamani C, et al: Retinoblastoma manifesting as orbital cellulitis. *Am J Ophthalmol* 112:442-449, 1991.

58. Shine BSF, Hungerford J, Vaghela B, Sheraidah GAK: Electrophoretic assessment of aqueous and serum neurone-specific enolase in retinoblastoma and ocular malignant melanoma. *Br J Ophthalmol* 74:427-430, 1990.

59. Smith JLS: Histology and spontaneous regression of retinoblastoma. *Trans Ophthalmol Soc UK* 94:953-967, 1974.

60. Takahashi T, Tamura S, Inoue M, et al: Retinoblastoma in a 26-year-old adult. *Ophthalmology* 90:179-183, 1983.
61. Tamboli A, Podgor MJ, Horm JW: The incidence of retinoblastoma in the United States: 1974 through 1985. *Arch Ophthalmol* 108:128-132, 1990.
62. Traboulsi EI, Zimmerman LE, Manz HJ: Cutaneous malignant melanoma in survivors of heritable retinoblastoma. *Arch Ophthalmol* 106:1059-1061, 1988.
63. Weiss AH, Karr DJ, Kalina RE, et al: Visual outcomes of macular retinoblastoma after external beam radiation therapy. *Ophthalmology* 101:1244-1249, 1994.
64. Wiggs JL, Dryja TP: Editorial: Predicting the risk of hereditary retinoblastoma. *Am J Ophthalmol* 106:346-351, 1988.

Leukemic Choroidopathy

65. Blodi FC: The difficult diagnosis of choroidal melanoma. *Arch Ophthalmol* 69:253-256, 1963.
66. Burns CA, Blodi FC, Williamson BK: Acute lymphocytic leukemia and central serous retinopathy. *Trans Am Acad Ophthalmol Otolaryngol* 69:307-309, 1965.
67. Clayman HM, Flynn JT, Koch K, Israel C: Retinal pigment epithelial abnormalities in leukemic disease. *Am J Ophthalmol* 74:416-419, 1972.
68. Gass JDM: *Differential diagnosis of intraocular tumors; a stereoscopic presentation,* St. Louis, 1974, CV Mosby, p. 145.
69. Jakobiec F, Behrens M: Leukemic pigment epitheliopathy with report of a unilateral case. *J Pediatr Ophthalmol* 12:10-15, 1975.
70. Kincaid MC, Green WR, Kelley JS: Acute ocular leukemia. *Am J Ophthalmol* 87:698-702, 1979.
71. Schimmelpfennig W, Aur RJA: Leopardenfleck-Chorioretinopathie; erstes Anzeichen eines Rezidivs einer akuten lymphozytischen Leukämie. *Ophthalmologe* 89:430-431, 1992.
72. Stewart MW, Gitter KA, Cohen G: Acute leukemia presenting as a unilateral exudative retinal detachment. *Retina* 9:110-114, 1989.
73. Tang RA, Vila-Coro AA, Wall S, Frankel LS: Acute leukemia presenting as a retinal pigment epithelium detachment. *Arch Ophthalmol* 106:21-22, 1988.
74. Zimmerman LE, Thoreson HT: Sudden loss of vision in acute leukemia; a clinicopathologic report of two unusual cases. *Surv Ophthalmol* 9:467-473, 1964.

Leukemic Retinopathy and Optic Neuropathy

75. Allen RA, Straatsma BR: Ocular involvement in leukemia and allied disorders. *Arch Ophthalmol* 66:490-508, 1961.
76. Badelon I, Chaine G, Tolub O, Coscas G: Occlusion de la veine et de l'artere centrale de la retine par infiltration du nerf optique au cours d'une leucemie aigue lymphoblastique. *Bull Soc Ophtalmol Fr* 86:261-264, 1986.
77. Brown DM, Kimura AE, Ossoinig KC, Weiner GJ: Acute promyelocytic infiltration of the optic nerve treated by oral *trans*-retinoic acid. *Ophthalmology* 99:1463-1467, 1992.
78. Culler AM: Fundus changes in leukemia. *Trans Am Ophthalmol Soc* 49:445-473, 1951.
79. Cullis CM, Hines DR, Bullock JD: Anterior segment ischemia: classification and description in chronic myelogenous leukemia. *Ann Ophthalmol* 11:1739-1744, 1979.
80. Currie JN, Lessell S, Lessell IM, et al: Optic neuropathy in chronic lymphocytic leukemia. *Arch Ophthalmol* 106:654-660, 1988.
81. De Juan E, Green WR, Rice TA, Erozan YS: Optic disc neovascularization associated with ocular involvement in acute lymphocytic leukemia. *Retina* 2:61-64, 1982.
82. Delaney WV Jr, Kinsella G: Optic disk neovascularization in leukemia. *Am J Ophthalmol* 99:212-213, 1985.
83. Duke JR, Wilkinson CP, Sigelman S: Retinal microaneurysms in leukaemia. *Br J Ophthalmol* 52:368-374, 1968.
84. Ellis W, Little HL: Leukemic infiltration of the optic nerve head. *Am J Ophthalmol* 75:867-871, 1973.
85. Frank RN, Ryan SJ Jr: Peripheral retinal neovascularization with chronic myelogenous leukemia. *Arch Ophthalmol* 87:585-589, 1972.
86. Gass JDM: *Differential diagnosis of intraocular tumors: a stereoscopic presentation,* St. Louis, 1974, CV Mosby, pp. 159-176.
87. Glaser B, Smith JL: Leukaemic glaucoma. *Br J Ophthalmol* 50:92-94, 1966.
88. Guyer DR, Schachat AP, Vitale S, et al: Leukemic retinopathy; relationship between fundus lesions and hematologic parameters at diagnosis. *Ophthalmology* 96:860-864, 1989.
89. Hofman P, Le Tourneau A, Negre F, et al: Primary uveal B immunoblastic lymphoma in a patient with AIDS. *Br J Ophthalmol* 76:700-702, 1992.
90. Holt JM, Gordon-Smith EC: Retinal abnormalities in diseases of the blood. *Br J Ophthalmol* 53:145-160, 1969.
91. Horton JC, Garcia EG, Becker EK: Magnetic resonance imaging of leukemic invasion of the optic nerve. *Arch Ophthalmol* 110:1207-1208, 1992.
92. Inkeles DM, Friedman AH: Retinal pigment epithelial degeneration, partial retinal atrophy and macular hole in acute lymphocytic leukemia. *Albrecht von Graefes Arch Clin Exp Ophthalmol* 194:253-261, 1975.
93. Jampol LM, Goldberg MF, Busse B: Peripheral retinal microaneurysms in chronic leukemia. *Am J Ophthalmol* 80:242-248, 1975.
94. Johnston SS, Ware CF: Iris involvement in leukaemia. *Br J Ophthalmol* 57:320-324, 1973.
95. Karesh JW, Goldman EJ, Reck K, et al: A prospective ophthalmic evaluation of patients with acute myeloid leukemia: correlation of ocular and hematologic findings. *J Clin Oncol* 7:1528-1532, 1989.
96. Kuwabara T, Aiello L: Leukemic miliary nodules in the retina. *Arch Ophthalmol* 72:494-497, 1964.
97. Leonardy NJ, Rupani M, Dent G, Klintworth GK: Analysis of 135 autopsy eyes for ocular involvement in leukemia. *Am J Ophthalmol* 109:436-444, 1990.
98. Leveille AS, Morse PH: Platelet-induced retinal neovascularization in leukemia. *Am J Ophthalmol* 91:640-643, 1981.
99. Little HL: The role of abnormal hemorrheodynamics in the pathogenesis of diabetic retinopathy. *Trans Am Ophthalmol Soc* 74:573-636, 1976.
100. Mahneke A, Videbaek A: On changes in the optic fundus in leukaemia; aetiology, diagnostic and prognostic role. *Acta Ophthalmol* 42:201-210, 1964.
101. Mehta P: Ophthalmologic manifestations of leukemia. *J Pediatr* 95:156-157, 1979.
102. Minnella AM, Yannuzzi LA, Slakter JS, Rodriguez A: Bilateral perifoveal ischemia associated with chronic granulocytic leukemia. *Arch Ophthalmol* 106:1170-1171, 1988.
103. Morse PH, McCready JL: Peripheral retinal neovascularization in chronic myelocytic leukemia. *Am J Ophthalmol* 72:975-978, 1971.
104. Nikaido H, Mishima H, Ono H, et al: Leukemic involvement of the optic nerve. *Am J Ophthalmol* 105:294-298, 1988.
105. Ohkoshi K, Tsiaras WG: Prognostic importance of ophthalmic manifestations in childhood leukaemia. *Br J Ophthalmol* 76:651-655, 1992.

106. Robb RM, Ervin LD, Sallan SE: A pathological study of eye involvement in acute leukemia of childhood. *Trans Am Ophthalmol Soc* 76:90-101, 1978.

107. Rosenthal AR: Ocular manifestations of leukemia; a review. *Ophthalmology* 90:899-905, 1983.

108. Rosenthal AR, Egbert PR, Wilbur JR, Probert JC: Leukemic involvement of the optic nerve. *J Pediatr Ophthalmol* 12:84-93, 1975.

109. Schachat AP, Markowitz JA, Guyer DR, et al: Ophthalmic manifestations of leukemia. *Arch Ophthalmol* 107:697-700, 1989.

110. Swartz M, Schumann GB: Acute leukemic infiltration of the vitreous diagnosed by pars plana aspiration. *Am J Ophthalmol* 90:326-330, 1980.

111. Verbraak FD, van den Berg W, Bos PJM: Retinal pigment epitheliopathy in acute leukemia. *Am J Ophthalmol* 111:111-113, 1991.

112. Wiznia RA, Rose A, Levy AL: Occlusive microvascular retinopathy with optic disc and retinal neovascularization in acute lymphocytic leukemia. *Retina* 14:253-255, 1994.

113. Wood WJ, Nicholson DH: Corneal ring ulcer as the presenting manifestation of acute monocytic leukemia. *Am J Ophthalmol* 76:69-72, 1973.

114. Zimmerman LE, Thoreson HT: Sudden loss of vision in acute leukemia; a clinicopathologic report of two unusual cases. *Surv Ophthalmol* 9:467-473, 1964.

Hodgkin's Disease

115. Miller NR, Iliff WJ: Visual loss as the initial symptom in Hodgkin disease. *Arch Ophthalmol* 93:1158-1161, 1975.

116. Primbs GB, Monsees WE, Irvine AR Jr: Intraocular Hodgkin's disease. *Arch Ophthalmol* 66:477-482, 1961.

117. Siatkowski RM, Lam BL, Schatz NJ, et al: Optic neuropathy in Hodgkin's disease. *Am J Ophthalmol* 114:625-629, 1992.

Large-Cell Non-Hodgkin's Lymphoma (Reticulum Cell Sarcoma, Histocytic Lymphoma)

118. Antle CM, White VA, Horsman DE, Rootman J: Large cell orbital lymphoma in a patient with acquired immune deficiency syndrome; case report and review. *Ophthalmology* 97:1494-1498, 1990.

119. Appen RE: Posterior uveitis and primary cerebral reticulum cell sarcoma. *Arch Ophthalmol* 93:123-124, 1975.

120. Barr CC, Green WR, Payne JW, et al: Intraocular reticulum-cell sarcoma: clinicopathologic study of four cases and review of the literature. *Surv Ophthalmol* 19:224-239, 1975.

121. Blumenkranz MS, Ward T, Murphy S, et al: Applications and limitations of vitreoretinal biopsy techniques in intraocular large cell lymphoma. *Retina* 12(Suppl):S64-S70, 1992.

122. Chambers JD, Mosher ML Jr: Intraocular involvement in systemic lymphoma. *Surv Ophthalmol* 11:562-564, 1966.

123. Char DH, Ljung B-M, Deschênes J, Miller TR: Intraocular lymphoma: immunological and cytological analysis. *Br J Ophthalmol* 72:905-911, 1988.

124. Char DH, Ljung B-M, Miller T, Phillips T: Primary intraocular lymphoma (ocular reticulum cell sarcoma); diagnosis and management. *Ophthalmology* 95:625-630, 1988.

125. Char DH, Margolis L, Newman AB: Ocular reticulum cell sarcoma. *Am J Ophthalmol* 91:480-483, 1981.

126. Collyer R: Reticulum cell sarcoma of eye and orbit. *Can J Ophthalmol* 7:247-249, 1972.

127. Cooper EL, Riker JL: Malignant lymphoma of the uveal tract. *Am J Ophthalmol* 34:1153-1158, 1951.

128. DeAngelis LM: Primary central nervous system lymphoma: a new clinical challenge. *Neurology* 41:619-621, 1991.

129. DeAngelis LM, Yahalom J, Heinemann M-H, et al: Primary CNS lymphoma: combined treatment with chemotherapy and radiotherapy. *Neurology* 40:80-86, 1990.

130. Duker JS, Shields JA, Ross M: Intraocular large cell lymphoma presenting as massive thickening of the uveal tract. *Retina* 7:41-45, 1987.

131. Eby NL, Grufferman S, Flannelly CM, et al: Increasing incidence of primary brain lymphoma in the US. *Cancer* 62:2461-2465, 1988.

132. Erny BC, Egbert PR, Peat IM, et al: Intraocular involvement with subretinal pigment epithelial infiltrates by mycosis fungoides. *Br J Ophthalmol* 75:698-701, 1991.

133. Freeman LN, Schachat AP, Knox DL, et al: Clinical features, laboratory investigations, and survival in ocular reticulum cell sarcoma. *Ophthalmology* 94:1631-1639, 1987.

134. Gass JDM: *Differential diagnosis of intraocular tumors; a stereoscopic presentation,* St. Louis, 1974, CV Mosby, p. 160.

135. Gass JDM, Sever RJ, Grizzard WS, et al: Multifocal pigment epithelial detachments by reticulum cell sarcoma; a characteristic funduscopic picture. *Retina* 4:135-143, 1984.

136. Gass JDM, Trattler HL: Retinal artery obstruction and atheromas associated with non-Hodgkin's large cell lymphoma (reticulum cell sarcoma). *Arch Ophthalmol* 109:1134-1139, 1991.

137. Gass JDM, Weleber RG, Johnson DR: Non-Hodgkin's lymphoma causing fundus picture simulating fundus flavimaculatus. *Retina* 7:209-214, 1987.

138. Givner I: Malignant lymphoma with ocular involvement; a clinico-pathologic report. *Am J Ophthalmol* 39:29-32, 1955.

139. Goder G, Klein S, Königsdörffer E: Klinische und pathologische Besonderheiten des malignen Lymphoms der Netzhaut. *Klin Monatsbl Augenheilkd* 197:514-518, 1990.

140. Goldey SH, Stern GA, Oblon DJ, et al: Immunophenotypic characterization of an unusual T-cell lymphoma presenting as anterior uveitis; a clinicopathologic case report. *Arch Ophthalmol* 107:1349-1353, 1989.

141. Gray RS, Abrahams JJ, Hufnagel TJ, et al: Ghost-cell tumor of the optic chiasm; primary CNS lymphoma. *J Clin Neuro-Ophthalmol* 9:98-104, 1989.

142. Guyer DR, Green WR, Schachat AP, et al: Bilateral ischemic optic neuropathy and retinal vascular occlusions associated with lymphoma and sepsis; clinicopathologic correlation. *Ophthalmology* 97:882-888, 1990.

143. Hofman P, Le Tourneau A, Negre F, et al: Primary uveal B immunoblastic lymphoma in a patient with AIDS. *Br J Ophthalmol* 76:700-702, 1992.

144. Jensen OA, Johansen S, Kiss K: Intraocular T-cell lymphoma mimicking a ring melanoma. First manifestation of systemic disease; report of a case and survey of the literature. *Graefes Arch Clin Exp Ophthalmol* 232:148-152, 1994.

145. Johnson BL: Intraocular and central nervous system lymphoma in a cardiac transplant recipient. *Ophthalmology* 99:987-992, 1992.

146. Kaplan HJ, Meredith TA, Aaberg TM, Keller RH: Reclassification of intraocular reticulum cell sarcoma (histiocytic lymphoma); immunologic characterization of vitreous cells. *Arch Ophthalmol* 98:707-710, 1980.

147. Kattah JC, Suski ET, Killen JY, et al: Optic neuritis and systemic lymphoma. *Am J Ophthalmol* 89:431-436, 1980.

148. Kennerdell JS, Johnson BL, Wisotzkey HM: Vitreous cellular reaction; association with reticulum cell sarcoma of brain. *Arch Ophthalmol* 93:1341-1345, 1975.

149. Kim EW, Zakov ZN, Albert DM, et al: Intraocular reticulum cell sarcoma: a case report and literature review. *Graefes Arch Klin Exp Ophthalmol* 209:167-178, 1979.

150. Kirmani MH, Thomas EL, Rao NA, Laborde RP: Intraocular reticulum cell sarcoma: diagnosis by choroidal biopsy. *Br J Ophthalmol* 71:748-752, 1987.

151. Kohno T, Uchida H, Inomata H, et al: Ocular manifestations of adult T-cell leukemia/lymphoma; a clinicopathologic study. *Ophthalmology* 100:1794-1799, 1993.

152. Kumar SR, Gill PS, Wagner DG, et al: Human T-cell lymphotropic virus type I-associated retinal lymphoma; a clinicopathologic report. *Arch Ophthalmol* 112:954-959, 1994.

153. Lang GK, Surer JL, Green WR, et al: Ocular reticulum cell sarcoma; clinicopathologic correlation of a case with multifocal lesions. *Retina* 5:79-86, 1985.

154. Margolis L, Fraser R, Lichter A, Char DH: The role of radiation therapy in the management of ocular reticulum cell sarcoma. *Cancer* 45:688-692, 1980.

155. Matzkin DC, Slamovits TL, Rosenbaum PS: Simultaneous intraocular and orbital non-Hodgkin lymphoma in the acquired immune deficiency syndrome. *Ophthalmology* 101:850-855, 1994.

156. Michels RG, Knox DL, Erozan YS, Green WR: Intraocular reticulum cell sarcoma; diagnosis by pars plana vitrectomy. *Arch Ophthalmol* 93:1331-1335, 1975.

157. Michelson JB, Michelson PE, Bordin GM, Chisari FV: Ocular reticulum cell sarcoma; presentation as retinal detachment with demonstration of monoclonal immunoglobulin light chains on the vitreous cells. *Arch Ophthalmol* 99:1409-1411, 1981.

158. Minckler DS, Font RL, Zimmerman LE: Uveitis and reticulum cell sarcoma of brain with bilateral neoplastic seeding of vitreous without retinal or uveal involvement. *Am J Ophthalmol* 80:433-439, 1975.

159. Neuwelt EA, Frenkel EP, Gumerlock MK, et al: Developments in the diagnosis and treatment of primary CNS lymphoma; a prospective series. *Cancer* 58:1609-1620, 1986.

160. Parver LM, Font RL: Malignant lymphoma of the retina and brain; initial diagnosis by cytologic examination of vitreous aspirate. *Arch Ophthalmol* 97:1505-1507, 1979.

161. Ridley ME, McDonald HR, Sternberg P Jr, et al: Retinal manifestations of ocular lymphoma (reticulum cell sarcoma). *Ophthalmology* 99:1153-1161, 1992.

162. Saga T, Ohno S, Matsuda H, et al: Ocular involvement by a peripheral T-cell lymphoma. *Arch Ophthalmol* 102:399-402, 1984.

163. Schanzer MC, Font RL, O'Malley RE: Primary ocular malignant lymphoma associated with the acquired immune deficiency syndrome. *Ophthalmology* 98:88-91, 1991.

164. Siegel MJ, Dalton J, Friedman AH, et al: Ten-year experience with primary ocular "reticulum cell sarcoma" (large cell non-Hodgkin's lymphoma). *Br J Ophthalmol* 73:342-346, 1989.

165. Sloas HA, Starling J, Harper DG, Cupples HP: Update of ocular reticulum cell sarcoma. *Arch Ophthalmol* 99:1048-1052, 1981.

166. Stanton CA, Sloan DB III, Slusher MM, Greven CM: Acquired immunodeficiency syndrome-related primary intraocular lymphoma. *Arch Ophthalmol* 110:1614-1617, 1992.

167. Sullivan SF, Dallow RL: Intraocular reticulum cell sarcoma: its dramatic response to systemic chemotherapy and its angiogenic potential. *Ann Ophthalmol* 9:401-406, 1977.

168. Vogel MH, Font RL, Zimmerman LE, Levine RA: Reticulum cell sarcoma of the retina and uvea; report of six cases and review of the literature. *Am J Ophthalmol* 66:205-215, 1968.

169. Völcker HE, Naumann GOH: "Primary" reticulum cell sarcoma of the retina. *Dev Ophthalmol* 2:114-120, 1981.

170. Wagoner MD, Gonder JR, Albert DM, Canny CL: Intraocular reticulum cell sarcoma. *Ophthalmology* 87:724-727, 1980.

171. Weisenthal R, Frayer WC, Nichols CW, Eagle RC: Bilateral ocular disease as the initial presentation of malignant lymphoma. *Br J Ophthalmol* 72:248-252, 1988.

172. Wender A, Adar A, Maor E, Yassur Y: Primary B-cell lymphoma of the eyes and brain in a 3-year-old boy. *Arch Ophthalmol* 112:450-451, 1994.

173. Whitcup SM, de Smet MD, Rubin BI, et al: Intraocular lymphoma; clinical and histopathologic diagnosis. *Ophthalmology* 100:1399-1406, 1993.

174. Wilson DJ, Braziel R, Rosenbaum JT: Intraocular lymphoma; immunopathologic analysis of vitreous biopsy specimens. *Arch Ophthalmol* 110:1455-1458, 1992.

175. Ziemianski MC, Godfrey WA, Lee KY, Sabates FN: Lymphoma of the vitreous associated with renal transplantation and immunosuppressive therapy. *Ophthalmology* 87:596-601, 1980.

Angioendotheliomatosis

176. Al-Hazzaa SAF, Green WR, Mann RB: Uveal involvement in systemic angiotropic large cell lymphoma; microscopic and immunohistochemical studies. *Ophthalmology* 100:961-965, 1993.

177. Elner VM, Hidayat AA, Charles NC, et al: Neoplastic angioendotheliomatosis; a variant of malignant lymphoma immunohistochemical and ultrastructural observations of three cases. *Ophthalmology* 93:1237-1245, 1986.

Lymphocytic Lymphoma

178. Kattah JC, Suski ET, Killen JY, et al: Optic neuritis and systemic lymphoma. *Am J Ophthalmol* 89:431-436, 1980.

179. Lewis RA, Clark RB: Infiltrative retinopathy in systemic lymphoma. *Am J Ophthalmol* 79:48-52, 1975.

Burkitt's Lymphoma

180. Feman SS, Niwayama G, Hepler RS, Foos RY: "Burkitt tumor" with intraocular involvement. *Surv Ophthalmol* 14:106-111, 1969.

181. Karp LA, Zimmerman LE, Payne T: Intraocular involvement in Burkitt's lymphoma. *Arch Ophthalmol* 85:295-298, 1971.

182. Zimmerman LE: Lymphoid tumors. *In:* Boniuk M, editor: *Ocular and adnexal tumors; new and controversial aspects,* St. Louis, 1964, CV Mosby, pp. 429-446.

Mycosis Fungoides

183. Foerster HC: Mycosis fungoides with intraocular involvement. *Trans Am Acad Ophthalmol Otolaryngol* 64:308-313, 1960.

184. Gärtner J: Mycosis fungoides mit Beteiligung der Aderhaut. *Klin Monatsbl Augenheilkd* 131:61-69, 1957.

185. Hogan MJ: A case of intraocular mycosis fungoides. Read before the Verhoeff Society meeting, Armed Forces Institute of Pathology, Washington, DC, April 11, 1972.

186. Keltner JL, Fritsch E, Cykiert RC, Albert DM: Mycosis fungoides; intraocular and central nervous system involvement. *Arch Ophthalmol* 95:645-650, 1977.

187. Leitch RJ, Rennie IG, Parsons MA: Ocular involvement in mycosis fungoides. *Br J Ophthalmol* 77:126-127, 1993.

188. Wolter JR, Leenhouts TM, Hendrix RC: Corneal involvement in mycosis fungoides. *Am J Ophthalmol* 55:317-322, 1963.

Multiple Myeloma

189. Clarke E: Ophthalmological complications of multiple myelomatosis. *Br J Ophthalmol* 39:233-236, 1955.

190. Gudas PP Jr: Optic nerve myeloma. *Am J Ophthalmol* 71:1085-1089, 1971.

900

191. Langdon HM: Multiple myeloma with bilateral sixth nerve paralysis and left retrobulbar neuritis. *Trans Am Ophthalmol Soc* 37:223-228, 1939.

Lymphomatoid Granulomatosis

192. Kinyoun LJ, Kalina RE, Klein ML: Choroidal involvement in systemic necrotizing vasculitis. *Arch Ophthalmol* 105:939-942, 1987.
193. Pearson AD, Craft AW, Howe JM: Choroidal involvement in lymphomatoid granulomatosis. *Br J Ophthalmol* 75:688-689, 1991.
194. Tse DT, Mandelbaum S, Chuck DA, et al: Lymphomatoid granulomatosis with ocular involvement. *Retina* 5:94-97, 1985.

Metastatic Carcinoma and Cutaneous Malignant Melanoma to the Retina

195. De Bustros S, Augsburger JJ, Shields JA, et al: Intraocular metastases from cutaneous malignant melanoma. *Arch Ophthalmol* 103:937-940, 1985.
196. Duke JR, Walsh FB: Metastatic carcinoma to the retina. *Am J Ophthalmol* 47:44-48, 1959.
197. Flindall RJ, Fleming KO: Metastatic tumour of the retina. *Can J Ophthalmol* 2:130-132, 1967.
198. Font RL, Naumann G, Zimmerman LE: Primary malignant melanoma of the skin metastatic to the eye and orbit; report of ten cases and review of the literature. *Am J Ophthalmol* 63:738-754, 1967.
199. Friedman AH: Discussion of three papers. *Ophthalmology* 86:1355-1358, 1979.
200. Kennedy RJ, Rummel WD, McCarthy JL, Hazard JB: Metastatic carcinoma of the retina; report of a case and the pathologic findings. *Arch Ophthalmol* 60:12-18, 1958.
201. Klein R, Nicholson DH, Luxenberg MN: Retinal metastasis from squamous cell carcinoma of the lung. *Am J Ophthalmol* 83:358-361, 1977.
202. Koenig RP, Johnson DL, Monahan RH: Bronchogenic carcinoma with metastases to the retina. *Am J Ophthalmol* 56:827-829, 1963.
203. Letson AD, Davidorf FH: Bilateral retinal metastases from cutaneous malignant melanoma. *Arch Ophthalmol* 100:605-607, 1982.
204. Levy RM, de Venecia G: Trypsin digest study of retinal metastasis and tumor cell emboli. *Am J Ophthalmol* 70:778-782, 1970.
205. Leys AM, Van Eyck LM, Nuttin BJ, et al: Metastatic carcinoma to the retina; clinicopathologic findings in two cases. *Arch Ophthalmol* 108:1448-1452, 1990.
206. Liddicoat DA, Wolter JR, Wilkinson WC: Retinal metastasis of malignant melanoblastoma; a case report. *Am J Ophthalmol* 48:172-177, 1959.
207. Piro P, Pappas HR, Erozan YS, et al: Diagnostic vitrectomy in metastatic breast carcinoma in the vitreous. *Retina* 2:182-188, 1982.
208. Pollock SC, Awh CC, Dutton JJ: Cutaneous melanoma metastatic to the optic disc and vitreous. *Arch Ophthalmol* 109:1352-1354, 1991.
209. Riffenburgh RS: Metastatic malignant melanoma to the retina. *Arch Ophthalmol* 66:487-489, 1961.
210. Robertson DM, Wilkinson CP, Murray JL, Gordy DD: Metastatic tumor to the retina and vitreous cavity from primary melanoma of the skin; treatment with systemic and subconjunctival chemotherapy. *Ophthalmology* 88:1296-1301, 1981.
211. Smoleroff JW, Agatston SA: Metastatic carcinoma of the retina; report of a case, with pathologic observations. *Arch Ophthalmol* 12:359-365, 1934.

212. Striebel-Gerecke SU, Messmer EP, Landolt U: Retinale and vitreale Metastase eines kleinzelligen Bronchuskarzinoms. *Klin Monatsbl Augenheilkd* 200:535-536, 1992.
213. Tachinami K, Katayama T, Takeda N, et al: A case of metastatic carcinoma to the retina. *Acta Soc Ophthalmol Jpn* 96:1336-1340, 1992.
214. Takagi T, Yamaguchi T, Mizoguchi T, Amemiya T: A case of metastatic optic nerve head and retinal carcinoma with vitreous seeds. *Ophthalmologica* 199:123-126, 1989.
215. Uhler EM: Metastatic malignant melanoma of the retina. *Am J Ophthalmol* 23:158-162, 1940.
216. Young SE, Cruciger M, Lukeman J: Metastatic carcinoma to the retina: Case report. *Ophthalmology* 86:1350-1354, 1979.

Paraneoplastic Retinopathy Associated with Carcinoma (Cancer-Associated Retinopathy or CAR Syndrome)

217. Brain RL, Norris FH Jr: *The remote effects of cancer on the nervous system,* New York, 1965, Grune & Stratton, p. 24.
218. Buchanan TAS, Gardiner TA, Archer DB: An ultrastructural study of retinal photoreceptor degeneration associated with bronchial carcinoma. *Am J Ophthalmol* 97:277-287, 1984.
219. Cogan DG, Kuwabara T, Currie J, Kattah J: Paraneoplastische Retinopathie unter dem klinischen Bild einer Zapfendystrophie mit Achromatopsie. *Klin Monatsbl Augenheilkd* 197:156-158, 1990.
220. Grunwald GB, Klein R, Simmonds MA, Kornguth SE: Autoimmune basis for visual paraneoplastic syndrome in patients with small-cell lung carcinoma. *Lancet* 1:658-661, 1985.
221. Grunwald GB, Kornguth SC, Towfighi J, et al: Autoimmune basis for visual paraneoplastic syndrome in patients with small cell lung carcinoma; retinal immune deposits and ablation of retinal ganglion cells. *Cancer* 60:780-786, 1987.
222. Jacobson DM, Thirkill CE, Tipping SJ: A clinical triad to diagnose paraneoplastic retinopathy. *Ann Neurol* 28:162-167, 1990.
223. Keltner JL, Roth AM, Chang RS: Photoreceptor degeneration; possible autoimmune disorder. *Arch Ophthalmol* 101:564-569, 1983.
224. Keltner JL, Thirkill CE, Tyler NK, Roth AM: Management and monitoring of cancer-associated retinopathy. *Arch Ophthalmol* 110:48-53, 1992.
225. Klingele TG, Burde RM, Rappazzo JA, et al: Paraneoplastic retinopathy. *J Clin Neuro-Ophthalmol* 4:239-245, 1984.
226. Kornguth SE, Kalinke T, Grunwald GB, et al: Anti-neurofilament antibodies in the sera of patients with small cell carcinoma of the lung and with paraneoplastic syndrome. *Cancer Res* 46:2588-2595, 1986.
227. Kornguth SE, Klein RR, Appen R, Choate J: Occurrence of anti-retinal ganglion cell antibodies in patients with small cell carcinoma of the lung. *Cancer* 50:1289-1293, 1982.
228. Malik S, Furlan AJ, Sweeney PJ, et al: Optic neuropathy: a rare paraneoplastic syndrome. *J Clin Neuro-Ophthalmol* 12:137-141, 1992.
229. Matsui Y, Mehta MC, Katsumi O, et al: Electrophysiological findings in paraneoplastic retinopathy. *Graefes Arch Clin Exp Ophthalmol* 230:324-328, 1992.
230. Rizzo JF III, Gittinger JW Jr: Selective immunohistochemical staining in the paraneoplastic retinopathy syndrome. *Ophthalmology* 99:1286-1295, 1992.
231. Sawyer RA, Selhorst JB, Zimmerman LE, Hoyt WF: Blindness caused by photoreceptor degeneration as a remote effect of cancer. *Am J Ophthalmol* 81:606-613, 1976.
232. Thirkill CE, FitzGerald P, Sergott RC, et al: Cancer-associated retinopathy (CAR syndrome) with antibodies

reacting with retinal, optic-nerve, and cancer cells. *N Engl J Med* 321:1589-1594, 1989.

233. Thirkill CE, Keltner JL, Tyler NK, Roth AM: Antibody reactions with retina and cancer-associated antigens in 10 patients with cancer-associated retinopathy. *Arch Ophthalmol* 111:931-937, 1993.

234. Thirkill CE, Roth AM, Keltner JR: Cancer-associated retinopathy. *Arch Ophthalmol* 105:372-375, 1987.

235. Thirkill CE, Tait RC, Tyler NK, et al: Intraperitoneal cultivation of small-cell carcinoma induces expression of the retinal cancer-associated retinopathy antigen. *Arch Ophthalmol* 111:974-978, 1993.

236. Van Der Pol BAE, Planten JT: A non-metastatic remote effect of lung carcinoma. *Doc Ophthalmol* 67:89-94, 1987.

Paraneoplastic Chorioretinopathy Associated with Melanoma

237. Albert DM, Sober AJ, Fitzpatrick TB: Iritis in patients with cutaneous melanoma and vitiligo. *Arch Ophthalmol* 96:2081-2084, 1978.

238. Berson EL, Lessell S: Paraneoplastic night blindness with malignant melanoma. *Am J Ophthalmol* 106:307-311, 1988.

239. Donaldson RC, Canaan SA Jr, McLean RB, Ackerman LV: Uveitis and vitiligo associated with BCG treatment for malignant melanoma. *Surgery* 76:771-778, 1974.

240. Duke-Elder S, editor: *System of ophthalmology, vol. 9. Diseases of the uveal tract,* St. Louis, 1966, CV Mosby, p. 373.

241. Gass JDM: Acute Vogt-Koyanagi-Harada-like syndrome occurring in a patient with metastatic cutaneous melanoma. *In:* Saari K M, editor: *Uveitis update: proceedings of the First International Symposium on Uveitis held in Hanasaari, Espoo, Finland on May 16-19, 1984,* Amsterdam, 1984, Excerpta Medica, pp. 407-408.

242. Gass JDM: Vitiliginous chorioretinitis. *Arch Ophthalmol* 99:1778-1787, 1981.

243. Hertz KC, Gazze LA, Kirkpatrick CH, Katz SI: Autoimmune vitiligo; detection of antibodies to melanin-producing cells. *N Engl J Med* 297:634-637, 1977.

244. Rush JA: Paraneoplastic retinopathy in malignant melanoma. *Am J Ophthalmol* 115:390-391, 1993.

245. Weinstein JM, Kelman SE, Bresnick GH, Kornguth SE: Paraneoplastic retinopathy associated with antiretinal bipolar cell antibodies in cutaneous malignant melanoma. *Ophthalmology* 101:1236-1243, 1994.

12

Macular Dysfunction Caused by Vitreous and Vitreoretinal Interface Abnormalities

Diseases affecting primarily the vitreous and vitreoretinal interface are associated with a variety of macular lesions causing loss of central vision. These lesions may be detected ophthalmoscopically and biomicroscopically and should be differentiated from the other causes of macular dysfunction. In no other area of macular disease is the use of a fundus contact lens more important to detect and define the anatomic changes. Recently introduced techniques that may improve our ability in this regard are confocal laser tomographic analysis, laser biomicroscopy (Puliafito's technique), and kinetic ultrasonography.[8,57,71,106]

▼ ANATOMIC CONSIDERATIONS

The vitreous is a semisolid gel containing a hyaluronic acid network interspersed in a framework of randomly spaced collagen fibrils. The framework is most apparent histologically in the region of the pars plana, where it is strongly anchored to the ciliary epithelium in an area referred to as the vitreous base. Posterior to the pars plana the concentration of collagen and hyaluronic acid is greatest in the ill-defined outer part of the vitreous gel, referred to as the vitreous cortex, that lies along the inner retinal surface. The collagen fibrils, which are condensed to form an outer layer of the vitreous cortex, are adherent to the internal limiting membrane (basement membrane, or basal lamina of the Müller cells) of the retina (Figs. 12-1 and 12-2). The basal lamina thickness increases from the vitreous base posteriorly to where it reaches maximal thickness at the crest of the foveal clivus. From there it rapidly becomes thinner, reaching a thickness of 200 Å or less in the foveal center.[38] At the margin of the optic disc, the basal lamina abruptly thins to approximately 450 Å, where it covers the disc surface. Here the basal lamina is associated with multiple gaps associated with glial epipapillary membranes that are probably of developmental origin.[218] Attachment plaques or hemidesmosomes are evident electron microscopically along the vitreoretinal juncture in the peripheral and equatorial zones but are absent posteriorly except in the foveal area.[38] These findings indicate greater adherence of the basal lamina to the Müller cells in these zones with attachment plaques but do not necessarily reflect greater adherence of the vitreous to the basal lamina in these areas.[37] There is other evidence, however, to indicate greater adherence of cortical vitreous to the basal lamina in these areas including the central macular region.[72,104,116] Progressive liquefaction of the posterior vitreous occurs with aging, giving rise to a large optically empty cavity of liquified vitreous in the premacular area, referred to as the premacular bursa, or prefoveolar pocket (Fig. 12-3).[73,74,76,116,140-142] The thin layer of the posterior cortical vitreous gel lying on the inner surface of the macula is not visible biomicroscopically, and the anterior interface of the bursa may be visible and misinterpreted biomicroscopically as the posterior hyaloid of the separated vitreous. The degree of vitreoretinal adherence varies with age as well as location in the eye. Generally the adherence decreases with age. The attachment of the vitreous to the retina is greatest at those sites where the internal limiting membrane of the retinal is the thinnest (Fig. 12-1). These sites include the vitreous base, the major retinal vessels, the optic nerve head, the 1500-μm-diameter rim surrounding the fovea, and the 500-μm-diameter foveola. The latter two sites of attachment are probably important in the development of idiopathic age-related macular hole. Forces generated by movement of the vitreous and the premacular bursa as the eye moves also may play a role in the pathogenesis of posterior vitreous detachment, epiretinal membranes, and macular holes (Fig. 12-3).

FIG. 12-1   Vitreoretinal Attachment in the Macular Region.

The collagen fibrillae making up the vitreous cortex *(vc)* are adherent to the internal limiting membrane (basement membrane of Müller cells). This membrane is thick in the perifoveal area but extremely thin in the foveal region. *Arrow* indicates vitreocyte lying on the internal limiting membrane at the vitreoretinal interface.

FIG. 12-2   Vitreoretinal Interface at the Electron Microscopic Level.

The collagen fibrillae making up the vitreous cortex *(vc)* are adherent to the basement membrane *(bm,* basal lamina, internal limiting membrane) of the Müller cells *(M).* On separation of the vitreous, the collagen fibrillae realign to form the posterior hyaloid membrane *(phm).* Some of the vitreous cortex may remain adherent to the basement membrane *(arrow).*

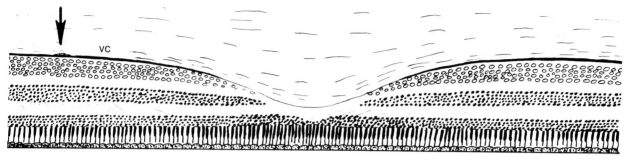

12-1

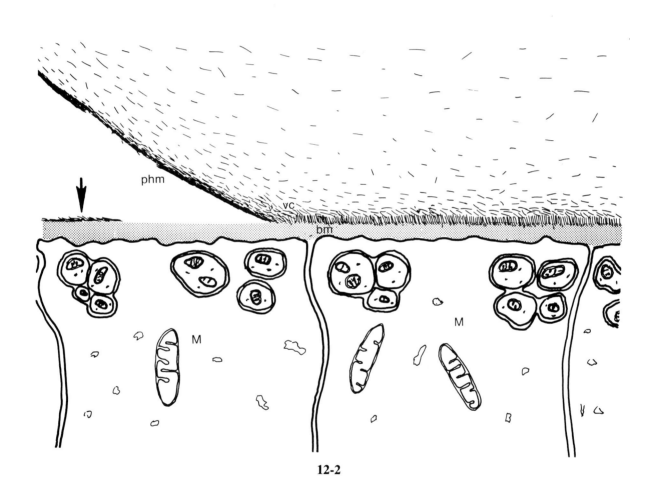

12-2

Kishi and coworkers found anatomic evidence that the prefoveolar vitreous cortex (PVC) may be focally condensed and tightly adherent to the inner surface of the foveolar retina.[72] They examined 59 eyes with spontaneous posterior vitreous detachment with scanning electron microscopy. In 44% of the eyes they found three patterns of vitreous remnants on the surface of the foveolar area. The most common pattern, type 1, found in one-half of these eyes, was a 500-μm-diameter disc of condensed cortical vitreous adherent to the foveolar retina (Fig. 12-4, *A*). In 30% of cases (type 2) a 500-μm-diameter ring of remnants was found adherent to the margin of the foveolar retina (Fig. 12-4, *B* and *C*). In some eyes they also noted a 1500-μm-diameter ring of vitreous remnants at the foveal margin (Fig. 12-4, *A*). Twenty percent of the eyes (type 3) showed a pseudocyst formation consisting of a focal 200- to 300-μm-diameter disc of contracted vitreous cortex bridging the foveolar area. These findings suggest that the structures of the PVC and the vitreoretinal interface in the foveolar area are probably different from that elsewhere in the macular area.

FIG. 12-3 Diagrams of Vitreous Structure in Older Adults.

A, Optically empty premacular bursa, sites of maximum vitreoretinal attachment *(larger arrows* indicate greater attachment) and dynamics of vitreous movement with gaze left and right (**B** and **C**).

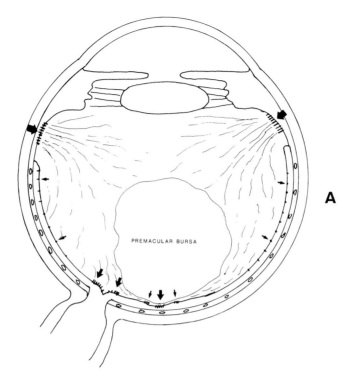

PREMACULAR BURSA

A

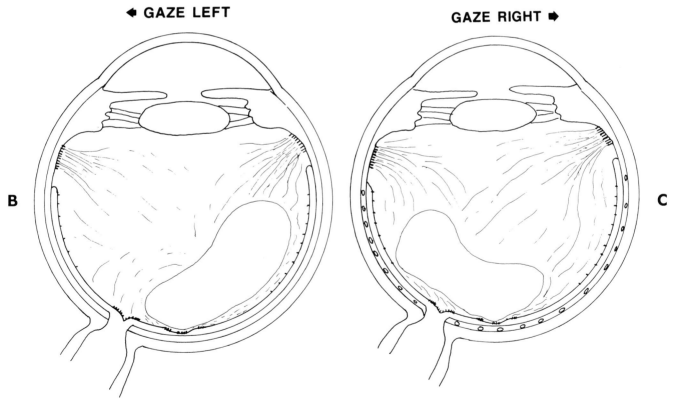

B

C

The cells that are part of the normal vitreous are widely scattered within the vitreous cortex along the surface of the retina and ciliary body. Their concentration is maximal within the vitreous base and near the posterior pole. These cells, termed "hyalocytes," show phagocytic properties, have a high metabolic activity, and may be responsible for both the formation and the maintenance of several vitreous components. They are probably mesenchymal cells. When properly stimulated, they are capable of proliferation and collagen formation. This capability of fibrous metaplasia may supplement the process of collapse, condensation, and shrinkage of the normal collagen framework in the production of pathologic vitreous membranes. Much of the posterior vitreous becomes liquefied by the seventh decade (synchysis senilis). This process of syneresis may be accompanied by spontaneous separation of the vitreous cortex from the retina, a process referred to as posterior vitreous detachment (PVD).* Following vitreous separation, there is condensation and realignment of the collagen molecules comprising the outer surface of the cortical vitreous to form a distinct membrane, the so-called posterior hyaloid membrane, which may be visible biomicroscopically and histologically (Fig. 12-2). Posterior vitreous detachment is present in over 25% of persons by the seventh decade and approximately 65% by the eighth decade. It is more common in women. Posterior vitreous detachment most frequently begins in the macular region following spontaneous dehiscence of the posterior hyaloid near the center of the macula.[30,39,87] It may, however, begin more peripherally. In most patients separation of the posterior hyaloid face from the retina occurs rapidly and smoothly and may or may not be accompanied by symptoms of photopsia and floaters. Slit-lamp examination reveals anterior displacement of the posterior hyaloid membrane. A

*References 30, 38, 39, 63, 108, 117, 132, 133.

FIG. 12-4   Vitreous Remnants on Inner Retinal Surface in the Fovea Following Spontaneous Vitreoretinal Separation.

A, Scanning electron micrograph showing 500 μm diameter disc of condensed vitreous cortex *(white arrow)* adherent to foveolar retina. Open arrow indicates 1500-μm-diameter ring of vitreous remnants at the margin of the foveal retina.

B, Scanning electron micrograph showing 500 μm diameter ring of vitreous cortical remnants *(white arrow)* at the margin of the foveola.

C, Higher magnification of open arrow shown in **B.** Note aligned collagen fibers of vitreous origin in contrast to smooth appearance of underlying internal limiting membrane.

(From Kishi and others.[72])

FIG. 12-5   Diagram Showing Stages of Posterior Vitreous Separation.

Top, Vitreofoveal detachment. *Arrow* indicates contracted and condensed prefoveolar vitreous cortex (pseudooperculum) suspended on the posterior surface *(arrowheads)* of the vitreous cortical gel.

Middle, Vitreomacular detachment. The posterior hyaloid *(arrowheads)* is separated from the macula but not the optic disc.

Bottom, Posterior vitreous detachment with hyaloid *(arrowheads)* separated from the retina and optic disc. *Arrows* indicate prepapillary condensation ring.

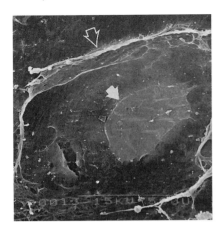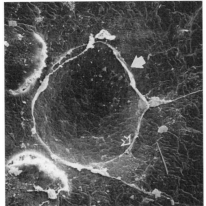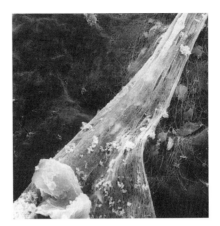

12-4

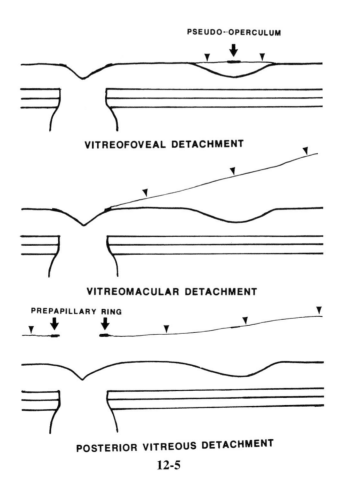

PSEUDO-OPERCULUM

VITREOFOVEAL DETACHMENT

VITREOMACULAR DETACHMENT

PREPAPILLARY RING

POSTERIOR VITREOUS DETACHMENT

12-5

909

gray-white ring of vitreous condensation (Weiss ring) that marks the site of previous vitreous attachment to the margins of the optic disc is usually visible and is the single most important biomicroscopic sign of posterior vitreous separation from the optic disc and macular area (Fig. 12-5). In cases where the posterior hyaloid face tears near the site of attachment to the crest of the fovea, a similar condensation ring may lie in front of the macula (Fig. 12-4). These condensation rings are often distorted and twisted. Posterior vitreous detachment usually occurs without producing any visible alterations in the retina. As the vitreous separates, traction on the inner surface of the optic disc, along the major vascular arcades, or near the vitreous base may occasionally produce a focal intraretinal, preretinal, or diffuse vitreous hemorrhage (Fig. 12-6, A and B).[22,113] Posterior vitreous detachment is the primary cause of peripheral retinal tears and rhegmatogenous retinal detachment.[37,38] Pathologic alterations in the vitreous gel unrelated to aging may be responsible for vitreous shrinkage and premature PVD. Patients with high myopia are more likely to develop PVD early.[144]

▼ VITREOUS TRACTION MACULOPATHIES

Changes in the vitreous gel may cause traction on the retinal surface and macular distortion through several different mechanisms, including anterior–posterior oriented vitreous traction caused by (1) incomplete PVD in which the vitreous remains attached focally to the macular surface; (2) vitreous gel condensation and shrinkage caused by inflammatory, vascular, and metabolic diseases in the absence of PVD; and (3) a peculiar form of traction maculopathy that is related to focal tangential contraction of the prefoveolar vitreous cortex, anterior displacement of the foveal retina, and idiopathic macular hole formation.

FIG. 12-6   Anatomic Changes in the Macula Caused by Traction Exerted by Incomplete Posterior Detachment of the Vitreous.

A, Transient macular distortion. *Arrow* indicates the area where vitreous remains adherent and is exerting traction on the retina.

B, Posterior vitreous detachment is complete. Note rarefaction of the posterior hyaloid anterior to the foveal area.

C, Macular traction, edema, degeneration, and detachment.

D, Paramacular traction, retinal vessel avulsion, and retinal detachment.

E, Juxtapapillary traction and retinal detachment.

F, Macular hole.

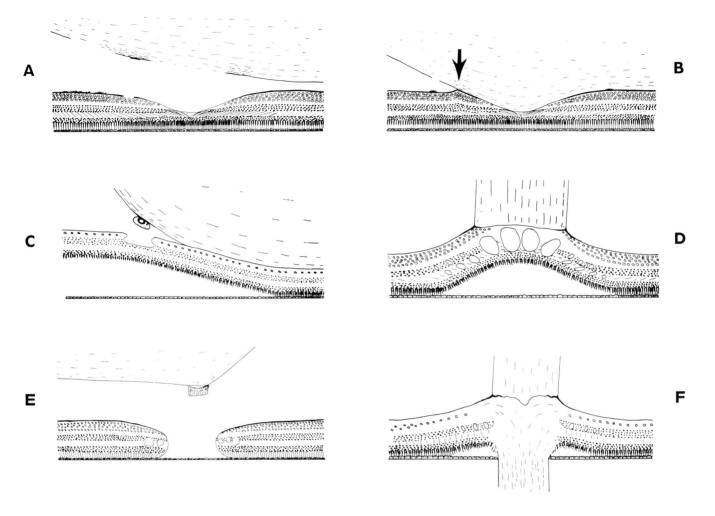

A

B

C

D

E

F

Traction maculopathy caused by incomplete posterior vitreous detachment

Approximately 30% of patients (average age of 60 years) who develop a symptomatic PVD will have evidence of vitreous hemorrhage or a peripheral retinal tear or both. This affects twice as many women as men. Ten percent to 15% of these patients will develop a PVD in the second eye, usually within 2 years. Vitreous hemorrhage that usually is caused by a demonstrable peripheral full- or partial-thickness retinal tear is the most frequent cause of transient loss of vision in patients after an acute PVD (Figs. 12-6, *D,* and 12-7, *A*). In most cases the macula is unaffected by the PVD. Small hemorrhages around the optic disc, along the major vascular arcades, and less frequently in the macula may be the only sign of microtrauma to the retina caused by the PVD (Fig. 12-7, *A* and *B*).[22,113] When the PVD is impeded by abnormal vitreoretinal adhesions in the macular area, traction and distortion of the macula may cause blurring of vision, metamorphopsia, and occasionally a scotoma (Figs. 12-6, *A,* and 12-7, *C* to *F* and *J* to *L*). Ophthalmoscopic and biomicroscopic examination reveals a partial PVD and tenting of the retina at the site of the vitreoretinal adhesion.[63,64,69,87,105] This site may be localized in the parafoveal region rather than directly in the foveal area. If the onset of symptoms is recent, the vitreoretinal adhesion may separate in a matter of days or weeks and visual function may be restored to normal (Fig. 12-7, *E, F,* and *L*). These patients, however, may subsequently develop evidence of epiretinal membrane (Fig. 12-7, *G*). In a few cases an epiretinal membrane may develop before PVD occurs (Fig. 12-8, *A* to *C*).

FIG. 12-7   Vitreous Traction Maculopathy.

A and **B,** This woman experienced sudden blurring of vision associated with a preretinal hemorrhage caused by posterior vitreous detachment and avulsion of a small capillary in the vicinity of the superotemporal retinal vein *(arrows).*

C to **G,** A 41-year-old man noted sudden onset of blurred vision and metamorphopsia in the right eye as a result of incomplete separation of the vitreous, which remained attached to the superior nasal portion of the macula *(arrow,* **C** and **D;** see Fig. 12-6, **A**). Fine retinal striae radiated outward from the macula. Visual acuity was 20/70. Angiography revealed no definite abnormality. Eight days later spontaneous separation of the vitreous was associated with a circular tear in the posterior hyaloid in the foveal area (**E** and **F**). The condensation of the edges of the hole in the posterior hyaloid indicated in the fundus painting (**F**) is not visible in **E** (see Fig. 12-6, **B**). Visual acuity returned to 20/25. The retinal wrinkles noted in **C** were no longer visible. Eighteen months later he developed metamorphopsia caused by contraction of an epiretinal membrane in the nasal half of the macula. Note the fine retinal folds radiating from the temporal edge of the membrane (**G**).

H, Paramacular vitreous traction causing retinal vessel avulsion *(arrow)* and serous detachment of the macula (see Fig. 12-6, **D**).

I, Vitreous traction on the optic disc and juxtapapillary retina was responsible for the misdiagnosis of papilledema in this patient (see Fig. 12-6, **E**).

J to **L,** Blurred vision in a 62-year-old woman with macular edema and detachment resulting from prolonged vitreous traction (see Fig. 12-6, **C**). Visual acuity was 20/200. *Arrows* indicate margin of the detachment. Angiography revealed evidence of cystoid macular edema (**K**). Twenty-nine months later the vitreous separated and visual acuity returned to 20/40 (**L**).

(**H** from Benson WE, Tasman W: *Arch Ophthalmol* 102:669, 1984; copyright 1984, American Medical Association.[10])

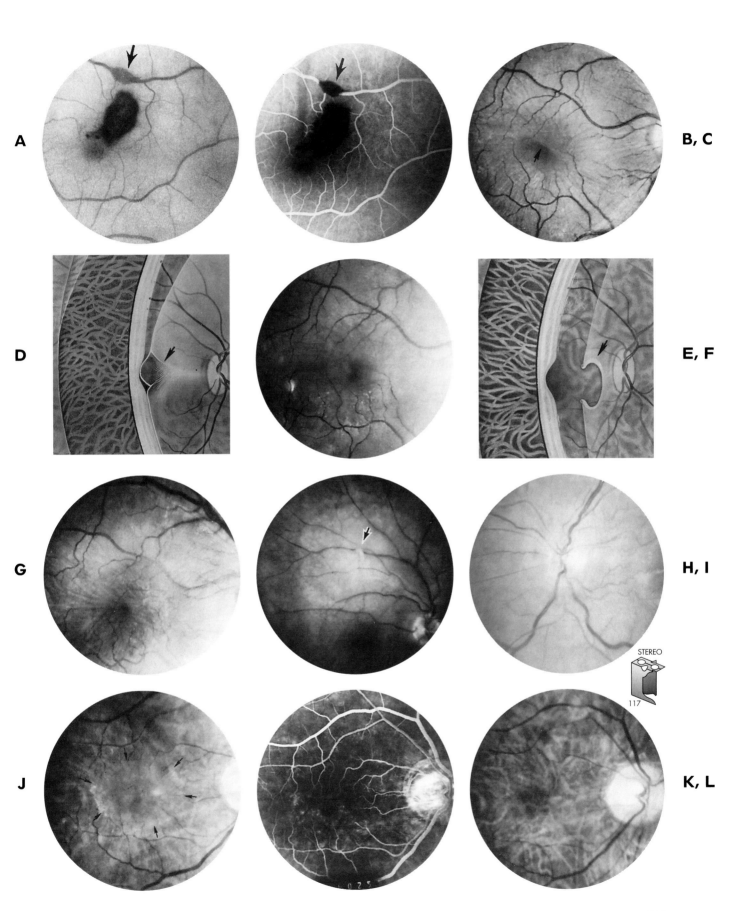

A

B, C

D

E, F

G

H, I

STEREO
117

J

K, L

913

In some patients vitreoretinal adhesion in the macular area is sufficiently dense that prolonged traction causes distortion, cystic edema, degeneration, and detachment of the macula. This may be caused by a linear area of attachment of the posterior hyaloid to the retinal surface (Fig. 12-7, *C*), a single condensed strand of vitreous attached to the paracentral retina, a cone-shaped mass of condensed vitreous with attachment to the entire foveal inner surface (Figs. 12-6, *C*, and 12-7, *J* and *L*), and paracentral traction at the major vascular arcades (Fig. 12-7, *A* and *H*). When the partly detached vitreous remains attached to the center of the macula, the retina is tented anteriorly, causing a localized tractional serous retinal detachment that is surrounded by radiating retinal folds (Figs. 12-6, *C*, and 12-7, *J* and *L*). Cystic changes are often evident centrally.[15] Prolonged vitreous traction may be associated with angiographic evidence of retinal capillary permeability alterations, and development of an epiretinal membrane in the area of vitreoretinal adhesion. Spontaneous separation of the adhesion may eventually occur (Fig. 12-7, *J* to *L*). Surgical separation of the vitreoretinal attachment may be required to reattach the macula (Fig. 12-8, *J* to *L*).* Lysis of vitreoretinal adhesions may be accomplished in some cases with Q-switched neodymium laser.[65]

Vitreous traction at the site of a major retinal vessel may cause not only a tractional retinal detachment that extends into the macula but also avulsion of the blood vessel (Figs. 12-6, *D*, and 12-7, *H*), vitreous hemorrhage, proliferative retinopathy (Fig. 12-8), and infrequently a full-thickness retinal hole.†

Vitreous traction on the optic nerve head and juxtapapillary retina may cause a fundus picture that simulates papilledema, optic disc capillary angioma, astrocytoma, or combined RPE and retinal hamartoma (Figs. 12-6, *E*; and 12-7, *I*; 12-8, *D* to *G*).[16]

In some cases with unusual adherence of the center of the fovea to the vitreous, a PVD that begins in the extramacular area may cause either a partial or full-thickness macular hole as it extends through the macular area (Figs. 12-6, *F*, and 12-8, *H*). This, however, is an infrequent mechanism for causing a macular hole (see discussion of senile macular hole in a subsequent section).

---

*References 88, 94, 108, 109, 126, 129, 130.
†References 10, 26, 36, 110, 137.

FIG. 12-8 Vitreous Traction Maculopathy Associated with Epiretinal Membrane Formation.

A to C, A 26-year-old patient initially was seen because of blurred vision caused by vitritis associated with an active focus of toxoplasmosis in the peripheral fundus. Three months later the vitreous cleared and visual acuity returned to 20/20. One month later he developed crinkling of the inner retinal surface caused by an epiretinal membrane (*arrows,* **A**). Seven weeks later he was seen because of metamorphopsia. The vitreous along with the epiretinal membrane had detached superiorly and was adherent to the center of the macula (*arrows,* **B**). Visual acuity was 20/30. One week later the vision had improved to 20/20. The vitreous detachment had extended further inferiorly. Six years later the condensed ball of epiretinal membrane (*arrow,* **C**) and the posterior hyaloid were still attached to the retina inferonasally.

D to G, This 65-year-old patient developed blurred vision associated with a macular pucker that appeared to have pulled free from its attachment to a branch retinal artery inferior to the macular inferiorly (*arrow,* **D**). Note the suggestion of a small vascular tuft (*arrow,* **D**). Seven months later the patient returned with a semiopaque angiomatous preretinal lesion resembling an astrocytoma (**E**). Angiography revealed a neovascular frond within this lesion (**F**). Over the next 6 months the tumor enlarged (**G**). Following photocoagulation the patient developed subretinal neovascularization.

H, Macular hole caused by vitreous traction. Note irregular inferior edge of hole where the flap has torn free. The operculum *(arrow)* was attached to the posterior hyaloid face.

I, In 1989, this 40-year-old man with high myopia noted a paracentral scotoma in the right eye. One year later his visual acuity was 20/25 bilaterally. There was an incomplete posterior vitreous detachment and adherence of the vitreous to a focal area of epiretinal membrane condensation and tractional retinal detachment. Angiography demonstrated evidence of mild underlying depigmentation of the pigment epithelium. Over the subsequent 4 years he developed a focal area of geographic atrophy beneath the focal area of tractional retinal detachment (**I**). The visual acuity was 20/30.

J to L, Macular detachment and hole caused by vitreous traction. Note in the *stereoscopic views* (**J** and **K**) the focal adherence of the vitreous strand to the edge of the hole. Because of persistence of the detachment a vitrectomy was done and the retina was reattached (**L**).

(**B** from Jaffe NS: Complications of acute posterior vitreous detachment, *Trans Am Acad Ophthalmol Otolaryngol* 71:641, 1967 [64]; **D** to **G**, courtesy of Dr. Robert Machemer.)

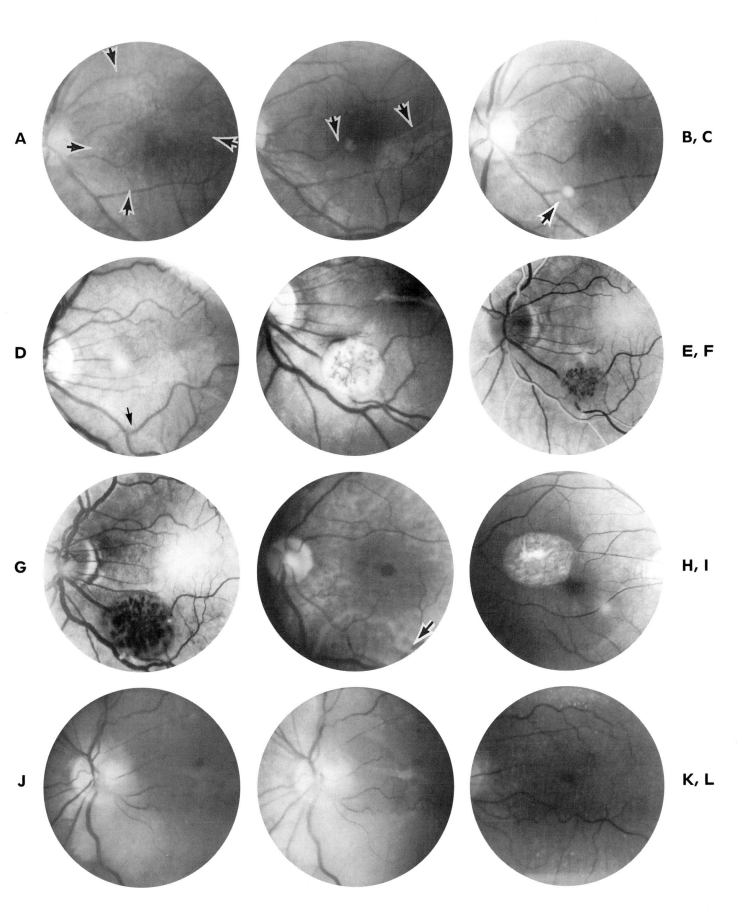

Traction maculopathy caused by spontaneous contraction of the prefoveolar vitreous cortex unassociated with a posterior vitreous detachment

Idiopathic age-related macular hole

Idiopathic age-related macular hole, referred to henceforth in this section as macular hole, affects predominantly older patients, more often women at a ratio of 2 or 3:1.[1] They often discover blurred vision and metamorphopsia when they cover the fellow normal eye.* Most patients report that both eyes were normal during their last eye examination 1 or 2 years previously. From the pathogenetic and therapeutic standpoint, it is important to differentiate idiopathic age-related macular hole from the less common causes of macular hole, such as trauma or macular traction resulting from incomplete posterior vitreous separation, transvitreal bands of vitreous condensation, or neighboring epiretinal membranes. An understanding of the structure of the vitreous, and aging changes in its structure discussed previously in this chapter, and the ultrastructure of the foveolar retina (Fig. 12-9) are important in considering the pathogenesis of age-related macular hole, which typically begins in eyes with an optically empty liquefied premacular vitreous and no evidence of posterior vitreous separation.

Table 12-1 and the diagrams in Figs. 12-10 and 12-11 summarize the characteristic biomicroscopic features and the presumed anatomic changes accompanying each of the stages of development of a macular hole.[47]

*References 2, 6, 45, 66, 79, 91, 95, 99, 102, 143, 145.

FIG. 12-9

Ultrastructure of the foveolar area lying between the small arrows shows a significant population of Müller cells (pale staining cells indicated by the *large arrow*) in the umbo region.

(From Hogan and others.[61])

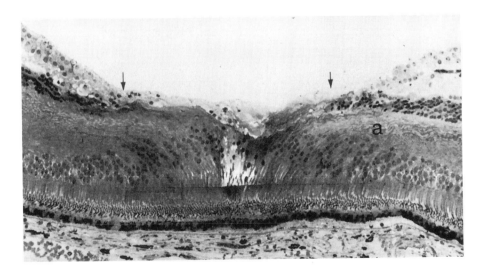

TABLE 12-1

BIOMICROSCOPIC CLASSIFICATION OF AGE-RELATED MACULAR HOLE

Stage	Biomicroscopic findings	Anatomic interpretation
1-A (impending hole)	Central yellow spot, loss of foveolar depression, no vitreofoveolar separation	Early serous detachment of foveolar retina
1-B (impending or occult hole)	Yellow ring with bridging interface, loss of foveolar depression, no vitreofoveolar separation	Small ring—serous foveolar detachment with lateral displacement of xanthophyll. Large ring—central occult foveolar hole with centrifugal displacement of foveolar retina and xanthophyll, with bridging contracted prefoveolar vitreous cortex. Cannot detect transition from impending to occult hole.
2	Eccentric oval, crescent, or horseshoe retinal defect inside edge of yellow ring	Hole (tear) in periphery of contracted prefoveolar vitreous cortex bridging round retinal hole, no loss of foveolar retina.
	Central round retinal defect with rim of elevated retina	
	With prefoveolar opacity	Hole with pseudo-operculum,* rim of retinal detachment, no posterior vitreous detachment from optic disc and macula
	Without prefoveolar opacity	Hole without pseudo-operculum or posterior vitreous detachment
3	Central round ≥ 400 μm diameter retinal defect, no Weiss's ring, rim of elevated retina	
	With prefoveolar opacity	Hole with pseudo-operculum, no posterior vitreous detachment from optic disc and periphery of macula
	Without prefoveolar opacity	Hole without pseudo-operculum, no posterior vitreous detachment from optic disc and macula
4	Central round retinal defect, rim of elevated retina, Weiss's ring	
	With small vitreous opacity near temporal edge of ring	Hole with pseudo-operculum, posterior vitreous detachment from optic disc and macula with mobile Weiss ring and pseudo-operculum†
	Without small opacity	Hole and posterior vitreous detachment from optic disc and macula without pseudo-operculum

*Pseudo-operculum contains no retinal receptors.
†Usually found near temporal border of Weiss's ring.

Stage 1-A impending macular hole

Although the earliest precipitating event responsible for the progression of changes leading to a macular hole has not been identified, the author believes that proliferation of Müller cells located in the center of the normal foveola (Figs. 12-9 and 12-10)[61] and their extension through the internal limiting membrane at the umbo into the outer part of the layer of formed prefoveolar vitreous cortex is most likely responsible for causing contraction, condensation, and partial loss of transparency of the outer part of vitreous cortex in the foveolar and perifoveolar region. Retinal astrocytes and vitreocytes would seem to be less likely candidates as cells responsible for inducing contracture of the prefoveolar vitreous cortex.[19,134] Tangential contraction of the outer part of the prefoveolar cortical vitreous causes anterior displacement and serous detachment of the foveolar retina (Figs. 12-10, *B*, and 12-11, *B*). Biomicroscopically a yellow spot appears centrally (Figs. 12-12, *A*, and 12-13, *A*). This spot is caused by greater visibility of the retinal xanthophyll, which is highly concentrated in the receptor cells and nerve fiber layer in the foveolar region. It is more apparent as the retina separates from the RPE. The patient, particularly if he or she has a macular hole in the fellow eye, may experience the abrupt onset of metamorphopsia unassociated with photopsia or floaters. The visual acuity may be almost normal. Distortion of the Amsler grid is usually present. Biomicroscopically, there is no evidence of a PVD but there is loss of the normal foveolar depression and the foveal reflex. Fluorescein angiography often shows a focal area of faint fluorescence centrally (Fig. 12-13, *B*).

Stage 1-B impending macular hole

As the foveal retina elevates to the level of the surrounding thick perifoveal retina (Figs. 12-10, *C*, and 12-11, *C*), the retinal receptor layer is put on stretch and thinning of the foveolar retina around the umbo causes a change in the biomicroscopic appearance from a yellow spot to a small donut-shaped yellow ring lesion (Figs. 11-12, *D*, and 12-14, *A*). Although a yellow spot occurs with foveal detachment from other causes, e.g., idiopathic central serous chorioretinopathy, the change from a spot to a ring is peculiar to patients developing a macular hole.[47]

Stage 1-B occult macular hole

Whereas the small central area of translucence in the center of the yellow spot may result from attenuation of the foveolar retina, it is probable

FIG. 12-10   Diagrams Illustrating Presumed Mechanism of Early Macular Hole Development.

A, Extension of Müller cells through the internal limiting membrane of retina into the outer part of the layer of gelatinous vitreous cortex *(vc)* to form a prefoveolar vitreoglial membrane *(arrows)*. The premacular bursa *(pmb)* contains liquefied vitreous. The dotted matrix indicates the area of highly concentrated retinal xanthophyll.

B, Stage 1-A impending macular hole. Condensation and tangential contraction of the prefoveolar vitreoglial membrane causes detachment of the foveolar retina. Separation of the foveolar retina from the pigment epithelium causes the xanthophyll to be visible biomicroscopically as a yellow spot.

C, Stage 1-B impending macular hole. Further contraction of the prefoveolar vitreoglial membrane elevates the foveolar retina to the level of the perifoveal retina and causes stretching and attenuation of the retinal receptor layer centrally and a change from a yellow spot to a small, yellow, doughnut-shaped ring biomicroscopically.

that the clearly defined yellow ring that develops soon afterward is caused by a break in the continuity of the receptor cell layer at the umbo, structurally the thinnest and weakest site in the retina. This is followed by centrifugal movement of the foveolar retinal receptor cells, their radiating nerve fibers, the Müller cells, and the xanthophyll beneath the internal limiting membrane of the retina and the contracted prefoveolar vitreous cortex (Fig. 12-11, *D* and *E*). Initially the internal limiting membrane of the foveolar retina and the thin layer of horizontally oriented Müller cell processes separating it from the retinal receptor cells may not be involved in the central retinal break. Regardless, as long as the contracted prefoveolar contracted vitreous cortex bridges the hole, it may be visible biomicroscopically as a semitranslucent interface. Thus the change from a stage 1-B impending hole to a stage 1-B occult hole cannot be detected biomicroscopically. Reactive proliferation of Müller cells and retinal astrocytes occurring within the area of the receptor cell dehiscence probably contribute to the opacification of the tissue bridging the defect and, in some cases, may cause ruffled edges of the retinal dehiscence surrounded by fine radiating retinal folds (Fig. 12-12, *G* and *H*).

Fluorescein angiography in stage 1-B lesions of all sizes usually shows hyperfluorescence of variable intensity centrally. Although a high intensity of fluorescence is more suggestive that a full-thickness hole is present, angiography is not reliable in this regard.

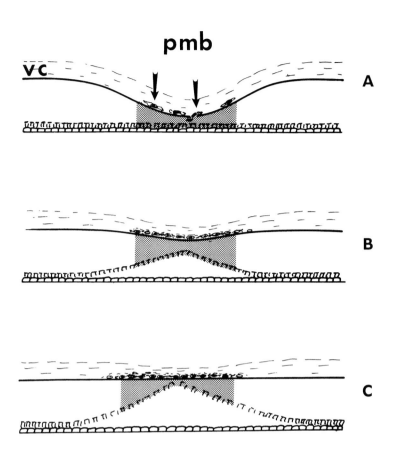

Stage 2 hole

Spontaneous vitreofoveal separation may occur soon after the central retinal dehiscence, and the contracted prefoveolar vitreous cortex becomes visible as a semitranslucent prehole opacity or operculum-like structure lying anterior to a small foveolar hole (Fig. 12-11, *F*). Initially the diameter of this opacity is often larger than that of the foveolar hole. In a few patients with early stage 1-B lesions, separation of the prefoveolar vitreous cortex may be accompanied by avulsion of part of the foveolar retina, resulting in a true operculum formation. Biomicroscopy, however, cannot determine the presence or absence of retinal tissue in the prehole opacity. In some patients the contracted prefoveolar vitreous cortex, either while it remains attached to and bridges the macular hole or after it separates from the perifoveolar retina, may be transparent and undetectable biomicroscopically. In such cases very small stage 2 holes without a prehole opacity may be evident. In most patients, however, the contracted vitreous cortex is semitransparent and remains attached to the inner retinal surface surrounding the retinal hole as the foveolar retina continues to retract centrifugally (Fig. 12-11, *E*). Biomicroscopically there is progressive enlargement of the yellow ring, which may become serrated along its inner margin that corresponds to the edge of the occult round retinal hole (Fig. 12-12, *H* to *K*). Eventually the first biomicroscopic evidence of a dehiscence may occur in the semitransparent vitreous cortex at the inner edge of the yellow ring (Figs. 12-11, *G,* and 12-12, *G*). In the area of the dehiscence, the serration of the yellow ring disappears, presumably because of relief of traction on the edge of the retinal hole, and the yellow pigmentation fades, possibly as a result of diffusion of xanthophyll out of the retina in this area. Over a period of days or weeks, further enlargement of the macular hole and additional contraction of the prefoveolar vitreous cortex cause a can opener–type 360-degree tear in the contracted prefoveolar vitreous cortex, separating it from the less condensed outer vitreous cortex at the edge of the retinal hole (Figs. 12-11, *H,* and 12-12, *G* to *L*). The contracted prefoveal vitreous cortex is visible biomicroscopically as an operculum-like opacity (pseudooperculum) suspended anterior to the hole on the posterior surface of the layer of transparent vitreous gel that bridges the hole and lies along the inner retinal surface in the macula. This prefoveolar opacity oscillates slightly with eye movements. It is usually not possible to detect biomicroscopically an interface caused by the layer

FIG. 12-11   Diagrams Illustrating the Presumed Anatomy of the Stages of Development of an Idiopathic Macular Hole.

A, Normal fovea. Layer of vitreous cortex (*vc*) lying on internal limiting membrane of retina.

B, Stage 1-A impending hole. Early contraction of outer part of vitreous cortex with foveolar detachment.

C, Stage 1-B impending hole.

D and **E,** Stage 1-B occult hole. Dehiscence of the retinal receptor layer at the umbo with centrifugal retraction of the retinal receptors.

F, Stage 2 hole with early separation of condensed prefoveolar vitreous cortex with formation of pseudo-operculum that is larger than the hole.

G, Stage 2 hole with tear in vitreous cortex at junction of the prefoveolar vitreous cortex and edge of macular hole.

H, Stage 3 hole with pseudo-operculum.

I, Stage 4 hole after posterior vitreous separation.

(From Gass.[47])

of transparent vitreous cortical gel surrounding the pseudooperculum.

Stage 3 hole

Centrifugal retraction of the foveolar retinal receptors continues until the hole becomes fully developed and its diameter in all but a few cases reaches 400 to 600 μm (Figs. 12-11, *H;* 12-12, *F* and *L;* and 12-13, *C, G, I,* and *K*). All stages of progressive enlargement of the hole are considered as stage 2 holes. Since the ultimate diameter of the hole is variable, for purposes of classification the author suggests that all holes less than 400 μm in diameter be considered stage 2 holes.

Stage 3 holes are associated with a mean visual acuity of 20/200 with a range from 20/40 to 5/200. The sharply outlined 400- to 600-μm-diameter hole is typically surrounded by a 1000- to 1500-μm-diameter gray rim of retinal detachment.[1,2,45,60,131] The patient describes metamorphopsia on the Amsler grid. A well-defined central scotoma, however, is usually difficult to demonstrate on the grid. Microperimetry using the scanning laser ophthalmoscope demonstrates an absolute scotoma corresponding with a macular hole, and a relative scotoma corresponding with the rim of retinal detachment surrounding the hole. With further refinement of the perimetric technique, it is probable that visual defects that extend beyond the area corresponding with the rim of detachment will be detected.[3,18a,120,121] Ninety-five percent of patients report a gap in a narrow slit beam of light (positive slit-beam sign) when the slit of light is directed through a fundus contact lens into the center of the

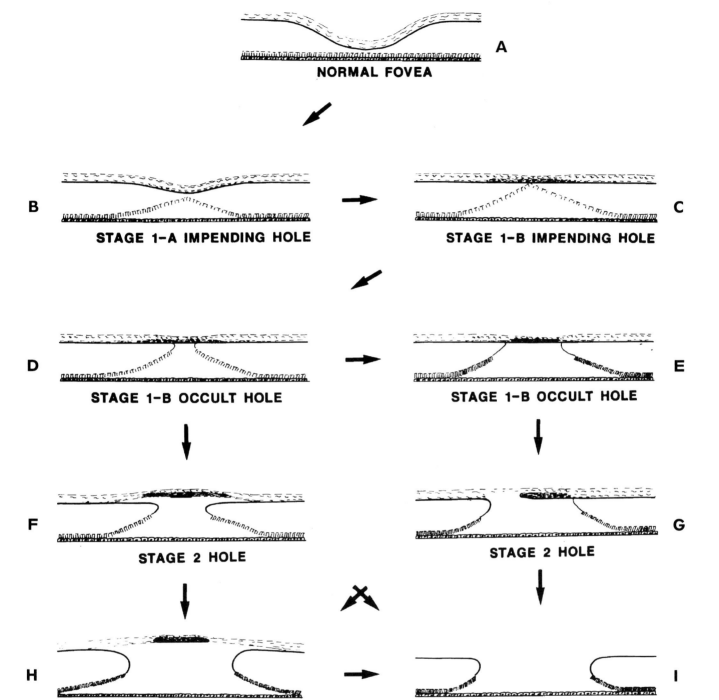

A

NORMAL FOVEA

B
STAGE 1-A IMPENDING HOLE

C
STAGE 1-B IMPENDING HOLE

D
STAGE 1-B OCCULT HOLE

E
STAGE 1-B OCCULT HOLE

F
STAGE 2 HOLE

G
STAGE 2 HOLE

H
STAGE 3 HOLE

I
STAGE 4 HOLE

macular hole. A 50-μm krypton or argon laser aiming spot placed within a stage 3 or 4 hole will not be seen in almost 100% of patients (positive laser beam sign). Thinning and depigmentation of the retinal pigment epithelium (RPE) develop within the area of the hole. A pigmented demarcation ring may occur (Fig. 12-16, F). Within most of the holes there are several yellow nodular opacities at the level of the RPE (Figs. 12-12, E, F, and I; 12-13, K; and 12-16, C and D). These opacities change in number and distribution from one examination to the other. The RPE and choroid surrounding the hole typically appear normal, although some patients may have drusen. Several small intraretinal cysts may be evident near the margin of the hole. In 10% to 20% of patients, fine crinkling of the inner retinal surface caused by an epiretinal membrane develops around the hole. The membrane occasionally may distort the contour of the hole (Fig. 12-13, K). An operculum-like structure (contracted prefoveolar vitreous cortex) is suspended on the posterior surface of the hyaloid membrane in front of the hole in 75% to 85% of cases (Figs. 12-12, B, F and L, and 12-13, C and I). In these cases there is no evidence of a PVD except in the foveal area.

Stage 4 hole

After separation of the vitreous from the entire macular surface and optic disc, irrespective of its diameter, the hole is designated stage 4 (Figs. 12-11, I; and 12-12, C). The operculum-like opacity can often be found attached to the mobile posterior hyaloid membrane near the temporal side of the Weiss ring.

Fluorescein angiography in patients with stages 2, 3, and 4 holes typically demonstrates prominent early hyperfluorescence caused primarily by the absence of xanthophyll in the area of the hole but is also caused by RPE thinning, depigmentation of the RPE, and slight loss of transparency of the retina immediately surrounding the hole.[45,47,49,50] In patients with a long-standing hole, the central zone of hyperfluorescence may be surrounded by a rim of faint fluorescence corresponding with the rim of retinal detachment and the underlying hypopigmented RPE (Fig. 12-13, L). In a few patients with a heavily pigmented choroid, the fluorescence may be minimal or absent. The yellow deposits within the depth of the hole and the operculum overlying the macular hole (Fig. 12-13, J and L) usually appear nonfluorescent or hypofluorescent.

If the anatomic interpretations summarized in Fig. 12-11 are correct, the implications include the

following: (1) most macular holes develop as the result of a central retinal dehiscence at the umbo, followed by centrifugal displacement of the relatively normal complement of retinal receptors; (2) this dehiscence occurs soon after the change from a yellow spot (stage 1-A impending hole) to a yellow ring lesion (stage 1-B impending hole), but in most cases it is not detectable with a thin slit beam as a defect in the center of the ring because of the presence of the semitranslucent condensed cortical vitreous bridging the hole (stage 1-B occult hole); (3) most of the prehole opacities overlying stage 2 and stage 3 holes are condensed prefoveal vitreous cortex (pseudoopercula), not opercula; and (4) following successful vitreous surgery, which includes tamponade of the hole with an intravitreal gas bubble and which is done within 1 year after commencement of hole formation, the anatomy of the central retina and its visual function may be restored to nearly normal levels in some patients as a result of retinal reattachment and centripetal repositioning of the retinal receptors. If these concepts of the anatomic changes occurring in macular hole development are correct, histopathologic examination of the prehole opacities should determine that most of them contain no retinal receptor cells but are composed of vitreous collagen, reactive Müller cell and astrocytic proliferation, and in some cases internal limiting membrane of the retina. Although retinal opercula have been described histopathologically in two eyes, one with

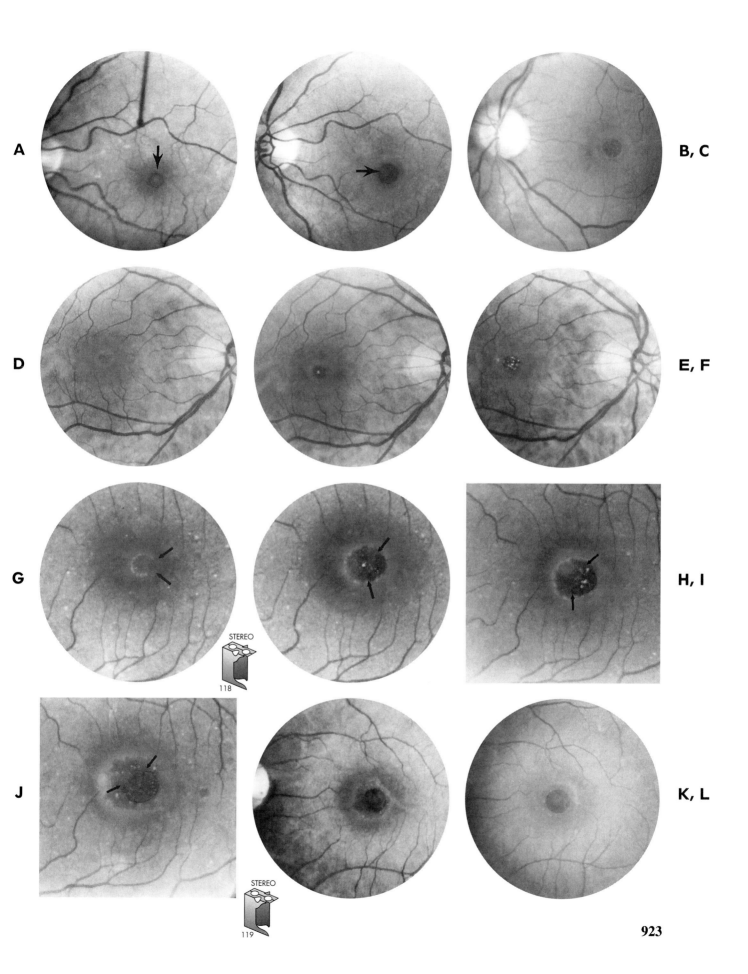

A

B, C

D

E, F

G

STEREO
118

H, I

J

STEREO
119

K, L

923

posttraumatic and the other with an idiopathic macular hole, it is uncertain whether the "opercula" contained retinal receptor cells.[40] Opercula have not been observed in most idiopathic macular holes studied histopathologically.

Spontaneous abortion of macular hole formation

In approximately 50% of cases, patients with stage 1-A and early stage 1-B lesions may experience rapid improvement in visual symptoms because of spontaneous separation of the vitreous from the fovea without developing a full-thickness macular hole (Fig. 12-14).[25,45,55,139] In such cases, the patient usually notices improvement in the symptoms and biomicroscopy may show several different pictures, all of which are accompanied by return of the foveal depression and a good visual prognosis.

VITREOFOVEAL SEPARATION AND PSEUDOOPERCULUM FORMATION

The foveal area returns to a normal appearance except for the presence of a semitranslucent, operculum-like structure or pseudooperculum (condensed, contracted prefoveal vitreous cortex) immediately in front of the fovea (Fig. 12-14, A to C). When viewed obliquely with a thin slit beam, the pseudooperculum in a few patients will cast a yellow shadow on the pigment epithelium.[51] Some patients with a pseudooperculum will notice a small scotoma when reading and a few will describe it as having a yellow color.

VITREOFOVEAL SEPARATION WITHOUT PSEUDOOPERCULUM FORMATION

After spontaneous vitreofoveal separation the fundus returns to a normal appearance and no pseudooperculum is evident.

FIG. 12-13 Angiographic Findings in Stages of Macular Hole Development.

A to C, A stage 1-A impending macular hole developed in a 62-year-old woman with a 4-day history of metamorphopsia in the left eye. She had previously developed a macular hole in the right eye (see **I** and **J**). Visual acuity in the left eye was 20/40. Note central yellow lesion (**A**). There were no cystic changes or evidence of a dehiscence in the retina. Angiography revealed slight fluorescence centrally (**B**). Twenty-six months later (**C**) a macular hole with an operculum was present and the patient's visual acuity was 20/70.

D to F, What appeared to be an inner lamellar macular hole (**D**) showed focal hyperfluorescence (**E**), suggesting the presence of an occult small stage 2 hole. Eight months later she showed evidence of the small stage 2 hole with a rim of retinal detachment.

G and H, Stage 3 macular hole in a 64-year-old woman with a visual acuity of 20/100. Note sharp margins of the hole, surrounding halo caused by retinal elevation and cystic degeneration of the retina, small yellow deposits that appear to lie on the surface of the RPE, and small pre-hole opacity lying just anterior to the retina and partly obscuring the underlying yellow deposits from view. The retinal vessels are within normal limits. Fluorescein angiography (**H**) revealed a circumscribed area of hyperfluorescence corresponding to the size of the retinal hole. This fluorescence faded within 1 hour. The parafoveal capillary bed was within normal limits.

I and J, Stage 3 macular hole with prehole opacity in a 62-year-old woman with a 3-year history of loss of vision in the right eye and a 4-day history of distortion of vision in the left eye (see **A** to **C**). Vision in the right eye was 20/200. Angiography (**J**) revealed hyperfluorescence corresponding to the area of the hole and obstruction of this fluorescence by the prehole opacity.

K and L, A long-standing macular hole and localized retinal detachment surrounded by an epiretinal membrane. Angiography showed that the white opacities within the hole were nonfluorescent (**L**). Note rim of hyperfluorescence around the hole showing evidence of loss of pigment from the RPE in the area of long-standing retinal detachment surrounding the hole.

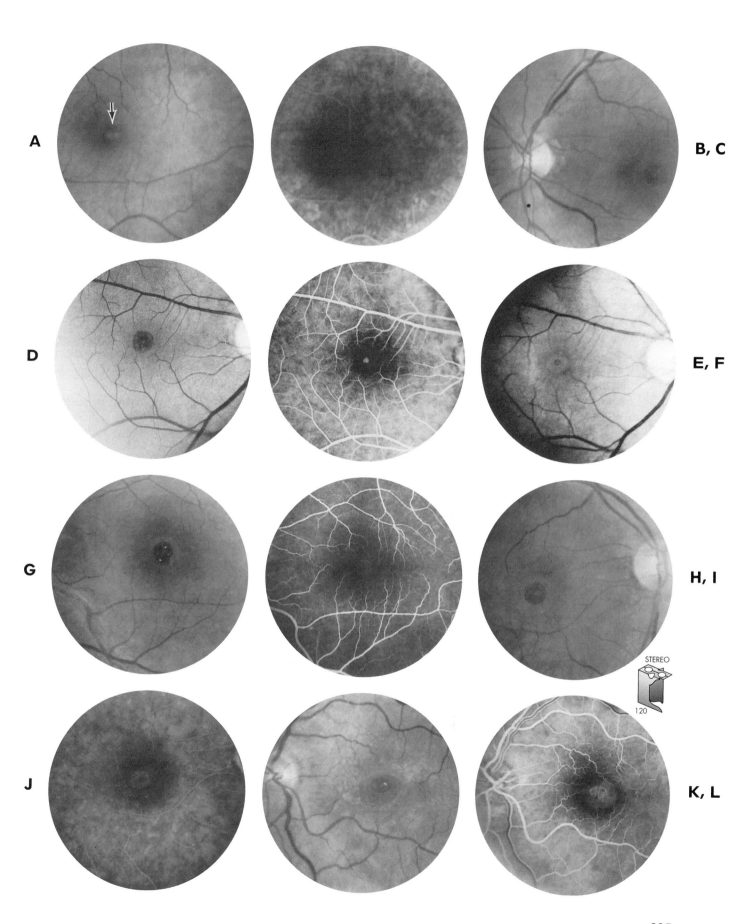

VITREOFOVEAL SEPARATION AND LAMELLAR HOLE FORMATION

Separation of the vitreous from the fovea in these patients is associated with a break in the continuity of the internal limiting membrane and the biomicroscopic appearance of one or more sharply defined reddish defects in the inner retinal surface in the foveolar area (Figs. 12-14, D to F and I and J, and 12-16, H). An operculum is usually evident overlying the defect. The defect may be minute and simulate that seen after sun gazing or in patients with no recognizable cause (Fig. 12-14, J).[18] Larger lamellar holes often have a scalloped border (Fig. 12-14, D). Unlike full-thickness holes there is no rim of retinal detachment. The visual acuity is usually 20/30 or better. Fluorescein angiography shows minimal or no fluorescence in the area of the lamellar hole (Fig. 12-14, E). The demonstration of a focus of bright fluorescence within the area of the lamellar hole suggests the possible presence of a full-thickness hole without a rim of detachment (Fig. 12-13, D to F). This type of full-thickness hole appears identical biomicroscopically to a lamellar hole, may be associated with visual acuity of 20/30 or better, and is likely to develop a rim of retinal detachment and be associated with visual loss at a later date. The visual prognosis for patients with a lamellar hole is excellent.

INCOMPLETE SEPARATION OF THE CONTRACTED PREFOVEOLAR VITREOUS CORTEX

A portion or all of the contracted prefoveolar vitreous cortex may remain as a small stellate opacity on the surface of the center of the foveolar retina and be associated with fine stellate retinal folds simulating X-linked foveomacular schisis (Fig. 12-14, K and L).[50]

It is important to use a fundus contact lens to look for signs of vitreofoveal separation not only in the symptomatic eye but also in the fellow eye of any patient with evidence of a macular hole in one eye. Fellow eyes with evidence of vitreofoveal separation probably have less than a 5% chance of developing a macular hole.[4,5,6,45] Some patients who have reportedly developed a hole after demonstration of a posterior vitreous detachment probably had small occult holes that developed at the time of PUD.[54] Others probably had residual vitreous cortex on the inner retinal surface centrally after separation of the vitreous from the optic disc and paracentral macular area.

FIG. 12-14   Aborted Stages of Development of a Macular Hole.

A to C, This woman with a macular hole in the fellow eye developed blurred vision and a stage 1-B lesion in the right eye (A and top part of C). Several weeks later her symptoms disappeared and her visual acuity and fundus returned to normal (B and bottom part of C). Arrow in C indicates pseudooperculum that was faintly visible biomicroscopically.

D to F, This man with a macular hole in his fellow eye developed metamorphopsia and blurred vision in the left eye caused by a stage 1-A impending macular hole. His symptoms improved spontaneously and examination revealed a large inner lamellar macular hole and prehole opacity (D). Note the sharply defined scalloped edges and absence of a rim of detachment. Angiography showed only faint fluorescence (E). Diagram F indicates the probable anatomy of this lesion. His visual acuity in this eye has remained 20/25 + for 5 years.

G to I, This woman noted blurred vision and metamorphopsia in the right eye associated with a stage 1-B lesion (G). She improved spontaneously and her visual acuity improved to 20/30. Note the pair of paracentral inner lamellar holes (arrow, I).

J, Note the small inner lamellar hole (arrow) associated with 20/20 visual acuity in this man with a stage 3 hole and 20/200 visual acuity in his fellow eye.

K and L, Radiating retina folds associated with stellate contracted prefoveolar vitreous cortex associated with 20/30 visual acuity in a woman who probably spontaneously aborted an impending macular hole.

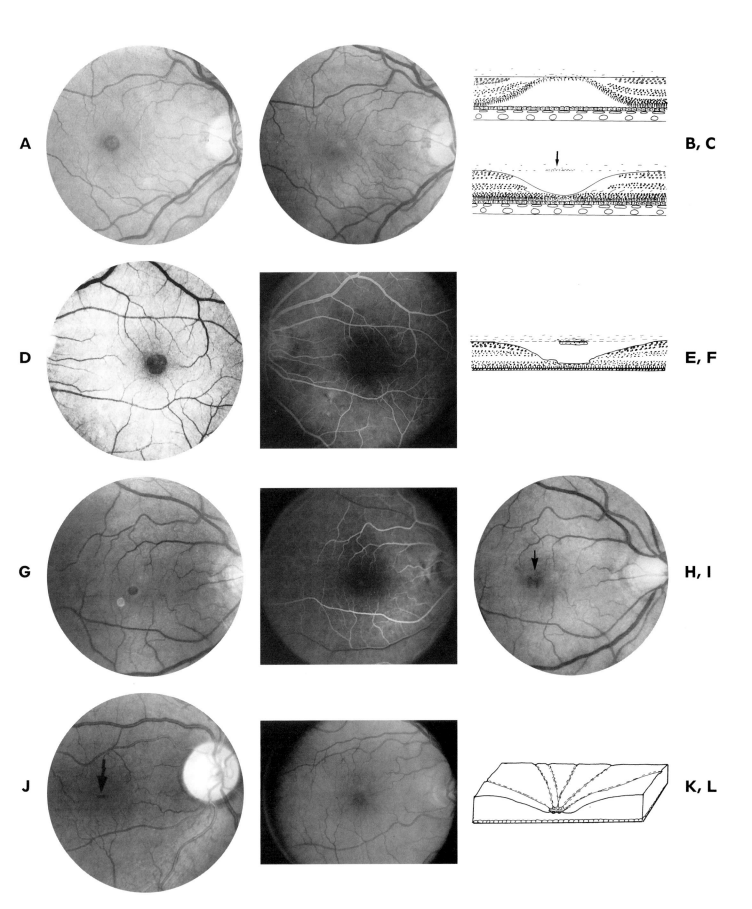

Natural course

The time course from the development of symptoms and stage 1 impending macular hole to a fully developed stage 3 or 4 hole varies but in most patients is within 6 months. In some patients the course may be complete within a matter of weeks, and in others hole formation may not have progressed beyond stage 2 several years later. The visual acuity usually stabilizes after the first 6 to 12 months at a mean level of 20/200.[58,67] A few patients with stage 3 and 4 holes may maintain excellent visual function of 20/40 to 20/50 for years.

Spontaneous reattachment of the retina surrounding the hole may occur (Figs. 12-15 and 12-16, G) and the biomicroscopic appearance may be identical with that of a lamellar macular hole. In some cases the hole may disappear and recovery of vision may be excellent.[11,59,146] Closure of a macular hole occurs occasionally as the result of development of an epiretinal membrane (Fig. 12-15).[84]

Approximately 25% of patients with a macular hole have evidence of posterior vitreous separation from the optic disc and macula in the fellow eye. The macula of the asymptomatic eye is usually normal but it may show evidence of previous spontaneous separation of the vitreous that is limited to the foveal area.[67] In addition, other minor changes may occur at the vitreoretinal interface, including epiretinal membrane formation, small irregular folds of the inner retinal surface, and absence of the foveal reflex. Fluorescein angiography in the "asymptomatic eye" is typically normal. The value of focal electroretinography in detecting predilection for hole development in the fellow eye is uncertain.[12] The only finding of definite prognostic significance in the fellow eye is the presence or absence of a PVD.[45,48,75,135] The reported risk for development of a hole in the normal fellow eye has varied from 1% to 22%.* The probable risk is between 10% and 15%. The presence of a PVD or

*References 1, 17, 32, 34, 45, 55, 56, 85, 99, 135, 143, 145, 146.

FIG. 12-15   Natural Course of Macular Hole.

A, Diagrams showing natural course of macular hole.

Stage 3 hole, Most macular holes remain at 400 to 600 μm in diameter with a mean visual acuity of 20/200.

Stage 4 hole, A posterior vitreous detachment occurs in some holes. An epiretinal membrane *(arrow)* often becomes apparent clinically around both stage 3 and stage 4 holes. The mean visual acuity is 20/200.

Spontaneous reattachment of the retina, This occasionally occurs and the visual acuity may improve remarkably. These holes are indistinguishable biomicroscopically from inner lamellar holes (see **B** and **C**). Angiography, however, typically shows hyperfluorescence in the former and not the latter.

Disappearance of the hole, The edges of the reattached retina may flatten and in some cases, not shown on the diagram, they may be drawn together, probably as the result of glial proliferation, in a way similar to that which occurs in patients following vitreous surgery.

Closure of the hole by overgrowth of an epiretinal membrane, Contracture or overgrowth of an epiretinal membrane surrounding the hole may result in its closure.

B and **C,** The rim of detachment in this stage 2 macular hole in **B** had spontaneously disappeared (**C**) when the patient returned for followup almost 3 years later. The patient's visual acuity was 20/200.

vitreofoveal separation probably reduces the risk of developing a hole to 1% or less. Possible explanations for the occasional patient with a PVD who develops a hole include: a tear in the posterior hyaloid at the time of PVD, leaving vitreous cortex attached to the central macular area, and a subclinical full-thickness microhole caused by traction during the PVD.[122] In most patients the second eye becomes involved within 2 years.[2] Those with bilateral involvement usually retain moderately useful central vision, and most can read successfully with high-power spectacles.

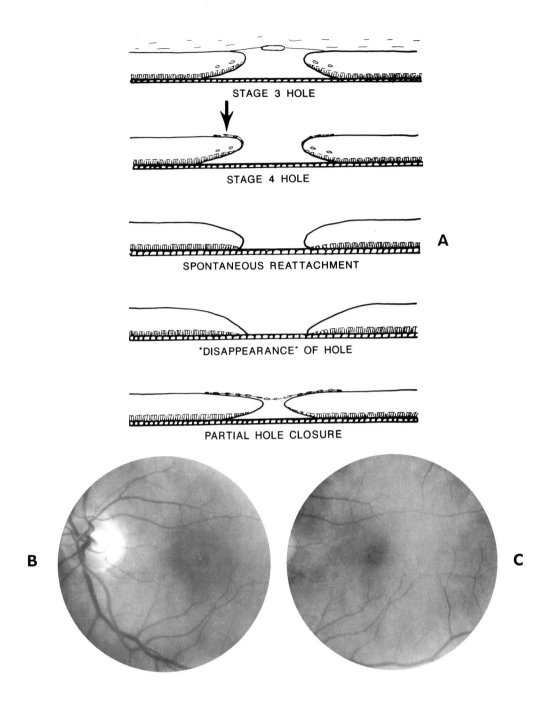

STAGE 3 HOLE

STAGE 4 HOLE

SPONTANEOUS REATTACHMENT

"DISAPPEARANCE" OF HOLE

PARTIAL HOLE CLOSURE

A

B

C

Pathology and pathogenesis

Immunocytochemical labeling and electron microscopic examination of vitreous removed at the time of surgery for impending macular holes has demonstrated cortical vitreous containing RPE and glial cells.[19,118,127] Histopathologic examination of a macular hole has failed to demonstrate any evidence of either retinal or choroidal vascular disease as a cause for the development of a macular hole (Fig. 12-16).[40,49,56,100] The edges of the hole are typically rounded, some cystic spaces in the outer plexiform and inner nuclear layers are often present, and there is frequently cellular proliferation from the edges of the hole onto the neighboring inner retinal surface (Fig. 12-16, E).[56] A cellular prehole opacity may occasionally be observed (Fig. 12-16, A and B). It is not known whether or not retinal receptor cells are included. Nodular proliferations of the RPE overlying an eosinophilic material probably account for the yellowish deposits noted biomicroscopically in the depth of the macular hole (Fig. 12-16, C and D). These appear to be identical in structure to the reactive, proliferative type of drusen noted histopathologically in eyes with long-standing retinal detachment. Proliferation of the RPE is probably caused by loss of the RPE's contact with the outer segments of the retina as well as its exposure to the vitreous.[40] There are two reports in which histopathologic examination of the second eye in patients with unilateral macular hole found cystic spaces in the outer plexiform layer in the paracentral macular area.[40,78] The fact that fluorescein angiography in asymptomatic second eyes, as well as in the affected eyes, shows no permeability alterations suggests that these cysts probably are not caused by abnormal retinal vascular permeability. In spite of these findings, which suggest that a slow process of cystic degeneration of the center of the fovea may predate the development of a macular hole, my observations suggest that macular hole development is not preceded by a gradual change in either the appearance of the macula or visual function. On the contrary, its formation

begins abruptly, although its full development usually occurs over a period of 2 to 3 months. There is no evidence to incriminate either the underlying RPE or the choroid in the pathogenesis of macular hole formation.[78,79,100] As discussed previously the primary tissues involved in macular hole formation involve the vitreoretinal interface region in the foveolar area. Electron microscopic study of a series of prefoveolar operculum-like structures collected at the time of macular hole surgery are needed to confirm the anatomic interpretation of the biomicroscopic stages of hole development suggested here by the author.[47]

The predilection for hole development to occur in women has suggested that ingestion of estrogenic compounds may be of importance in the pathogenesis of macular hole.[66,82,95]

FIG. 12-16 **Histopathology of an Idiopathic Senile Macular Hole.**

A, Gross photograph showing retinal "operculum" (arrow) suspended in front of the hole.

B, Photomicrograph of retinal "operculum" shown in **A** demonstrates glial cells but no definite evidence of retinal photoreceptor cells. This may be the balled-up nodule of contracted prefoveolar fibroglial membrane and not an operculum.

C, Histopathology of full-thickness macular hole with nodular proliferations of the RPE in the base of the hole (arrows).

D, High-power view of change in the RPE shown in **A** (arrows). Note that the underlying choroid is within normal limits.

E, High-power view of the edge of the hole shown in **C**. Note the extension of retinal glial cells (arrow) onto the anterior surface of the retina.

F, Long-standing macular hole with demarcation ring (arrows) composed of proliferated RPE cells.

G, Macular hole with reattachment of its edges.

H, Inner lamellar macular hole.

(**A** and **B** from Frangieh et al.[40] **G** and **H** from Guyer et al.[56])

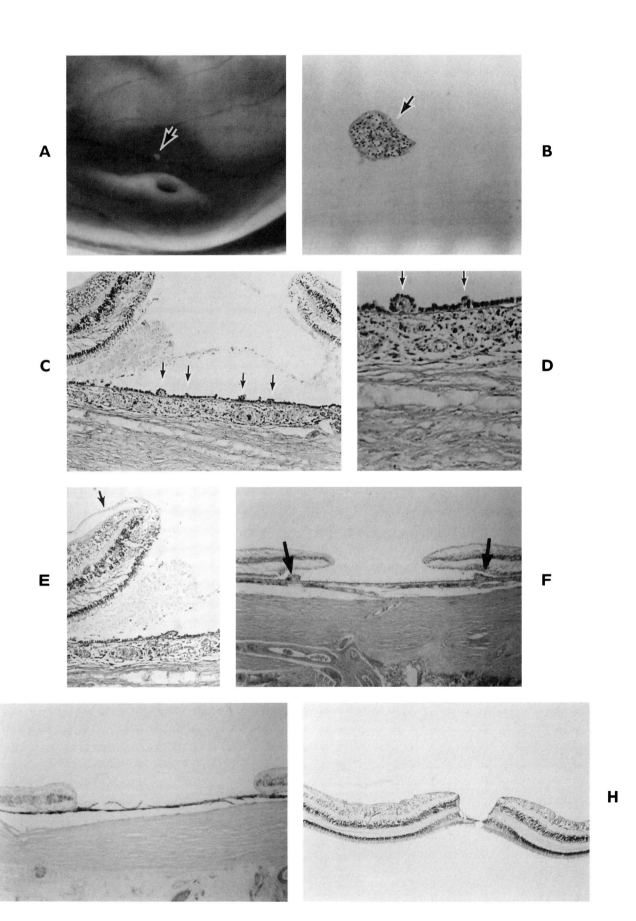

931

Differential diagnosis

Most patients referred to the author with a diagnosis of a stage 1-A impending hole have had a foveolar yellow lesion caused by one of the following: solitary drusen, small RPE detachment, idiopathic central serous chorioretinopathy, foveolar detachment with epiretinal membrane, bilateral idiopathic juxtafoveolar retinal telangiectasis, pattern dystrophy, cystoid macular edema, and solar maculopathy (Fig. 12-17).[50]

Lesions that may simulate a full-thickness macula hole includes an inner lamellar macular hole (Fig. 12-14, *D*), a hole in an epiretinal membrane (Figs. 12-17, *J*, to *L*; and 12-21, *A*), geographic atrophy of the RPE (Fig. 12-17, *G* to *I*), choroidal neovascularization, a small focal area of central serous chorioretinopathy, cystoid macular edema with a large central cyst (Fig. 12-17, *A* to *C*), focal retinal atrophy associated with bilateral juxtafoveal retinal telangiectasis (Fig. 12-17, *D* to *E*) and congenital optic pit, and a solitary macular cyst, a lesion that rarely occurs.[32,46,93,123] Features of a full-thickness macular hole that differentiate it from most simulating lesions are the presence of a halo of retinal detachment surrounding the hole, yellow deposits within the depth of the hole, and a zone of hyperfluorescence corresponding to the size of the hole during the early stages of angiography. Use of the slit-beam test (Watzke sign), 50-μm-size aiming beam laser perimetry, and fluorescein angiography are helpful adjuncts to contact lens examination in arriving at the correct diagnosis. Echography is capable of detecting posterior vitreous detachment and the presence of pseudoopercula but appears to be no better than contact lens examination in this regard.[27,33,136]

FIG. 12-17   Lesions Simulating a Macular Hole.

A to **C,** Idiopathic cystoid macular edema was associated with a large central cyst (**A** and **C**) that was mistaken for a macular hole in this man. Angiography revealed the correct diagnosis (**B**).

D to **F,** Bilateral idiopathic juxtafoveolar telangiectasis was the cause of the focal atrophy of the retina (**D** and **F**) that was incorrectly diagnosed as a macular hole, before the angiogram (**E**) was obtained.

G to **I,** Geographic atrophy of the outer retina and RPE caused by age-related macular degeneration (**G** and **I**) and focal hyperfluorescence (**H**) was responsible for the incorrect diagnosis of a macular hole in this elderly patient.

J to **L,** This patient who had a macular hole in the right eye had no complaints in the left eye. Visual acuity was 20/20. A circular rim of condensed vitreous lying on the inner retinal surface centrally (**J**) and minimal evidence of crinkling of the inner retinal surface suggested the presence of an occult perifoveolar epiretinal membrane (**L**). There was no evidence of posterior vitreous detachment. She soon developed a posterior vitreous separation, mild visual blurring, and definite evidence of a pericentral epiretinal membrane (**K**).

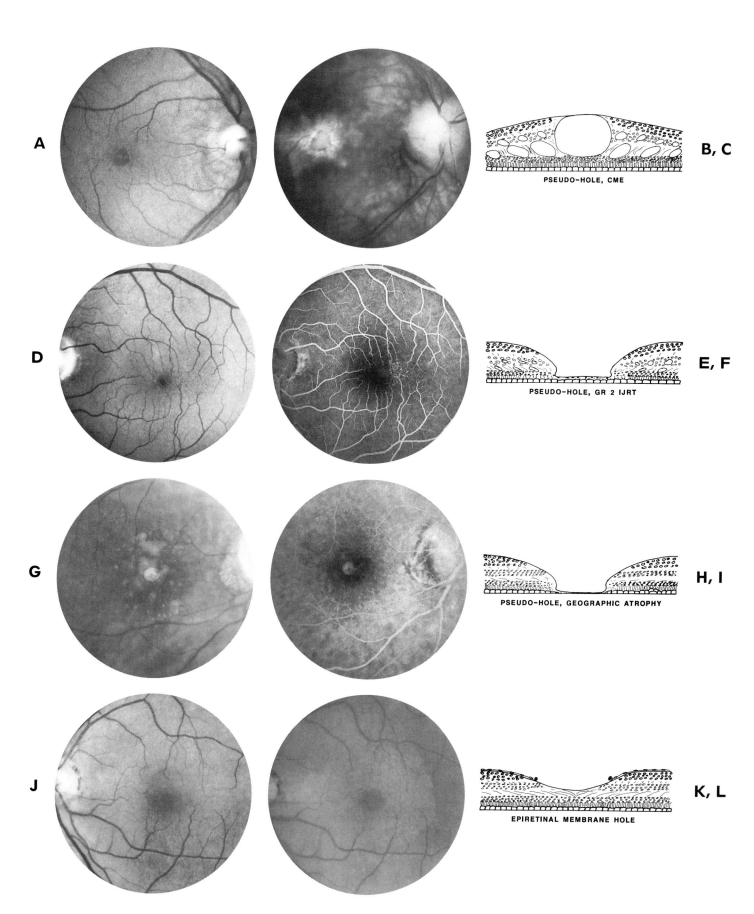

A

B, C

PSEUDO-HOLE, CME

D

E, F

PSEUDO-HOLE, GR 2 IJRT

G

H, I

PSEUDO-HOLE, GEOGRAPHIC ATROPHY

J

K, L

EPIRETINAL MEMBRANE HOLE

933

Treatment

In 1988 surgical separation of the prefoveolar vitreous cortex was suggested as a possible treatment to prevent hole formation in patients with stage 1 impending macula holes.[45] Uncontrolled pilot studies of vitreous surgery for treatment of impending macular holes suggested that the surgery might be of benefit.* The criteria used for an impending hole by these authors, however, were not confined to those of a stage 1 impending hole as defined by this author.[45] Furthermore, there are many lesions that may simulate a stage 1 hole and misdiagnosis of an impending hole is frequent.[50] A randomized, multicenter, clinical trial to evaluate the effectiveness of surgical peeling of the vitreous for treatment of an impending macular hole in one eye in patients with a stage 3 or 4 hole in the fellow eye was organized in 1988.[24] The results of this study of 62 patients showed that approximately 40% of eyes in both groups developed a full-thickness hole. The study was discontinued before definite conclusions could be reached because of a dramatic drop in patient recruitment coinciding with enthusiastic reports concerning treatment of full-thickness holes. With the following available information: (1) that 40% to 60% of stage 1 holes spontaneously abort, (2) that there is a high incidence of misdiagnosis of stage 1 holes, and (3) the apparent favorable results of surgery for full-thickness holes, it is probably prudent to observe patients with a stage 1 impending hole, particularly when the fellow eye is normal.

Kelly and Wendel in 1991,[70] Glaser and colleagues in 1992,[52] Poliner and Tornambe in 1992,[107] and others,[97,111,124,125,126,138] in uncontrolled pilot studies, reported successful closure of macular holes and visual improvement using pars plana vitrectomy, intraocular gas, and 1 to 2 weeks of face-down positioning (Fig. 12-18). Glaser's group used a tissue growth factor, TGF-Beta, to stimulate proliferation of glial cells to seal the hole. Some surgeons have used the patient's serum in lieu of TGF-Beta.[86] The visual results obtained by all of these investigators were similar in those eyes with successful reattachment of the retina. Approximately 70% obtained improvement of two lines of visual acuity or better, and 20% to 40% regained 20/40 or better. These same authors, who originally obtained only approximately a 50% reattachment rate, have reported at recent meetings successful reattachment in 90% to 95% of cases and return of acuity to 20/40 or better in

*References 20, 44, 68, 92, 97, 127, 128, 130.

FIG. 12-18   Diagram of Surgical Repair of Macular Hole.

A, Preoperative appearance of stage 3 hole. *Arrow* indicates contracted vitreous cortex (pseudooperculum) attached to the layer of vitreous gel lying between the liquefied vitreous (premacular bursa) and the retinal hole.

B, Postoperative appearance after vitrectomy, surgical peeling of cortical vitreous, and intravitreal gas injection. With the patient in the face-down position, the bubble compresses the edges of the hole against the RPE.

C to E, Enlarged views to show that proliferation and contraction of retinal glial cells causes centripetal movement of the retina and closure of the hole.

approximately 50% of cases (Fig. 12-19, *A* to *F*). The success of surgery appears to be primarily related to the patient's ability to maintain the face-down position postoperatively rather than the surgical technique employed. Reoperation of eyes with failed macular hole surgery may result in visual improvement.[29,62] Surgical complications have included retinal tears with and without retinal detachment; retinal vascular occlusion; light toxicity pigment epitheliopathy; cataract; acute permanent loss of temporal visual field, probably caused by damage to the nasal part of the optic disc during fluid–gas exchange; and reopening of the macular hole.* A controlled clinical trial randomizing patients with full-thickness holes to surgery or to observation is under way, and over 150 patients have been randomized.[41]

Following successful reattachment of the retina after surgery for a macular hole, the macula may return to a nearly normal appearance, the hyperfluorescence corresponding with the hole preoperatively often disappears, and a central scotoma may no longer be demonstrable.[121,134] A few patients may regain 20/20 visual acuity.[11] These surgical results were difficult to explain on the basis of the initial anatomic interpretation of the biomicroscopic stages of hole development.[45] The prehole opacity seen in 75% to 80% of patients was originally thought to represent an operculum containing the foveolar retina; this operculum was thought to be derived from a circumferential tear occurring in the periphery of a stage 1-B lesion, and significant improvement of vision even with reattachment of the retina around the hole was thought unlikely. Evidence now strongly suggests that nearly all macular holes begin as an occult central foveolar dehiscence at the umbo and that hole

*References 21, 28, 29, 52, 70, 80, 97a, 107.

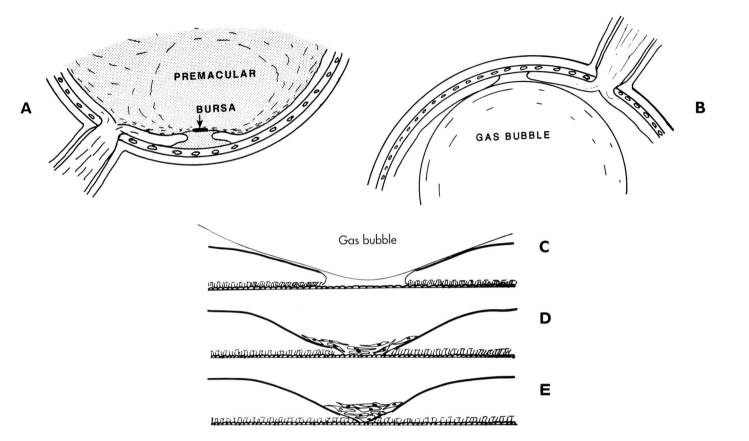

development is the result of centrifugal sliding and retraction of the receptors away from the center of the hole analogous to the opening of a lens diaphragm. It is understandable that surgical reattachment of the retina around the hole, when accompanied by reactive glial cell proliferation and contraction, may result in "closure of the lens diaphragm" and return of the foveal retina to its near-normal anatomic position and function in some patients (Figs. 12-18 and 12-19). The disappearance of the focal hyperfluorescence corresponding with the hole, and of the absolute central scotomas that occur in some patients after successful macular hole surgery, is further evidence in support of the concept of centripetal movement of the paracentral retinal receptors and the xanthophyll.[134]

Limited histopathologic information also supports this mechanism of hole formation and closure (Fig. 12-19, D to G). Funata and coworkers examined histopathologically both eyes of a patient whose visual acuity improved from 20/400 to 20/30 in the left eye and from 20/400 to 20/40 in the right eye after surgery for a retinal hole.[42] They found successful reattachment of the retina in both eyes. Closure of the hole in the right eye was associated with glial proliferation and probable centripetal inward drawing of the retinal receptors (Fig. 12-19, D to F). In the left eye retinal reattachment was unassociated with gliosis. Madreperla et al. reported their findings in another patient whose preoperative visual acuity was 20/80 and postoperative acuity was 20/40.[89] One month postoperatively the patient died and histopathologic examination showed closure of the hole and close approximation of the retinal receptors centrally by proliferating Müller cells (Fig. 12-19, G).

The criteria for recommending surgery for a macular hole are still evolving. Until recently most patients undergoing surgery have had symptoms for a year or less, visual acuity of 20/70 or worse, and a large stage 2 or stage 3 or 4 macular hole. If results of a randomized study and other reports confirm those already available, the criteria for surgery will probably be broadened to include early stage 2 holes and holes of longer duration. Although the likelihood for progression to a stage 2 hole is probably directly related to the diameter of the stage 1-B yellow ring and the level of visual acuity loss, there is no reliable information or method at this time to determine which stage 1-B lesions will progress to hole formation.[45]

The patient considering surgery for a macular hole in one eye and having normal function in the fellow eye should be aware of the following: (1) chances of developing a hole in the fellow eye are 10% to 15% and probably less than 5% in the presence of vitreofoveal separation; (2) surgery, even if successful, probably will not improve their overall visual function; and (3) treatment usually involves two operations, including cataract surgery.[31,162]

Laser treatment to the edge of macular holes has had minimal success in improving visual function.[90,114] The treatment has no rationale as far as preventing further retinal detachment in patients with senile macular holes is concerned since the detachment involves only the central macular area and is unlikely to cause extensive detachment in these patients with relatively emmetropic eyes.[67]

There is less chance for visual improvement following surgical treatment of macular holes associated with other diseases, such as diabetic retinopathy, or for holes caused by trauma.[35]

Macular or paramacular holes do not cause rhegmatogenous retinal detachment unless they are associated with a posterior staphyloma and high myopia,[119] or with vitreous bands causing traction on the surface of the posterior retina. In such cases the detachment infrequently extends beyond the equator. Treatment of such holes requires either one or a combination of permanent or temporary scleral buckling techniques; for example, the Klotti clip; vitrectomy; intravitreal injection of air or gas; and cryotherapy, diathermy, or photocoagulation.*

Macular holes may develop in several clinical settings, some of which are unusual, e.g., Best's disease,[96,112] adult vitelliform foveomacular dystrophy,[103] high myopia with posterior staphyloma,[119] posterior microphthalmos,[83] congenital arteriove-

*References 14, 53, 77, 82, 98, 115.

FIG. 12-19   Surgical Repair of Macular Hole.

A to **D,** Preoperative appearance of stage 3 macular hole (**A**). Visual acuity, 20/80. Angiogram showed fluorescence centrally. Postoperative appearance (**B**). Visual acuity, 20/20. The hole was no longer evident. Angiogram (**D**) showed a ring of persistent fluorescence.

D to **E,** Preoperative appearance of a stage 3 hole (**D**). Visual acuity was 20/200. Postoperative appearance (**E**). Visual acuity was 20/40. Histopathologic examination of the eye obtained at autopsy shows closure of hole by proliferating glial cells (*arrow,* **F**).

G, Histopathology of a macula hole following surgical repair shows reapproximation of the hole edges (*arrows*) by Müller cell proliferation.

(**A** to **D,** courtesy Dr. William E. Smiddy; **E** to **G** from Funata et al.[42]; **H** from Madreperla et al.[89])

nous aneurysm,[101] hypertensive retinopathy,[23] and following commencement of topical pilocarpine therapy,[9,43] pneumatic retinopexy,[7] and Nd-YAG posterior capsulotomy.[13] Macular holes occurring in association with rhegmatogenous retinal detachment caused by peripheral retinal tears, trauma, myopia, contraction of an epiretinal membrane, and solar retinopathy are discussed elsewhere in this text.

Idiopathic traction maculopathy unassociated with posterior vitreous detachment

There is some evidence to suggest that subtle changes may occasionally occur in the vitreous body, causing it to contract and to exert anterior traction on the retinal surface posteriorly without any biomicroscopic evidence of posterior separation of discrete vitreous bands attached to the inner retinal surface. This traction may be associated with cystoid macular edema and angiographic evidence of retinal capillary leakage in the macular area or serous detachment of the sensory retina. (See discussion of diabetic traction maculopathy, p. 520, and congenial pit of the optic nerve head, p. 982.)

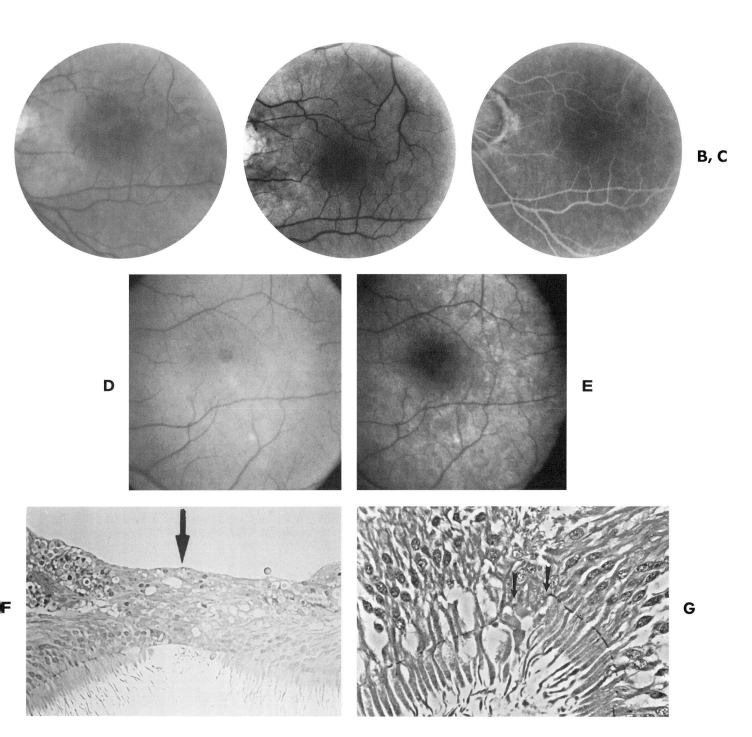

B, C

D

E

F

G

937

▼ MACULAR DYSFUNCTION CAUSED BY EPIRETINAL MEMBRANE CONTRACTION

After partial or complete posterior vitreous detachment (PVD), a translucent or semitranslucent fibrocellular membrane may become apparent ophthalmoscopically and biomicroscopically on the inner retinal surface in the macular area (Fig. 12-7, C to G). In approximately 25% of cases similar membranes may develop before development of a PVD (Fig. 12-8, A to C). The contraction or shrinkage of this epiretinal membrane may occur and produce varying degrees of distortion, intraretinal edema, and degeneration of the underlying retina (Figs. 12-20 and 12-21).[158,169,171,181,240]

Epiretinal membranes may be classified according to the severity of retinal distortion, associated biomicroscopic changes, and associated ocular disorders.

Classification of epiretinal membranes according to severity of retinal distortion

Grade 0: "cellophane maculopathy"

In cellophane maculopathy the membrane may be completely translucent and may be unassociated with any distortion of the inner retinal surface. The only ophthalmoscopic or biomicroscopic clue to its presence is a "cellophane" light reflex coming from the inner retinal surface.

Grade 1: "crinkled cellophane maculopathy"

Following contraction or shrinkage of the epiretinal membrane, the underlying inner retinal surface may be gathered into a series of small irregular folds. These alterations produce an irregular, iridescent light reflex, which may be likened to that stemming from the surface of cellophane that has been rolled into a ball and reopened into a sheet containing many fine irregular crinkles on its surface (Figs. 12-7, G; 12-8, A; and 12-20, A, C, and F). Biomicroscopically, details of the underlying small retinal vessels may be indistinct. Fine, superficial radiating retinal folds extend outward from the margins of the contracted membrane and are often the most prominent sign indicating the presence of an epiretinal membrane (Fig. 12-20, C and D). The membrane is often centered in the perifoveal area but may occasionally extend across the full width of the macula. The wrinkling may be sufficient to produce tortuosity of the fine macular capillaries. If the area of membrane contraction is sufficiently large, it produces tortuosity of the underlying paramacular vessels and displaces the surrounding retinal vessels to-

FIG. 12-20 Epiretinal Membrane.

A, Diagram showing crinkled cellophane maculopathy associated with fine irregular wrinkles of the inner retinal layers.

B, Diagram showing macular pucker. Coarse retinal folds often associated with retinal edema, cystic degeneration, and localized detachment.

C to E, This patient developed metamorphopsia caused by a small juxtafoveolar epiretinal membrane *(arrows).* Note retinal folds radiating outward from the region of the membrane. Some of these pass through the macula. Fundus painting (**D**) of the same patient illustrating the relationship of the epiretinal membrane *(arrow)* to the underlying retina. Angiography revealed mild tortuosity of the retinal vessels in the region of the membrane (**E**).

F, Semitranslucent epiretinal membrane causing distortion of the macula of this 55-year-old patient, who had no other evidence of intraocular disease. Contraction of the membrane has pulled the paramacular vessels toward the horizontal raphe.

G, Epiretinal membrane lying in the central area of the macula in this 14-year-old girl, who had no other evidence of ocular disease. Note retinal folds radiating outward from the macula.

H, Prominent epiretinal membrane in a 40-year-old man whose visual acuity was 20/20.

I to K, Epiretinal membrane causing macular pucker in a 72-year-old man who had no other evidence of intraocular disease. Visual acuity was 20/400. Several small holes with an appearance similar to Swiss cheese were present in the retina superior to the macula *(arrow,* **I**). Beneath these holes was a small amount of subretinal fluid. This patient has been observed for approximately 8 years with no change. Angiography revealed marked central displacement of the paramacular retinal vessels (**J**), early leakage of dye from the retinal capillaries, and an irregular pattern of fluorescein staining in the retina (**K** and **L**). The typical cystoid pattern is not apparent because of the marked distortion of the retinal architecture.

ward the fovea (Fig. 12-20, *F*). Some patients show multiple focal areas of preretinal membrane contraction in the posterior pole. Cystoid macular edema, retinal hemorrhages, retinal exudates, and disturbances of the RPE are typically absent except in those cases in which the vitreoretinal interface changes are either secondary to or incidental to other choroidal and retinal diseases. Vitreous degenerative changes and a PVD are often present. Inflammatory cells are usually not present. When seen they suggest that an underlying inflammatory disease is present and that the inflammation is more likely the cause of rather than the result of the epiretinal membrane. Many patients with grade 1 membranes have normal acuity and are asymptomatic. Some patients are seen because of a mild visual disturbance in one eye. The patient is often

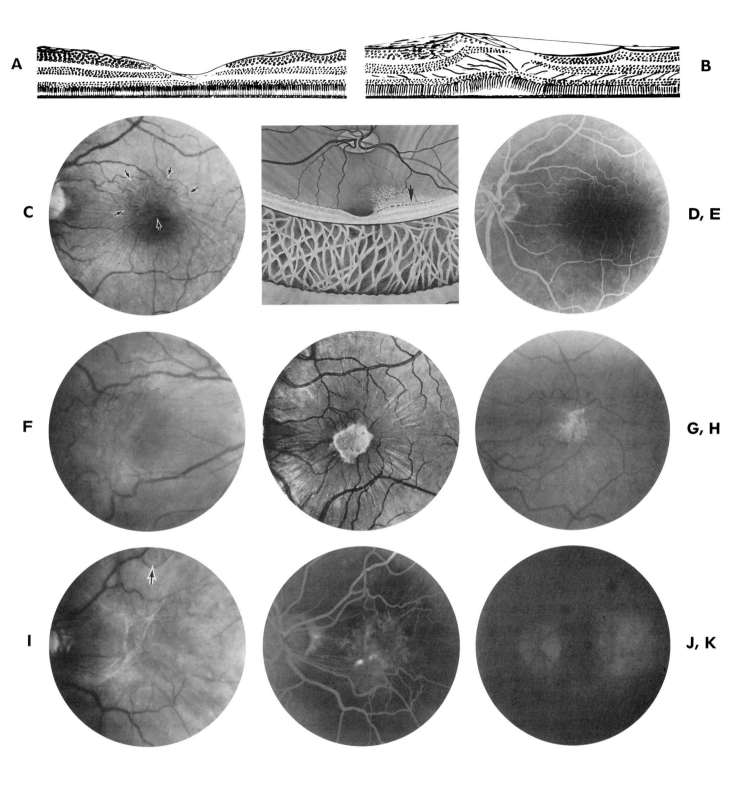

unable to date the onset of his visual complaint. His acuity is typically reduced to a level no worse than 20/40. Metamorphopsia is demonstrable in patients with reduced acuity. The reduction in acuity caused by an epiretinal membrane is primarily related to the distortion produced in the outer retinal layers and not to the size or degree of translucency of the membrane. Visual acuity may be unaffected in some patients with prominent centrally located membranes (Fig. 12-20, *H*). This latter type of membrane probably is caused by centripetal sliding of the contracting membrane along the internal limiting membrane.

Grade 2: "macular pucker"

The epiretinal membrane may be sufficiently dense to be visible as a distinct grayish membrane on the inner retinal surface (Figs. 12-20, *B, G* to *I,* and 12-23, *A*). It may partly obscure the underlying retinal vessels. In such cases the degree of retinal distortion and crinkling is usually marked, and gross puckering of the macula may be present (Figs. 12-20, *I;* 12-23, *A* and *C* to *E;* and 12-24, *C*). Retinal edema, small retinal hemorrhages, cotton-wool exudates, and localized serous detachment of the retina may accompany prominent preretinal vitreous membrane formation and contraction. A PVD is present in over 90% of cases.

Soon after the development of severe macular distortion, angiography usually shows leakage of dye from the underlying retinal vessels and evidence of retinal edema (Fig. 12-20, *J* and *K*). Because of retinal distortion, the pattern of dye staining is irregular and not typical of cystoid macular edema. In a matter of weeks or months there is usually a reduction in the amount of retinal edema and dye leakage. Visual acuity is usually significantly affected. It may be less than 20/200 if the macula is severely puckered. In many instances patients are unable to date the onset of their symptoms. In others, they may suddenly experience central photopsia and loss of central vision (Fig. 12-24, *C*). Metamorphopsia is usually demonstrable in these cases in which the entire thickness of the retina is affected by wrinkling.

Epiretinal membranes responsible for puckering of the retina may be eccentrically located in the paracentral region, including the area of the optic disc, in which case loss of macular function is primarily caused by tractional displacement as well as distortion of the foveal area (Fig. 12-23, *C* to *E*). Contraction of a juxtapapillary epiretinal membrane may occasionally be mistaken for papilledema or juxtapapillary combined RPE and retinal hamartoma.

940

FIG. 12-21 **Spontaneous Contraction of a Perifoveolar Epiretinal Membrane Causing a Picture Simulating a Macular Hole.**

A to C, Hole in epiretinal membrane simulating a macular hole in an asymptomatic 64-year-old woman who had 20/15 visual acuity and normal Amsler grid, static, and kinetic perimetric findings in this eye. Note the fine crinkling of the inner retinal surface surrounding the hole in an epiretinal membrane and the fine retinal folds radiating outward from the macular area (**A**). Angiography showed no abnormality (**B**). Diagram (**C**) shows fibrocellular epiretinal membrane *(arrow, above)* before contraction, and after contraction *(below)* and formation of a pseudo–macular hole. The membrane surrounds but does not cover the foveal area. **B,** Following spontaneous contraction of the epiretinal membrane. Shortening of the cells making up the epiretinal membrane produces an anterior and central displacement of the inner retinal layers to produce the clinical picture of a pseudo–macular hole. Note there is minimal or no distortion of the outer retinal layers or the RPE.

D to F, Spontaneous partial closure of a hole in an epiretinal membrane occurred in this 69-year-old woman with a 2-month history of floaters in the right eye. Visual acuity in the right eye was 20/25 and in the left eye was 20/20. A posterior vitreous detachment and a few cells in the anterior and posterior vitreous in the right eye were present. Note the oval hole surrounded by an epiretinal membrane (**D**). Fluorescein angiography was normal. Fifteen months later visual acuity in the right eye was 20/50. Further contraction of the epiretinal membrane has narrowed the oval hole in the membrane to a horizontal slit that is now displaced temporal to the center of the macula (**E**). Diagram (**F**) illustrates the contraction of the epiretinal membrane and partial closure of the pseudo-macular hole.

G to I, Anterior herniation of the foveolar retina following spontaneous contraction of a perifoveolar epiretinal membrane (**G** and **I**) was misinterpreted as a macular hole. Following surgical excision of the membrane the visual acuity improved from 20/400 to 20/60 (**H**). Diagram (**I**) illustrates the progression of an epiretinal membrane *(above)* to retinal herniation *(below)* after contraction of the epiretinal membrane.

J to L, This 57-year-old woman complained of mild blurring of the right eye. Visual acuity in the right eye was 20/25 and J-1. Vision in the left eye was 20/20 and J-1. Note the pseudo–macular hole (**J**) surrounded by an epiretinal membrane. Fifteen months later the patient was asymptomatic. Visual acuity was 20/15. The epiretinal membrane had spontaneously peeled from the retinal surface (**K**). Diagram (**L**) shows epiretinal membrane before *(above)* and after *(arrow, below)* peeling.

(**A** and **B** from Gass[166] and **G** to **I** from Smiddy and Gass.[123])

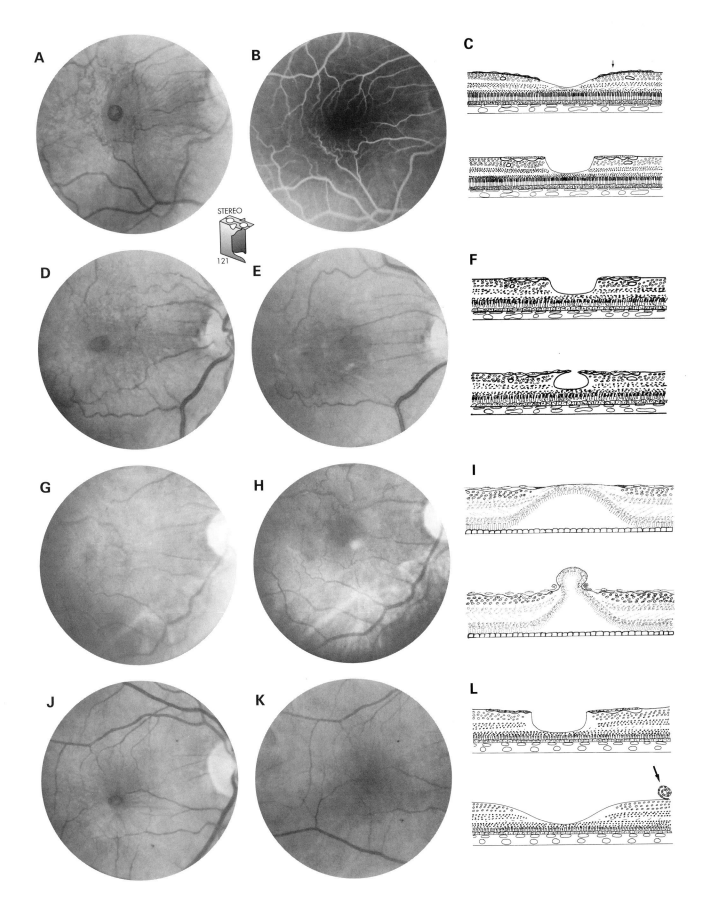

Classification of epiretinal membranes according to associated biomicroscopic findings

Foveolar hole in epiretinal membrane simulating a macular hole (pseudo-macular hole)

Spontaneous contraction of an epiretinal membrane that surrounds but does not cover the foveolar area may produce a biomicroscopic appearance simulating a full-thickness macular hole (Figs. 12-17, *J* to *L;* 12-21; and 12-22).[149,165,166,198] Most of these membranes probably develop before posterior vitreous detachment and fail to cover the foveolar area because of the unusual degree of vitreoretinal adherence there. The patient usually has no complaints, and visual acuity is normal or nearly normal. Biomicroscopy reveals crinkling of the inner retinal surface surrounding the hole in the epiretinal membrane and a punched-out appearance in the area of the hole. As the slit beam is moved across the hole, there is usually a light reflex that is evidence of retinal tissue in the base of the hole. The foveal reflex is usually absent. Fluorescein angiography is generally normal (Fig. 12-21, *B*) but may show a very faint zone of hyperfluorescence corresponding with the pseudohole. This zone of hyperfluorescence is typically much less prominent than the finely granular area of hyperfluorescence seen with a full-thickness hole (Fig. 12-13, *I* to *L*). The presence of the semitransparent perifoveolar epiretinal membrane probably causes the foveolar area to appear faintly hyperfluorescent by contrast to the perifoveolar area. Features of a full-thickness macular hole, including the halo of marginal detachment, yellow deposits within the hole, and a translucent operculum in front of some holes, are not seen in a pseudo–macular hole. The visual prognosis in these patients is good. In a few patients additional contraction of an eccentrically located perifoveal epiretinal membrane may distort the foveal area (Fig. 12-21, *D* and *E*). In others the epiretinal membrane may peel free from the inner retinal surface (Figs. 12-21, *J* to *L*). Teardrop-shaped or slitlike pseudo–macular holes frequently accompany a severe macular pucker. Contraction of a pericentral epiretinal membrane that remains firmly adherent to the inner retinal surface may cause an anterior herniation of the foveolar retinal through the hole in the membrane (Fig. 12-21, *G* to *I*).[123,243] This lesion may also be mistaken for a full-thickness macular hole. Bonnett and Fleury noted development of this foveolar prolapse in three eyes that developed recurrent epiretinal membrane following surgical peeling of an epiretinal membrane.[154]

FIG. 12-22   Pseudo–Macular Holes and Macular Holes Associated with Epiretinal Membranes.

A to **C,** Hole in partly detached epiretinal membrane (**A** and **C**) simulating a macular hole and rim of retinal detachment in an asymptomatic man whose visual acuity was 20/25. Angiography showed minimal fluorescence centrally (**B**). Diagram shows hole in partly detached epiretinal membrane (*arrows,* **C**).

D to **F,** Hole in perifoveolar epiretinal membrane that is detached along with the posterior hyaloid (*stereoscopic view,* **D** and **E**) simulating a macular hole. Diagram (**F**) shows presumed anatomy of the lesion.

G to **L,** Contraction of epiretinal membrane associated with a full-thickness macular hole and retinal detachment. Note small hole (*arrow,* **G**) on June 12, 1970. Epiretinal membrane covers most of the inferonasal part of the hole. By July 27, 1970, the membrane has contracted further and uncovered a one-third disc diameter hole (**H**). On December 4, 1970, the patient noted further loss of vision caused by rhegmatogenous retinal detachment (**I**). Arrows indicate outer retinal folds. Note absence of the epiretinal membrane and hyperfluorescence that confirms a full-thickness hole (*arrow,* **J**). No other hole was present. By February 9, 1971, the epiretinal membrane had regrown across the hole (*arrow,* **K**). The retinal detachment persisted. Photocoagulation was placed on the macular hole. Ten months later the epiretinal membrane had retracted inferiorly, the macular hole was closed, and the retinal detachment had resolved (**L**).

942

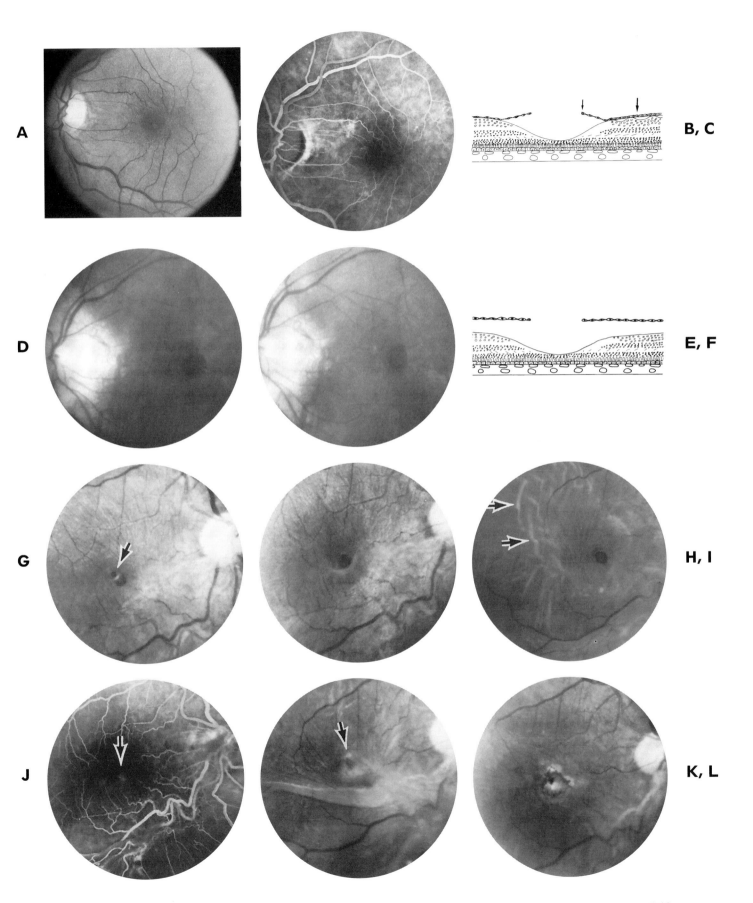

Epiretinal membrane formation associated with full-thickness macular hole

Occasionally vitreous contraction on the retinal surface around the foveal area may be sufficient to mechanically cause a full-thickness hole in the macula (Fig. 12-22, *G* to *I*) or in the paracentral region (Fig. 12-20, *J*). Macular holes produced by this mechanism are typically oval or irregular in shape. They simulate closely a hole that involves the epiretinal membrane alone (pseudo–macular hole). Angiography in the former case, however, shows striking hyperfluorescence corresponding with the full-thickness hole (Fig. 12-22, *J*). It is usually impossible to determine whether the macular hole occurred before the development of an epiretinal membrane or developed as a complication of the membrane. Mild degrees of crinkled cellophane retinopathy often accompany a full-thickness macular hole (Fig. 12-13, *K*).

Pigmentation of epiretinal membranes

Hyperpigmentation of an idiopathic epiretinal membrane may occur spontaneously in the absence of a retinal hole (Fig. 12-23, *C* and *D*).[169] Pigmented epiretinal membranes caused by a proliferation of RPE cells may occur, usually in the extramacular region, in as many as 3% of patients following repair of rhegmatogenous retinal detachment.[217] Similar pigmented membranes may occur in the maculae of patients with peripheral retinal holes.[158,183,188,217,238] They also have been observed overlying photocoagulation scars.[238] Proliferation of pigmented as well as nonpigmented RPE cells has been demonstrated histopathologically in epiretinal membranes.[158,196] In some cases, pigmentation of epiretinal membranes may be caused by the incorporation of macrophages containing either melanin or hemosiderin.

Choroidal neovascularization underlying epiretinal membranes

I have observed the development of choroidal neovascularization in two patients several years

FIG. 12-23   Macular Pucker.

A and **B**, Macular pucker with partial separation and rolled edge of epiretinal membrane (*arrow*, **A**). Note marked distortion and displacement of the retinal vessels toward the horizontal raphe (**B**).

C and **D**, Delayed pigmentation occurring in an idiopathic epiretinal membrane in a healthy woman who was 57 years old when seen initially in 1965 because of recent loss of vision in the right eye. Her visual acuity was 20/400. She had a nonpigmented macular pucker (**C**). She was observed at yearly intervals until 1975, during which time her visual acuity improved to 20/70 and the epiretinal membrane became progressively pigmented (**D**). There were no holes in the retina.

E and **F**, This patient was referred to the Bascom Palmer Eye Institute for surgical removal of an idiopathic epiretinal membrane in the right eye (**E**). There was no biomicroscopic evidence of choroidal neovascularization. Angiography, however, unexpectedly revealed its presence (**F**).

G to **I**, Idiopathic juxtapapillary pucker and retinal neovascularization in a 35-year-old man who noted metamorphopsia of 2 years' duration. His visual acuity was 20/25. Note capillary dilation and leakage (**H** and **I**) within the area of the epiretinal membrane, whose peripheral edges have contracted toward the papillomacular bundle.

after they developed an idiopathic macular pucker. An unsuspected choroidal neovascular membrane (CNVM) was discovered by fluorescein angiography beneath the pucker of another patient referred for surgical peeling of the epiretinal membrane (Fig. 12-23, *E* and *F*). In these three patients there was no evidence of any abnormality in the macula of the opposite eye or of any other cause for the choroidal neovascularization in the affected eye. Stereoscopic fluorescein angiograms should be obtained in all patients scheduled for surgical peeling of opacified epiretinal membranes to exclude the presence of occult choroidal neovascularization.

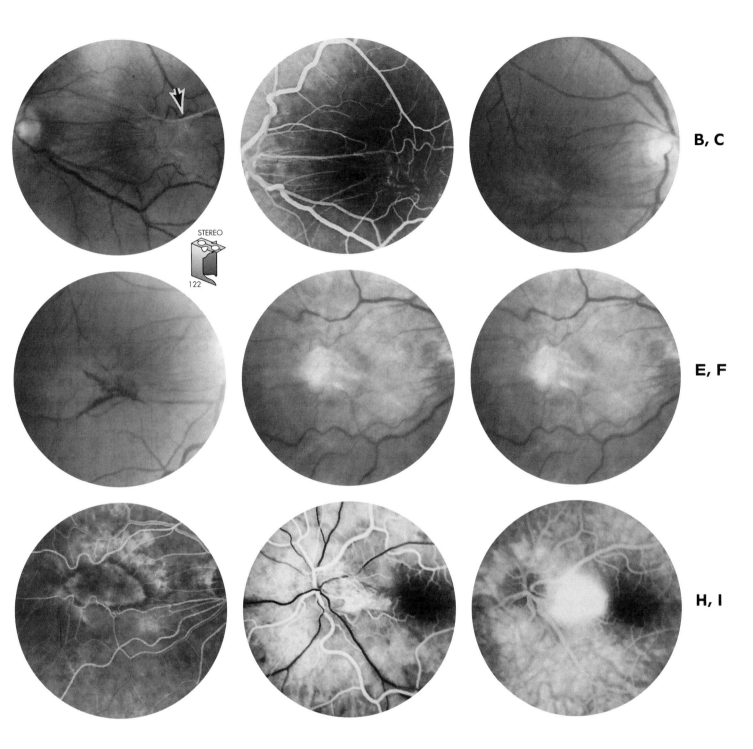

B, C

E, F

H, I

STEREO
122

945

Spontaneous separation of an epiretinal membrane

Occasionally the peripheral portions of the contracting membrane detach from or slide along the retinal surface and curl up into a roll or ridge at one edge of the membrane (Figs. 12-21, *J* to *L;* 12-23, *A;* and 12-24, *C* and *D*).* This process of spontaneous peeling of a preretinal membrane often stops along the course of a major retinal vessel, where the vitreoretinal adhesion may be maximum. In some instances the membrane may spontaneously detach from the entire macular surface and remain as an adherent localized mass in the extramacular region (Figs. 12-8, *A* to *C,* and 12-24, *D*). Distortion of the macula may disappear and visual function improve in such instances. Spontaneous detachment of more peripherally located epiretinal membranes that are the cause of tractional retinal detachment may also occur.[155]

---

*References 149, 160, 168, 169, 181, 202, 232, 240.

FIG. 12-24 Spontaneous Separation and Movement of Epiretinal Membranes.

A and **B,** Note partial peeling and superotemporal displacement of an epiretinal membrane *(arrows)* that occurred over 5 years in this 44-year-old man.

C and **D,** Spontaneous detachment of the epiretinal membrane occurred in this 66-year-old man who developed acute loss of vision, photopsia, and metamorphopsia caused by macular pucker (**C**) 28 months after cataract extraction. Eleven months after his initial examination, his visual acuity had returned to 20/30 and the condensed remnant of the membrane remained attached to the retina in the papillo-macular bundle area (**D**).

E to **H,** This woman with a history of a scleral buckle in the left eye developed loss of central vision caused by an epiretinal membrane in the macula (**E**). On the buckle inferiorly she had an angiomatous proliferation of capillaries in the retina. Angiography revealed mild tortuosity of the retinal vessels in the area of the pucker (**F**) and staining of the peripheral neovascular lesion. Several months following laser treatment of the neovascular lesion (**G**), she noted spontaneous improvement in the vision and the epiretinal membrane in the left macula had peeled off the central macular area (**H**).

I to **L,** This 11-year-old boy developed loss of central vision in the right eye caused by a pucker (**I**). Angiography revealed tortuosity and central displacement of the macular retinal vessels (stereo, **J** and **K**). Following surgical excision of the membrane (**L**) the visual acuity improved from 20/200 to 20/25.

(**I** to **L,** courtesy Dr. Patrick E. Rubsamen.)

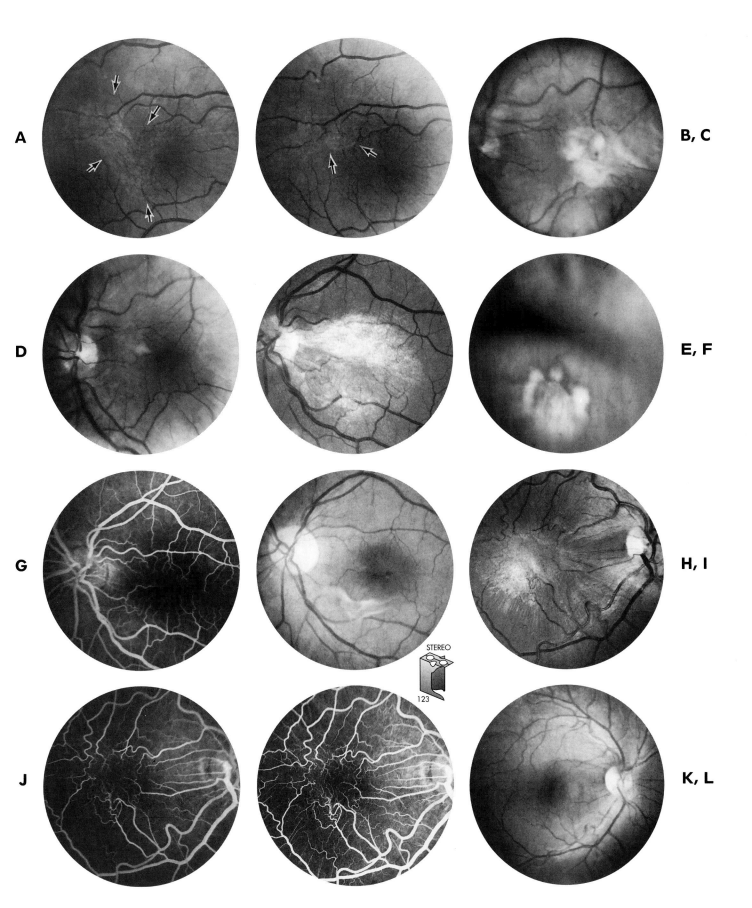

A

B, C

D

E, F

G

STEREO
123

H, I

J

K, L

947

Classification of epiretinal membranes according to associated disorders

Idiopathic epiretinal membranes

Crinkled cellophane maculopathy and macular pucker may occur in healthy patients without evidence of other intraocular disease.* These membranes usually occur in one eye of patients 50 years of age or older. Both sexes are affected equally. Bilateral loss of central vision from severe pucker occurs infrequently. The peripheral fundus should be examined to rule out peripheral tears or retinal vascular lesions. In 90% of the patients a PVD is present.[224]

Macular dysfunction caused by an epiretinal membrane is occasionally seen in asymptomatic children and young adults in the absence of any history to explain their presence (Fig. 12-20, *G*, and 12-24, *I* to *L*).† These membranes in younger patients are generally nonprogressive and are frequently centered over major retinal vessels.

Retinal vascular diseases

Epiretinal membrane formation occurs frequently in association with retinal vascular diseases causing intraretinal exudation, such as diabetes, hypertension (see Fig. 6-15, *H* and *L*), venous obstruction, telangiectasis, angiomatosis (see Fig. 10-22, *A* to *F*), and aphakic cystoid edema (see pp. 478, 486).[164] Macular distortion caused by the development of an epiretinal membrane may occasionally occur early following photocoagulation of retinal vascular diseases, particularly when the treatment is done in the paramacular area (see Fig. 14-17, *A* to *C*).

---

*References 168, 169, 181, 219, 222, 224, 240, 241.
†References 151, 168, 186, 209, 228, 234, 241.

Retinal tears and rhegmatogenous retinal detachment

Crinkled cellophane maculopathy and macular pucker are frequently encountered in patients either before or after treatment for either a peripheral retinal hole or a rhegmatogenous retinal detachment.[150,159,172,220,236] Macular pucker is a major cause of poor central vision after successful repair of a retinal detachment.[159,175,192,233,236] It typically occurs 8 to 16 weeks following surgery. Its development is probably determined primarily by the events occurring at the time of vitreous contraction and retinal hole formation rather than by the type of treatment used. Nevertheless, various authors have incriminated a variety of factors in its pathogenesis, including preoperative findings of macular detachment, vitreous hemorrhage, low visual acuity, rolled edges of retinal holes, star folds, equatorial folds, cryotherapy, age greater than 30 years,[192] and multiple operations,[153,175,192,233,236] as well as intraoperative complications such as loss of vitreous and multiple attempts at subretinal fluid drainage.[233] Focal areas of epiretinal membrane formation in the periphery of the fundus identical to that occurring in the macula are responsible for the star-shaped retinal folds that may accompany detachment. Macular pucker and star-shaped folds represent mild forms of the more severe disorder of periretinal proliferation (massive vitreous retraction), which is caused by cellular proliferation, predominantly that of RPE cells and astrocytes, on both the anterior and posterior surfaces of the retina.[194,195]

Approximately 20% of patients who develop a macular pucker after a scleral buckling procedure will experience improvement in visual acuity.[175] Part of this improvement is caused by relaxation or partial peeling of the epiretinal membrane, and part is caused by partial resolution of the intraretinal edema, which is more likely to be severe early after its development, particularly in aphakic patients.

Vitreous inflammatory diseases

Any disease producing an inflammatory cellular infiltrate in the vitreous, such as toxoplasmosis retinitis (Fig. 12-8, *A* to *C*), uveitis, trauma, intraocular tumor, or tapetoretinal dystrophies, may be associated with development of epiretinal membranes in the macula.

Pathology and pathogenesis

Histopathologically, epiretinal membranes are composed of a fibrocellular sheet that varies in thickness from a single layer of collagen and interspersed cells (Fig. 12-25, *A*) to a thicker layer of fibrocellular proliferation that often bridges coarse folds on the retinal surface (Fig. 12-25, *B*). The latter is often associated with intraretinal edema.* The precise morphologic identification of the cells of origin of epiretinal membranes by either electron or light microscopy is difficult because of the ability of astrocytes, hyalocytes, fibrocytes, macrophages,[183,184] and RPE cells to change into cells with a similar appearance and function.† Most epiretinal membranes are composed of a variety of cell types, including one or more of the following: RPE cells, fibrous astrocytes, fibrocytes, and macrophages. Several, and perhaps all, cell types have the capability of developing myofibroblastic properties that are probably responsible for the contractile properties of epiretinal and vitreous membranes.‡ Epiretinal membranes can be produced experimentally by a variety of techniques, including intravitreal injection of blood, carbon particles, fibroblasts, and RPE cells.§

The stimuli for epiretinal membrane formation are poorly understood. A PVD appears to be one important stimulus.[177,181,220] Approximately 75% of epiretinal membranes are found in eyes with a PVD.[177,219,242] These membranes are particularly prone to develop in eyes following transient vitreomacular traction soon after separation of the vitreous from the retina and within weeks or several months after vitreous detachment and

rhegmatogenous retinal detachment.[220] Two different mechanisms for epiretinal membrane formation and contraction after vitreous detachment have been proposed. One mechanism is the proliferation and contraction of fibrous astrocytes that extend from the retina and optic nerve through either preexisting dehiscences in the internal limiting membrane of the retina and optic nerve head, or dehiscences caused by vitreous separation. These dehiscences are most likely to occur on the optic nerve head or along the major retinal vessels where the internal limiting membrane is attenuated. These fibrocellular membranes are composed of a syncytium of cells with small, spindle-shaped nuclei and scanty cytoplasm arranged in either a single or a multilayered fashion along the inner retinal surface (Fig. 12-25, *A*). Contraction and interaction of the cells rather than contraction of the extracellular component of the membrane are probably most important in causing retinal wrinkling.[170] Electron microscopic studies of idiopathic epiretinal membranes have demonstrated that RPE cells and fibrous astrocytes are the predominant cell type composing these membranes.[226] Membranes in younger patients, ones in patients with a history of recent development of symptoms, and recurrent membranes are more likely to contain RPE cells with myoblastic differentiation as well as myofibroblasts.[191,209,228] Other cell types that occasionally predominate are fibrocytes and myofibroblasts.

Contraction of vitreous cortical remnants and proliferation and fibrous metaplasia of hyalocytes left on the inner retinal surface after PVD constitute another postulated mechanism for the development of epiretinal membranes (Fig. 12-2.)[168,181,187,200] This mechanism may be more common in those membranes that are confined to the central macular area and those that histologically are hypocellular.[158] Kishi and Shimizu noted oval defects in the detached posterior hyaloid membrane anterior to the macula in most eyes seen with epiretinal membranes.[187] They interpreted this as a tear in the hyaloid membrane that probably occurred before development of epiretinal membranes in the macula. They postulated that the cortical vitreous remaining on the macular surface acted as a scaffold for the influx of cellular elements responsible for the epiretinal membrane.

---

*References 158, 164, 166, 172, 173, 176, 183, 188, 189.
†References 152, 157, 171, 178, 179, 182-185, 190, 193, 196, 197, 200, 207, 208, 210, 214, 215, 217, 225, 227.
‡References 180, 182, 184, 227, 237, 239.
§References 148, 191, 206, 213, 214, 231.

Prognosis

Patients with macular distortion caused by contraction of an epiretinal membrane usually show little or no progression of distortion after their initial examination.[168,169,224] A few patients, however, experience a progressive loss of visual function over a period of months or years.[184,235] The infrequency with which the distortion worsens suggests that membrane contraction usually occurs rapidly and is self-limiting. Angiographic evidence of retinal capillary permeability is more likely to be present soon after contraction of the epiretinal membrane has occurred, and in eyes with membranes that are more likely to progress.[147] Approximately 50% of patients maintain good visual acuity, and in over 80% the visual function is either stable or improves. Fewer than 10% show a decline in visual acuity. Spontaneous peeling of the membrane occasionally results in dramatic visual improvement (Figs. 12-8, *A* to *C;* 12-21, *J* to *L;* and 12-24, *C* and *D*).[167,174,209,221,226] Spontaneous separation of a preretinal membrane in the macula is particularly likely to occur following laser or cryotherapy of a peripheral retinal angioma (Figs. 10-22, *A* to *F,* and 10-24, *E* to *H*).[167,221]

Treatment

In the absence of any evidence of intravitreal inflammation, there is no reason to believe that corticosteroid treatment is beneficial in treating patients with intraretinal edema that may accompany a severe pucker. Surgical peeling of epiretinal membranes from the macular surface has been successfully accomplished (Fig. 12-24, *I* to *L*).* The best surgical candidates are those patients with 20/100 acuity or worse, and a short duration of macular puckering. Approximately 75% of patients experience two lines of visual acuity improvement after surgery. Surgical complications include cataract (approximately 50% to 75% within 2 years), peripheral retinal tears, retinal detachment, posterior retinal tears, photic maculopathy, anterior ischemic optic neuropathy, and endophthalmitis.† Regrowth of epiretinal tissue occurs in a small percentage of cases. Photocoagulation of the epiretinal membrane is contraindicated.

FIG. 12-25 Histopathology of Macular Distortion Caused by Epiretinal Membranes.

A, Photomicrograph of crinkled cellophane maculopathy showing fine wrinkling of the inner retinal surface resulting from contraction of an epiretinal membrane. A fine fibrocellular membrane *(arrow)* lies on the surface of the folded internal limiting membrane.

B, Photomicrograph showing macular pucker, cystoid macular edema, and degeneration secondary to contraction of an epiretinal membrane. The membrane is artifactitiously detached near the large retinal folds *(arrow).*

---

*References 161, 163, 199, 201, 203-205, 211, 212, 216, 223, 226, 230.
†References 156, 201, 203, 205, 211, 212, 223.

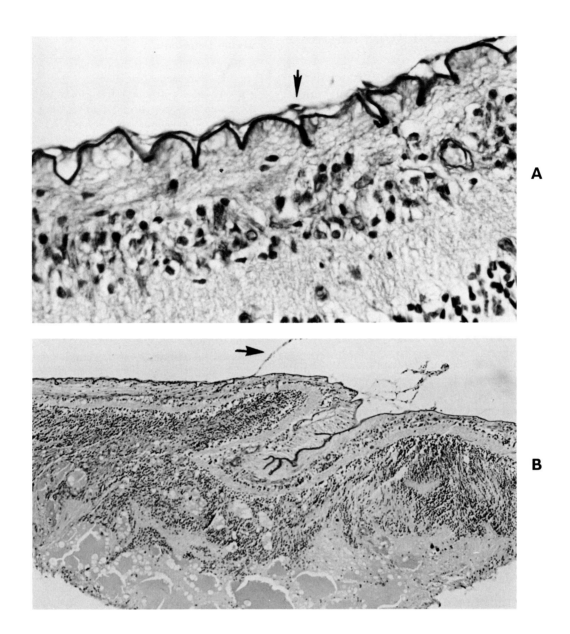

A

B

▼ RETINAL CHANGES ASSOCIATED WITH RHEGMATOGENOUS RETINAL DETACHMENT

Rhegmatogenous retinal detachment is one of the most important disorders of the vitreoretinal interface, and it may cause or be associated with a variety of abnormalities in the macular area. Approximately 30% to 40% of patients in whom retinal detachment includes the macula will regain good visual acuity after successful reattachment.* Most patients who fail to regain good visual acuity will show biomicroscopic and fluorescein angiographic lesions that account for the loss.[251,257,266] In some, however, usually those with macular detachment of 2 months' or longer duration, the macular area will show minimal changes, and visual loss is probably caused by failure of regeneration and realignment of photoreceptors.[254]

Epiretinal membrane

Epiretinal membranes may be present before the development of a retinal detachment but often become apparent only during the postoperative course. Preoperatively, patients with detachment and epiretinal membranes in the macular area will usually show a stellate arrangement of multiple, white, retinal folds (Fig. 12-26, A and B). These are often accompanied by peripheral star folds, meridional folds, and rolled edges of retinal tears. Postoperatively, epiretinal membranes are the most frequently recognized abnormality in the macula.[251,257] Approximately 5% of patients undergoing scleral buckling procedures will develop severe macular pucker that may or may not be associated with massive periretinal proliferation and failure of standard scleral buckling procedures. Vitrectomy and surgical removal of these membranes are successful in salvaging the sight in some of these patients.

Cystoid macular edema

Cystoid macular edema may be present either when the patient is seen initially with a retinal detachment (Fig. 12-26, C) or postoperatively. It occurs most frequently but not exclusively in

---

*References 250, 252, 253, 256, 262, 263, 265, 272, 281, 286

FIG. 12-26 Macular Changes in Rhegmatogenous Retinal Detachment.

A, Early stellate pattern of retinal folds indicative of the presence of epiretinal membrane.

B, Advanced stellate retinal folds in a patient who developed massive periretinal proliferation.

C, Cystoid macular edema (arrows).

D to **F,** Seventeen-year-old myopic girl with recent onset of rhegmatogenous retinal detachment and multiple peripheral retinal tears. Note cloudiness of subretinal fluid and angiographic evidence of leaking retinal blood vessels.

G to **I,** Long-standing superior rhegmatogenous retinal detachment and outer retinal cyst (arrow, **H**) in a 56-year-old man who was asymptomatic until several days before admission, when he noted loss of central vision caused by extension of the detachment into the macula. Angiography showed early hyperfluorescence caused by attenuation of the RPE and late staining caused by retinal capillary leakage in the area of long-standing detachment (**I**).

J, Subretinal fibrous proliferative bands and fenestrated membranes in a patient with long-standing retinal detachment.

K and **L,** Subretinal fibrous strands (arrows) associated with a long-standing inferior rhegmatogenous retinal detachment that spontaneously reattached. Similar findings were present in the opposite eye.

(**G** to **I** from Gass.[165])

aphakic eyes. Cystoid macular edema and epiretinal membranes are the most frequent macular findings in patients with poor acuity after buckling procedures (see p. 482).

In most patients with rhegmatogenous retinal detachment, fluorescein angiography shows no evidence of retinal vascular permeability alterations. In long-standing retinal detachment, however, angiography may demonstrate evidence of capillary dilation, increased permeability, and areas of capillary nonperfusion. In myopic children with recent onset of detachment, angiography may demonstrate large areas of diffuse leakage of dye (Fig. 12-26, D to F).[257]

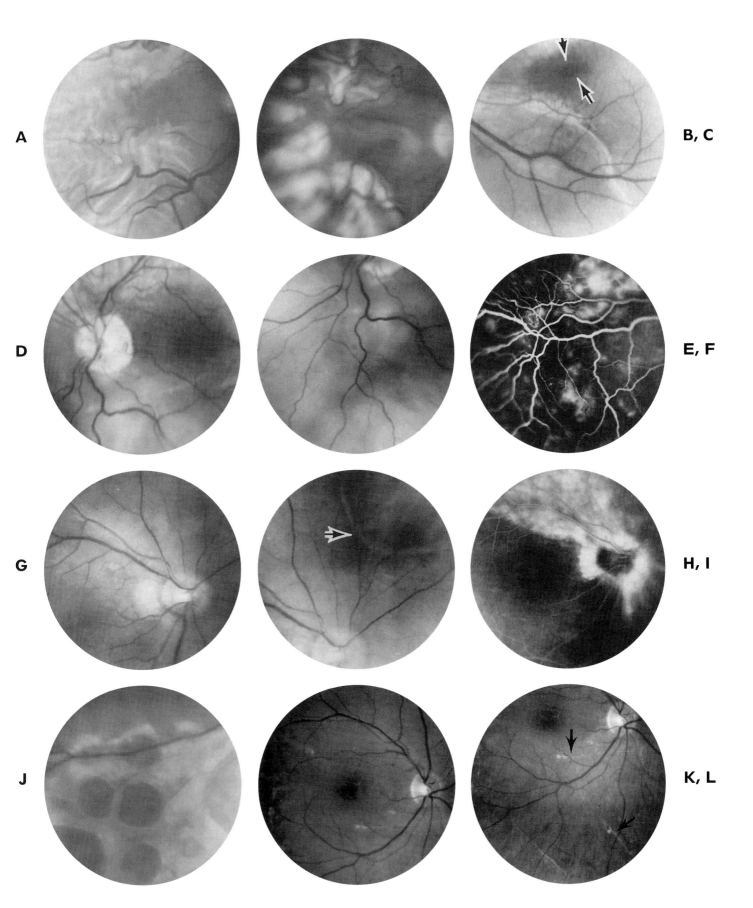

A

B, C

D

E, F

G

H, I

J

K, L

Macular and paramacular holes

Rhegmatogenous detachments caused by holes in the macula or paramacular region usually occur in highly myopic patients with posterior staphylomata or in patients with direct vitreous traction on the posterior retina.[119,273,279] In most cases these detachments are confined to the posterior half of the eye, and they infrequently extend out to the ora serrata. When the detachment is confined to the macula in patients with a posterior staphyloma and myopia, the detachment may be caused by traction rather than a hole, and spontaneous reattachment may occur.[248] See discussion in Chapter 3, pp. 126-129.

Approximately 0.5% to 1% of patients with rhegmatogenous retinal detachment and a peripheral retinal hole will also have a macular hole.[249,273] During the course of surgery or immediately following surgery a macular hole may develop in another 1% to 2% of patients.[249] Fluorescein angiography may be helpful in differentiating macular holes from macular cysts, pseudo–macular hole caused by an epiretinal membrane (Fig. 12-21, A and B), or partial-thickness macular holes (see Figs. 6-22 and 6-23).

Macular holes in nonmyopic eyes without evidence of vitreous traction do not require treatment at the time of surgery for retinal detachment caused by peripheral retinal tears.[276] A variety of techniques has been employed in the repair of retinal detachments caused by macular and paramacular holes in patients with myopic staphylomata or posterior vitreous traction (Fig. 12-8, J to L).*

Pigment epithelial atrophy, demarcation lines, and subretinal neovascularization

With prolonged retinal detachment (usually beyond a period of 6 months), the RPE becomes partly depigmented within the area of detachment (Figs. 12-26, G to I, and 12-27, K), and it may proliferate along the junction of detached and attached retina to form a demarcation line (Figs. 12-27, A, F, and K; and 12-28, A to D). A series of these lines may occur as the detachment spreads over a period of months or years. They may eventually extend into the macular area (Fig. 12-27, L). Similar demarcation lines may occur along the posterior border of a chronic choroidal detachment (Fig. 12-28, F). These RPE changes are more easily detected with fluorescein angiography (Figs. 12-26, I, and 12-27, K).[244,257] Angiography is helpful in differentiating a long-standing

*References 14, 53, 54, 57, 81, 98, 115, 261, 275.

954

FIG. 12-27 Complications of Long-Standing Rhegmatogenous Retinal Detachment.

A to F, This young myopic woman presented with bilateral inferior retinal detachments and prominent pigmented demarcation lines that extended only to the peripheral macular region in both eyes. A scleral buckling procedure was done in the left eye. The patient elected to have reinforcement of the demarcation lines with laser photocoagulation rather than surgery in the right eye (A). She had no further trouble for 10 years, when she developed evidence of intraretinal neovascularization and angiomatous formation within the area of retinal detachment in the area indicated by the *arrow* in A. No further treatment was done until 2 years later when the retinal tumor enlarged (B) and caused symptomatic vitreous cells and mild cystoid macular edema (stereo, C, D, and F). Following argon laser treatment of the angiomatous lesion (B), the lipid exudate disappeared and the vitreous cells and CME improved.

G to L, Retinal angiomatous proliferation (*arrows,* I to K) and yellow intraretinal and subretinal exudation developed in a 24-year-old woman with long-standing bilateral inferior rhegmatogenous retinal detachments and demarcation lines (G and H). The retina reattached after cryotherapy of the angiomatous proliferation and retinal holes. Note the hyperfluorescence on the detachment side of the demarcation line *(arrow)* in the left eye (L). The demarcation line in the left eye was reinforced using argon laser.

retinal detachment from retinoschisis. The latter condition is not associated with RPE changes unless it is associated with retinal detachment from holes developing in the outer and usually the inner layer of retinoschisis (Fig. 12-29).[257]

I have seen three patients with loss of central vision caused by choroidal neovascularization at the edge of a demarcation line lying adjacent to the foveal area (Fig. 12-28, A to D).[258,268,271]

Subretinal fibrosis

A light gray fenestrated sheet or multiple opaque strands may be present on the posterior surface of the detached retina in approximately 3% of patients with a rhegmatogenous detachment (Fig. 12-26, J).[270,278,284,285] Subretinal strands are frequently arranged in a reticular or other geometric pattern. In some cases they may be separated from the posterior retinal surface. They are most often seen in long-standing detachment and are often associated with demarcation lines. They result from fenestrations developing in large, thin fibrocellular sheets growing on the back surface of the retina. In contrast to epiretinal membranes, these usually do not affect the incidence of surgical success.[284] Occasionally, however, one or more of these strands may remain taut after scleral buckling and prevent complete reattachment of the macula.

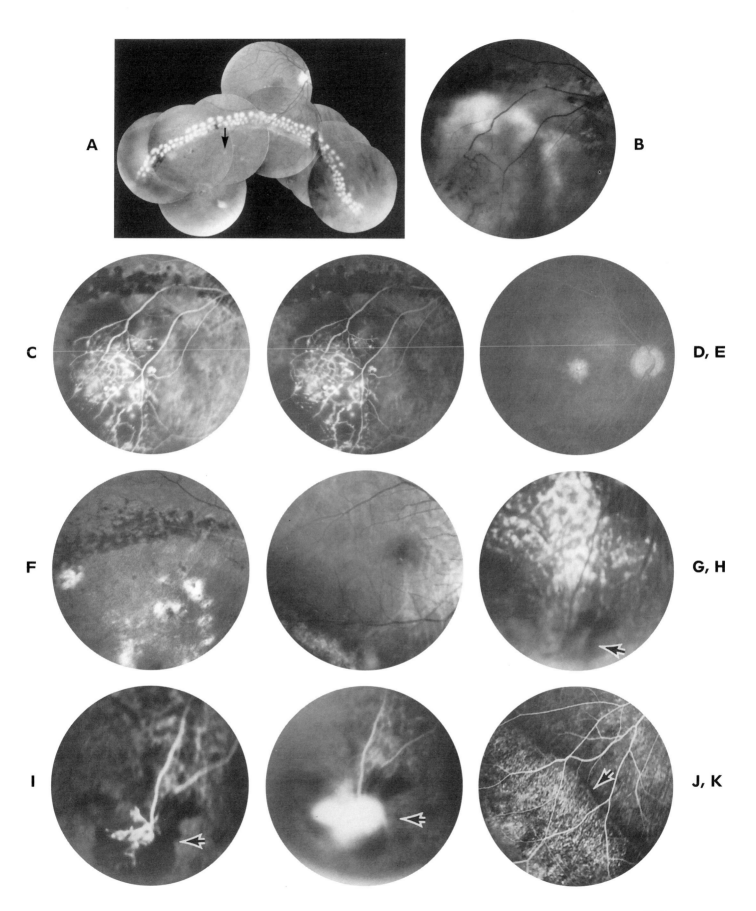

Gravitation of subretinal pigment following cryotherapy

RPE pigment liberated at the time of vigorous cryotherapy, usually to superotemporal holes in patients with retinal detachments involving the macula, may gravitate within the subretinal fluid to the macular area. This pigment deposit may remain static or may become diminished to some degree. It is probably not associated with any significant morbidity in regard to visual recovery.* This granular, polymorphic deposition of pigment should be distinguished from the pigmentation caused by proliferation and fibrous metaplasia of the RPE on the inner retinal surface (Fig. 12-28, K and L).

Lesions simulating serous detachments of the retinal pigment epithelium

Early in the postoperative course following successful repair of a retinal detachment, the physician may notice one or more lesions with the biomicroscopic features of serous detachments of the RPE in the macular region or elsewhere in the fundus (Fig. 12-28, G to I).[246,267] Angiographically, however, these lesions do not show staining with fluorescein, and they probably represent focal areas of cloudy serous detachment of the sensory retina. They vary in size from one-fourth to four disc diameters. Several months or a year may be required before resolution occurs. When these lesions are large and solitary, they are most likely to be misdiagnosed as serous detachments of the RPE. When they are multiple they may be mistaken for multifocal areas of choroiditis.[287] Similar lesions have been observed in experimental retinal detachment.[269]

Retinal neovascularization and angiomatous proliferation caused by chronic retinal detachment

Long-standing rhegmatogenous retinal detachment may cause retinal vascular occlusion and focal proliferation of preretinal as well as intraretinal capillaries that may simulate a capillary hemangioma (Fig. 12-27, A to F).[247,255] These lesions may cause intraretinal and subretinal exudation and occasionally vitreous hemorrhage. Similar proliferative vascular lesions as well as choroidal neovascularization may occur at drainage sites made during scleral buckling procedures.[259,260]

---

*References 245, 251, 264, 277, 280, 282.

FIG. 12-28 Macular Complications Associated with Long-Standing Retinal Detachment.

A to **C,** Subretinal neovascularization (*arrow,* **B**) developed within a pigmented demarcation line in a patient who had previous successful surgery for a long-standing retinal detachment.

D and **E,** This patient was followed for 8 years with recurrent subfoveal bleeding caused by subretinal neovascularization occurring within a demarcation line (**D**). Eight years after the photograph in **D** she returned with evidence of intraretinal vascular proliferation and exudation temporal to the macula (**E**) occurring within the area of intraretinal migration of RPE caused by long-standing retinal detachment.

F, Angiographic evidence of demarcation lines (*arrows*) caused by long-standing choroidal and retinal detachment.

G, Sharply circumscribed puddle of subretinal fluid simulating serous RPE detachment after successful scleral buckling operation.

H to **J,** Similar large puddle of cloudy subretinal fluid (*arrows,* **H** and **I**) remained for 3 to 4 weeks after a successful buckling operation. Note the multiloculated appearance superiorly (**I**). Angiography showed no evidence of RPE detachment (**J**).

K and **L,** Pigmented epiretinal membranes causing macular pucker in two patients following scleral buckling procedures.

Submacular hemorrhage during surgery

Choroidal hemorrhage occurring at the time of drainage of the subretinal fluid is the most common cause of subretinal blood extending into the macular area. It may occur occasionally, however, because of spontaneous rupture of an occult CNVM in the macular or juxtapapillary area. Many patients who have spread of subretinal blood into the macula from adjacent sources (e.g., CNVMs or choroidal ruptures) regain good acuity after clearing of the blood. This is less likely to occur, however, in patients with rhegmatogenous retinal detachment.

Post–scleral buckle macular folds

Retinal folds extending into the macular area may be the cause of a poor visual result after a scleral buckling procedure. These may be either radial or curvilinear folds at the posterior edge of a radial buckle that was placed too far posteriorly; radial folds extending from a drainage site associated with retinal incarceration; or folds caused by posterior slippage of the retina following the use of intraocular gas in the repair of a large retinal tear (see Fig. 4-6, C).[274,283]

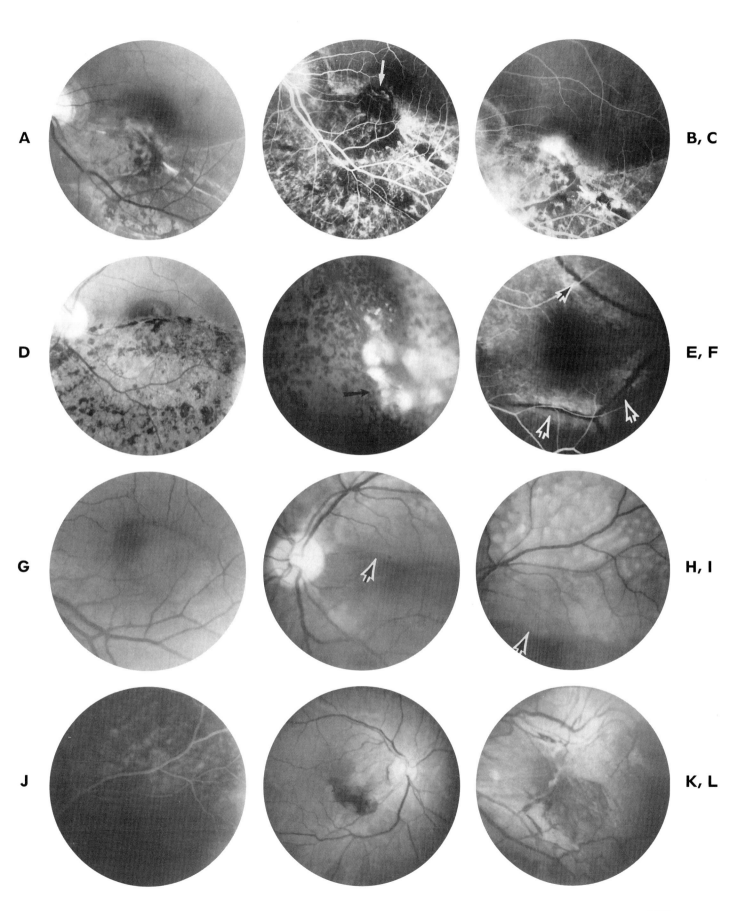

A

B, C

D

E, F

G

H, I

J

K, L

957

▼ DEGENERATIVE RETINOSCHISIS

Degenerative retinoschisis is present in approximately 1% to 4% of healthy adult patients.* It most frequently involves the inferotemporal peripheral fundus and is often bilateral. Anatomically, the splitting of the retina usually occurs at the outer plexiform layer but it may occur more superficially (Fig. 12-29, *A*). It typically is seen clinically as a sharply circumscribed, smooth, nonmobile elevation of the inner retina extending posteriorly from the ora serrata (Fig. 12-29, *B* and *C*). It is not associated with changes in the RPE, which is in contact with the retinal receptor layer in the area of the split retina. The outer layer is difficult to see without scleral depression. Retinoschisis in most patients is asymptomatic and nonprogressive.[291] Posterior extension of retinoschisis into the macular area occurs rarely and is most likely to develop in patients with the reticular form of degenerative retinoschisis, in which there is an extremely thin inner retinal layer (Fig. 12-29, *B* and *C*).[292,298] It has been estimated that the chance of retinal detachment developing in a patient with retinoschisis is 0.04%.[292]

---

*References 290, 292, 294, 296, 298, 299.

FIG. 12-29   Degenerative Retinoschisis.

A, Photomicrograph showing split at the level of the nerve fiber layer *(arrow)* and extensive cystoid degeneration of the peripheral retina.

B and **C,** Stereoscopic angiograms of a large area of retinoschisis that extends posteriorly into the temporal portion of the macula in this 52-year-old man, who also had retinoschisis in the other eye. Note there is no evidence of RPE degeneration in the area of the retinoschisis.

D to **G,** In November of 1975, bilateral retinoschisis was noted in this asymptomatic 68-year-old woman. In the left eye it extended almost to the macula (**D**). One year later she lost central vision in the left eye because of macular detachment caused by a large posterior outer wall tear at the posterior edge of the retinoschisis. A scleral buckle supplemented with postoperative photocoagulation (**E** and **F**) was used in closing the tear *(arrows)*. Ten years later her visual acuity was 20/30 (**G**).

H and **I,** Spontaneous collapse of degenerative retinoschisis in this middle-aged woman. The retinoschisis was present in June of 1979 (**H**) and had disappeared in September of 1979 (**I**).

(**A,** courtesy Dr. Robert Y. Foos.)

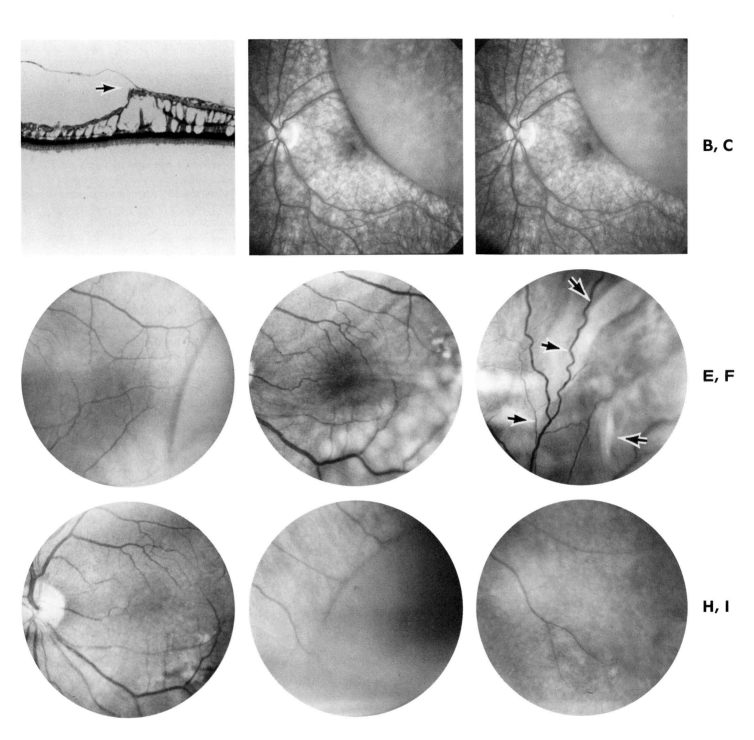

B, C

E, F

H, I

959

Schisis-detachment

There is some predilection for large areas of posterior extension of schisis to develop large outer wall holes and a shallow retinal detachment that may slowly extend into the macula (Fig. 12-30).[288,297,299] Before posterior extension of the retinal detachment beyond the edge of the schisis, the detachment may be difficult to detect. The presence of hypopigmentation of the RPE around the outer retinal holes or one or more pigmented demarcation lines indicate retinal detachment (Fig. 12-30, *B* and *G*). The retinal detachment extending into the macula may be shallow and it may be possible to close the communication between the macular detachment and the outer wall holes with one or more sessions of moderately intense laser photocoagulation across the neck of the detachment along the posterior edge of the schisis as well as along the edge of the outer wall holes (Fig. 12-30, *C* to *J*).[288] In other cases, it may be necessary to employ vitrectomy and intravitreal gas injection to achieve resolution of the detachment.[288,289,297,299] Schisis detachment, when confined to the peripheral fundus, rarely progresses and requires no treatment.[291] The author believes, however, that posterior extension of schisis to near the macula, particularly when associated with large outer wall holes, constitutes a threat to central vision and should be delimited with several rows of laser photocoagulation without waiting to demonstrate progression.

Unlike patients with sex-linked juvenile retinoschisis, there is no evidence of any specific macular abnormality in patients with degenerative retinoschisis. Detailed macular function tests in these patients are comparable to those in unaffected patients.[296]

Fluorescein angiography shows no abnormality in the background choroidal fluorescence in the area of retinoschisis (Fig. 12-29, *B* and *C*) as long as there is no hole or detachment in the outer retinal layer. In some cases there may be evidence of retinal capillary dilation, leakage, and dropout in the inner retinal layers.

The pathogenesis of degenerative retinoschisis is unknown, but chronic vitreous traction on the peripheral retina that is predisposed to cystic degenerative changes, particularly on the temporal side, is probably important.

Spontaneous reattachment of the inner layer occasionally occurs (Fig. 12-29, *H* and *I*). No

treatment is indicated unless a retinal detachment associated with inner and outer retinal holes develops, or unless there is demonstrated progression of schisis or a schisis detachment with outer wall holes into the macular area.

Retinoschisis is most likely to be mistaken for a localized rhegmatogenous retinal detachment. The typical configuration of the elevated inner retinal surface, absence of evidence of visible and angiographic changes in the underlying RPE, and presence of an absolute scotoma are features suggesting retinoschisis. The presence of a demarcation line is strong evidence of a rhegmatogenous detachment, which in the presence of schisis may be difficult to identify. Angiographic evidence of depigmentation of the RPE peripheral to the demarcation line indicates present or past retinal detachment in that area.

FIG. 12-30   Senile Schisis-Detachment.

A and **B,** This woman had peripheral retinoschisis with large outer retinal holes *(arrows).* There was no evidence of extension of the shallow retinal detachment surrounding the holes posterior to the zone of schisis.

C to **J,** Extension of fluid from within the schisis cavity through holes in the outer retinal layer *(arrow,* **C**) into the subretinal space in the macula occurred in a 66-year-old man who noted loss of vision in the right eye. His visual acuity was 20/60. He had a large bullous area of peripheral retinoschisis temporally, associated with several large holes *(small arrows,* **D** and **E**) in the outer retinal layer posteriorly. A shallow serous retinal detachment extended from the edge of the outer retinal holes into the center of the macula *(large arrow,* **D** and **F**). Angiography revealed a large area of early hyperfluorescence indicative of RPE depigmentation within the areas of the outer retinal holes *(arrows,* **G**) and in a zone of long-standing shallow retinal detachment that extended from the posterior edge of the holes into the temporal macula **(H).** Argon green laser was used to treat the edge of the outer retinal holes and along the posterior edge of the schisis **(I)** in an effort to close the neck of the detachment. Because of incomplete closure the same area was retreated several months later, and was successful in reattaching the retina in the macular area **(J).** His acuity returned to 20/30.

(**A** and **B,** courtesy Dr. Gerald A. Brooksby; **C** to **K** from Ambler et al.[288])

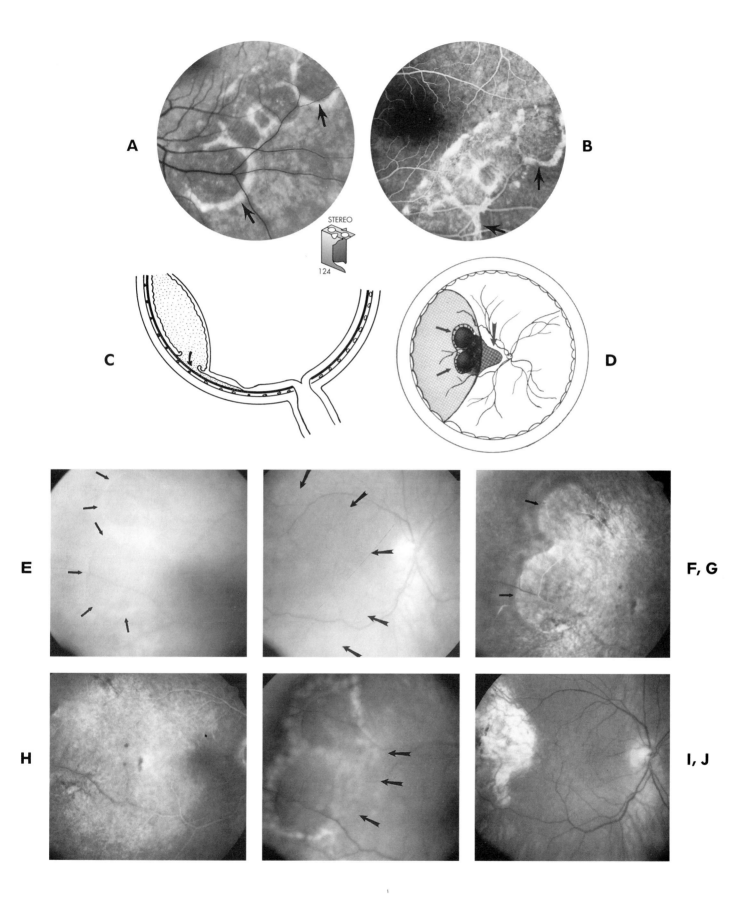

▼ AMYLOIDOSIS

Loss of vision caused by accumulation of amyloid in the vitreous may occur in primary familial amyloidosis with or without systemic involvement* and occasionally in patients with neither systemic nor familial involvement. The amyloid is probably produced in the retinal vessels and secreted into the vitreous. Early, it may produce prominent perivascular sheathing and localized vitreous veils.[319] Later, as the vitreous becomes more opacified, it has been described biomicroscopically as having a cotton-wool, glass-wool, or cobweb appearance (Fig. 12-31, *A*). It may be misdiagnosed as inflammatory exudate or resolving retinal blood. Cotton-wool spots unassociated with hypertension occurred in one patient.[307]

Histopathologically, amyloid may be demonstrated within and surrounding retinal vessels as well as within large choroidal vessels and the choriocapillaris (Fig. 12-31, *E*).[309,317]

Vitreous deposits in amyloidosis occur primarily in patients with dominantly inherited amyloidosis associated with peripheral neuropathy and cardiomyopathy (Fig. 12-31, *B* and *C*).[301,312] Most of these patients have a mutant form of the protein transthyretin.[313-315] This mutation may be present in patients with vitreous opacification and no family history of the disorder.[316] Patients with vitreous opacities should be checked for the transthyretin mutation even when they have no definite family history of amyloidosis. Additional means of diagnosis include biopsy of affected organs, including the eye, or rectum.

Familial oculoleptomeningeal amyloidosis is characterized by hemiplegic migraine, periodic obtundation, psychosis, seizures, carpal-tunnel syndrome, intracerebral hemorrhage, myelopathy, deafness, peripheral neuropathy, visual loss associated with retinal and vitreous infiltration with amyloid, and systemic organ involvement (Fig. 12-31, *G* to *L*).[306,318] The retinal lesions resemble cotton-wool patches but histologically are amyloid infiltration of the retina (Fig. 12-31, *G* and *I*).

Crawford reported cotton-wool exudates in a patient with nonfamilial systemic amyloidosis and no evidence of systemic hypertension.[304] Histologically, these retinal lesions were swollen, degenerated, necrotic axons in the nerve fiber layer unassociated with amyloid deposits in either the retina or the vitreous.

Vitrectomy is the only effective means of restoring vision in patients with amyloidosis (Fig. 12-31, *D* and *E*).[305,309,315] Removal of as much of the vitreous framework as possible is indicated since recurrence of the amyloid deposits may occur.[303,308]

---

*References 300-304, 306, 307, 309-313, 318, 319.

FIG. 12-31 Primary Amyloidosis.

A to **F,** Slit-lamp photograph of this 62-year-old man who experienced painless progressive loss of vision for several years because of amyloid deposition *(arrow)* in the vitreous of both eyes (**A**). His past medical history was positive for severe peripheral neuropathy and the carpal-tunnel syndrome. Note the atrophy of the skin and muscles of the hands and feet (**B** and **C**). His family history was negative. An open-sky lensectomy and vitrectomy were done. His visual acuity improved from counting fingers at 1 foot to 20/30. Note the remnants of amyloid on the optic disc *(arrow,* **D**) and on the retinal surface temporal to the macula *(arrow,* **E**). He subsequently died of a coronary thrombosis. Photomicrograph (**F**) showing amyloid deposits occluding much of the choriocapillaris and within the wall of the large choroidal vessels *(arrows)*.

G and **H,** This 51-year-old woman with dominantly inherited oculoleptomeningeal amyloidosis had a 20-year history of progressive peripheral neuropathy, carpal-tunnel syndrome, hyperreflexia, dysarthria, nystagmus, and memory loss. Visual acuity was 20/25 bilaterally. In the perimacular area she had numerous superficial gray-white lesions that stained angiographically (**G** and **H**). One year later she developed visual loss, vitreous opacification and thickening of the tongue. Visual acuity improved from 20/400 to 20/40 in both eyes following vitrectomy. The vitreous exhibited dichroism and stained positively for amyloid.

I to **L,** The 28-year-old son of the patient in **G** and **H** had a history of hemiplegic migraine and seizures beginning in his teenage years. He died at age 29 years from complications of intracerebral hemorrhage. Pathologic examination of the eyes revealed birefringent amyloid deposits in the blood vessel walls and perivascular spaces of the retina *(arrows,* **I** [Congo red stain] and **J** [polarized light]), extensive amyloid deposition in the leptomeninges and the blood vessel walls within the leptomeninges *(arrows,* **K** and **L** [Congo red stain]). Other organ involvement included the heart, alimentary tract, skeletal muscle, and nerves.

(**D** and **E** from Kasner et al.[309]; **J** to **L** from Uitti et al.[318])

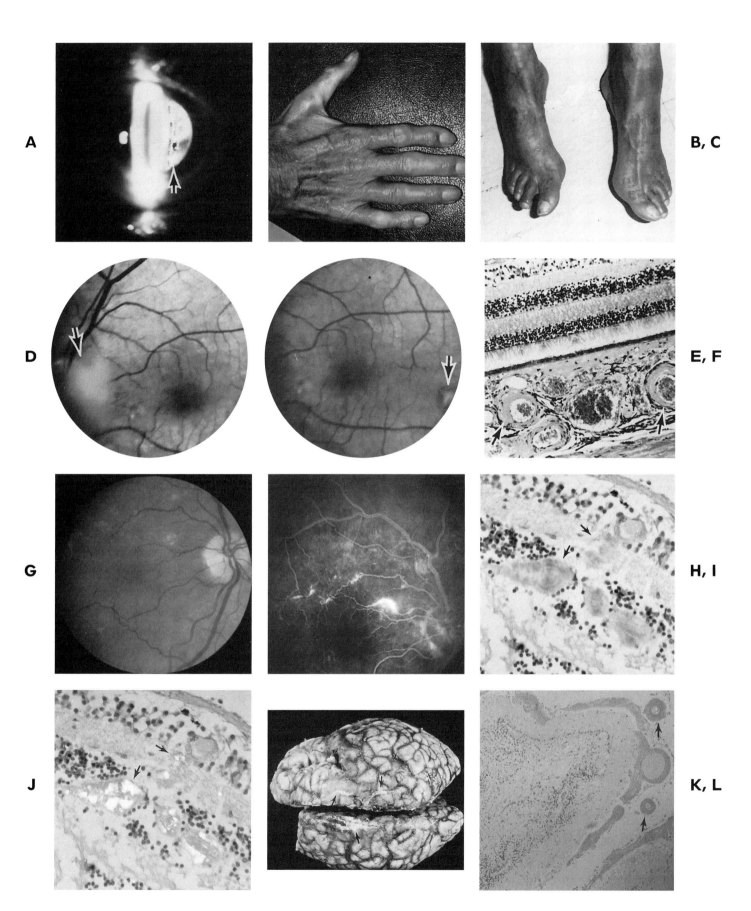

A

B, C

D

E, F

G

H, I

J

K, L

▼ VITREOUS CYSTS

Vitreous cysts may arise in otherwise normal eyes, in diseased eyes, or in association with remnants of the hyaloid system.[320-325] Those occurring in normal or diseased eyes are typically round or lobulated, partly pigmented or nonpigmented, translucent structures lying free in the vitreous cavity (Fig. 12-32, *A* and *B*). The cyst wall in most cases is probably composed of retinal pigment epithelial cells.[323] Cysts associated with the hyaloid system are usually sessile, nonpigmented, gray cysts attached to the surface of the optic disc (Fig. 12-32, *C*). Most free-floating cysts probably remain unchanged for many years, cause no symptoms, and require no treatment.[325] They occasionally interfere with visual function, and in such cases aspiration of the cyst or disruption with laser may provide symptomatic relief.[320,324]

▼ ASTEROID HYALOSIS

Asteroid hyalosis is a degenerative disease of the vitreous of unknown cause.[326-333] It is characterized by the development of white or yellow-white spherical or disk-shaped bodies composed of calcium soap within the collagen framework of the vitreous (Fig. 12-32, *D* and *F*). They develop initially in the vicinity of the retinal blood vessels and may eventually be present in such large numbers throughout the vitreous that visualization of the ocular fundus is not possible. In spite of this, however, the patient's visual function is only minimally affected. Fluorescein angiography may provide an excellent view of the fundus when it is obscured ophthalmoscopically (Fig. 12-32, *D* and *E*).[328] Histopathologically, the asteroid bodies have a crystalline appearance and they stain positively with fat and acid mucopolysaccharides that are unaffected by pretreatment with hyaluronidase.[331]

FIG. 12-32 Vitreous Cysts.

A, Irregular, translucent, pigmented, free-floating vitreous cyst.

B, Free-floating pigmented cyst located just inferior to the macula.

C, Nonpigmented cyst attached to the optic nerve head.

Asteroid Hyalosis.

D and **E,** Asteroid bodies were sufficiently concentrated that a view of the fundus details was difficult in this patient, who was complaining of visual loss in the left eye (**D**). Angiography (**E**), however, provided a clear view of evidence of age-related macular degeneration and subfoveal neovascularization.

F, Gross eye specimen showing asteroid bodies suspended in the vitreous framework.

G, Histopathology of asteroid hyalosis showing spherical and ovoid PAS-positive amorphous bodies suspended in the vitreous framework.

Ultrastructurally they are composed primarily of multilaminar membranes typical of complex lipids, particularly phospholipids, and are associated with calcium phosphate complexes lying in a homogeneous background matrix.[332,333]

Asteroid hyalosis typically develops in later life and most often affects only one eye. Its association with diabetes mellitus is a subject of debate.[326,329] Vitrectomy is rarely needed to restore vision but may be necessary in the occasional patient who has unexplained visual loss.[328,331]

▼ METASTATIC CARCINOMA AND MELANOMA TO THE VITREOUS

See Chapter 11.

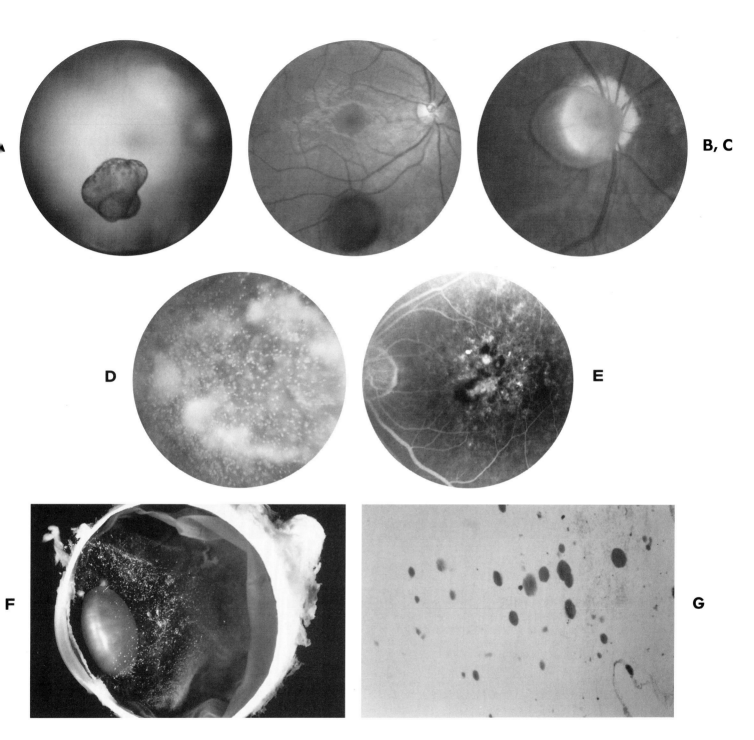

A

B, C

D

E

F

G

REFERENCES
Anatomic Considerations and Vitreous Traction Maculopathies

1. Aaberg TM: Macular holes; a review. *Surv Ophthalmol* 15: 139-162, 1970.

2. Aaberg TM, Blair CJ, Gass JDM: Macular holes. *Am J Ophthalmol* 69:555-562, 1970.

3. Acosta F, Lashkari K, Reynaud X, et al: Characterization of functional changes in macular holes and cysts. *Ophthalmology* 98:1820-1823, 1991.

4. Akiba J, Quiroz MA, Trempe CL: Role of posterior vitreous detachment in idiopathic macular holes. *Ophthalmology* 97:1610-1613, 1990.

5. Akiba J, Yoshida A, Trempe CL: Risk of developing a macular hole. *Arch Ophthalmol* 108:1088-1090, 1990.

6. Avila MP, Jalkh AE, Murakami K, et al: Biomicroscopic study of the vitreous in macular breaks. *Ophthalmology* 90:1277-1283, 1983.

7. Avins LR, Krummenacher TR: Macular holes after pneumatic retinopexy. *Arch Ophthalmol* 106:724-725, 1988.

8. Bartsch D-U, Intaglietta M, Bille JF, et al: Confocal laser tomographic analysis of the retina in eyes with macular hole formation and other focal macular diseases. *Am J Ophthalmol* 108:277-287, 1989.

9. Benedict WL, Shami M: Impending macular hole associated with topical pilocarpine. *Am J Ophthalmol* 114:765-766, 1992.

10. Benson WE, Tasman W: Rhegmatogenous retinal detachments caused by paravascular vitreoretinal traction. *Arch Ophthalmol* 102:669-670, 1984.

11. Bidwell AE, Jampol LM: Macular holes and excellent visual acuity. *Arch Ophthalmol* 106:1350-1351, 1988.

12. Birch DG, Jost BF, Fish GE: The focal electroretinogram in fellow eyes of patients with idiopathic macular holes. *Arch Ophthalmol* 106:1558-1563, 1988.

13. Blacharski PA, Newsome DA: Bilateral macular holes after Nd:YAG laser posterior capsulotomy. *Am J Ophthalmol* 105:417-418, 1988.

14. Blodi CF, Folk JC: Treatment of macular hole retinal detachments with intravitreal gas. *Am J Ophthalmol* 98:811, 1984.

15. Boniuk M: Cystic macular edema secondary to vitreoretinal traction. *Surv Ophthalmol* 13:118-121, 1968.

16. Bonnet M: Hyperfluorescence papillaire par tardif du vitré. *J Fr Ophtalmol* 14:529-536, 1991.

17. Bronstein MA, Trempe CL, Freeman HM: Fellow eyes of eyes with macular holes. *Am J Ophthalmol* 92:757-761, 1981.

18. Cairns JD, MacCombe MF: Microholes of the fovea centralis. *Aust NZ J Ophthalmol* 16:75-79, 1988.

18a. Callanan DG, Blodi BA, Lubinski WP, et al: S (blue) cone perimetry in macular holes before and after vitrectomy. ARVO Abstract 1415. Invest Ophthalmol Vis Sci, 34:990, 1993.

19. Campochiaro PA, Van Niel E, Vinores SA: Immunocytochemical labeling of cells in cortical vitreous from patients with premacular hole lesions. *Arch Ophthalmol* 110:371-377, 1992.

20. Chambers RB, Davidorf FH, Gresak P, Stief WC IV: Modified vitrectomy for impending macular holes. *Ophthalmic Surg* 22:730-734, 1991.

21. Charles S: Retinal pigment epithelial abnormalities after macular hole surgery. *Retina* 13:176, 1993.

22. Cibis GW, Watzke RC, Chua J: Retinal hemorrhages in posterior vitreous detachment. *Am J Ophthalmol* 80:1043-1046, 1975.

23. Cohen SM, Gass JDM: Macular hole following severe hypertensive retinopathy. *Arch Ophthalmol* 112:878-879, 1994.

24. de Bustros S: Editorial: Early stages of macular holes; to treat or not to treat. *Arch Ophthalmol* 108:1085, 1990.

25. de Bustros S, The Vitrectomy for Prevention of Macular Hole Study Group: Vitrectomy for prevention of macular holes; results of a randomized multicenter clinical trial. *Ophthalmology* 101:1055-1059, 1994.

26. de Bustros S, Welch RB: The avulsed retinal vessel syndrome and its variants. *Ophthalmology* 91:86-88, 1984.

27. Dugel PU, Smiddy WE, Byrne SF, et al: Macular hole syndromes; echographic findings with clinical correlation. *Ophthalmology* 101:815-821, 1994.

28. Duker JS: Retinal pigment epitheliopathy after macular hole surgery. *Ophthalmology* 100:1604-1605, 1993.

29. Duker JS, Wendel R, Patel AC, Puliafito CA: Late re-opening of macular holes after initially successful treatment with vitreous surgery. *Ophthalmology* 101:1373-1378, 1994.

30. Eisner G: *Biomicroscopy of the peripheral fundus: an atlas and textbook,* Berlin, New York, 1973, Springer, p. 45.

31. Fine SL: Editorial: Vitreous surgery for macular hole in perspective. Is there an indication? *Arch Ophthalmol* 109:635-636, 1991.

32. Fish RH, Anand R, Izbrand DJ: Macular pseudoholes; clinical features and accuracy of diagnosis. *Ophthalmology* 99:1665-1670, 1992.

33. Fisher YL, Slakter JS, Friedman RA, Yannuzzi LA: Kinetic ultrasound evaluation of the posterior vitreoretinal interface. *Ophthalmology* 98:1135-1138, 1991.

34. Fisher YL, Slakter JS, Yannuzzi LA, Guyer DR: A prospective natural history study and kinetic ultrasound evaluation of idiopathic macular holes. *Ophthalmology* 101:5-11, 1994.

35. Flynn HW Jr: Macular hole surgery in patients with proliferative diabetic retinopathy. *Arch Ophthalmol* 112:877-878, 1994.

36. Folk JC, Ma C, Blodi CF, Han DP: Occlusion of bridging or avulsed retinal vessels by repeated photocoagulation. *Ophthalmology* 94:1610-1613, 1987.

37. Foos RY: Subhyaloid hemorrhage illustrating a mechanism of macular hole formation. *Arch Ophthalmol* 110:598, 1992.

38. Foos RY: Vitreoretinal juncture; topographical variations. *Invest Ophthalmol* 11:801-808, 1972.

39. Foos RY, Wheeler NC: Vitreoretinal juncture: synchysis senilis and posterior vitreous detachment. *Ophthalmology* 89:1502-1512, 1982.

40. Frangieh GT, Green WR, Engel HM: A histopathologic study of macular cysts and holes. *Retina* 1:311-336, 1981.

41. Freeman WR: Editorial: Vitrectomy surgery for full-thickness macular holes. *Am J Ophthalmol* 116:233-235, 1993.

42. Funata M, Wendel RT, de la Cruz Z, Green WR: Clinicopathologic study of bilateral macular holes treated with pars plana vitrectomy and gas tamponade. *Retina* 12:289-298, 1992.

43. Garlikov RS, Chenoweth RG: Macular hole following topical pilocarpine. *Ann Ophthalmol* 7:1313-1316, 1975.

44. Gass JDM: Discussion of Glaser BM, Michels RG, Kuppermann BD, et al: Transforming growth factor-β_2 for the treatment of full-thickness macular holes; a prospective randomized study. *Ophthalmology* 99:1173, 1992.

45. Gass JDM: Idiopathic senile macular hole; its early stages and pathogenesis. *Arch Ophthalmol* 106:629-639, 1988.

46. Gass JDM: Lamellar macular hole: a complication of cystoid macular edema after cataract extraction: clinicopathologic case report. *Trans Am Ophthalmol Soc* 73:231-250, 1975; also *Arch Ophthalmol* 94:793-800, 1976.

47. Gass JDM: Reappraisal of biomicroscopic classification of stages of development of a macular hole. *Am J Ophthalmol* 119:752-759, 1995.

48. Gass JDM: Risk of developing macular hole. *Arch Ophthalmol* 109:610-611, 1991.

49. Gass JDM: *Stereoscopic atlas of macular diseases; diagnosis and treatment,* ed. 2, St. Louis, 1977, CV Mosby, p. 334.

50. Gass JDM, Joondeph BC: Observations concerning patients with suspected impending macular holes. *Am J Ophthalmol* 109:638-646, 1990.

51. Gass JDM, Van Newkirk M: Xanthic scotoma and yellow foveolar shadow caused by a pseudo-operculum after vitreo-foveal separation. *Retina* 12:242-244, 1992.

52. Glaser BM, Michels RG, Kuppermann BD, et al: Transforming growth factor-β$_2$ for the treatment of full-thickness macular holes; a prospective randomized study. *Ophthalmology* 99:1162-1172, 1992.

53. Gonvers M, Machemer R: A new approach to treating retinal detachment with macular hole. *Am J Ophthalmol* 94:468-472, 1982.

54. Gordon LW, Glaser BM, Darmakusuma I, et al: Full-thickness macular hole formation in eyes with a pre-existing complete posterior vitreous detachment. *Ophthalmology* 102:1702-1705, 1995.

55. Guyer DR, de Bustros S, Diener-West M, Fine SL: Observations on patients with idiopathic macular holes and cysts. *Arch Ophthalmol* 110:1264-1268, 1992.

56. Guyer DR, Green WR, de Bustros S, Fine SL: Histopathologic features of idiopathic macular holes and cysts. *Ophthalmology* 97:1045-1051, 1990.

57. Hee MR, Puliafito CA, Wong C, et al: Optical coherence tomography of macular holes. *Ophthalmology* 102:748-756, 1995.

58. Hikichi T, Trempe CL: Relationship between floaters, light flashes, or both, and complications of posterior vitreous detachment. *Am J Ophthalmol* 117:593-598, 1994.

59. Hikichi T, Trempe CL: Resolution of an absolute scotoma after spontaneous disappearance of idiopathic full-thickness macular hole. *Am J Ophthalmol* 118:121-122, 1994.

60. Hikichi T, Trempe CL: Risk of decreased visual acuity in full-thickness idiopathic macular holes. *Am J Ophthalmol* 116:708-712, 1993.

61. Hogan MJ, Alvarado JA, Weddell JE: *Histology of the human eye; an atlas and textbook,* Philadelphia, 1971, WB Saunders, pp. 491-492.

62. Ie D, Glaser BM, Thompson JT, et al: Retreatment of full-thickness macular holes persisting after prior vitrectomy; a pilot study. *Ophthalmology* 100:1787-1793, 1993.

63. Jaffe NS: Complications of acute posterior vitreous detachment. *Arch Ophthalmol* 79:568-571, 1968.

64. Jaffe NS: Vitreous traction at the posterior pole of the fundus due to alterations in the vitreous posterior. *Trans Am Acad Ophthalmol Otolaryngol* 71:642-651, 1967.

65. Jagger JD, Hamilton AMP, Polkinghorne P: Q-switched neodymium YAG laser vitreolysis in the therapy of posterior segment disease. *Graefes Arch Clin Exp Ophthalmol* 228:222-225, 1990.

66. James M, Feman SS: Macular holes. *Albrecht von Graefes Arch Klin Exp Ophthalmol* 215:59-63, 1980.

67. Johnson RN, Gass JDM: Idiopathic macular holes; observations, stages of formation, and implications for surgical intervention. *Ophthalmology* 95:917-924, 1988.

68. Jost BF, Hutton WL, Fuller DG, et al: Vitrectomy in eyes at risk for macular hole formation. *Ophthalmology* 97:843-847, 1990.

69. Kanski JJ: Complications of acute posterior vitreous detachment. *Am J Ophthalmol* 80:44-46, 1975.

70. Kelly NE, Wendel RT: Vitreous surgery for idiopathic macular holes; results of a pilot study. *Arch Ophthalmol* 109:654-659, 1991.

71. Kiryu J, Shahidi M, Ogura Y, et al: Illustration of the stages of idiopathic macular holes by laser biomicroscopy. *Arch Ophthalmol* 113(9):1156-1160, 1995.

72. Kishi S, Demaria C, Shimizu K: Vitreous cortex remnants at the fovea after spontaneous vitreous detachment. *Int Ophthalmol* 9:253-260, 1986.

73. Kishi S, Shimizu K: Posterior precortical vitreous pocket. *Arch Ophthalmol* 108:979-982, 1990.

74. Kishi S, Shimizu K: Reply to letter by JGF Worst. *Arch Ophthalmol* 109:1060, 1991.

75. Kishi S, Yokozuka K, Kamei Y: The state of the vitreous in idiopathic macular holes. *Acta Soc Ophthalmol Jpn* 95:678-685, 1991.

76. Kishi S, Yokozuka K, Tobe K: Bursa premacularis. *Acta Soc Ophthalmol Jpn* 92:1881-1888, 1988.

77. Klöti R: Erfahrungen mit der Silberklemme bei Makulaloch-bedingten Netzhautablösungen. *Ophthalmologica* 161:210-216, 1970.

78. Kornzweig AL, Feldstein M: Studies of the eye in old age. II. Hole in the macula: a clinico-pathologic study. *Am J Ophthalmol* 33:243-247, 1950.

79. Kruis JA, Bastiaensen LAK, Hoefnagels KLJ: Senile idiopathic macular holes. *Doc Ophthalmol* 55:81-89, 1983.

80. Lansing MB, Glaser BM, Liss H, et al: The effect of pars plana vitrectomy and transforming growth factor-beta 2 without epiretinal membrane peeling on full-thickness macular holes. *Ophthalmology* 100:868-872, 1993.

81. Laqua H: Die Behandlung der Ablatio mit Maculaforamen nach der Methode von Gonvers und Machemer. *Klin Monatsbl Augenheilkd* 186:13-17, 1985.

82. Larsson L, Österlin S: Posterior vitreous detachment; a combined clinical and physicochemical study. *Graefes Arch Clin Exp Ophthalmol* 223:92-95, 1985.

83. Lee S, Ai E, Lowe M, Wang T: Bilateral macular holes in sporadic posterior microphthalmos. *Retina* 10:185-188, 1990.

84. Lewis H, Cowan GM, Straatsma BR: Apparent disappearance of a macular hole associated with development of an epiretinal membrane. *Am J Ophthalmol* 102:172-175, 1986.

85. Lewis ML, Cohen S, Smiddy WE, Gass JDM: Bilaterality of idiopathic macular holes. *Graefes Arch Clin Exp Ophthalmol* 234:241-245, 1996.

86. Liggett PE, Alfaro DV, Horio B, et al: Autologous serum as a tissue adhesive in the treatment of idiopathic macular holes. *Ophthalmology* 100(Suppl):73, 1993.

87. Linder B: Acute posterior vitreous detachment and its retinal complications; a clinical biomicroscopic study. *Acta Ophthalmol Suppl* 87, 1966.

88. Machemer R, Williams JM Sr: Pathogenesis and therapy of traction detachment in various retinal vascular diseases. *Am J Ophthalmol* 105:170-181, 1988.

89. Madreperla SA, Geiger GL, Funata M, et al: Clinicopathologic correlation of a macular hole treated by cortical vitreous peeling and gas tamponade. *Ophthalmology* 101:682-686, 1994.

90. Makabe R: Kryptonlaserkoagulation bei idiopathischem Makulaloch. *Klin Monatsbl Augenheilkd* 196:202-204, 1990.

91. Margherio RR, Schepens CL: Macular breaks. I. Diagnosis, etiology, and observations. *Am J Ophthalmol* 74:219-232, 1972.

92. Margherio RR, Trese MT, Margherio AR, Cartright K: Surgical management of vitreomacular traction syndromes. *Ophthalmology* 96:1437-1445, 1989.

93. Martinez J, Smiddy WE, Kim J, Gass JDM: Differentiating macular holes from macular pseudoholes. *Am J Ophthalmol* 117:762-767, 1994.

94. McDonald HR, Johnson RN, Schatz H: Surgical results in the vitreomacular traction syndrome. *Ophthalmology* 101:1397-1403, 1994.

95. McDonnell PJ, Fine SL, Hillis AI: Clinical features of idiopathic macular cysts and holes. *Am J Ophthalmol* 93:777-786, 1982.

96. Mehta M, Katsumi O, Tetsuka S, et al: Best's macular dystrophy with a macular hole. *Acta Ophthalmol* 69:131-134, 1991.

97. Mein CE, Flynn HW Jr: Recognition and removal of the posterior cortical vitreous during vitreoretinal surgery for impending macular hole. *Am J Ophthalmol* 111:611-613, 1991.

97a. Melberg NS, Thomas MA: Visual field loss after pars plana vitrectomy with air/fluid exchange. Am J Ophthalmol 120:386-388, 1995.

98. Miyake Y: A simplified method of treating retinal detachment with macular hole. *Am J Ophthalmol* 97:243-245, 1984.

99. Morgan CM, Schatz H: Idiopathic macular holes. *Am J Ophthalmol* 99:437-444, 1985.

100. Morgan CM, Schatz H: Involutional macular thinning; a pre-macular hole condition. *Ophthalmology* 93:153-161, 1986.

101. Muñoz FJ, Rebolleda G, Cores FJ, Bertrand J: Congenital retinal arteriovenous communication associated with a full-thickness macular hole. *Acta Ophthalmol* 69:117-120, 1991.

102. Murakami K: Biomicroscopic observation of macular breaks. *Hokkaido Igaku Zasshi* 60:335-341, 1985.

103. Noble KG, Chang S: Adult vitelliform macular degeneration progressing to full-thickness macular hole. *Arch Ophthalmol* 109:325, 1991.

104. Nork TM, Gioia VM, Hobson RR, Kessel RH: Subhyaloid hemorrhage illustrating a mechanism of macular hole formation. *Arch Ophthalmol* 109:884-885, 1991.

105. Novak MA, Welch RB: Complications of acute symptomatic posterior vitreous detachment. *Am J Ophthalmol* 97:308-314, 1984.

106. Ogura Y, Shahidi M, Mori MT, et al: Improved visualization of macular hole lesions with laser biomicroscopy. *Arch Ophthalmol* 109:957-961, 1991.

107. Poliner LS, Tornambe PE: Retinal pigment epitheliopathy after macular hole surgery. *Ophthalmology* 99:1671-1677, 1992.

108. Reese AB, Jones IS, Cooper WC: Macular changes secondary to vitreous traction. *Am J Ophthalmol* 64:544-549, 1967.

109. Reese AB, Jones IS, Cooper WC: Vitreomacular traction syndrome confirmed histologically. *Am J Ophthalmol* 69:975-977, 1970.

110. Robertson DM, Curtin VT, Norton EWD: Avulsed retinal vessels with retinal breaks; a cause of recurrent vitreous hemorrhage. *Arch Ophthalmol* 85:669-672, 1971.

111. Ruby AJ, Williams DF, Grand MG, et al: Pars plana vitrectomy for treatment of stage 2 macular holes. *Arch Ophthalmol* 112:359-364, 1994.

112. Schachat AP, de la Cruz Z, Green WR, Patz A: Macular hole and retinal detachment in Best's disease. *Retina* 5:22-25, 1985.

113. Schachat AP, Sommer A: Macular hemorrhages associated with posterior vitreous detachment. *Am J Ophthalmol* 102:647-649, 1986.

114. Schocket SS, Lakhanpal V, Xiaoping M, et al: Laser treatment of macular holes. *Ophthalmology* 95:574-582, 1988.

115. Schulenburg WE, Cooling RJ, McLeod D: Management of retinal detachments associated with macular breaks. *Trans Ophthalmol Soc UK* 103:360-364, 1983.

116. Sebag J: Age-related changes in human vitreous structure. *Graefes Arch Clin Exp Ophthalmol* 225:89-93, 1987.

117. Sebag J: Age-related differences in the human vitreoretinal interface. *Arch Ophthalmol* 109:966-971, 1991.

118. Sebag J: Tissue analysis from two patients with premacular hole lesions. *Arch Ophthalmol* 111:22, 1993.

119. Siam A-L: Macular hole with central retinal detachment in high myopia with posterior staphyloma. *Br J Ophthalmol* 53:62-63, 1969.

120. Sjaarda RN, Frank DA, Glaser BM, et al: Assessment of vision in idiopathic macular holes with macular microperimetry using the scanning laser ophthalmoscope. *Ophthalmology* 100:1513-1518, 1993.

121. Sjaarda RN, Frank DA, Glaser BM, et al: Resolution of an absolute scotoma and improvement of relative scotoma after successful macular hole surgery. *Am J Ophthalmol* 116:129-139, 1993.

122. Smiddy WE: Atypical presentations of macular holes. *Arch Ophthalmol* 111:626-631, 1993.

123. Smiddy WE, Gass JDM: Masquerades of macular holes. *Ophthalmic Surg* 26:16-24, 1995.

124. Smiddy WE, Glaser BM, Green WR, et al: Transforming growth factor beta; a biologic chorioretinal glue. *Arch Ophthalmol* 107:577-580, 1989.

125. Smiddy WE, Glaser BM, Thompson JT, et al: Transforming growth factor-β2 significantly enhances the ability to flatten the rim of subretinal fluid surrounding macular holes; preliminary anatomic results of a multicenter prospective randomized study. *Retina* 13:296-301, 1993.

126. Smiddy WE, Green WR, Michels RG, de la Cruz Z: Ultrastructural studies of vitreomacular traction syndrome. *Am J Ophthalmol* 107:177-185, 1989.

127. Smiddy WE, Michels RG, de Bustros S, et al: Histopathology of tissue removed during vitrectomy for impending idiopathic macular holes. *Am J Ophthalmol* 108:360-364, 1989.

128. Smiddy WE, Michels RG, Glaser BM, de Bustros S: Vitrectomy for impending idiopathic macular holes. *Am J Ophthalmol* 105:371-376, 1988.

129. Smiddy WE, Michels RG, Glaser BM, de Bustros S: Vitrectomy for macular traction caused by incomplete vitreous separation. *Arch Ophthalmol* 106:624-628, 1988.

130. Smiddy WE, Michels RG, Green WR: Morphology, pathology, and surgery of idiopathic vitreoretinal macular disorders; a review. *Retina* 10:288-296, 1990.

131. Smith RG, Hardman Lea SJ, Galloway NR: Visual performance in idiopathic macular holes. *Eye* 4:190-194, 1990.

132. Tabotabo MM, Karp LA, Benson WE: Posterior vitreous detachment. *Ann Ophthalmol* 12:59-61, 1980.

133. Tasman WS: Posterior vitreous detachment and peripheral retinal breaks. *Trans Am Acad Ophthalmol Otolaryngol* 72:217-224, 1968.

134. Thompson JT, Hiner CJ, Glaser BM, et al: Fluorescein angiographic characteristics of macular holes before and after vitrectomy with transforming growth factor beta-2. *Am J Ophthalmol* 117:291-301, 1994.

135. Trempe CL, Weiter JJ, Furukawa H: Fellow eyes in cases of macular hole; biomicroscopic study of the vitreous. *Arch Ophthalmol* 104:93-95, 1986.

136. Van Newkirk MR, Gass JDM, Callanan D, et al: Follow-up and ultrasonographic examination of patients with macular pseudo-operculum. *Am J Ophthalmol* 117:13-18, 1994.

137. Vine AK: Avulsed retinal veins without retinal breaks. *Am J Ophthalmol* 98:723-727, 1984.

138. Wendel RT, Patel AC, Kelly NE, et al: Vitreous surgery for macular holes. *Ophthalmology* 100:1671-1676, 1993.

139. Wiznia RA: Reversibility of the early stages of idiopathic macular holes. *Am J Ophthalmol* 107:241-245, 1989.

140. Worst J: Extracapsular surgery in lens implantation (Binkhorst lecture). Part IV: Some anatomical and patho-physiological implications. *Am Intra-Ocular Implant Soc J* 4:7-14, 1978.

141. Worst JGF: Cisternal systems of the fully developed vitreous body in the young adult. *Trans Ophthalmol Soc UK* 97:550-554, 1977.

142. Worst JGF: Posterior precortical vitreous pocket. (Letter) *Arch Ophthalmol* 109:1058-1059, 1991.

143. Yaoeda H: Clinical observation on macular hole. *Acta Soc Ophthalmol Jpn* 71:1723-1736, 1967.

144. Yonemoto J, Ideta H, Sasaki K, et al: The age of onset of posterior vitreous detachment. *Graefes Arch Clin Exp Ophthalmol* 232:67-70, 1994.

145. Yoshioka H: Clinical studies on macular hole. III. On the pathogenesis of the senile macular hole. *Acta Soc Ophthalmol Jpn* 72:575-584, 1968.

146. Yuzawa M, Watanabe A, Takahashi Y, Matsui M: Observation of idiopathic full-thickness macular holes; follow-up observation. *Arch Ophthalmol* 112:1051-1056, 1994.

Macular Dysfunction Caused by Epiretinal Membrane Contraction

147. Akiba J, Yoshida A, Trempe CL: Prognostic factors in idiopathic preretinal macular fibrosis. *Graefes Arch Clin Exp Ophthalmol* 229:101-104, 1991.

148. Algvere P, Kock E: Experimental epiretinal membranes induced by intravitreal carbon particles. *Am J Ophthalmol* 96:345-353, 1983.

149. Allen AW Jr, Gass JDM: Contraction of a perifoveal epiretinal membrane simulating a macular hole. *Am J Ophthalmol* 82:684-691, 1976.

150. Appiah AP, Hirose T: Secondary causes of premacular fibrosis. *Ophthalmology* 96:389-392, 1989.

151. Barr CC, Michels RG: Idiopathic nonvascularized epiretinal membranes in young patients: report of six cases. *Ann Ophthalmol* 14:335-341, 1982.

152. Bellhorn MB, Friedman AH, Wise GN, Henkind P: Ultrastructure and clinicopathologic correlation of idiopathic preretinal macular fibrosis. *Am J Ophthalmol* 79:366-373, 1975.

153. Bishara SA, Buzney SM: Dispersion of retinal pigment epithelial cells from experimental retinal holes. *Graefes Arch Clin Exp Ophthalmol* 229:195-199, 1991.

154. Bonnet M, Fleury J: Pseudo-trou maculaire tardif après pelage chirurgical d'une membrane prémaculaire. *J Fr Ophtalmol* 15:123-130, 1992.

155. Byer NE: Spontaneous disappearance of early postoperative preretinal retraction; a sequel of retinal detachment surgery. *Arch Ophthalmol* 90:133-135, 1973.

156. Cherfan GM, Michels RG, de Bustros S, et al: Nuclear sclerotic cataract after vitrectomy for idiopathic epiretinal membranes causing macular pucker. *Am J Ophthalmol* 111:434-438, 1991.

157. Cherfan GM, Smiddy WE, Michels RG, et al: Clinicopathologic correlation of pigmented epiretinal membranes. *Am J Ophthalmol* 106:536-545, 1988.

158. Clarkson JG, Green WR, Massof D: A histopathologic review of 168 cases of preretinal membrane. *Am J Ophthalmol* 84:1-17, 1977.

159. Cleary PE, Leaver PK: Macular abnormalities in the reattached retina. *Br J Ophthalmol* 62:595-603, 1978.

160. Curtin VT: Pathologic changes following retinal detachment surgery. *In: Symposium on retina and retinal surgery: transactions of the New Orleans Academy of Ophthalmology,* St. Louis, 1969, CV Mosby, pp. 147-170.

161. de Bustros S, Rice TA, Michels RG, et al: Vitrectomy for macular pucker; use after treatment of retinal tears or retinal detachment. *Arch Ophthalmol* 106:758-760, 1988.

162. de Bustros S, Thompson JT, Michels RG, et al: Nuclear sclerosis after vitrectomy for idiopathic epiretinal membranes. *Am J Ophthalmol* 105:160-164, 1988.

163. de Bustros S, Thompson JT, Michels RG, et al: Vitrectomy for idiopathic epiretinal membranes causing macular pucker. *Br J Ophthalmol* 72:692-695, 1988.

164. Gass JDM: A fluorescein angiographic study of macular dysfunction secondary to retinal vascular disease. III. Hypertensive retinopathy. *Arch Ophthalmol* 80:569-582, 1968.

165. Gass JDM: Fluorescein angiography: an aid to the retinal surgeon. *In:* Pruett RC, Regan CDJ: *Retina Congress; 25th Anniversary meeting of the Retina Service, Massachusetts Eye and Ear Infirmary,* New York, 1972, Appleton-Century-Crofts, pp. 181-201.

166. Gass JDM: Lamellar macular hole: a complication of cystoid macular edema after cataract extraction: clinicopathologic case report. *Trans Am Ophthalmol Soc* 73:231-250, 1975; also *Arch Ophthalmol* 94:793-800, 1976.

167. Gass JDM: Photocoagulation of macular lesions. *Trans Am Acad Ophthalmol Otolaryngol* 75:580-582, 1971.

168. Gass JDM: *Stereoscopic atlas of macular diseases; a funduscopic and angiographic presentation,* St. Louis, 1970, CV Mosby, p. 215.

169. Gass JDM: *Stereoscopic atlas of macular diseases; diagnosis and treatment,* ed. 2, St. Louis, 1977, CV Mosby, p. 344.

170. Glaser BM, Cardin A, Biscoe B: Proliferative vitreoretinopathy; the mechanism of development of vitreoretinal traction. *Ophthalmology* 94:327-332, 1987.

171. Gloor BP: Cellular proliferation on the vitreous surface after photocoagulation. *Albrecht von Graefes Arch Klin Exp Ophthalmol* 178:99-113, 1969.

172. Gloor BP: On the question of the origin of macrophages in the retina and the vitreous following photocoagulation (autoradiographic investigations by means of ^{3}H-thymidine). *Albrecht von Graefes Arch Klin Exp Ophthalmol* 190:183, 1974.

173. Green WR, Kenyon KR, Michels RG, et al: Ultrastructure of epiretinal membranes causing macular pucker after retinal re-attachment surgery. *Trans Ophthalmol Soc UK* 99:63-77, 1979.

174. Greven CM, Slusher MM, Weaver RG: Epiretinal membrane release and posterior vitreous detachment. *Ophthalmology* 95:902-905, 1988.

175. Hagler WS, Aturaliya U: Macular puckers after retinal detachment surgery. *Br J Ophthalmol* 55:451-457, 1971.

176. Hamilton CW, Chandler D, Klintworth GK, Machemer R: A transmission and scanning electron microscopic study of surgically excised preretinal membrane proliferations in diabetes mellitus. *Am J Ophthalmol* 94:473-488, 1982.

177. Hirokawa H, Jalkh AE, Takahashi M, et al: Role of the vitreous in idiopathic preretinal macular fibrosis. *Am J Ophthalmol* 101:166-169, 1986.

178. Hiscott PS, Grierson I, McLeod D: Retinal pigment epithelial cells in epiretinal membranes; an immunohistochemical study. *Br J Ophthalmol* 68:708-715, 1984.

179. Hiscott PS, Grierson I, Trombetta CJ, et al: Retinal and epiretinal glia—an immunohistochemical study. *Br J Ophthalmol* 68:698-707, 1984.

180. Hui Y-N, Goodnight R, Zhang X-J, et al: Glial epiretinal membranes and contraction; immunohistochemical and morphological studies. *Arch Ophthalmol* 106:1280-1285, 1988.
181. Jaffe NS: Macular retinopathy after separation of vitreoretinal adherence. *Arch Ophthalmol* 78:585-591, 1967.
182. Jiang DY, Hiscott PS, Grierson I, McLeod D: Growth and contractility of cells from fibrocellular epiretinal membranes in primary tissue culture. *Br J Ophthalmol* 72:116-126, 1988.
183. Kampik A, Green WR, Michels RG, Nase PK: Ultrastructural features of progressive idiopathic epiretinal membrane removed by vitreous surgery. *Am J Ophthalmol* 90:797-809, 1980.
184. Kampik A, Kenyon KR, Michels RG, et al: Epiretinal and vitreous membranes; comparative study of 56 cases. *Arch Ophthalmol* 99:1445-1454, 1981.
185. Kenyon KR, Michels RG: Ultrastructure of epiretinal membrane removed by pars plana vitreoretinal surgery. *Am J Ophthalmol* 83:815-823, 1977.
186. Kimmel AS, Weingeist TA, Blodi CF, Wells KK: Idiopathic premacular gliosis in children and adolescents. *Am J Ophthalmol* 108:578-581, 1989.
187. Kishi S, Shimizu K: Oval defect in detached posterior hyaloid membrane in idiopathic preretinal macular fibrosis. *Am J Ophthalmol* 118:451-456, 1994.
188. Laqua H: Pigmented macular pucker. *Am J Ophthalmol* 86:56-58, 1978.
189. Laqua H, Machemer R: Clinical-pathological correlation in massive periretinal proliferation. *Am J Ophthalmol* 80:913-929, 1975.
190. Laqua H, Machemer R: Glial cell proliferation in retinal detachment (massive periretinal proliferation). *Am J Ophthalmol* 80:602-618, 1975.
191. Lean JS: Origin of simple glial epiretinal membranes in an animal model. *Graefes Arch Clin Exp Ophthalmol* 225:421-425, 1987.
192. Lobes LA Jr, Burton TC: The incidence of macular pucker after retinal detachment surgery. *Am J Ophthalmol* 85:72-77, 1978.
193. Machemer R: Pathogenesis and classification of massive periretinal proliferation. *Br J Ophthalmol* 62:737-747, 1978.
194. Machemer R, Aaberg TM, Freeman HM, et al: An updated classification of retinal detachment with proliferative vitreoretinopathy. *Am J Ophthalmol* 112:159-165, 1991.
195. Machemer R, Laqua H: Pigment epithelium proliferation in retinal detachment (massive periretinal proliferation). *Am J Ophthalmol* 80:1-23, 1975.
196. Machemer R, van Horn D, Aaberg TM: Pigment epithelial proliferation in human retinal detachment with massive periretinal proliferation. *Am J Ophthalmol* 85:181-191, 1978.
197. Maguire AM, Smiddy WE, Nanda SK, et al: Clinicopathologic correlation of recurrent epiretinal membranes after previous surgical removal. *Retina* 10:213-222, 1990.
198. Mandelcorn MS, Lipton N: Epi-macular holes: a cause of decreased vision in the elderly. *Can J Ophthalmol* 12:182-187, 1977.
199. Margherio RR, Cox MS Jr, Trese MT, et al: Removal of epimacular membranes. *Ophthalmology* 92:1075-1083, 1985.
200. Maumenee AE: Further advances in the study of the macula. *Arch Ophthalmol* 78:151-165, 1967.
201. McDonald HR, Verre WP, Aaberg TM: Surgical management of idiopathic epiretinal membranes. *Ophthalmology* 93:978-983, 1986.
202. Messner KH: Spontaneous separation of preretinal macular fibrosis. *Am J Ophthalmol* 83:9-11, 1977.
203. Michels RG: Vitrectomy for macular pucker. *Ophthalmology* 91:1384-1388, 1984.
204. Michels RG: Vitreous surgery for macular pucker. *Am J Ophthalmol* 92:628-639, 1981.
205. Michels RG, Gilbert HD: Surgical management of macular pucker after retinal reattachment surgery. *Am J Ophthalmol* 88:925-929, 1979.
206. Miller B, Miller H, Ryan SJ: Experimental epiretinal proliferation induced by intravitreal red blood cells. *Am J Ophthalmol* 102:188-195, 1986.
207. Mittleman D, Green WR, Michels RG, de la Cruz Z: Clinicopathologic correlation of an eye after surgical removal of an epiretinal membrane. *Retina* 9:143-147, 1989.
208. Morino I, Hiscott P, McKechnie N, Grierson I: Variation in epiretinal membrane components with clinical duration of the proliferative tissue. *Br J Ophthalmol* 74:393-399, 1990.
209. Mulligan TG, Daily MJ: Spontaneous peeling of an idiopathic epiretinal membrane in a young patient. *Arch Ophthalmol* 110:1367-1368, 1992.
210. Newsome DA, Rodrigues MM, Machemer R: Human massive periretinal proliferation; in vitro characteristics of cellular components. *Arch Ophthalmol* 99:873-880, 1981.
211. Pesin SR, Olk RJ, Grand MG, et al: Vitrectomy for premacular fibroplasia; prognostic factors, long-term follow-up, and time course of visual improvement. *Ophthalmology* 98:1109-1114, 1991.
212. Poliner LS, Olk RJ, Grand MG, et al: Surgical management of premacular fibroplasia. *Arch Ophthalmol* 106:761-764, 1988.
213. Radke ND, Tano Y, Chandler D, Machemer R: Simulation of massive periretinal proliferation by autotransplantation of retinal pigment epithelial cells in rabbits. *Am J Ophthalmol* 91:76-87, 1981.
214. Rentsch FJ: Preretinal proliferation of glial cells after mechanical injury of the rabbit retina. *Albrecht von Graefes Arch Klin Exp Ophthalmol* 188:79-90, 1973.
215. Rentsch FJ: The ultrastructure of preretinal macular fibrosis. *Albrecht von Graefes Arch Clin Exp Ophthalmol* 203:321-337, 1977.
216. Rice TA, de Bustros S, Michels RG, et al: Prognostic factors in vitrectomy for epiretinal membranes of the macula. *Ophthalmology* 93:602-610, 1986.
217. Robertson DM, Buettner H: Pigmented preretinal membranes. *Am J Ophthalmol* 83:824-829, 1977.
218. Roth AM, Foos RY: Surface structure of the optic nerve head. 1. Epipapillary membranes. *Am J Ophthalmol* 74:977-985, 1972.
219. Roth AM, Foos RY: Surface wrinkling retinopathy in eyes enucleated at autopsy. *Trans Am Acad Ophthalmol Otolaryngol* 75:1047-1058, 1971.
220. Sabates NR, Sabates FN, Sabates R, et al: Macular changes after retinal detachment surgery. *Am J Ophthalmol* 108:22-29, 1989.
221. Schwartz PL, Trubowitsch G, Fastenberg DM, Stein M: Macular pucker and retinal angioma. *Ophthalmic Surg* 18:677-679, 1987.
222. Scudder MJ, Eifrig DE: Spontaneous surface wrinkling retinopathy. *Ann Ophthalmol* 7:333-341, 1975.
223. Shea M: The surgical management of macular pucker in rhegmatogenous retinal detachment. *Ophthalmology* 87:70-74, 1980.
224. Sidd RJ, Fine SL, Owens SL, Patz A: Idiopathic preretinal gliosis. *Am J Ophthalmol* 94:44-48, 1982.
225. Singh AK, Glaser BM, Lemor M, Michels RG: Gravity-dependent distribution of retinal pigment epithelial cells dispersed into the vitreous cavity. *Retina* 6:77-80, 1986.

226. Sivalingam A, Eagle RC Jr, Duker JS, et al: Visual prognosis correlated with the presence of internal-limiting membrane in histopathologic specimens obtained from epiretinal membrane surgery. *Ophthalmology* 97:1549-1552, 1990.

227. Smiddy WE, Maguire AM, Green WR, et al: Idiopathic epiretinal membranes; ultrastructural characteristics and clinicopathologic correlation. *Ophthalmology* 96:811-821, 1989.

228. Smiddy WE, Michels RG, Gilbert HD, Green WR: Clinicopathologic study of idiopathic macular pucker in children and young adults. *Retina* 12:232-236, 1992.

229. Sramek SJ, Wallow IH, Stevens TS, Nork TM: Immunostaining of preretinal membranes for actin, fibronectin, and glial fibrillary acidic protein. *Ophthalmology* 96:835-841, 1989.

230. Stallman JB, Meyers SM: Spontaneous disappearance of white retinal changes after dissection of epiretinal macular membranes. *Retina* 8:165-168, 1988.

231. Stern WH, Fisher SK, Anderson DH, et al: Epiretinal membrane formation after vitrectomy. *Am J Ophthalmol* 93:757-772, 1982.

232. Sumers KD, Jampol LM, Goldberg MF, Huamonte FU: Spontaneous separation of epiretinal membranes. *Arch Ophthalmol* 98:318-320, 1980.

233. Tanenbaum HL, Schepens CL, Elzeneiny I, Freeman HM: Macular pucker following retinal detachment surgery. *Arch Ophthalmol* 83:286-293, 1970.

234. Tetsumoto K, Nakahashi K, Tsukahara Y, et al: Two cases of idiopathic preretinal macular fibrosis in children. *Acta Soc Ophthalmol Jpn* 94:875-881, 1990.

235. Thomas EL, Michels RG, Rice TA, et al: Idiopathic progressive unilateral vitreous fibrosis and secondary traction retinal detachment. *Retina* 2:134-144, 1982.

236. Uemura A, Ideta H, Nagasaki H, et al: Macular pucker after retinal detachment surgery. *Ophthalmic Surg* 23:116-119, 1992.

237. Wallow IHL, Greaser ML, Stevens TS: Actin filaments in diabetic fibrovascular preretinal membrane. *Arch Ophthalmol* 99:2175-2181, 1981.

238. Wallow IHL, Miller SA: Preretinal membrane by retinal pigment epithelium. *Arch Ophthalmol* 96:1643-1646, 1978.

239. Wallow IHL, Stevens TS, Greaser ML, et al: Actin filaments in contracting preretinal membranes. *Arch Ophthalmol* 102:1370-1375, 1984.

240. Wise GN: Clinical features of idiopathic preretinal macular fibrosis. *Am J Ophthalmol* 79:349-357, 1975.

241. Wise GN: Congenital preretinal macular fibrosis. *Am J Ophthalmol* 79:363-365, 1975.

242. Wiznia RA: Posterior vitreous detachment and idiopathic preretinal macular gliosis. *Am J Ophthalmol* 102:196-198, 1986.

243. Zarbin MA, Michels RG, Green WR: Epiretinal membrane contracture associated with macular prolapse. *Am J Ophthalmol* 110:610-618, 1990.

Retinal Changes Associated with Rhegmatogenous Retinal Detachment

244. Aaberg TM, Machemer R: Correlation of naturally occurring detachments with long-term retinal detachment in the owl monkey. *Am J Ophthalmol* 69:640-650, 1970.

245. Abraham RK, Shea M: Significance of pigment dispersion following cryoretinopexy: scotomata and atrophy. *Mod Probl Ophthalmol* 8:455-461, 1969 (*Biblio Ophthalmol* No. 79).

246. Avins LR, Hilton GF: Lesions simulating serous detachment of the pigment epithelium; occurrence after retinal detachment surgery. *Arch Ophthalmol* 98:1427-1429, 1980.

247. Bonnet M: Peripheral neovascularization complicating rhegmatogenous retinal detachments of long duration. *Graefes Arch Clin Exp Ophthalmol* 225:59-62, 1987.

248. Bonnet M, Semiglia R: Evolution spontanée du décollement de la rétine du pôle postérieur du myope fort. *J Fr Ophtalmol* 14:618-623, 1991.

249. Brown GC: Macular hole following rhegmatogenous retinal detachment repair. *Arch Ophthalmol* 106:765-766, 1988.

250. Chisholm IA, McClure E, Foulds WS: Functional recovery of the retina after retinal detachment. *Trans Ophthalmol Soc UK* 95:167-172, 1975.

251. Cleary PE, Leaver PK: Macular abnormalities in the reattached retina. *Br J Ophthalmol* 62:595-603, 1978.

252. Davidorf FH, Havener WH, Lang JR: Macular vision following retinal detachment surgery. *Ophthalmic Surg* 6(4):74-81, 1975.

253. Davies EWG, Gundry MF: Failure of visual recovery following retinal surgery. *Mod Probl Ophthalmol* 12:58-63, 1974.

254. Enoch JM, Van Loo JA Jr, Okun E: Realignment of photoreceptors disturbed in orientation secondary to retinal detachment. *Invest Ophthalmol* 12:849-853, 1973.

255. Felder KS, Brockhurst RJ: Retinal neovascularization complicating rhegmatogenous retinal detachment of long duration. *Am J Ophthalmol* 93:773-776, 1982.

256. Friberg TR, Eller AW: Prediction of visual recovery after scleral buckling of macula-off retinal detachments. *Am J Ophthalmol* 114:715-722, 1992.

257. Gass JDM: Fluorescein angiography: an aid to the retinal surgeon. *In:* Pruett RC, Regan CDJ, editors: *Retina Congress; 25th Anniversary meeting of the Retina Service, Massachusetts Eye and Ear Infirmary,* New York, 1972, Appleton-Century-Crofts, pp. 181-201.

258. Gass JDM: *Stereoscopic atlas of macular diseases; diagnosis and treatment,* ed. 3, St. Louis, 1987, CV Mosby, pp. 716-717.

259. Goldbaum MH, Weidenthal DT, Krug S, Rosen R: Subretinal neovascularization as a complication of drainage of subretinal fluid. *Retina* 3:114-117, 1983.

260. Gottlieb F, Fammartino JJ, Stratford TP, Brockhurst RJ: Retinal angiomatosis mass; a complication of retinal detachment surgery. *Retina* 4:152-157, 1984.

261. Greco GM, Bonavolonta G: Treatment of retinal detachments due to macular holes. *Retina* 7:177-179, 1987.

262. Grupposo SS: Visual acuity following surgery for retinal detachment. *Arch Ophthalmol* 93:327-330, 1975.

263. Gundry MF, Davies EWG: Recovery of visual acuity after retinal detachment surgery. *Am J Ophthalmol* 77:310-314, 1974.

264. Hilton GF: Subretinal pigment migration; effects of cryosurgical retinal reattachment. *Arch Ophthalmol* 91:445-450, 1974.

265. Isernhagen RD, Wilkinson CP: Visual acuity after the repair of pseudophakic retinal detachments involving the macula. *Retina* 9:15-21, 1989.

266. Jarrett WH, Brockhurst RJ: Unexplained blindness and optic atrophy following retinal detachment surgery. *Arch Ophthalmol* 73:782-791, 1965.

267. Lobes LA Jr, Grand MG: Subretinal lesions following scleral buckling procedure. *Arch Ophthalmol* 98:680-683, 1980.

268. Lopez PF, Aaberg TM, Lambert HM, et al: Choroidal neovascularization occurring within a demarcation line. *Am J Ophthalmol* 114:101-102, 1992.

269. Machemer R: Experimental retinal detachment in the owl monkey. II. Histology of retina and pigment epithelium. *Am J Ophthalmol* 66:396-410, 1968.

270. Machemer R: Surgical approaches to subretinal strands. *Am J Ophthalmol* 90:81-85, 1980.

271. Matsumura M, Yamakawa R, Yoshimura N, et al: Subretinal strands; tissue culture and histological study. *Graefes Arch Clin Exp Ophthalmol* 225:341-345, 1987.

272. McPherson AR, O'Malley RE, Butner RW, Beltangady SS: Visual acuity after surgery for retinal detachment with macular involvement. *Ann Ophthalmol* 14:639-645, 1982.

273. Morita H, Ideta H, Ito K: Causative factors of retinal detachment in macular holes. *Retina* 11:281-284, 1991.

274. Pavan PR: Retinal fold in macula following intraocular gas; an avoidable complication of retinal detachment surgery. *Arch Ophthalmol* 102:83-84, 1984.

275. Rashed O, Sheta S: Evaluation of the functional results after different techniques for treatment of retinal detachments due to macular holes. *Graefes Arch Clin Exp Ophthalmol* 227:508-512, 1989.

276. Riordan-Eva P, Chignell AH: Full thickness macular breaks in rhegmatogenous retinal detachment with peripheral retinal breaks. *Br J Ophthalmol* 76:346-348, 1992.

277. Shea M: Complications of cryotherapy in retinal detachment surgery. *Can J Ophthalmol* 3:109-115, 1968.

278. Sternberg P Jr, Machemer R: Subretinal proliferation. *Am J Ophthalmol* 98:456-462, 1984.

279. Stirpe M, Michels RG: Retinal detachment in highly myopic eyes due to macular holes and epiretinal traction. *Retina* 10:113-114, 1990.

280. Sudarsky RD, Yannuzzi LA: Cryomarcation line and pigment migration after retinal cryosurgery. *Arch Ophthalmol* 83:395-401, 1970.

281. Tani P, Robertson DM, Langworthy A: Prognosis for central vision and anatomic reattachment in rhegmatogenous retinal detachment with macula detached. *Am J Ophthalmol* 92:611-620, 1981.

282. Theodossiadis GP, Kokolakis SN: Macular pigment deposits in rhegmatogenous retinal detachment. *Br J Ophthalmol* 63:498-506, 1979.

283. van Meurs JC, Humalda D, Mertens DAE, Peperkamp E: Retinal folds through the macula. *Doc Ophthalmol* 78:335-340, 1991.

284. Wallyn RH, Hilton GF: Subretinal fibrosis in retinal detachment. *Arch Ophthalmol* 97:2128-2129, 1979.

285. Wilkes SR, Mansour AM, Green WR: Proliferative vitreoretinopathy; histopathology of retroretinal membranes. *Retina* 7:94-101, 1987.

286. Wilkinson CP: Visual results following scleral buckling for retinal detachments sparing the macula. *Retina* 1:113-116, 1981.

287. Woldoff HS, Dooley WJ Jr: Multifocal choroiditis after retinal detachment surgery. *Ann Ophthalmol* 11:1182-1184, 1979.

Degenerative Retinoschisis

288. Ambler JS, Gass JDM, Gutman FA: Symptomatic retinoschisis-detachment involving the macula. *Am J Ophthalmol* 112:8-14, 1991.

289. Ambler JS, Meyers SM, Zegarra H, Gutman FA: The management of retinal detachment complicating degenerative retinoschisis. *Am J Ophthalmol* 107:171-176, 1989.

290. Byer NE: Clinical study of senile retinoschisis. *Arch Ophthalmol* 79:36-44, 1968.

291. Byer NE: Long-term natural history study of senile retinoschisis with implications for management. *Ophthalmology* 93:1127-1136, 1986.

292. Byer NE: The natural history of senile retinoschisis. *Mod Probl Ophthalmol* 18:304-311, 1977.

293. DiSclafani M, Wagner A, Humphery W, Valone J Hr: Pigmentary changes in acquired retinoschisis. *Am J Ophthalmol* 105:291-293, 1988.

294. Gass JDM: Fluorescein angiography: an aid to the retinal surgeon. *In:* Pruett RC, Regan CDJ, editors: *Retina Congress; 25th Anniversary meeting of the Retina Service, Massachusetts Eye and Ear Infirmary,* New York, 1972, Appleton-Century-Crofts, pp. 181-201.

295. Göttinger W: *Senile retinoschisis; morphological relationship of the formation of the spaces within the peripheral retina to senile retinoschisis and schisis detachment,* Stuttgart, 1978, Georg Thieme.

296. Hauch TL, Straatsma BR, Andersen E, Shahinian J: Macular function in typical and reticular retinoschisis. *Retina* 1:293-295, 1981.

297. Sneed SR, Blodi CF, Folk JC, et al: Pars plana vitrectomy in the management of retinal detachments associated with degenerative retinoschisis. *Ophthalmology* 97:470-474, 1990.

298. Straatsma BR, Foos RY: Typical and reticular degenerative retinoschisis. *Am J Ophthalmol* 75:551-575, 1973.

299. Sulonen JM, Wells CG, Barricks ME, et al: Degenerative retinoschisis with giant outer layer breaks and retinal detachment. *Am J Ophthalmol* 99:114-121, 1985.

Amyloidosis

300. Ando E, Ando Y, Maruoka S, et al: Ocular microangiopathy in familial amyloidotic polyneuropathy, type I. *Graefes Arch Clin Exp Ophthalmol* 230:1-5, 1992.

301. Andrade C: A peculiar form of peripheral neuropathy; familial atypical generalized amyloidosis with special involvement of the peripheral nerves. *Brain* 75:408-427, 1952.

302. Bene C, Kranias G: Ocular amyloidosis: Clinical points learned from one case. *Ann Ophthalmol* 22:101-102, 1990.

303. Biswas J, Badrinath SS, Rao NA: Primary nonfamilial amyloidosis of the vitreous; a light microscopic and ultrastructural study. *Retina* 12:251-253, 1992.

304. Crawford JB: Cotton wool exudates in systemic amyloidosis. *Arch Ophthalmol* 78:214-216, 1967.

305. Ferry AP, Lieberman TW: Bilateral amyloidosis of the vitreous body; report of a case without systemic or familial involvement. *Arch Ophthalmol* 94:982-991, 1976.

306. Goren H, Steinberg MC, Farboody GH: Familial oculoleptomeningeal amyloidosis. *Brain* 103:473-495, 1980.

307. Hamburg A: Unusual cause of vitreous opacities; primary familial amyloidosis. *Ophthalmologica* 162:173-177, 1971.

308. Irvine AR, Char DH: Recurrent amyloid involvement in the vitreous body after vitrectomy. *Am J Ophthalmol* 82:705-708, 1976.

309. Kasner D, Miller GR, Taylor WH, et al: Surgical treatment of amyloidosis of the vitreous. *Trans Am Acad Ophthalmol Otolaryngol* 72:410-418, 1968.

310. Monteiro JG, Martins AFF, Figueira A, et al: Ocular changes in familial amyloidotic polyneuropathy with dense vitreous opacities. *Eye* 5:99-105, 1991.

311. Okayama M, Goto I, Ogata J, et al: Primary amyloidosis with familial vitreous opacities; an unusual case and family. *Arch Intern Med* 138:105-111, 1978.

312. Rukavina JG, Block WD, Jackson CE, et al: Primary systemic amyloidosis: a review and an experimental, genetic, and clinical study of 29 cases with particular emphasis on the familial form. *Medicine* 35:239-334, 1956.

313. Sandgren O, Holmgren G, Lundgren E: Vitreous amyloidosis associated with homozygosity for the transthyretin methionine-30 gene. *Arch Ophthalmol* 108:1584-1586, 1990.

314. Sandgren O, Holmgren G, Lundgren E, Steen L: Restriction fragment length polymorphism analysis of mutated transthyretin in vitreous amyloidosis. *Arch Ophthalmol* 106:790-792, 1988.

315. Schwartz MF, Green WR, Michels RG, et al: An unusual case of ocular involvement in primary systemic nonfamilial amyloidosis. *Ophthalmology* 89:394-401, 1982.

316. Skinner M, Harding J, Skare I, et al: A new transthyretin mutation associated with amyloidotic vitreous opacities; asparagine for isoleucine at position 84. *Ophthalmology* 99:503-508, 1992.

317. Ts'o MOM, Bettman JW Jr: Occlusion of choriocapillaris in primary nonfamilial amyloidosis. *Arch Ophthalmol* 86:281-286, 1971.

318. Uitti RJ, Donat JR, Rozdilsky B, et al: Familial oculoleptomeningeal amyloidosis; report of a new family with unusual features. *Arch Neurol* 45:1118-1122, 1988.

319. Wong VG, McFarlin DE: Primary familial amyloidosis. *Arch Ophthalmol* 78:208-213, 1967.

Vitreous Cysts

320. Awan KJ: Biomicroscopy and argon laser photocystotomy of free-floating vitreous cysts. *Ophthalmology* 92:1710-1711, 1985.

321. Flynn WJ, Carlson DW: Pigmented vitreous cyst. *Arch Ophthalmol* 112:1113, 1994.

322. Lusky M, Weinberger D, Kremer I: Vitreous cyst combined with bilateral juvenile retinoschisis. *J Pediatr Ophthalmol Strabismus* 25:75-76, 1988.

323. Orellana J, O'Malley RE, McPherson AR, Font RL: Pigmented free-floating vitreous cysts in two young adults; electron microscopic observations. *Ophthalmology* 92:297-302, 1985.

324. Ruby AJ, Jampol LM: Nd:YAG treatment of a posterior vitreous cyst. *Am J Ophthalmol* 110:428-429, 1990.

325. Steinmetz RL, Straatsma BR, Rubin ML: Posterior vitreous cyst. *Am J Ophthalmol* 109:295-297, 1990.

Asteroid Hyalosis

326. Bergren RL, Brown GC, Duker JS: Prevalence and association of asteroid hyalosis with systemic disease. *Am J Ophthalmol* 111:289-293, 1991.

327. Feist RM, Morris RE, Witherspoon CD, et al: Vitrectomy in asteroid hyalosis. *Retina* 10:173-177, 1990.

328. Hampton GR, Nelsen PT, Hay PB: Viewing through the asteroids. *Ophthalmology* 88:669-672, 1981.

329. Luxenberg M, Sime D: Relationship of asteroid hyalosis to diabetes mellitus and plasma lipid levels. *Am J Ophthalmol* 67:406-413, 1969.

330. Renaldo DP: Pars plana vitrectomy for asteroid hyalosis. *Retina* 1:252-254, 1981.

331. Rodman HI, Johnson FB, Zimmerman LE: New histopathological and histochemical observations concerning asteroid hyalitis. *Arch Ophthalmol* 66:552-563, 1961.

332. Streeten BW: Vitreous asteroid bodies; ultrastructural characteristics and composition. *Arch Ophthalmol* 100:969-975, 1982.

333. Topilow HW, Kenyon KR, Takahashi M, et al: Asteroid hyalosis; biomicroscopy, ultrastructure, and composition. *Arch Ophthalmol* 100:964-968, 1982.

13

Optic Nerve Diseases that May Masquerade as Macular Diseases

Diseases that primarily affect the optic nerve may occasionally involve secondarily the macular area or may be mistaken for retinal diseases. Some of the most frequent of these diseases are discussed in this chapter.

▼ OPTIC DISC ANOMALIES ASSOCIATED WITH SEROUS DETACHMENT OF THE MACULA

Serous detachment of the sensory retina may occur in association with one or a combination of developmental anomalies of the optic nerve head. This spectrum of anomalies includes pit, coloboma, morning glory deformity, and juxtapapillary staphyloma.

Congenital pit of the optic disc and serous detachment of the macula

Usually between the ages of 20 and 40 years, patients with congenital pit of the optic nerve head may develop serous detachment of the macula (Figs. 13-1 to 13-3).* The detachment usually extends in a teardrop fashion from the disc margin in the vicinity of the optic pit, which in most cases is located along the temporal margin of the optic disc. Pits and detachment are uncommon at the nasal margin of the optic disc (Fig. 13-2, *A* to *D*). The optic disc diameter in the affected eye is usually larger than in the nonaffected eye.[10,23] An optic pit may occur bilaterally in 10% to 15% of cases and may be inherited as an autosomal dominant abnormality.[10,24,57,62] Pits may be associated with a coloboma of the optic nerve head, and details of the pit may be difficult or impossible to identify (Fig. 13-2, *K* and *L*). Some patients with severe colobomatous malformation of the optic disc may develop extensive retinal detachment (see discussion below). Optic pits located in the center of the optic disc are not associated with macular detachment. The optic pit is often covered with a gray membrane that frequently has one or more holes within it, particularly in patients with macular detachments. Most authors agree that there typically is no posterior vitreous detachment in eyes with a pit and serous detachment of the macula.[8,10,24,25] Occasionally, condensed vitreous strands may extend from the surface of the optic pit into the anterior vitreous. In some patients a cloudy precipitate may occur on the posterior surface of the detached retina (Fig. 13-1, *A* and *G*). When this

*References 1, 3, 5, 8, 10-12, 16, 18, 19, 22, 23, 25, 27, 32, 34, 36, 38, 42, 45, 46, 50, 54, 56, 58, 64.

FIG. 13-1   Congenital Pit of the Optic Disc Causing Serous Macular Detachment.

A to F, This 27-year-old woman complained of blurred vision that fluctuated in the right eye for several weeks. Serous detachment of the retina extended to the margin of the optic disc pit (*arrow,* **A** and **B**). Note subretinitic precipitates forming concentric lines of demarcation temporally. The diameter of the optic disc was about twice that of the normal eye. Arteriovenous-phase angiograms showed the relative absence of capillary filling in the area of the pit (*arrow,* **C**). One hour after dye injection, note absence of dye in the subretinal fluid and staining in the area of the pit (**D**). Xenon photocoagulation was placed along the temporal edge of the optic disc as well as in the optic pit (**E**). Seven months later the detachment had not resolved. Six and one-half years later the patient returned with approximately 20/200 vision in the right eye. There was no longer any serous detachment of the macula (**F**).

G to I, Long-standing, large, serous retinal detachment associated with an optic pit. There was yellow exudate on the posterior surface of the detached retina centrally. Note in the early angiogram hypofluorescence of the pit (*arrow,* **H**), the small zone of marked hyperfluorescence adjacent to the pit, and the larger area of slight hyperfluorescence in the area of the detachment. This hyperfluorescence becomes less intense later (**I**) and was caused by depigmentation of the RPE secondary to the long-standing detachment.

J to L, This 29-year-old woman who was known to have an optic pit and normal visual function in the right eye since 10 years of age presented with a 4-month history of blurred vision in the right eye. Visual acuity was 20/50. There was a moundlike elevation of the inner retinal surface (*arrowheads*) that extended from the optic pit throughout the macular area. There was a smaller sharply circumscribed zone of what appeared to be detachment of the retinal receptors from the pigment epithelium (*arrows,* **J**) that did not extend to the optic pit. The patient could see a 50-μm krypton red laser aiming beam throughout the area of inner retinal elevation, including the central area of retinal detachment, both before and even after placement of two rows of krypton red photocoagulations along the temporal edge of the optic pit. Seven months later the elevation of the inner retinal surface and retinal detachment were no longer present. There was a pattern of radiating lines resembling foveomacular schisis centrally (**K**). Twenty-six months after treatment her visual acuity was 20/20 and the macula appeared normal (**L**).

(**A to E** from Gass.[23])

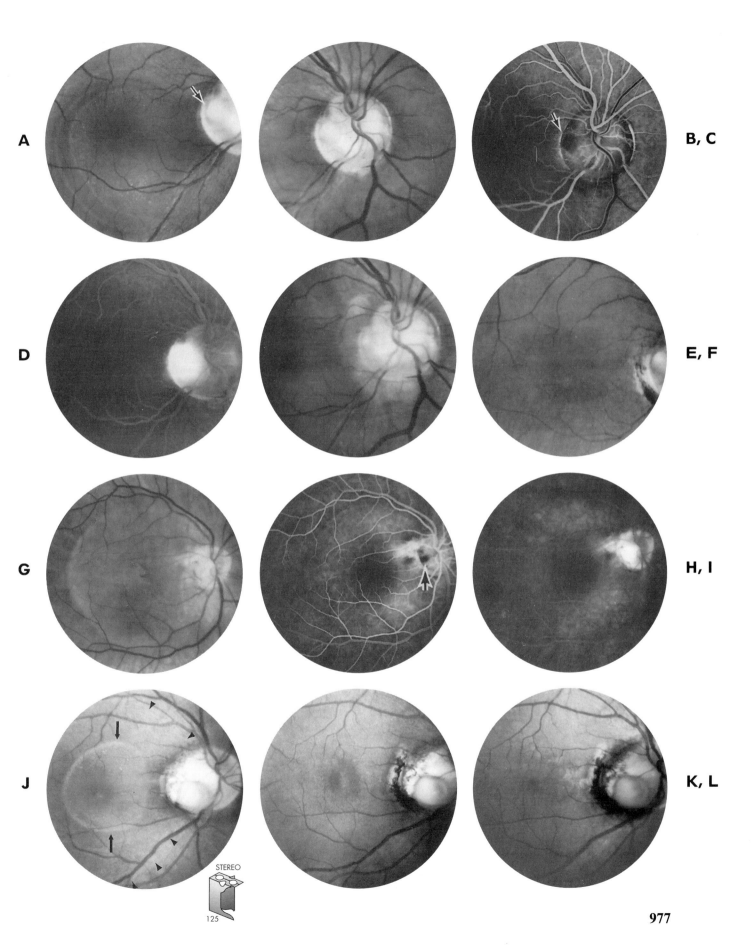

A

B, C

D

E, F

G

H, I

J

STEREO

125

K, L

977

occurs, the area of detachment may be misdiagnosed as a solid tumor (Fig. 13-3, *E*).[19,23] Some patients develop a central area of sharply defined retinal detachment with a surrounding larger, less well-defined area of elevation of the inner retinal surface, suggesting the presence of retinoschisis (Fig. 13-1, *J* to *L*).[45,46] Unlike retinoschisis, however, there is not complete loss of retinal function in the area of pseudoschisis in patients with an optic pit. There has been no satisfactory anatomic explanation for this peculiar configuration of retinal elevation seen biomicroscopically in these patients. With prolonged retinal detachment, depigmentation of the retinal pigment epithelium (RPE) occurs in the area of the detachment (Figs. 13-1, *G* to *I*, and 13-3, *A* to *D*). Cystic retinal degeneration, marked thinning of the foveolar portion of the retina, and rarely full-thickness macular hole formation and rhegmatogenous retinal detachment may occur (Fig. 13-2, *E* and *F*).[5,64,72] Subretinal neovascularization may arise near the optic pit.[10,36]

In patients with a recent onset of macular detachment, angiography shows no abnormalities in the macular area (Fig. 13-1, *C* and *D*).[8,23] In early-phase angiograms the pit appears hypofluorescent (Fig. 13-1, *C* and *H*). In later phases, in most patients, there is evidence of staining in the area of the pit with no evidence of perfusion of dye into the subretinal fluid (Fig. 13-1, *D* and *I*). Absence of staining of the pit has been associated with absence of retinal detachment, recent macular detachment, and no cilioretinal arteries emanating from the pit.[8,71] Staining of the subretinal fluid occasionally occurs.[10] Patients with loss of pigment caused by prolonged retinal detachment show hyperfluorescence corresponding with the areas of depigmentation during the early phases of angiography (Figs. 13-1, *H;* 13-2, *F, I,* and *J;* and 13-3, *B* and *C*).[23] This is often seen in the papillomacular bundle region adjacent to the optic disc in patients with no previous history of macular detachment. Angiography shows no evidence of either choroidal or retinal capillary permeability alterations. The failure to demonstrate angiographically either retinal or choroidal permeability alterations in the presence of a serous macular detachment should always alert the clinician to the possibility of an optic pit or a more peripheral lesion to account for the detachment.

FIG. 13-2 Congenital Pit and Juxtapapillary Coloboma of the Optic Disc.

A to D, A congenital pit in the nasal part of the nerve head caused a serous retinal detachment *(arrows)* nasally (**A**) that subsequently spread to the macular area (**B** and **C**) in this boy. A midphase angiogram showed marked hyperfluorescence within the pit *(arrows,* **D**).

E and **F,** Serous detachment of the macula and macular hole secondary to a congenital pit *(arrow,* **E**) of the optic nerve in a 39-year-old woman with a 2-month history of blurred vision in the right eye. Visual acuity in the right eye was 20/200. Fluorescein angiography showed evidence of depigmentation of the RPE *(arrows,* **F**) in the area of the serous detachment. Note the mottled-background hyperfluorescence apparent in the area of the macular hole. This angiogram suggests the probability that the serous detachment of the right macula had been present much longer than 2 months.

G to I, This 15-year-old boy with a large optic disc pit developed a peculiar vitelliform deposit in the subretinal space over a 6-month period (**G** and **H**). He had a positive scotoma, but his visual acuity was 20/20 on both occasions. There was early mottled hyperfluorescence centrally and the late staining of the pit (**I**).

J, Coloboma with "double disc" deformity in a 5-year-old, otherwise normal child.

K and **L,** Morning glory deformity of the right optic nerve and extensive retinal detachment in the right eye (**K**) that developed in a 21-year-old woman noted to have the optic disc deformity since age 6 years. Her visual acuity was finger counting only in the right eye. The retina was reattached following a vitrectomy (**L**). There was no retinal hole, and the source of the subretinal fluid presumably was via a pitlike deformity hidden within the disc anomaly.

Presently there is limited information concerning the natural course of eyes with an optic pit before or after development of serous macular detachment.[10,22,64,67] It is probable that only a small percentage of eyes with a pit ever develop serous retinal detachment. Spontaneous reattachment of the macula occurs in 25% or more of patients with optic pits.[8,11,22,67] With a prolonged delay in reattachment, cystic degeneration and partial- or full-thickness hole formation may occur.[5,64] Long-term followup of untreated eyes suggests that in approximately 50% to 75% of eyes the visual acuity will be reduced to 20/100 or worse within 5 to 9 years.[10,64]

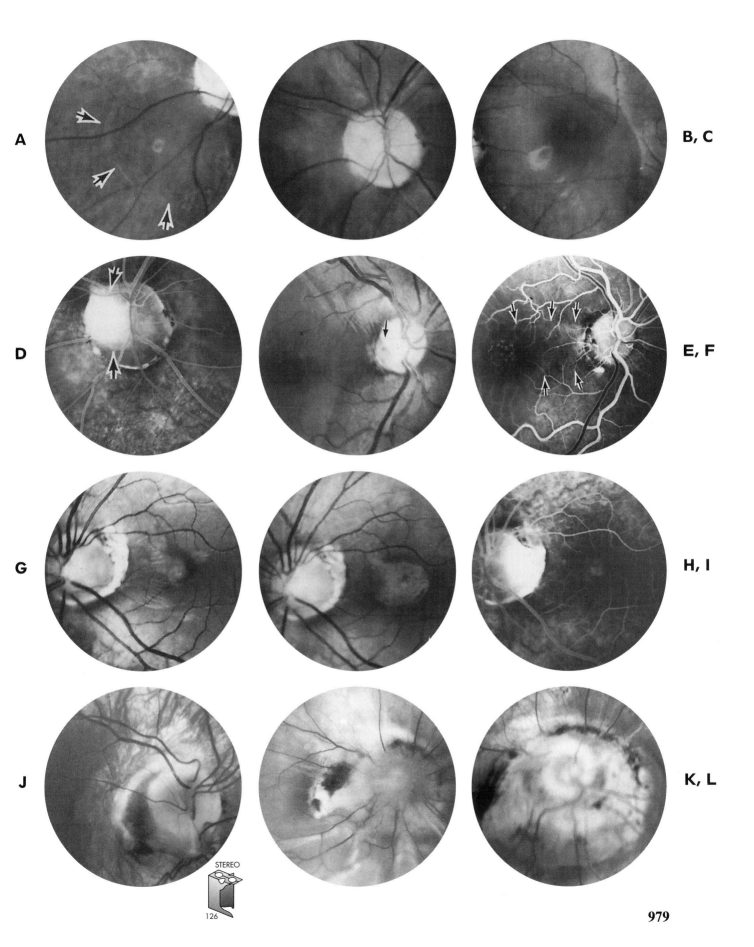

Histopathologically, an optic pit consists of herniation of dysplastic retina into a collagen-lined pocket extending posteriorly through a defect in the lamina cribrosa into the subarachnoid space (Fig. 13-3, *E* and *F*).

The pathogenesis of the detachment appears to involve the passage of fluid from the area of the pit into the subretinal space. The failure of intravascular fluorescein to diffuse into the subretinal fluid in all but a few cases suggests that it is derived from either the cerebrospinal fluid[23,54] or the vitreous (Fig. 13-3, *G*).[10,11] Chang and associates[14] reported metrizamide cisternographic evidence of communication of the subretinal and subarachnoid spaces in a child with a colobomatous malformation of the optic nerve and extensive retinal detachment. Other studies involving radioisotope cisternography[57] and intrathecal fluorescein,[38] as well as attempts to displace subretinal fluid into the subarachnoid space by elevating the intraocular pressure,[23] have failed to demonstrate evidence of direct communication between the subarachnoid space and subretinal space. One patient with an optic pit experienced two episodes of increased intracranial pressure caused by pseudotumor cerebri without developing a retinal detachment.[27] Direct communication between the vitreous cavity and subretinal space via the optic pit has been demonstrated in collie dogs (Fig. 13-3, *G*).[11] This communication could not be demonstrated in a human eye with an optic pit.[40]

FIG. 13-3 Congenital Pit of the Optic Disc.

A to **D,** In 1975 this 21-year-old man presented with blurred vision in the right eye caused by serous macular detachment (*arrows,* **A**) associated with an oval pit of the optic disc. His visual acuity was 20/70. Note in the stereoangiogram (**B** and **C**) the focal thinning of the retina and attenuation of the RPE at the temporal margin of the optic disc. The retina reattached spontaneously within several years, and 8 years later his visual acuity was 20/30. There are radiating pericentral retinal folds simulating X-linked schisis (**D**).

E and **F,** Histopathology of serous detachment of the retina in a 29-year-old woman with an optic disc pit. The eye was enucleated because of a misdiagnosis of a choroidal melanoma, presumably caused by some opacification of the subretinal fluid. Note the cystic degeneration of the detached retina (*arrow,* **E**). **F** shows details of the pit, indicating three possible routes (**1** to **3**) by which fluid from the vitreous (*v*) or the subarachnoid space (*ss*) might pass into the subretinal space (*srs*). The neuroectodermal portion of the pit (*n*) is separated from its surrounding fibrous capsule (*f*) by a multiloculated space (*s*).

G, Photomicrograph of optic pit in collie dog. *Arrows* indicate communication of vitreous cavity with subretinal space.

(**E** from Ferry[19]; **F** from Gass[23]; **G** from Brown G.C. et al.: Arch. Ophthalmol. 97:1341, 1979; copyright 1979, American Medical Association.[11])

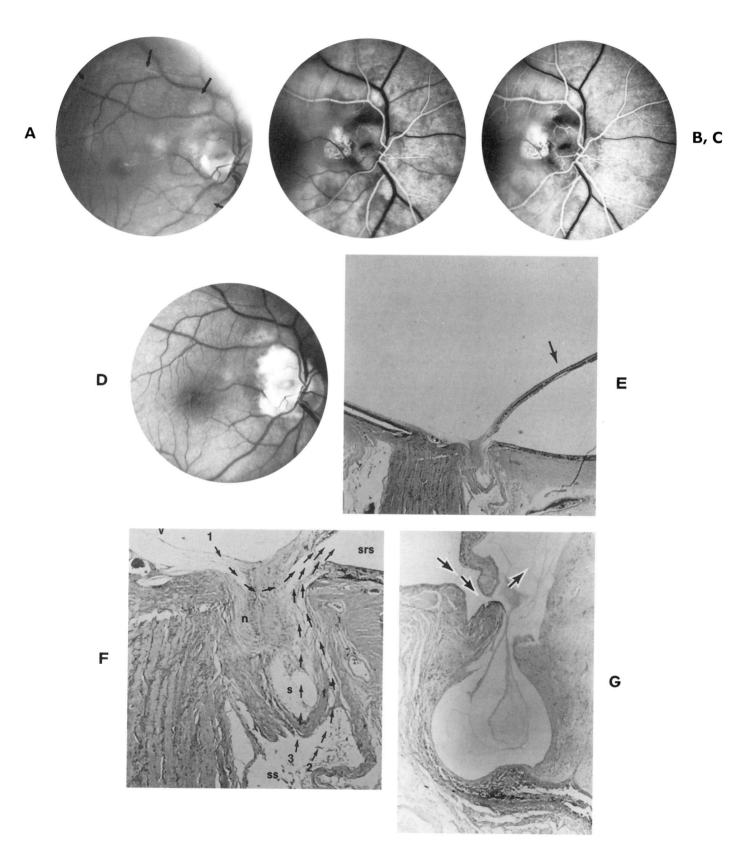

A

B, C

D

E

F

G

981

In general, attempts to close the neck of the detachment at the margin of the optic disc with photocoagulation, as well as photocoagulation of the optic pit itself, have been unsuccessful in causing prompt resolution of the macular detachment (Figs. 13-1, *A* to *F,* and *J* to *L*).[8,9,23,49,67] Several authors have reported resolution that may require several months or longer after photocoagulation.[5,9,34,69,70] Redetachment may occur weeks or months later.[58,77] The absence of posterior vitreous separation in patients with macular detachment suggests that traction of the formed vitreous in these patients on the anterior surface of the retina throughout the macular area may be important in causing the passive movement of either fluid vitreous or of CSF fluid through a defect within or at the margin of the optic pit into the subretinal space. In older patients whose posterior vitreous is extensively liquefied full-thickness holes in the macula and elsewhere in the posterior fundus do not cause retinal detachment in the absence of biomicroscopic evidence of focal vitreous traction. Some authors have reported successful reattachment of the macula using a combination of one or more of the following: pars plana vitrectomy, intravitreal gas tamponade, and photocoagulation.* No technique of treatment has proved uniformly successful in reattaching the retina. Until more information is available concerning the natural course and results of treatment, the author recommends the following: observation for at least a month after the onset detachment; if no improvement in the detachment occurs, photocoagulation across the neck of the detachment; if no response occurs within 6 to 8 weeks, repeat the laser treatment; if no improvement in the detachment occurs, consider intravitreal gas tamponade with or without pars plana vitrectomy. Use of prophylactic treatment either adjacent to the pit or as a coarse scatter pattern of laser in the macula to prevent detachment might be considered in the rare patient with a strong family history of detachment associated with optic nerve pit, and particularly in the second eye if the first eye has permanent loss of acuity from this complication.

*References 3, 16, 24, 58, 63, 77.

Acquired pits of the optic nerve

Pitlike changes in the optic nerve head may be acquired and may be the cause of unexplained loss of paracentral and occasionally central visual field loss. These pits typically develop in the inferotemporal quadrant in older patients with normal intraocular pressure or glaucoma.[35,43,48,53] There is an increased incidence of acquired pits in patients with low-tension glaucoma (74%) versus patients with typical glaucoma (15%).[35] Development of the pit may be preceded by the appearance on one or more occasions of a flame-shaped hemorrhage on the optic disc. The typical field defect in normotensive eyes extends from the blind spot to near fixation in a pistol-shaped configuration and has a steep central margin. Because patients with acquired pits and with low-tension glaucoma have significantly greater amounts of field loss than those with elevated IOP without pits, it is probable that optic nerves predisposed to developing pits are more susceptible to damage from the damaging effects of intraocular pressure. Whereas there are structural differences in the lamina cribrosa in patients with and without low-tension glaucoma,[52] the pathogenesis of the acquired pit of the optic disc is still not clear.[4]

Coloboma, juxtapapillary staphyloma, and morning glory deformity

A coloboma of the optic nerve head involves a defect in its structure occurring as a result of malclosure of the ocular fissure. It may be mild, in which case there is a defect in the optic nerve substance, usually inferiorly. This defect may be more extensive and involve the juxtapapillary choroid and retina. It may be associated with a pit deformity and with a juxtapapillary staphyloma. This latter term refers to an out-pouching of the ocular wall around the optic nerve head. This out-pouching may occur with little or no abnormality in the structure and function of the eye, or with varying degree of dysplasia of the nerve. If the coloboma or staphyloma if filled with glial tissue, the retinal blood vessels may exit from this tissue in a pattern that has suggested to some a morning glory (Fig. 13-2, *K*). These more severe anomalies of the optic disc may be associated with serous macular detachment; with other ocular abnormalities, including microphthalmos, lens coloboma, persistent primary hyperplastic vitreous, orbital cyst,* and occasionally intracranial abnormalities.[30,55] A pit deformity may or may not be present and is often obscured clinically by the other anomalies (Fig. 13-2, *K* and *L*). In some cases these anomalies may be combined to form a mass lesion simulating a capillary angioma, astrocytoma, combined retinal–RPE hamartoma, or melanoma in

the region of the optic disc.[15] Some patients may manifest clinical evidence of communication between the vitreous and retrobulbar ocular cysts via the optic disc anomalies.[21,61] In patients with these severe disc anomalies the retinal detachment begins in the juxtapapillary area, often on the temporal side.* The detachment, unlike that occurring with a pit alone, may extend to involve most of the fundus (Fig. 13-2, *K* to *L*). These detachments, like those associated with a pit, may resolve spontaneously.[7] The pathogenesis of the detachment occurring with all of these anomalies is probably similar in most cases, although this is controversial. In the morning glory deformity and juxtapapillary staphyloma, the detachment has been attributed to retinal breaks in the vicinity of the anomaly,[2,31,73] to communication between the subarachnoid and subretinal space,[14,23,44] to communication between the vitreous and subretinal space,[31] to communication with both the vitreous and subarachnoid space,[33] to vitreoretinal traction,[29] and to exudation from blood vessels within the anomaly,[39] the orbital tissue,[44] and juxtapapillary choriocapillaris.[44] Vitreoretinal traction is probably important in all cases, and successful repair of the detachment has been accomplished by vitrectomy, intravitreal gas, and thermal treatment at the edge of the anomaly.[2,31] Choroidal neovascularization may occur at the edge of any of these anomalies.[10,17,36,65,76]

---

*References 6, 7, 13, 21, 37, 57, 60.

*References 2, 6, 7, 13, 14, 28, 29, 31, 33, 39, 44, 51, 57, 65, 66.

Transient obscuration of vision secondary to peripapillary staphyloma

Peripapillary staphyloma is a rare congenital anomaly in which the normal or nearly normal optic nerve head lies in the depth of an excavation in the fundus (Fig. 13-4). It is usually present in only one eye. If the staphyloma does not involve the macula, the visual acuity may be normal (Fig. 13-4, A and C). In adulthood these patients may complain of transient obscurations of vision that in some cases may be associated with intermittent dilation of the retinal veins.[26,47,59] Figure 13-4, A, illustrates a mild degree of peripapillary staphylomatous formation that was initially misinterpreted as a choroidal hemangioma in a young woman with transient obscurations of vision.[59]

Peripapillary staphylomata may occasionally be associated with contractile movements of the walls of the staphyloma (Fig. 13-4, D).[41,75] These contractions are unassociated with the patient's respiration or pulse rate. There is some histopathologic evidence to suggest that the presence of atavistic smooth muscle in and around peripapillary staphylomata may be responsible for this contraction and, further, may be responsible for the transient obscuration of vision (Fig. 13-4, E and F).[74] Contractile movements have also been described in patients with choroidal coloboma and morning glory syndrome.[15,20,51] In 1962 Longfellow and coworkers reported a young man with unilateral intermittent blindness associated with marked dilation of the retinal veins of undetermined cause.[47] He had minimal abnormality of the optic nerve head, but the clinical findings otherwise suggest the possibility of an anomalous smooth muscle sphincter around the retrobulbar optic nerve.

FIG. 13-4   Peripapillary Staphyloma.

A and B, Peripapillary staphyloma in the right eye of a 31-year-old woman complaining of transient obscurations of vision in this eye. Note the circular area of depigmentation and excavation surrounding the optic disc (A). There was slight narrowing of the retinal vessels adjacent to the optic disc. Visual acuity in the right eye was 20/20 and in the left eye was 20/15. The left fundus was normal (B).

C, More fully developed peripapillary staphyloma in a 17-year-old girl with a 3-year history of intermittent episodes of complete amaurosis in the left eye.

D, Marked peripapillary staphyloma, the walls of which contracted about every minute to form a cavity approximately two-thirds of the diameter shown.

E and F, Photomicrographs of a cross-section of the dysplastic optic nerve just behind the eye of a patient with a peripapillary staphyloma. Note the dysplastic nerve surrounded by a ring of smooth muscle (arrows). Contraction of similar atavistic muscle is apparently responsible for the spontaneous contraction noted in the patient (D).

(A and B from Seybold and Rosen[59]; C courtesy Dr. A.R. Frederick Jr; D from Wise et al.[75]; E and F courtesy Dr. William H. Spencer.)

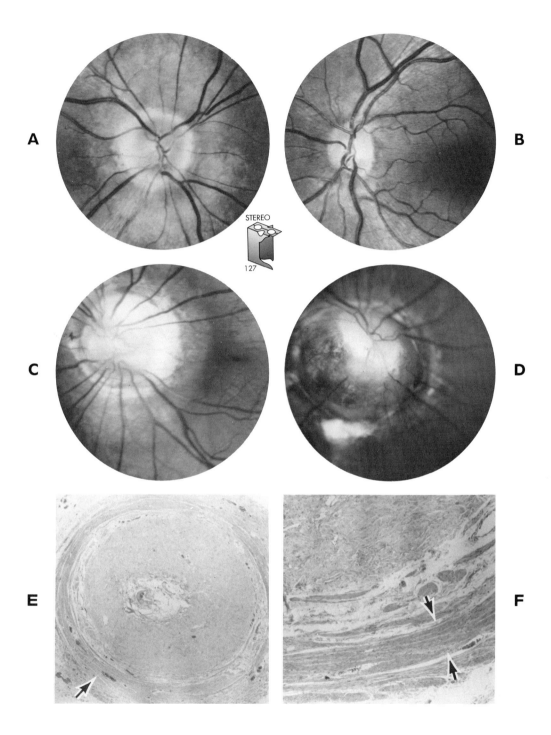

▼ OPTIC DISC HYPOPLASIA AND TILTED DISC SYNDROME

Mild dysplasia of the optic nerve must be considered in patients with unexplained visual loss.[85,87,88] There is considerable variation in the size of the normal optic disc. The disk diameter is often directly related to the eye size and refractive error. Some anomalies of the disc either may be overlooked or misinterpreted as papilledema. Failure to recognize a disc anomaly in a patient with a visual defect may cause initiation of an unnecessarily extensive evaluation for a retinal, retrobulbar, or intracranial lesion.

Moderate or severe hypoplasia of the optic disc is often associated with a visual defect (Fig. 13-5).[80,99] Ophthalmoscopic clues to its presence include reduction in the disc diameter, a low disc/artery ratio, and the peripapillary double ring sign (Fig. 13-5, *A* and *B*). This sign consists of a yellow-gray peripapillary halo delineated by an outer ring corresponding to the juncture between the sclera and lamina cribrosa and an inner ring caused by the termination of the RPE.[80,92] The diagnosis of mild degrees of hypoplasia may be difficult or impossible. Several techniques for measuring and defining optic disc hypoplasia have been described.[80,96,103] Romano, using photogrametric methods, found no overlap between the horizontal diameters of normal and hypoplastic discs.[96] The range in diameters for hypoplastic discs was 1.8 to 3.27 mm, with a mean of 2.64 mm, as compared to a range of 3.44 to 4.7 mm and a mean of 3.88 mm for normal discs. Zeki and others used the ratio of the distance from the edge of the disc to the center of the fovea to disk diameter to define optic disc hypoplasia; a ratio of 3 to 1 or greater characterizes a hypoplastic optic disc.[103] Disc hypoplasia may be unilateral or bilateral (Fig. 13-5, *C* to *E*). In bilateral cases the eye with the smaller disc often has a better Snellen acuity, indicating that factors other than size determine the visual function, e.g., macular hypoplasia, high refractive error, amblyopia, central scotoma, and optic atrophy.[103] A hypoplastic disc with a large central cup may have a disc diameter of normal size.[95] Hypoplastic optic discs may occasionally be supplied largely by cilioretinal arteries.[78] Disc hypoplasia may be associated with other extraocular or intraocular anomalies (e.g., aniridia)[90]; it may be segmental[85]; and it may be associated with normal visual acuity (Fig. 13-5, *C* to *E*).[81] Superior segmental disc hypoplasia may occur as a sign of maternal diabetes.[89,94]

FIG. 13-5   Hypoplasia and Dysplasia of the Optic Disc.

A, Marked hypoplasia of the optic disc in an infant.

B, Photomicrograph of severe optic disc hypoplasia.

C to E, Unilateral optic disc hypoplasia in left eye (**D**) of a young woman who had normal visual acuity in both eyes but an afferent pupillary defect and a peculiar visual field defect in the left eye (**E**). Compare with normal right disc (**C**).

F, Tilted optic disc was present bilaterally in this patient, who had superotemporal visual field defects in both eyes.

G to I, Septooptic dysplasia in a 17-year-old girl who was the product of full-term normal pregnancy and delivery. She had neonatal jaundice caused by Rh incompatibility. She was of short stature. She had nystagmus and concentric field constriction. Her visual acuity, right eye, was 20/60 and, left eye, no light perception. An MRI (**I**) showed evidence of aplasia of the septum pellucidum.

(**C** to **E**, courtesy Dr. Joel S. Glaser.)

Optic nerve hypoplasia can result from an insult to the embryo at any level of the optic pathway.[93] Evidence for a neuroendocrine disorder should be sought in any child presenting with bilateral optic disc hypoplasia, because of the frequent association of hypothalamic and pituitary dysfunction, partial or complete absence of the septum pellucidum, midbrain abnormalities, hypotonia, hydrocephalus, porencephaly, and orthopedic deformities (de Morsier's syndrome) (Fig. 13-5, *G* to *I*).*

The tilted disc syndrome has the following features: the long axis of the oval optic disc is obliquely directed; the upper and temporal portion of the disc lies anterior to the inferonasal portion; the retinal vessels emerge from the disc tissue in the upper and temporal aspect rather than nasally (situs inversus); there is an RPE conus in the direction of the tilt, as well as a large area of hypopigmentation and staphylomatous ectasia inferonasal to the optic disc; myopic astigmatism is present; and visual field depression occurs bitemporally (not truly hemianoptic) (Fig. 13-5, *F*).[82,100] Central vision may or may not be affected. The asymmetry of the disc elevation with the ill-defined margins superiorly may be mistaken for papilledema. Visual loss may be caused occasionally by choroidal neovascularization.[98] The disc anomaly may occur in association with other, nonocular anomalies.[91]

---

*References 79, 83, 84, 86, 91, 97, 101, 102, 104.

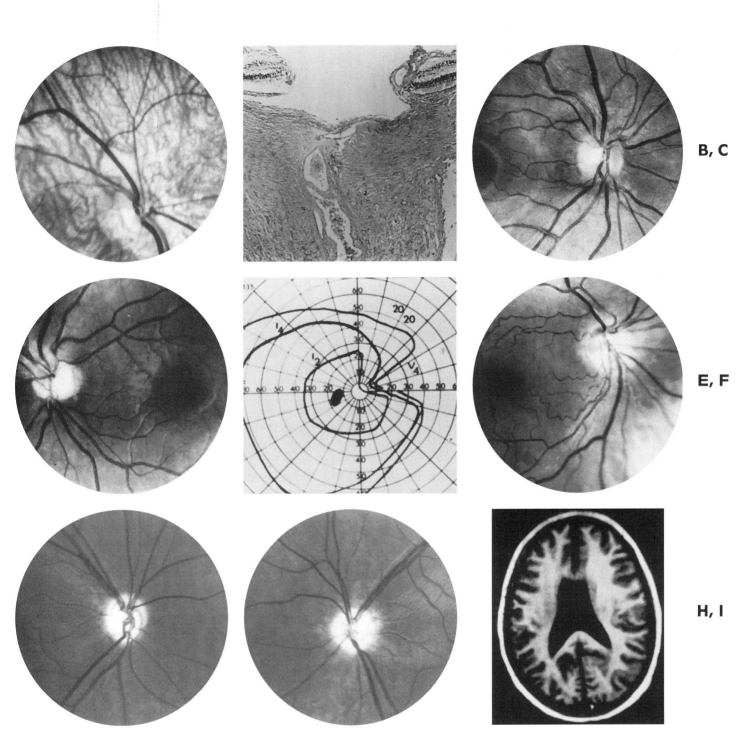

B, C

E, F

H, I

▼ DRUSEN (HYALINE BODIES) OF THE OPTIC NERVE HEAD

Drusen are discrete, multiple, amorphous, partly calcified, extracellular deposits in the prelaminar portion of the optic nerve.* In small numbers they may be present deep within a normal-appearing optic nerve head. In larger numbers in children and young adults, they cause a swollen nerve head that may simulate papilledema (Fig. 13-6, *A* and *B*).[123] As they become larger, more calcified, and associated with atrophy of surrounding nerve fibers, they become visible as discrete crystalline structures later in life (Fig. 13-6, *E*). When buried, they are most easily detected by retroillumination biomicroscopically. Although a "lumpy, bumpy" appearance to a swollen disc suggests the presence of drusen, a similar picture occasionally occurs in papilledema.[109] They frequently occur in small discs and may be associated with anomalous branching and tortuosity of the retinal vessels (Fig. 13-6, *A* and *B*).[124,135,140,149]

In some patients drusen may cause slow progressive loss of visual fields (characteristically inferonasal) in a nerve fiber distribution (Fig. 13-6, *C* and *D*).[128,130,142,150] Drusen may be associated with abnormal visual evoked potentials.[148,150] In a few patients drusen of the optic disc may lead to severe loss of central vision.[123,129] Drusen may also cause acute visual loss presumably resulting from acute swelling of the optic nerve head induced by the drusen's interfering with the blood supply of the nerve (Fig. 13-7, *G*).† This swelling may be evident ophthalmoscopically and accompanied by a few flame-shaped hemorrhages and cotton-wool patches, a picture suggesting anterior ischemic optic neuropathy.[117,118,129,131,274] In others the swelling of the optic nerve may be less apparent and cause obstruction of the central retinal vessels.[106,107,110,136,138] Optic disc drusen may also cause loss of vision associated with subretinal exudation and hemorrhage derived from peripapillary choroidal neovascularization (Figs. 13-6, *E*, and 13-7, *A* to *F*).‡ Bleeding into the subretinal space may occur adjacent to the optic disc in the absence of angiographic evidence of subretinal neovascularization (Fig. 13-6, *E*).[119]

Other fundus findings that have occurred in association with drusen of the optic nerve head include retinitis pigmentosa,[115,140] retinal hemorrhages,[108] angioid streaks[127] (see Fig. 3-32, *I*),

*References 107, 108, 111-113, 121, 126, 137, 143.
†References 106, 109, 110, 117, 118, 129, 131, 133, 147, 148, 274.
‡References 119, 120, 134, 141, 146, 154.

FIG. 13-6   Hyaline Bodies of the Optic Disc.

A and **B,** Asymmetric distribution of optic disc hyaline bodies in a 14-year-old girl whose condition was misdiagnosed as papilledema. Note the congenital tortuosity of the retinal vessels and the relatively small, less involved left optic disc.

C and **D,** Optic disc pallor and swelling caused by hyaline bodies in this 35-year-old woman with hypertension. Note marked autofluorescence of drusen **(D).** Visual acuity in both eyes was 20/15. She had loss of the inferior visual field in both eyes.

E, Subretinal hemorrhage *(arrow)* caused by calcified hyaline bodies.

F, Photomicrograph of a calcified hyaline body located anteriorly to the lamina cribrosa. Note multiple dilated capillaries *(arrows)* near the margins of the hyaline body.

subfoveal choroidal neovascularization,[153] chronic papilledema associated with pseudotumor cerebri,[139,140] and chorioretinal folds (see Chapter 4). Disc drusen have been reported in children with primary megacephaly.[122] Drusen bodies of the optic nerve head occur commonly, and therefore many associated findings may be coincidental.[132] The association of drusen and chorioretinal folds probably is not coincidental. Most chorioretinal folds are probably acquired and are caused by some subclinical inflammatory process causing shrinking and flattening of the posterior sclera. This process also causes narrowing of the optic canal and in turn may predispose the optic nerve head to drusen accumulation and other complications such as ischemic optic neuropathy and obstruction of the central retinal vessels. In some patients hyaline bodies are inherited as an autosomal dominant trait.[138,149,152]

Fluorescein angiography is helpful in identifying alterations in the normal optic nerve vascular pattern as well as in identifying subretinal neovascularization associated with drusen.[117,145] By virtue of their autofluorescence drusen near the surface of the optic disc can be detected with fundus photography using appropriate filters (Fig. 13-6, *C* and *D*). I have not found this technique helpful in detecting drusen that were not visible biomicroscopically.

Ultrasonography is also helpful in detecting optic disc drusen, particularly when they are buried in an optic disc that appears normal clinically, or in cases of unexplained optic disc swelling.[106] Failure to demonstrate calcified bodies in the optic nerve head of infants and children with a swollen optic nerve head may not exclude the presence of drusen. It is possible, although not proven histo-

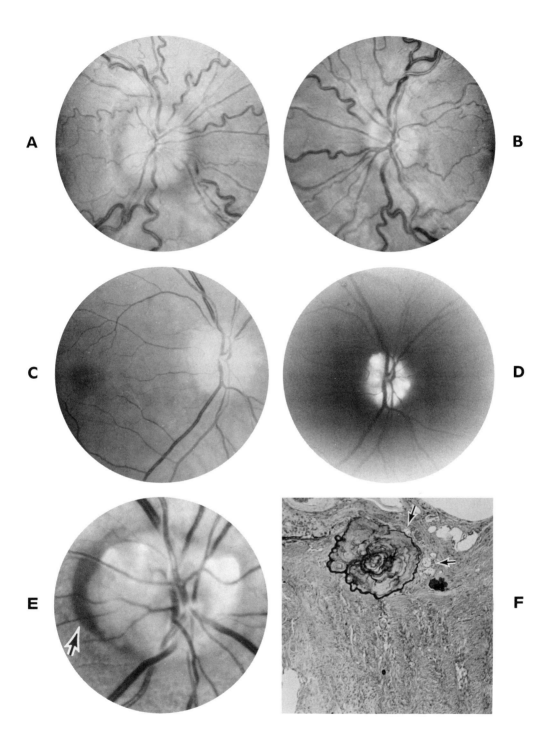

pathologically, that drusen may be relatively non-calcified hyaline structures in young patients. The calcification caused by drusen anterior to the level of the lamina cribrosa should not be confused with that located several millimeters posterior to the lamina cribrosa.[144] The cause of this latter focal calcification is uncertain. In some patients the calcification may be located in the walls or lumen of the central retinal artery, where it may develop as a degenerative change in association with atheromatous disease, or it may be a calcific embolus derived from the aortic valve. These focal retrolaminar calcifications may be found in some eyes with central retinal artery occlusion. Computed tomography is also capable of detecting buried drusen.[105,114]

Histopathologically, drusen are calcified extracellular bodies located anterior to the lamina cribrosa (Fig. 13-6, *F*).* They are associated with small scleral canal, crowding of nerve fibers, partial optic atrophy, elevation of the disc margins, cytoid bodies, dilated capillaries, juxtapapillary subretinal hemorrhage, subretinal neovascularization, retinal scarring, and calcification. Histochemically they are composed of a mucoprotein matrix containing acid mucopolysaccharides, ribonucleic acid, and occasionally iron.[107,112,113] Their pathogenesis has been ascribed to RPE migration, hyaline degeneration of the neuroglia, accumulation of degenerative products of axons, and coalescing intracellular deposits of glial cells,[125] transudative vasculopathy,[143] and axoplasmic transport alterations.[149] It is probable that a congenital, and less commonly an acquired, small optic nerve scleral canal that is small and crowded with nerve fibers is responsible for a local disturbance of axoplasmic transport and drusen formation.[124,149] Tso found ultrastructural evidence to suggest that optic disc drusen are the result of abnormal intracellular metabolism and calcification of mitochondria.[151] The mitochondria are extruded into the extracellular space, where they are nidi for continued buildup of calcific deposits. Acquired causes of chronic crowding of the optic nerve fibers such as idiopathic chorioret-

*References 107, 112, 113, 116, 121, 125, 143, 149.

FIG. 13-7 Hyaline Bodies of the Optic Disc.

A to **F,** Serous and hemorrhagic disciform detachment of the left macula (**B**) secondary to hyaline bodies of the optic disc in a 4-year-old boy with a 3-week history of left esotropia. Visual acuity in the right eye was 20/30 and in the left eye was 20/200. Note swollen optic disc in both eyes (**A** and **B**) and the gray, type 2, subretinal neovascular membrane (*arrows,* **B**) extending temporally from the left optic disc. Fluorescein angiography revealed evidence of perfusion and staining of the neovascular membrane extending from the temporal edge of the left optic disc (**C** and **D**). Xenon photocoagulation was placed over the area of subretinal neovascularization (**E**). Note that the photocoagulation was not carried into the center of the foveal area. Two months following photocoagulation note the atrophy of the RPE that extends into the central macular area (**F**). The patient's visual acuity was approximately 6/200.

G to **I,** Acute optic neuropathy with disc edema, peripapillary exudation, and exudative macular detachment in the right eye (**G**) of a 31-year-old man complaining of rapid loss of vision. His left optic disc was small and contained hyaline bodies (*arrow,* **H**). Two months later visual acuity had improved and hyaline bodies were evident in the right disc (*arrows,* **I**).

inal folds (see Chapter 4) and pseudotumor cerebri may also be a factor in drusen formation.[139,140]

The long-term visual prognosis for most patients with drusen of the optic disc is probably good. The natural course of those patients who develop juxtapapillary subretinal neovascularization is variable, and some patients may retain central vision in spite of peripapillary subretinal hemorrhage.[119,137]

The biomicroscopic diagnosis of drusen of the optic disc is relatively secure if the calcified bodies are visible within the elevated optic nerve head. Occasionally noncalcified drusenlike changes are caused by papilledema.[109] The differential diagnosis of juxtapapillary choroidal neovascularization associated with a swollen optic disc includes the presumed ocular histoplasmosis syndrome, angioid streaks, idiopathic choroidal neovascularization, sarcoidosis, papilledema with pseudotumor cerebri, and congenital pit of the optic disc.

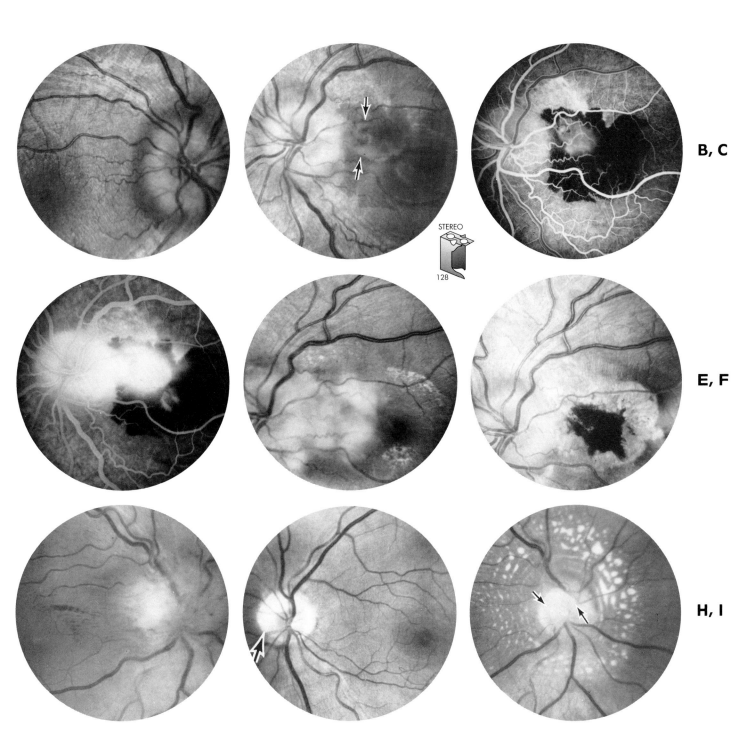

B, C

STEREO
128

E, F

H, I

▼ HEREDITARY OPTIC NEUROPATHIES

The heredodegenerative optic neuropathies must be considered in patients with insidious as well as rapid loss of central vision.

Dominant optic atrophy

Patients with dominant optic atrophy note the insidious onset of mildly progressive loss of visual acuity, usually beginning before 10 years of age.[155,158,161,167-169,173] Visual loss is bilateral but may be asymmetric. Many patients are unable to recall the time of onset of the disease, and some may be asymptomatic. Although the optic atrophy is dominantly inherited, a positive family history may not be obtained (Fig. 13-8). Interfamilial and intrafamilial variations in acuity loss may occur (range of 20/30 to 20/400). The characteristic field defect is a cecocentral scotoma. Depression of the temporal isopters may simulate a bitemporal hemianopia. Constriction of peripheral isopters is rare. Tritan dyschromatopsia is the characteristic color defect in dominant optic atrophy. A generalized dyschromatopsia, however, may be present in some cases. Temporal optic disc pallor, often with a triangular area of temporal excavation, is characteristic (Fig. 13-8, A and B). Although uncertainties remain concerning the pathogenesis of the frequently encountered West Indian optic atrophy, it is probable that many cases are examples of dominant optic atrophy (Fig. 13-8, B and C; see discussion of nutritional amblyopia in a subsequent section).

Weleber and Miyake described familial optic atrophy associated with "negative" electroretinograms in two families with loss of central vision occurring in the second and third decades of life, optic atrophy, defective color vision, mild to moderate myopia, and pericentral or central scotomas.[193]

Leber's hereditary optic neuropathy

Leber's hereditary optic neuropathy (LHON) is a maternally inherited disease that is characterized by acute, severe, bilateral visual loss in healthy young persons, usually males.[164,170,191] The central visual loss is acute or subacute at onset, painless, and accompanied by large cecocentral scotomata and dyschromatopsia. Central vision deteriorates progressively, first in one eye then in the other typically with an interval of days to weeks. Intervals of as long as 8 years have been reported.[176] Transient worsening with exercise or warming as occurs in other optic neuropathies (Uhthoff's

FIG. 13-8 Familial Optic Neuropathy.

A, This young girl had mild visual loss and a cecocentral scotoma in both eyes. Her sibling had similar findings. Note the segmental area of optic atrophy temporally.

B and **C,** This 49-year-old Jamaican man had poor vision in his left eye since sustaining trauma to that eye at 30 years of age. He was asymptomatic in the right eye but was referred because his best corrected vision in the eye was 20/70. There was a wedge-shaped area of temporal pallor in both optic discs (**B**) and posttraumatic scarring in the left macula. Angiography in the right eye (**C**) revealed no evidence of abnormality in the macula. He had bilateral cecocentral scotomata. It is probable that a familial optic atrophy that developed in early childhood was responsible for subnormal acuity in the right eye.

D to **G,** Dominant optic atrophy affected four generations of the family of this 8-year-old boy (**D** and **E**) and his 25-year-old father (**F** and **G**). The son's visual acuity was 20/40 bilaterally. The father gave a history of slow loss of vision since childhood. His visual acuity was 20/200 in both eyes.

symptom) may occur.[176,182,186] All levels of visual acuity loss have been reported, but it commonly declines to levels worse than 20/200 bilaterally, usually over several weeks to several months.[176,180] Although these patients are typically between the ages of 18 and 30 years at onset, visual loss may not occur until the sixth decade or beyond, when the clinical picture may be mistaken for anterior ischemic optic neuropathy.[157,176] Color vision is affected early, and visual fields examination reveals a central or cecocentral scotoma.[176,182] Biomicroscopy reveals circumpapillary telangiectatic microangiopathy, swelling of the nerve fiber layer around the disc (pseudoedema), and absence of fluorescein leakage (Fig. 13-9).[171,186] Most patients show no improvement but partial or even complete recovery may occur 5 to 10 years after onset of visual loss.[176,189] Dilation of the optic nerve sheaths with cerebrospinal fluid has been demonstrated by ultrasonography (30-degree test) and histopathologically.[159,187] Visual dysfunction is the only manifestation of LHON in most patients. Although other neurologic disorders are occasionally reported, the best established link is between LHON and cardiac conduction abnormalities.[183,184] A similar optic neuropathy has been reported with skeletal abnormalities,[176] and in association with Charcot-Marie-Tooth disease, a hereditary disease of peripheral nerves in at least two families.[174,175] Uemura and coworkers have identified mild but distinct biochemical and elec-

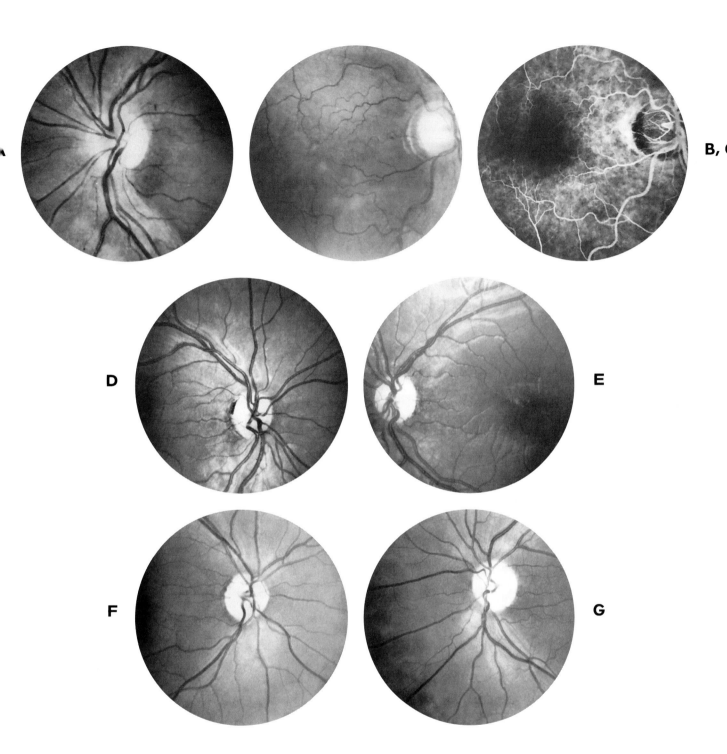

tron microscopic changes in muscle biopsy in patients with LHON.[190] Wallace and others, in 1988, identified a mitochondrial replacement mutation in 9 of 11 families with members diagnosed with LHON.[192]

When Leber's hereditary optic neuropathy appears for the first time in a family, the diagnosis is often delayed or missed. In the acute stage, circumpapillary telangiectatic microangiopathy, swelling of the nerve fiber layer around the optic disc (pseudoedema), and absence of staining on fluorescein angiography are characteristic (Fig. 13-9).[182,186] Progressive enlargement of the blind spot until it reaches fixation characterizes the early progression of field loss. Many asymptomatic family members with Leber's disease have peripapillary microangiopathy.[171,179,180] These vascular changes may be evident angiographically and occur years before the acute phase of the disease.[181,188] They include progressive arteriovenous shunting that starts in the inferior arcuate nerve fibers and that may be associated occasionally with preretinal hemorrhages. Acute visual loss is accompanied by dilation of the branches of the central retinal artery and peripapillary telangiectatic capillaries. These changes disappear as atrophy of the optic nerve develops (Fig. 13-9, *D*). Unlike dominant optic atrophy, the atrophy often progresses to involve the entire optic disc. Retinal arterial narrowing and increased circulation time occur. Angiography is probably useful in excluding Leber's disease in asymptomatic individuals.[181] Acquired red–green deficiency characterized by a deutanlike discrimination defect is characteristic and may be detected in some asymptomatic carriers. Electroretinography and dark adaptation are usually normal in these patients.[168] Visual loss typically stabilizes soon after onset, but some patients may show either improvement or worsening. There is no effective treatment for the disease. Since the primary locus of the disease appears to be in the intraocular rather than the retrobulbar area, Leber's hereditary vascular neuroretinopathy has been suggested as a more appropriate name.[180] Leber's hereditary optic neuropathy is strictly maternally inherited and passes to future generations only through women. An affected male never has affected offspring, whereas a woman may have affected children although she herself is visually normal.

Leber's hereditary optic neuropathy is associated with four different point mutations of mitochondrial DNA that appear to be pathogenetic for the disease.* These mutations affect nucleotide positions 3460, 11778, 14484, and 15257. The clinical findings are similar except patients with 14484 are more likely to experience visual recovery than patients with the other three mutations.[164] Patients with 15257, who also have an associated mutation at 15812, are less likely to recover vision than those without this association.[166] Patients with the 15257 mutation also have a higher incidence of spinal cord and peripheral neurologic symptoms than patients with the other mutations. Molecular genetic testing is of practical value in confirming the diagnosis of atypical cases or in patients presenting with optic atrophy, in the absence of a

*References 159, 162-165, 172, 177, 178, 185, 187, 189, 192.

FIG. 13-9 Leber's Optic Neuropathy.

A to D, One year previously this 18-year-old man developed blurred vision in the right eye. The diagnosis at that time was retrobulbar neuritis. Neurologic evaluation was negative. He gave a 2-week history of blurred vision in the left eye. Visual acuity in the right eye was 6/200 and in the left eye was 20/300. There was segmental atrophy of the right optic disc. There was telangiectasis and tortuosity of the capillaries of the left optic disc and juxtapapillary retina **(A).** Angiography demonstrated the pattern of these abnormal vessels (*arrows,* **B**), which showed no evidence of late staining **(C).** Fourteen years later visual acuity in the right eye was 20/400 and in the left eye was 20/200. Both optic discs showed temporal pallor **(D).** The telangiectatic vessels were less apparent.

E and F, A 38-year-old man with acute Leber's optic neuropathy. Note the telangiectatic tortuous retinal vessels (*arrows*).

G to J, This 14-year-old boy, with a family history of Leber's optic neuropathy, presented because of rapid loss of vision of 3 weeks' duration. At age 12 years his visual acuity was 20/20 and genetic analysis of his blood was positive for Leber's disease. His visual acuity at the time of these photographs was 20/200 in the right eye and 9/200 left eye. The right optic disc was hyperemic **(G);** the left optic disc showed temporal pallor. There was generalized tortuosity of the retinal veins. Note the dilation and tortuosity of the small juxtapapillary venules (*arrows,* **G** and **H**). Several months later the both optic discs showed temporal pallor **(I and J)** and the visual acuity was 3/200.

K and L, Optic atrophy in two siblings of the patient illustrated in **G to J.**

family history, and after the characteristic telangiectasis is no longer evident.[165,166] The proportion of mutant mitochondrial DNA molecules was found to shift markedly across generations and within tissues of an individual. Therefore, successful determination of the mitochondrial DNA genotype of a family or patient with Leber's optic neuropathy requires testing of more than one family member and more than one tissue from each individual.[172] Molecular genetic tests are 100% specific but only 50% sensitive for the diagnosis of LHON. It may be prudent to advise carriers to avoid exposure to toxins such as tobacco smoke and excessive alcohol intake since they may further compromise mitochondrial energy metabolism.[156,163]

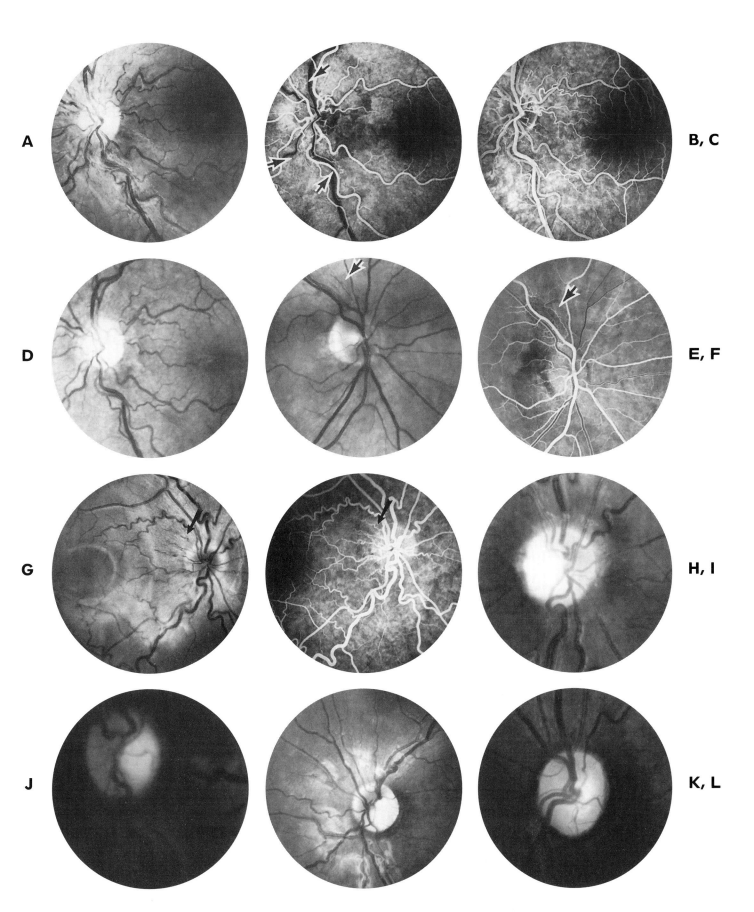

A

B, C

D

E, F

G

H, I

J

K, L

▼ LEBER'S IDIOPATHIC STELLATE NEURORETINITIS AND MULTIFOCAL RETINITIS

In 1916 Theodor Leber described the clinical syndrome characterized by unilateral loss of vision, optic disc swelling, macular star, and spontaneous resolution of unknown cause in otherwise healthy patients (Figs. 13-10 and 13-11).[208] In two-thirds of the patients seen at the Bascom Palmer Eye Institute, a viral-like illness has preceded the onset of symptoms.[116,199,204] In most patients the visual acuity ranges from 20/50 to 20/200 and an afferent pupillary defect is present.[199] During the first week after the onset of symptoms, the macular star is usually preceded by mild swelling of the optic disc and peripapillary exudative detachment of the retina (Fig. 13-10, A).* In a few patients the swelling of the disc may be more marked and may be associated with splinter hemorrhages. One or more focal white retinal lesions may occur (Figs. 13-10, G to I, and 3-11, E to I).† These focal areas of retinitis may cause occlusion of either a branch retinal artery or a vein.[196,201] In some patients the multifocal retinitis is unassociated with optic disc involvement. Vitreous cells are present in 90% of cases.[199] Anterior uveitis is present in a few patients. Within several days or weeks, the peripapillary exudate begins to subside and a macular star appears and becomes more prominent as the disc and peripapillary swelling disappears (Fig. 13-10, D and I).[116,199,204] Within the first several weeks the visual acuity begins to improve, and with a few exceptions it eventually returns to normal. The macular star usually disappears within 6 to 12 months. A few patients may be left with mild pallor of the optic disc and mild pigmentary changes in the center of the macula. The focal areas of retinitis resolve spontaneously usually within several weeks.

Fluorescein angiography shows evidence of abnormal capillary permeability, particularly from the capillaries deep within the optic disc, not only during the early phase of the disease (Fig. 13-10, B) but even after the disc has returned to its normal appearance (Fig. 13-10, D and F).[116,204] Ten percent to 15% of patients may show mild leakage of dye from the optic disc in the opposite eye (Fig. 13-11, D). Focal white retinal lesions, if present, usually show evidence of staining (Fig. 13-11, H and I). Angiography shows no abnormality of capillary permeability in the area of the macular star. It may demonstrate a mild window defect in the RPE,

FIG. 13-10   Leber's Idiopathic Stellate Neuroretinitis.

A to C, A 38-year-old woman developed blurred vision in the right eye 11 days after an episode of headaches, vomiting, and diarrhea. Note the oval, yellowish exudate in the center of the macula and the fine macular star, which is more prominent nasally than temporally (A). There is some exudative detachment of the peripapillary retina. The left fundus was normal. Angiography showed definite leakage of dye from the optic disc and no evidence of abnormality in the macular area (B). Angiography of the left eye was normal (C).

D to F, This 31-year-old man gave a 1-month history of decreased vision in his left eye. Visual acuity was 20/50. Note the faint yellowish material in the center of the macula and the macular star, which is more prominent nasally (D). The optic disc is within normal limits. Angiography of the right eye was normal (E). Angiography of the left eye (F) showed marked fluorescence of the optic disc compared to the right eye (E).

G to I, This 29-year-old man noted fever, nausea, vomiting, and rapid loss of vision in the left eye of 2 days' duration. He admitted sleeping with cats. His visual acuity was 20/30 right eye and 20/300 left eye. Note the peripapillary focal areas of retinitis in both eyes (arrows, G and H) and the swollen left optic disc (H). Four days later he had developed a macular star (I). His titer for Rochalimaea was positive 1:20. He was treated with doxycycline, 100 mg tid, for 2 weeks. Two months later his visual acuity was 20/20 bilaterally.

J to L, Swollen optic disc and macular star in a 19-year-old man complaining of recent loss of vision in the right eye that began 1 week after the onset of an upper respiratory infection. Visual acuity was 20/200. The left eye was normal. Medical evaluation was negative. Six years later the fundus was normal. Visual acuity was 20/25.

particularly in those patients following resolution of a prominent macular star. Loss of visual function primarily results from changes in the optic nerve head and not the macula. Laboratory investigations done at the time of visual loss are usually normal. Patients may show mild spinal fluid pleocytosis (Fig. 13-11, E to I).

There is mounting evidence that cat-scratch disease is one of the causes of this syndrome.* (See Chapter 7, pp. 604, 700.) This association has occurred in at least five patients seen at the Bascom Palmer Eye Institute. In one patient, Leptospira organisms were cultured from the spinal fluid.

---

*References 116, 197, 199, 202, 204, 206, 208, 210-212.
†References 116, 197, 199, 203, 205, 207.

*References 116, 194-196, 198-200, 204, 214, 215.

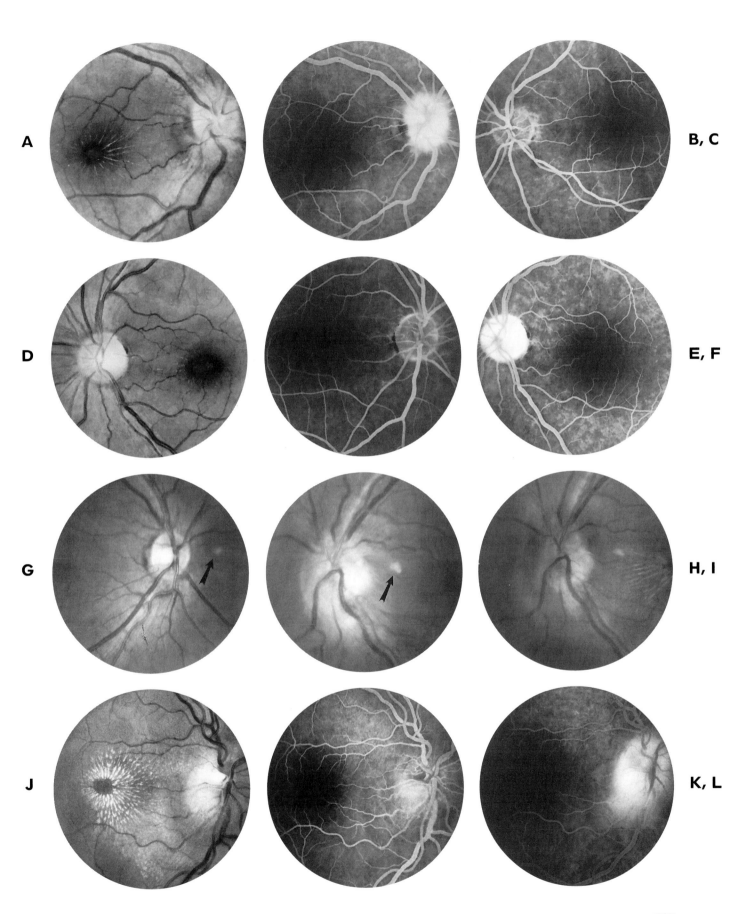

Histopathologically, the macular star is caused by the microglial ingestion of the lipid-rich exudate lying in the outer plexiform layer of Henle. Figure 13-11, *J,* depicts diagrammatically the probable pathogenesis of a macular star. A protein- and lipid-rich exudate leaks from the capillaries in the depth of the optic disc and extends beneath the retina in the peripapillary region as well as along the plane of the outer plexiform layer into the macular region.[116,204] With reabsorption of the serous component of the exudate in the macular region the lipid and protein precipitate in the outer plexiform layer and are engulfed by macrophages. This creates the fine stellate pattern of yellow exudate that is characteristic of a macular star. Stellate maculopathy is caused by a variety of diseases affecting the permeability of the capillaries in the depth of the optic nerve head. Retinal vascular diseases usually cause a more irregular and coarser deposition of yellowish exudate in the inner nuclear as well as the outer plexiform layers in the macular region.

The differential diagnosis of patients with an optic disc swelling and a macular star includes hypertensive retinopathy (see Figs. 6-14, *A,* and 6-15, *A*), diabetic optic neuropathy (see Fig. 6-41, *J*) and diseases associated with optic neuritis, such as sarcoidosis, bacterial septic optic neuritis, Lyme disease, and luetic optic neuritis.[209] A macular star infrequently accompanies diffuse unilateral subacute neuroretinitis and is rarely if ever seen in patients with optic neuritis secondary to demyelinating diseases.[199] The possibility of septic retinitis caused by pyogenic bacteria, cat-scratch disease, toxoplasmosis, or fungi is greater in those patients who manifest multifocal retinitis. The differential diagnosis in those presenting with a branch retinal artery or vein inclusion expands to include idiopathic recurrent branch retinal artery disease and Eales' disease. (See Chapter 6, pp. 458, 534.) Management of these patients depends upon the ocular findings and the presence or absence of signs and symptoms of systemic disease. Many of these patients are afebrile and the antecedent illness has resolved by the time of their eye examination. A general physical examination, routine blood counts, and serology to exclude syphilis may be all that is necessary. Those with multifocal retinitis, and particularly those who are febrile, should have appropriate evaluation including blood cultures to exclude systemic septic disease. Serologic testing for exposure to *Bartonella,* skin test for cat-scratch disease, and biopsy of enlarged lymph nodes may be appropriate in those patients exposed to cats.

FIG. 13-11 Leber's Idiopathic Stellate Neuroretinitis with Angiographic Evidence of Involvement of the Asymptomatic Eye.

A to **D,** This 9-year-old girl noted rapid loss of vision in the right eye. Note the macular star and slight swelling and pallor of the optic disc (**A**). The left fundus appeared normal (**B**). Visual acuity was 20/200 in the right eye and 20/20 in the left eye. Angiography revealed staining of the temporal half of the right optic disc (**C**) and the superonasal quadrant of the left optic disc (**D**).

E to **I,** This 14-year-old girl had a history of an upper respiratory infection before the onset of visual loss in the left eye. She also had a 6-month history of intermittent fever of unknown origin. Her visual acuity was 20/50 in the left eye. Note swelling of the left optic disc (**E**) and small white retinal lesions in the left fundus (*arrows,* **E** and **F**) and one that was unnoticed in the asymptomatic right eye until review of her angiographic study (*arrows,* **G** and **H**). The white lesions in the left eye as well as of the optic disc stained (**I**). Spinal fluid examination revealed pleocytosis. Spinal fluid and blood cultures were negative.

J, Diagram depicting the pathogenesis of a macular star. Lipid-rich exudate leaking from capillaries within the depth of the optic nerve head (*small arrows*) extends into the subretinal space surrounding the optic nerve head as well as along the outer plexiform layer into the macular region. Reabsorption of the serous portion of the exudate leaves a concentrated lipid exudate (*large arrows*) in the outer plexiform layer of Henle and causes a macular star that is usually more prominent in the nasal half of the macula.

The *Bartonella* bacillus can be identified with the Warthin-Starry stain.

The visual prognosis for patients with idiopathic stellate neuroretinitis and multifocal retinitis is good, and no treatment is required. An occasional patient will have a recurrence in the opposite eye months or years later.

Purvin and Chioran recently reported seven young adults (mean age of 27 years) who developed multiple episodes of monocular neuroretinitis, macular star formation, dense arcuate visual field defects, and in some cases severe permanent visual loss.[213] Both eyes were eventually affected in five patients. Laboratory studies were not revealing and the disorder appeared nonresponsive to systemic corticosteroids. Except for the presence of a macular star, their cases seem to share more in common with anterior ischemic optic neuropathy in young patients. (See discussion of idiopathic anterior ischemic optic neuropathy in the young, p. 1006.)

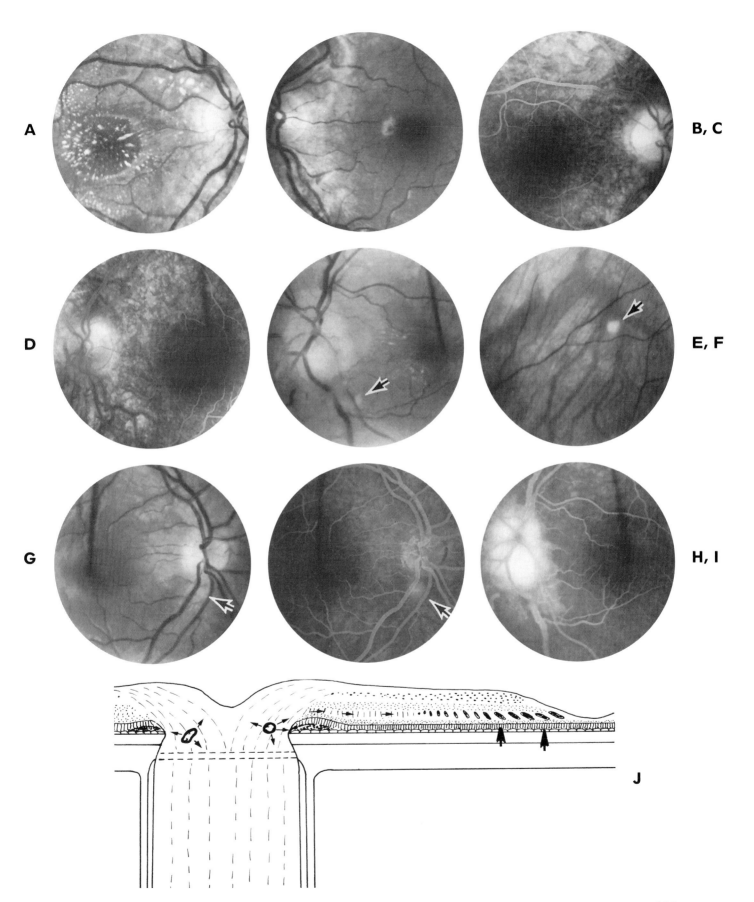

A

B, C

D

E, F

G

H, I

J

999

▼ NEURORETINOPATHY AND PROGRESSIVE FACIAL HEMIATROPHY

Progressive facial hemiatrophy (Parry-Romberg syndrome) is a disorder of unknown cause that is characterized by progressive unilateral atrophy of the skin, muscles, and bony structures of the face, usually in preadolescent patients.[216-223] It may extend down into the neck, shoulders, trunk, and extremities. All of the facial structures on one side may be involved (Fig. 13-12, *D* and *H*), or there may be only a linear depression in the scalp and forehead (*coup de sabre*) (Fig. 13-12, *A*). Vitiligo, poliosis, nevus flammeus, and moles are often present on the affected side. Ptosis, trichiasis, lagophthalmos, ectropion, neuroparalytic keratitis, canalicular obstruction, dacryocystitis, extraocular muscle palsies, enophthalmos, Horner's syndrome, heterochromia of the iris, uveitis, optic atrophy, and pigmentary disturbances of the fundi may occur. The brain may show evidence of hemiatrophy, and homolateral migraine or contralateral epilepsy may be present. This syndrome is not usually associated with visual loss. Visual loss, however, may be caused by either ipsilateral neuroretinopathy characterized by acute visual loss, optic disc swelling, peripapillary exudation, and macular star, or retinal telangiectasis and exudative retinal detachment (Fig. 13-12, *A* to *I;* see also Fig. 6-28, *I* to *L*).[216-220] Ultrasonography may demonstrate some enlargement of the affected optic nerve. The optic foramina are normal radiographically. Optic atrophy may occur as the peripapillary and macular exudation clears, but no patient has demonstrated progressive loss of visual field. Retinal vascular abnormalities have been reported previously in this disorder.[217,219,220] The pathogenesis of the acute neuroretinopathy and retinal vasculopathy is unknown.

FIG. 13-12   Acute Neuroretinopathy and Progressive Facial Hemiatrophy (Parry-Romberg Syndrome).

A to **C,** This 21-year-old woman, who had developed a linear depression of the forehead and scalp beginning at 4 years of age (**A**), had a 6-week history of acute visual loss in the ipsilateral eye caused by stellate exudative neuroretinopathy (**B**). Her visual acuity was 5/200. Optic foramina roentgenograms were normal. Three and one-half years later, the optic disc was pale (**C**) and her visual acuity was 20/80.

D to **G,** This 8-year-old boy developed progressive loss of vision in the left eye on the same side that he had facial hemiatrophy (**D**) that began at 6 years of age. His visual acuity was 10/400. He had a stellate exudative neuroretinopathy (**E**). Angiography revealed capillary dilation (**F**) and late staining in the area of the swollen optic disc. It also showed evidence of some dilation and leakage of the peripheral retinal capillaries (**G**). Computed tomography revealed normal optic canals. Echography and computed tomography showed some evidence of distention of the left optic nerve sheath.

H and **I,** This 13-year-old boy with progressive facial hemiatrophy (**H**), left deafness, congenital bowel defect, and hypospadias developed loss of vision in the right eye because of peripheral retinal telangiectasis and exudative retinal detachment (**I**). A similar exudative detachment was present in his opposite eye. Cryotherapy was successful in reattaching the retina in both eyes.

(**H** and **I** from Gass.[217])

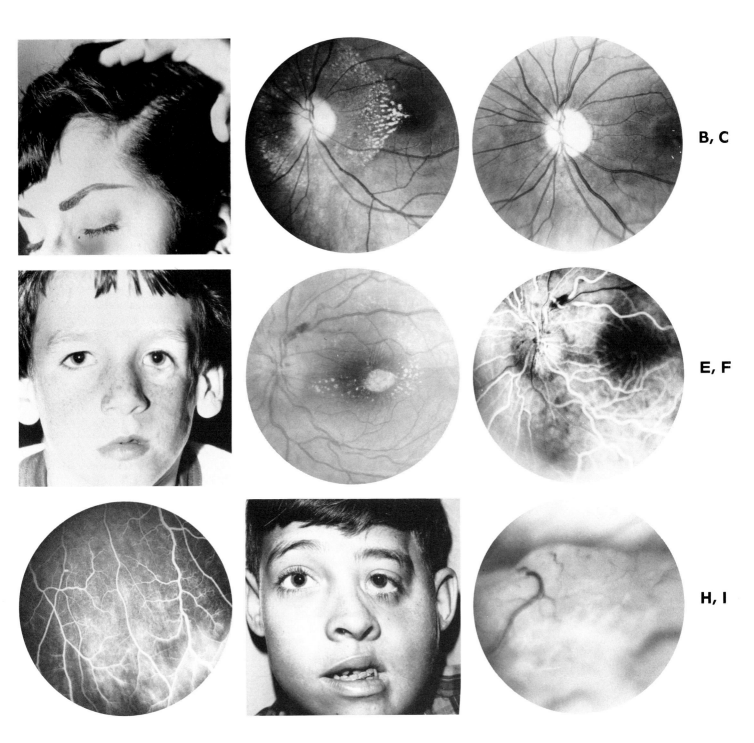

B, C

E, F

H, I

▼ ANTERIOR ISCHEMIC OPTIC NEUROPATHY

The term "anterior ischemic optic neuropathy" (AION) is used to describe swelling, ischemia, and varying degrees of infarction of the anterior part of the optic nerve caused by reduction in blood flow to the nerve (Figs. 13-13 and 13-14). The optic nerve head, by virtue of its closely arranged nerve fibers within the nonexpansile intrascleral canal, is ideally situated for ischemia to occur. Primary vascular insufficiency or secondary vascular insufficiency caused by any process that promotes stasis of axoplasmic flow and nerve fiber swelling can cause ischemia. Anterior ischemic optic neuropathy typically affects older patients, and the acute loss of vision may be mistakenly attributed to a macular disorder, for example, macular degeneration if pigment epithelial changes are present, or to cystoid macular edema in the aphakic patient (Fig. 13-13, *H* and *I*). For pathogenetic as well as therapeutic reasons, these patients can be subdivided into two major subgroups: (1) a nonarteritic group (those without evidence of arteritis) and (2) an arteritic group (those with giant-cell arteritis). The nonarteritic group may be subdivided into an idiopathic group, those with no identifiable cause, and those with a probable cause. Functionally, ophthalmoscopically, and fluorescein angiographically, all subgroups may present similar findings. The visual prognosis, however, is not the same for all groups.

Idiopathic ("nonarteritic") anterior ischemic optic neuropathy (n-AION)

Over 50% of patients with n-AION are generally healthy patients whose age is 45 years or older (mean of 69 years) and who experience an acute, usually moderate loss of vision in one eye (20/50 to 20/200).* Optic disc swelling accompanied by one or several flame-shaped hemorrhages is usually evident (Fig. 13-13). The swelling may or may not be pallid. It may be more pronounced in the superior half of the optic disc. A lower altitudinal or arcuate field defect that often is maximum at the time of presentation but that may progress during the first few weeks of the disease is present.[269,293] Fluorescein angiography usually demonstrates a delay of perfusion of the optic disc blood vessels, minimal alterations of choroidal filling, and staining of the optic disc (Fig. 13-13, *B* and *C*).[227] In

---

*References 230, 233, 240-242, 244, 255, 271, 281.

FIG. 13-13   Nonarteritic Anterior Ischemic Neuropathy.

A to C, This 57-year-old woman with noncongestive thyroid exophthalmos noted rapid loss of vision in the left eye. Her visual acuity was 4/200. The left optic disc was swollen, and a flame-shaped hemorrhage was present at its margin (**A**). Angiography showed a marked increase in retinal circulation time and late staining of the disc (**B** and **C**). She had an inferior attitudinal visual field defect. The acuity remained 20/200 in spite of intensive oral corticosteroid treatment for 2 months. She received X-ray irradiation to the left orbit. Her acuity 1 year later was 20/40.

D and E, Acute visual loss and an inferior attitudinal field defect occurred in the left eye of this healthy elderly patient with optic disc swelling and juxtapapillary hemorrhages (**D**). Two months later note the pallor of the inferior half of the optic disc (**E**).

F and G, This 67-year-old patient with marked inferior tilting of both optic discs developed acute visual loss and an inferior attitudinal field defect in the right eye. Note the pale swelling of the upper part of the disc (**F**) and the juxtapapillary subretinal hemorrhage. Several months later the blood resolved and there was remarkably little pallor of the optic disc (**G**).

H and I, This 67-year-old hypertensive patient experienced visual loss caused by ischemic optic neuropathy (**H**) soon after uneventful cataract extraction. Cystoid macular edema was suspected, but angiography revealed staining of the optic disc and no evidence of retinal capillary leakage in the macula. He subsequently developed optic atrophy (**I**). A similar course of events occurred in his left eye.

---

some cases there is a delay in the retinal artery appearance time, and an increased retinal circulation time, that presumably is caused by compression of the central retinal vessels by the swelling of the ischemic nerve fibers in the region of the lamina cribrosa. This compression occasionally may be sufficient to cause a fundus picture of central retinal artery or vein occlusion (Fig. 13-14, *A* to *C*). The disc swelling resolves in several weeks. The disc becomes pale and usually shows minimal cupping. Spontaneous improvement of visual acuity occurs in 10% to 35% of cases.[224,228,261,282,294] Recurrence of n-AION in the same eye is infrequent.[233,234,252] Possible explanations for the infrequent recurrences in n-AION include loss of nerve fibers after n-AION, providing more space for surviving nerve fibers to swell, and shunting of blood from the area of infarction to the surviving part of the nerve.[237,252,271] Focal engorgement and swelling of the nonischemic segment of the optic disc may simulate a capillary angioma.[287]

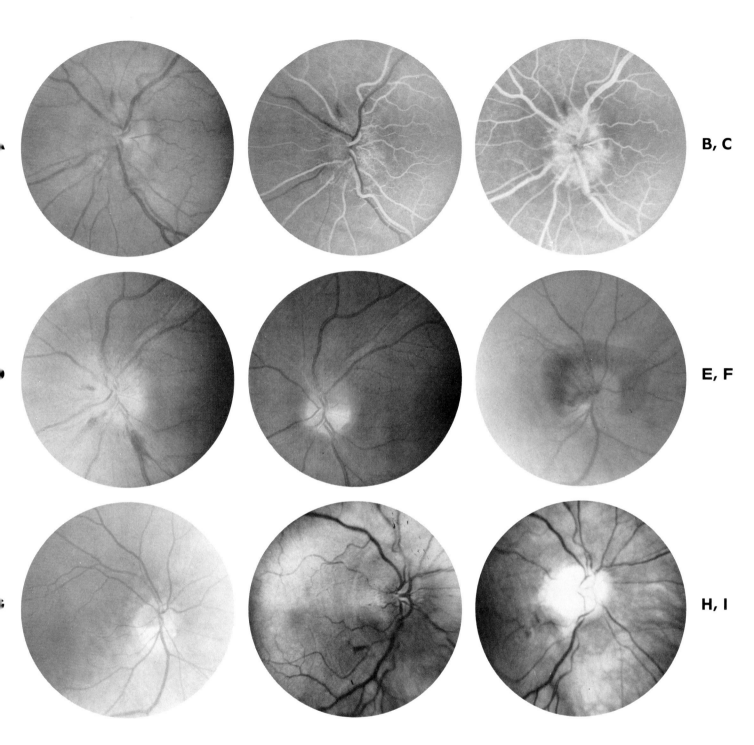

B, C

E, F

H, I

Approximately 40% of patients will develop n-AION in the opposite eye.[232] Although it has been presumed that most of these patients probably have an arteriosclerotic disorder, there is minimal evidence to support this view. These patients have no greater incidence of cardiovascular or cerebrovascular disease than a matched group of patients.[236,246,281,284] Idiopathic or n-AION occurs at a younger age in smokers (mean age 51 years) compared to nonsmokers (mean age 64 years).[238] The frequency of involvement in the upper half of the optic disc,[230,241,281] the rarity of second attacks of AION in the same eye,[233] and the small cup/disc ratio* suggest that structural factors are important in the pathogenesis of idiopathic AION.

Associated disorders that may precipitate nonarteritic AION include diabetes, malignant hypertension (Fig. 13-14, *A* to *C*), uremia,[253,270] eclampsia,[229,260] migraine,[252] embolism,[272,279,291] hemodynamic shock,[256,263] anemia (Fig. 13-14, *G* and *H*),[251] papilledema, orbital inflammation (Fig. 13-13, *A* to *C*), cataract extraction (Fig. 13-13, *H* and *I*),[247,248,254,288] elevation of intraocular pressure,[265,267,292] congenital anomalies of the optic disc (Fig. 13-13, *F* and *G*), and optic disc drusen.[276] Subretinal neovascularization occasionally occurs.[249] Familial n-AION has been reported.[239] HLA-A29 may be a risk factor for development of n-AION.[262]

Histopathologic evidence suggests that vascular insufficiency causing acute ischemic swelling of a segment of the nerve fibers immediately posterior to the lamina cribrosa is responsible for the clinical picture of n-AION.[280] The reason for the susceptibility of the superior segments of the optic nerve to ischemic damage is uncertain.

---

*References 230, 231, 233, 236, 244, 266, 274, 277.

FIG. 13-14 Anterior Ischemic Optic Neuropathy.

A to **C,** Hemorrhagic nonarteritic AION associated with a branch retinal artery occlusion in a severely hypertensive 40-year-old patient. Note ischemic whitening of the retina superotemporally (**B**) and delayed retinal perfusion in the area (**C**).

D to **F,** Arteritic AION in a 68-year-old woman with cranial arteritis. She presented because of blurred vision in the left eye. She previously lost vision in the right eye. Note the marked pallor of the swollen optic disc (**D**), the vertical zone of delayed choroidal perfusion (*arrows,* **E**), and late staining of the optic disc (**F**). Several months later the optic disc was atrophic.

G and **H,** Nonarteritic ischemic optic neuropathy caused by acute blood loss occurred in this 47-year-old woman who experienced massive extravasation of blood into the body tissues associated with liposuction. On the first postoperative day she noted roaring in the ear and no light perception in the right eye. The right optic disc was swollen and pale (**G**). The left eye was normal (**H**). Her hemoglobin was 5.5, and hematocrit was 16. Magnetic resonance imaging of the brain was normal. She was treated with prednisone, 80 mg daily, and received 2 units of blood. Her vision improved to light perception only.

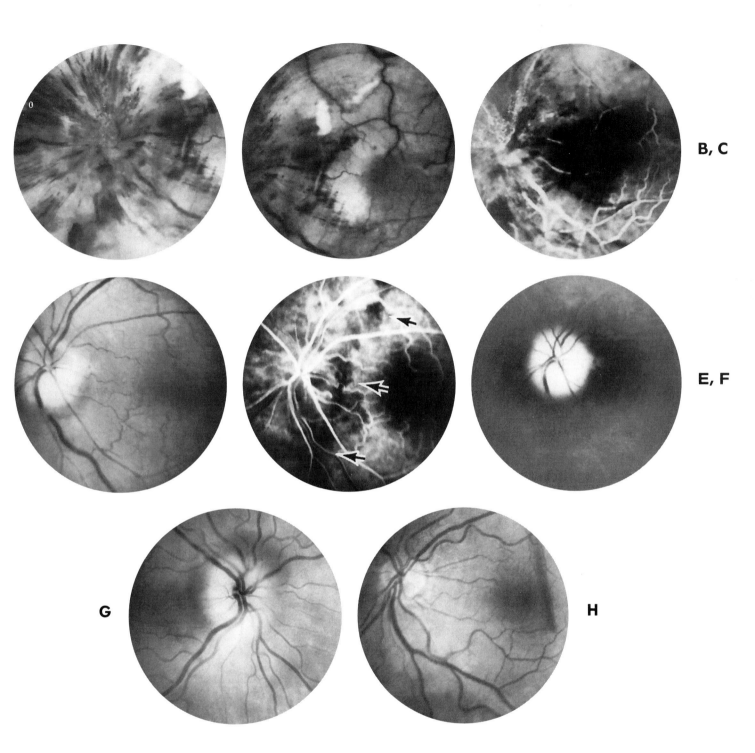

B, C

E, F

G

H

Idiopathic anterior ischemic optic neuropathy in the young (AIONY)

Idiopathic AION in the young is a rare entity characterized by recurrent episodes of acute visual loss associated with segmental pallid swelling of the optic nerve that frequently causes severe and permanent visual loss in otherwise healthy young adults with a mean age of onset of 25 years.[252,264] The fundus picture and visual field changes during the acute stage are identical to those in n-AION. This similarity includes the small optic disc size. Medical evaluation is negative. The cause is unknown.

It is important therapeutically to differentiate n-AION and AIONY from arteritic AION. The blood sedimentation rate is usually within normal limits in n-AION and AIONY and is usually greatly elevated in most cases of arteritic AION.

There is no effective treatment for n-AION or AIONY. Optic nerve sheath decompression was suggested as effective in the treatment of the acute progressive stage of n-AION.[245,285,289,290] Evidence, however, including the results of a controlled clinical trial, indicates that the procedure is ineffective and may be harmful for the treatment of n-AION.* The rate of operative complications, which include central retinal artery occlusion associated with optic nerve sheath decompression, may be as high as 40%.[278] Treatment of the associated systemic disorders in patients with nonarteritic AION, for example, corticosteroids or X-ray irradiation in orbital inflammatory disease (Fig. 13-13, *A* to *C*), or hemodialysis in patients with uremia, may improve the prognosis for return of vision.[253,270] Patients with evidence of arteritic AION require prompt treatment with high doses of corticosteroids (see next subsection).

---

*References 250, 257-259, 275, 283, 294, 304.

Arteritic anterior ischemic optic neuropathy (a-AION)

Giant-cell arteritis (temporal arteritis, cranial arteritis) is a systemic disease that is characterized by arthralgias, headaches, fever, weight loss, jaw claudication, and, frequently, acute severe visual loss in one eye that is often followed by severe loss in the second eye in elderly patients, usually 60 years of age or older.[226,268] The visual loss is generally more profound than in n-AION, and the optic disc pallor is usually more striking (Fig. 13-14, *D* to *F*, and see Fig. 6-13, *L*). Cotton-wool patches and flame-shaped hemorrhages may be present. Other findings may include hypotony, extraocular muscle palsies, and central retinal arterial as well as choroidal arterial occlusion (see Fig. 6-13). Fluorescein angiography demonstrates delayed perfusion of the choroid and optic disc.[273,286] The Westergren sedimentation rate is usually 100 mm or greater. Increased plasma viscosity, decreased red cell filterability, and decreased hematocrit are other findings in these patients.[235] The sedimentation rate and temporal artery biopsy findings are important in differentiating a-AION from n-AION.[226,235] Systemic corticosteroids should be instituted promptly if giant-cell arteritis is suspected. Monitoring changes in the blood sedimentation rate or C-reactive protein is used to adjust the corticosteroid dosage.[243]

Development or progression of visual loss occurs rarely in patients with giant-cell arteritis after the initiation of glucocorticoid therapy.[225,232] In a retrospective study of 245 patients with giant-cell arteritis seen over a 5-year period at the Mayo Clinic, Aiello and coworkers found that 14% had permanent loss of vision in one or both eyes.[225] In all but two of the patients, visual loss occurred before institution of corticosteroid therapy. Visual loss progressed after corticosteroid therapy in three patients. After 5 years the probability of developing visual loss after initiation of oral glucocorticoid treatment was determined to be 1% (Kaplan-Meier), and the probability of additional loss in patients who had a visual deficit at the time therapy was begun was 13%.

▼ IDIOPATHIC OPTIC NEURITIS AND PAPILLITIS

The results of the Optic Neuritis Treatment Trial, which enrolled 448 patients, indicate that this disorder is characterized by acute visual loss, often associated with pain, in predominantly females (77%) with a mean age of 32 years. The optic disc is swollen in approximately one-third of cases. Macular star figures occur rarely.[299] The patients demonstrate a wide variety of visual field defects. Magnetic resonance imaging (MRI) of the brain showed evidence of demyelinization in approximately 50% of cases. MRI, serologic studies (ANA, FTA-ABS), chest X-ray examination and lumbar puncture are of limited value in defining a cause for visual loss other than optic neuritis associated with demyelinating disease.[298] The MRI is more likely to be positive in patients with severe visual loss. Patients with retrobulbar neuritis are more likely to show evidence of multiple sclerosis than those with papillitis. Eliciting either Uhthoff's symptom (transient blurring of vision during exercise, hot shower or bath, or while under emotional stress) or Lhermitte's sign (sudden or transient electric-like shocks radiating down the spine or extremities, particularly with neck flexion) is evidence in patients with unexplained visual loss suggesting retrobulbar neuritis and multiple sclerosis. If clinical signs and symptoms are typical for optic neuritis other workup is unlikely to be fruitful. If the features are atypical such as progression of visual loss beyond 1 week, evidence of vitritis, presence of a macular star figure or iritis, age more than 45 years, or absence of pain, other diagnoses should be considered. In most patients the visual acuity and visual field return to normal within a year.[297] In those patients who at the onset of visual symptoms have MRI evidence of multiple sclerosis (MS)-like lesions, intravenous therapy with corticosteroids reduces the chances of the patient's developing new clinical signs of MS during the subsequent 2 years.[295,300] This restraining effect of cortisone wears off after 2 years. Oral administration of corticosteroids has no effect on visual outcome and increases the risk of recurrent optic neuritis.[295,296]

▼ TRAUMATIC OPTIC NEUROPATHY

Blunt injuries, particularly to the forehead, may cause loss of vision and no funduscopic changes as a result of injury to the optic nerve, even when the trauma seems trivial.[301,302,304] The optic nerve is most vulnerable to injury at either end of the optic canal. Shearing forces caused by abrupt deceleration of the skull probably cause injury to small nutrient blood vessels as well as contusion necrosis to the nerve. Immediate loss of vision to no light perception on impact portends a poor prognosis for recovery; a short lucid interval before deterioration suggests a potentially reversible process. Direct injury to the nerve may result from a fracture through the bony canal that severs or compresses the nerve. The value of corticosteroids and surgical decompression in both types of injury is uncertain.[303] Optic disc pallor usually appears several weeks after the injury.

▼ RADIATION-INDUCED OPTIC NEUROPATHY

See Chapter 6, p. 528.

▼ OPTIC NERVE MENINGIOMAS

Patients with meningiomas confined to the orbital portion of the optic nerve are typically women (70% to 80%) who are seen between the ages of 35 and 60 years because of transient obscurations of vision or mild visual loss in one eye (Fig. 13-16).* The visual acuity is usually normal or only mildly affected. Mild proptosis is present in 50% to 75% of cases and is easily overlooked. Ophthalmoscopic examination typically reveals mild optic disc edema and some dilation of the retinal veins (Fig. 13-15, *A*). Other evidence of central retinal vein obstruction is infrequently present.[323] Enlargement of the blind spot is the characteristic field defect initially. Over a period of months or years visual loss, increased papilledema (Fig. 13-15, *D* and *G*), refractile bodies and pallor of the optic disc, mild retinal vein dilation, and in 20% to 40% of cases optic disc shunt or collateral vessels develop (Fig. 13-15, *B* and *D*).† These changes are usually accompanied by contraction of the peripheral isopters. Juxtapapillary retinal and chorioretinal folds may be present (Fig. 13-15, *A*, *G*, *H*, and *K*). Extension of the tumor into the inner eye is rare (Fig. 13-15, *J*).[307,310,314,329] In the presence of optic disc edema, fluorescein angiography shows capillary dilation and leakage of the optic disc vessels. Later, after optic atrophy has occurred, dilation of the capillaries and leakage are usually no longer apparent. The pattern of dye filling the dilated venous loops on the optic disc suggests, at least in some cases, that these vessels may not be shunting venous blood from the retina into the juxtapapillary venous system but instead are hypertrophied collateral channels transporting venous blood from the retrobulbar meningioma into the central retinal vein.[306] Histopathologic examination in one case demonstrated communication between the retinal veins and the choroidal veins.[324] Primary optic nerve meningiomas occasionally occur bilaterally,[311,315,333] and may be associated with neurofibromatosis type 2 along with cranial nerve schwannomas.[308] Meningiomas as well as acoustic neuromas may be caused by loss of tumor suppressor genes on chromosome 22.[308]

Computed tomography and ultrasonography are invaluable in demonstrating the enlargement of the perioptic dural sheaths and in excluding tumor extension into the optic canals. Magnetic resonance imaging (MRI) plus fat saturation after gadolinium-diethylenepentaacetic acid is helpful in detecting intracranial extension of optic nerve meningioma that is not easily imaged with MRI alone.[320,334] The differential diagnosis includes optic nerve glioma, papilledema, and optic nerve cysts. In some cases an occult meningioma may be the cause of the cyst.[322] Whereas optic disc pallor and collateral venous channels are highly suggestive of a meningioma, they occasionally are caused by other disorders such as central retinal vein occlusion, hydrocephalus, and perioptic neuritis.[309,312] Visual loss typically occurs slowly over a period of months or years, and surgical extirpation of the meningioma is usually associated with profound visual loss. Therefore, in patients with good visual function and no evidence of extraorbital extension of the meningioma, observation for evidence of progressive visual loss or extraorbital extension is usually recommended before either surgical or irradiation treatment are consid-

FIG. 13-15   Meningioma of the Optic Disc.

A to **C**, Blurred vision, papilledema, and chorioretinal folds in this 46-year-old woman were caused by a meningioma of the left optic nerve (**A**). Note resolution of the edema and folds and the development of dilated venous loops (*arrows*, **B**) that occurred spontaneously over a 32-month period. Angiography showed evidence that venous blood in these loops as well as that in the retina was draining into the central retinal vein. The patient had 3600 R of X-ray irradiation to the right orbit. Note the reduced prominence of the venous loops 18 months later (**C**). Visual acuity was 20/20.

D to **F**, This 14-year-old boy developed blurred vision 4 months previously after being struck on chin with broom stick. He was treated for 4 weeks with 100 mg prednisone daily. His visual acuity was bare hand movements, right eye, and 20/20, left eye. He had 2 mm of right proptosis. Orbital MRI showed a mass that failed to enhance with gadolinium. Optociliary shunt vessels (*arrows*, **D**) suggested a meningioma that was confirmed on biopsy of an enlarged optic nerve. Angiography (**E** and **F**) shows the venous nature of shunt vessels. He received 4500 cGy irradiation. The fundus changes stabilized but there was no visual improvement.

G and **H**, Meningioma of the optic nerve in this 56-year-old woman with juxtapapillary chorioretinal folds (**G**) that are evident angiographically (**H**).

I, Photomicrograph of meningioma of the optic nerve. Note compression of the optic nerve (*arrows*) by the tumor.

J and **K**, Meningioma of the optic nerve with anterior extension into the subretinal space (*arrow*, **J**). Note the evidence of choroidal folds (*arrows*, **K**) adjacent to the subretinal tumor.

(**J** from Dunn and Walsh.[310])

---

*References 305, 306, 311, 319, 320, 323, 332-334.
†References 306, 313, 316, 317, 324-326, 328.

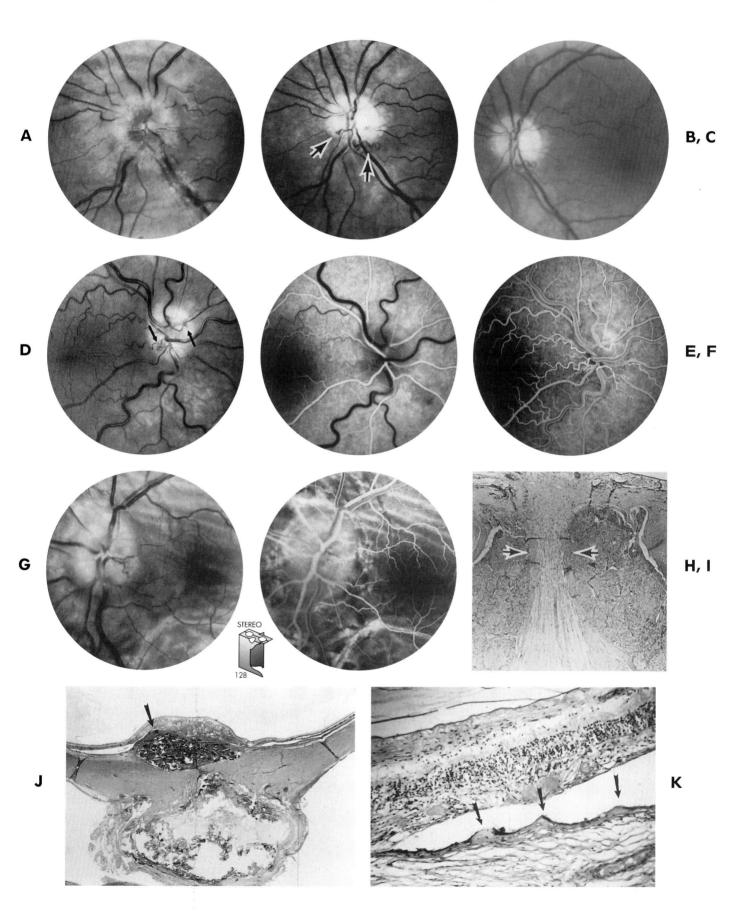

ered.[311,319,321,331-333] Some patients achieve at least temporary restoration of vision following irradiation treatment.[319,327] Optic nerve meningiomas in children and young adults are more aggressive and these patients require closer followup.[318,330,333]

▼ OPTIC NERVE GLIOMAS

Optic nerve gliomas cause insidious loss of vision, proptosis, and optic atrophy that are often discovered in children during a routine eye examination. The tumor may involve one or both optic nerves and may involve the chiasm. When both nerves are affected the patient is likely to have other manifestations of type 1 neurofibromatosis, for example, Leisch iris nodules and bright lesions demonstrated throughout the brain with gadolinium-enhanced MRI.[335,336,339] The latter lesions have uncertain pathology and consequences. Radiologic studies may reveal enlargement of the optic foramen on the affected side or evidence of J-shaped sella turcica in the case of chiasmal involvement. Optic nerve gliomas have a variable histopathogic appearance and growth potential. Most neural tumors of the anterior visual pathways are generally benign and are classified as pilocystic astrocytomas. Some, however, may exhibit aggressive growth and rarely may invade the eye.[337] Those with less growth potential frequently occur in association with other manifestations of neurofibromatosis.[340] The management of these tumors is controversial.[338,340]

▼ VISUAL LOSS SECONDARY TO PAPILLEDEMA CAUSED BY INCREASED INTRACRANIAL PRESSURE

Although transient obscuration of vision is a frequent complaint of patients with papilledema and increased intracranial pressure, most of them have normal visual acuity during the early stages. Those with chronic papilledema, particularly patients with pseudotumor cerebri, may develop loss of visual field and visual acuity in as many as 50% of cases.[344,347,348] Persons at high risk of visual loss are those with high-grade or atrophic papilledema, peripapillary subretinal hemorrhage,[342] anemia, high myopia, and old age.[357] The primary cause of visual loss is progressive atrophy and degeneration of the nerve fibers.[361] Other less frequent causes include juxtapapillary subretinal neovascularization,[349,350,355-357,366] preretinal hem-

FIG. 13-16   Choroidal Folds Associated with Unilateral Papilledema of Unknown Cause.

A to C, This apparently healthy 55-year-old man presented with visual complaints in the left eye. His right eye was normal **(B).** In the left eye he had papilledema and horizontally oriented chorioretinal folds (*arrows,* **A**). He noted further decline in his acuity and returned 5 days later. His visual acuity was 20/60. The papilledema had lessened. The chorioretinal folds were unchanged. **(C)** Neurologic evaluation including CAT scan was negative.

Nutritional Amblyopia.

D to F, Nutritional amblyopia misdiagnosed as macular degeneration in this 66-year-old man, who complained of loss of central vision of over 16 months' duration. His visual acuity was 20/100. There were mild RPE changes biomicroscopically **(D and E).** Angiography, however, was normal **(F).** He had bilateral cecocentral scotomata. He was treated with oral and intramuscular injections of B complex vitamins and within several months experienced dramatic improvement of vision to 20/30 and J-1+ in both eyes.

G and H, This 73-year-old man, with a history of nontropical sprue and lifelong amblyopia in the left eye, noted the development of a paracentral scotoma in the right eye 6 months previously. He was eating a wheat-free diet. Visual acuity in the right eye was 20/40 and in the left eye 20/400. He had a cecocentral scotoma in the right eye. His pupils and right fundus were normal except for a small, one clock-hour sector of pallor temporally in the optic disc (*arrow,* **G**). The left optic disc was hypoplastic **(H).** The diagnosis was possible nutritional amblyopia or focal ischemic optic atrophy.

orrhage,[355,359] central retinal vein occlusion,[349] serous macular detachment,[346] macular star,[345,355] macular pigmentation,[343] anterior ischemic optic neuropathy,[346] and chorioretinal folds (Fig. 13-16, *A* and *C*).[344,345,353,355,358] The latter three findings are not usually associated with visual loss when they occur in patients with papilledema. Occasionally the patient may be aware of a temporal scotoma associated with enlargement of the blind spot.[360] In such cases, particularly if the optic disc swelling is unilateral, visual field testing may yield a blind spot enlargement far larger than can be explained on the basis of the papilledema. (See discussion of idiopathic blind spot enlargement syndrome and acute zonal occult outer retinopathy, Chapter 7.

Treatment for papilledema associated with pseudotumor cerebri consists of oral diuretics, weight loss, and occasional use of corticosteroids.[352,365] In patients with visual loss who fail to

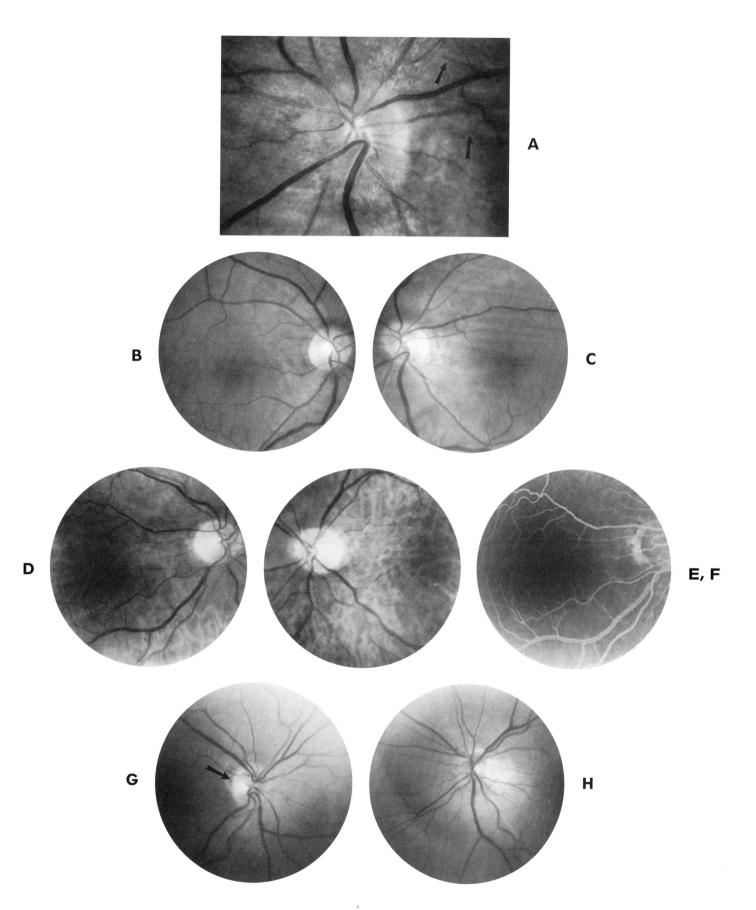

respond to medical therapy, optic nerve sheath decompression is an effective form of treatment.* It probably should be done initially in only one eye since in some patients this will result in resolution of papilledema bilaterally.[354] Recurrences may occur.[363]

▼ NUTRITIONAL AMBLYOPIA

Insidious and slowly progressive loss of central vision associated with central and cecocentral visual field defects may be caused by dietary deficiency of one or several vitamins as well as by exposure to toxins or adverse reaction to pharmaceuticals.[369,371,374] Initially the visual loss is not usually associated with fundus changes (Fig. 13-16, D and E). Evanescent dilation and tortuosity of small retinal vessels within the arcuate areas of the nerve fiber layer similar to that described in Leber's optic neuropathy, however, have been described during the early phase of acute malnutrition optic neuropathy.[371] Temporal disc pallor and atrophy of the papillomacular nerve fiber layer eventually occur (Fig. 13-16, G). Demonstration of a cecocentral scotoma, particularly to red test objects, with preservation of peripheral fields is the typical finding. Deficiency of the B complex vitamins (predominantly thiamin) is probably more important than either chronic use of alcohol or tobacco alone in causing visual loss. There are only a few well-documented cases of toxic amblyopia in smokers with no history of alcohol ingestion or nutritional deficiency.[377] A reliable dietary history is often best obtained from a friend or relative of the patient. Most of these patients show improvement of vision following institution of a balanced diet and B complex vitamin supplementation (Fig. 13-16, D to F).

A peculiar optic neuropathy, referred to as West Indian Jamaican optic neuropathy, is characterized by the rapid development of visual loss and optic atrophy in predominantly young West Indian Blacks.[368,375] Vision is usually reduced to 20/200 levels, and dense central scotoma and temporal disc pallor are characteristic. Nerve deafness, ataxia, and spasticity may accompany ocular involvement in a few instances.[375] It is uncertain whether this amblyopia has an infectious, toxic, hereditary, or nutritional basis.

An epidemic of optic neuropathy, characterized by bilateral subacute visual loss, dyschromatopsia, central or cecocentral scotomas, and in some patients peripheral neuropathy, occurring primarily in men, was identified in Cuba in 1992. Cigarette smoking, rum drinking, and vitamin deficiencies were identified as risk factors. In spite of the features in common with Leber's hereditary optic neuropathy, mitochondrial DNA mutations were found infrequently in these patients.[372,373]

To exclude the diagnosis of Leber's hereditary optic neuropathy, all patients suspected of having nutritional or tobacco–alcohol amblyopia should have mitochondrial testing.[370,376]

REFERENCES
Optic Disc Anomalies Associated with Serous Detachment of the Macula

1. Akiba J, Kakehashi A, Hikichi T, Trempe CL: Vitreous findings in cases of optic nerve pits and serous macular detachment. *Am J Ophthalmol* 116:38-41, 1993.
2. Akiyama K, Azuma N, Hida T, Uemura Y: Retinal detachment in morning glory syndrome. *Ophthalmic Surg* 15:841-843, 1984.
3. Alexander TA, Billson FA: Vitrectomy and photocoagulation in the management of serous detachment associated with optic nerve pits. *Aust J Ophthalmol* 12:139-142, 1984.
4. Anderson DR: Discussion of Javitt JC, Spaeth GL, Katz LJ, et al: Acquired pits of the optic nerve; increased prevalence in patients with low-tension glaucoma. *Ophthalmology* 97: 1043-1044, 1990.
5. Annesley W, Brown G, Bolling J, et al: Treatment of retinal detachment with congenital optic pit by krypton laser photocoagulation. *Graefes Arch Clin Exp Ophthalmol* 225:311-314, 1987.
6. Beyer WB, Quencer RM, Osher RH: Morning glory syndrome; a functional analysis including fluorescein angiography, ultrasonography, and computerized tomography. *Ophthalmology* 89:1362-1364, 1982.
7. Bochow TW, Olk RJ, Knupp JA, Smith ME: Spontaneous reattachment of a total retinal detachment in an infant with microphthalmos and an optic nerve coloboma. *Am J Ophthalmol* 112:347-348, 1991.
8. Bonnet M: Serous macular detachment associated with optic nerve pits. *Graefes Arch Clin Exp Ophthalmol* 229:526-532, 1991.
9. Brockhurst RJ: Optic pits and posterior retinal detachment. *Trans Am Ophthalmol Soc* 73:264-291, 1975.
10. Brown GC, Shields JA, Goldberg RE: Congenital pits of the optic nerve head. II. Clinical studies in humans. *Ophthalmology* 87:51-65, 1980.
11. Brown GC, Shields JA, Patty BE, Goldberg RE: Congenital pits of the optic nerve head. I. Experimental studies in collie dogs. *Arch Ophthalmol* 97:1341-1344, 1979.
12. Calhoun FP: Bilateral coloboma of the optic nerve associated with holes in the disk and a cyst of the optic sheath. *Arch Ophthalmol* 3:71-79, 1930.
13. Cennamo G, Liguori G, Pezone A, Iaccarino G: Morning glory syndrome associated with marked persistent hyperplastic primary vitreous and lens colobomas. *Br J Ophthalmol* 73: 684-686, 1989.
14. Chang S, Haik BG, Ellsworth RM, et al: Treatment of total retinal detachment in morning glory syndrome. *Am J Ophthalmol* 97:596-600, 1984.

*References 341, 343, 351, 354, 362-364, 367.

15. Cogan DG: Coloboma of optic nerve with overlay of peripapillary retina. *Br J Ophthalmol* 62:347-350, 1978.

16. Cox MS, Witherspoon CD, Morris RE, Flynn HW: Evolving techniques in the treatment of macular detachment caused by optic nerve pits. *Ophthalmology* 95:889-896, 1988.

17. Dailey JR, Cantore WA, Gardner TW: Peripapillary choroidal neovascular membrane associated with an optic nerve coloboma. *Arch Ophthalmol* 111:441-442, 1993.

18. Farpour H, Babel J: Les fossettes papillaires; diagnostic différentiel, anomalies vasculaires et cas limites. *Ann Oculist* 201:1-17, 1968.

19. Ferry AP: Macular detachment associated with congenital pit of the optic nerve head; pathologic findings in two cases simulating malignant melanoma of the choroid. *Arch Ophthalmol* 70:346-357, 1963.

20. Foster JA, Lam, S: Contractile optic disc coloboma. *Arch Ophthalmol* 109:472-473, 1991.

21. Friberg TR, McLellan TG: Vitreous pulsations, relative hypotony, and retrobulbar cyst associated with a congenital optic pit. *Am J Ophthalmol* 114:767-769, 1992.

22. Gass JDM: Discussion of paper by Brockhurst RJ: Optic pits and posterior retinal detachment. *Trans Am Ophthalmol Soc* 73:288-289, 1975.

23. Gass JDM: Serous detachment of the macula secondary to congenital pit of the optic nervehead. *Am J Ophthalmol* 67:821-841, 1969.

24. Gass JDM: *Stereoscopic atlas macular diseases; diagnosis and treatment,* ed. 3, St. Louis, 1987, CV Mosby, pp. 728-733.

25. Gordon R, Chatfield RK: Pits in the optic disc associated with macular degeneration. *Br J Ophthalmol* 53:481-489, 1969.

26. Graether JM: Transient amaurosis in one eye with simultaneous dilation of retinal veins; in association with a congenital anomaly of the optic nerve head. *Arch Ophthalmol* 70:342-345, 1963.

27. Grimson BS, Mann JD, Pantell JP: Optic nerve pit during papilledema. *Arch Ophthalmol* 100:99-100, 1982.

28. Haik BG, Greenstein SH, Smith ME, et al: Retinal detachment in the morning glory anomaly. *Ophthalmology* 91:1638-1647, 1984.

29. Hamada S, Ellsworth RM: Congenital retinal detachment and the optic disk anomaly. *Am J Ophthalmol* 71:460-464, 1971.

30. Hanson MR, Price RL, Rothner AD, Tomsak RL: Developmental anomalies of the optic disc and carotid circulation; a new association. *J Clin Neuro-Ophthalmol* 5:3-8, 1985.

31. Harris MJ, de Bustros S, Michels RG, Joondeph HC: Treatment of combined traction-rhegmatogenous retinal detachment in the morning glory syndrome. *Retina* 4:249-252, 1984.

32. Hendrikse F, Deutman AF: Central serous detachment with optic pit treated by gas injection and laser coagulation. *Lasers Light Ophthalmol* 2:249-252, 1989.

33. Irvine AR, Crawford JB, Sullivan JH: The pathogenesis of retinal detachment with morning glory disc and optic pit. *Retina* 6:146-150, 1986.

34. Jack MK: Central serous retinopathy with optic pit treated with photocoagulation. *Am J Ophthalmol* 67:519-521, 1969.

35. Javitt JC, Spaeth GL, Katz LJ, et al: Acquired pits of the optic nerve; increased prevalence in patients with low-tension glaucoma. *Ophthalmology* 97:1038-1043, 1990.

36. Jay WM, Pope J Jr, Riffle JE: Juxtapapillary subretinal neovascularization associated with congenital pit of the optic nerve. *Am J Ophthalmol* 97:655-658, 1984.

37. Jensen PE, Kalina RE: Congenital anomalies of the optic disk. *Am J Ophthalmol* 82:27-31, 1976.

38. Kalina RE, Conrad WC: Intrathecal fluorescein for serous macular detachment. *Arch Ophthalmol* 94:1421, 1976.

39. Kindler P: Morning glory syndrome: Unusual congenital optic disk anomaly. *Am J Ophthalmol* 69:376-384, 1970.

40. Kirchhof B, Arnold G, Kirchhof E: Zur Genese der Grubenpapille. Mikroskopische Untersuchungen bei einem Neugeborenen. *Klin Monatsbl Augenheilkd* 188:310-312, 1986.

41. Kral K, Svarc D: Contractile peripapillary staphyloma. *Am J Ophthalmol* 71:1090-1092, 1971.

42. Kranenburg EW: Crater-like holes in the optic disc and central serous retinopathy. *Arch Ophthalmol* 64:912-924, 1960.

43. Lichter PR, Henderson JW: Optic nerve infarction. *Am J Ophthalmol* 85:302-310, 1978.

44. Lin CCL, Tso MOM, Vygantas CM: Coloboma of optic nerve associated with serous maculopathy; a clinicopathologic correlative study. *Arch Ophthalmol* 102:1651-1654, 1984.

45. Lincoff H, Lopez R, Kreissig I, et al: Retinoschisis associated with optic nerve pits. *Arch Ophthalmol* 106:61-67, 1988.

46. Lincoff H, Yannuzzi L, Singerman L, et al: Improvement in visual function after displacement of the retinal elevations emanating from optic pits. *Arch Ophthalmol* 111:1071-1079, 1993.

47. Longfellow DW, Davis FS Jr, Walsh FB: Unilateral intermittent blindness with dilation of retinal veins; undetermined etiology. *Arch Ophthalmol* 67:554-555, 1962.

48. Morgan OG: Acquired hole in the disk. *Br J Ophthalmol* 45:437-439, 1951.

49. Mustonen E, Varonen T: Congenital pit of the optic nerve head associated with serous detachment of the macula. *Acta Ophthalmol* 50:689-698, 1972.

50. Petersen HP: Pits or crater-like holes in the optic disc. *Acta Ophthalmol* 36:435-443, 1958.

51. Pollock S: The morning glory disc anomaly: contractile movement, classification, and embryogenesis. *Doc Ophthalmol* 65:439-460, 1987.

52. Quigley HA, Hohman RM, Addicks EM, et al: Morphologic changes in the lamina cribrosa correlated with neural loss in open-angle glaucoma. *Am J Ophthalmol* 95:673-691, 1983.

53. Radius RL, Maumenee AE, Green WR: Pit-like changes of the optic nerve head in open-angle glaucoma. *Br J Ophthalmol* 62:389-393, 1978.

54. Regenbogen L, Stein R, Lazar M: Macular and juxtapapillary serous retinal detachment associated with pit of optic disc. *Ophthalmologica* 148:247-251, 1964.

55. Rosenberg LF, Burde RM: Progressive visual loss caused by an arachnoidal brain cyst in a patient with an optic nerve coloboma. *Am J Ophthalmol* 106:322-325, 1988.

56. Rubinstein K, Ali M: Complications of optic disc pits. *Trans Ophthalmol Soc UK* 98:195-200, 1978.

57. Savell J, Cook JR: Optic nerve colobomas of autosomal-dominant heredity. *Arch Ophthalmol* 94:395-400, 1976.

58. Schatz H, McDonald HR: Treatment of sensory retinal detachment associated with optic nerve pit or coloboma. *Ophthalmology* 95:178-186, 1988.

59. Seybold ME, Rosen PN: Peripapillary staphyloma and amaurosis fugax. *Ann Ophthalmol* 9:1139-1141, 1977.

60. Shami M, McCartney D, Benedict W, Barnes C: Spontaneous retinal reattachment in a patient with persistent hyperplastic primary vitreous and an optic nerve coloboma. *Am J Ophthalmol* 114:769-771, 1992.

61. Slamovits TL, Kimball GP, Friberg TR, Curtin HD: Bilateral optic disc colobomas with orbital cysts and hypoplastic optic nerves and chiasm. *J Clin Neuro-Ophthalmol* 9:172-177, 1989.

62. Slusher MM, Weaver RG Jr, Greven CM, et al: The spectrum

of cavitary optic disc anomalies in a family. *Ophthalmology* 96:342-347, 1989.

63. Snead MP, James N, Jacobs PM: Vitrectomy, argon laser, and gas tamponade for serous retinal detachment associated with an optic disc pit: a case report. *Br J Ophthalmol* 75:381-382, 1991.

64. Sobol WM, Blodi CF, Folk JC, Weingeist TA: Long-term visual outcome in patients with optic nerve pit and serous retinal detachment of the macula. *Ophthalmology* 97:1539-1542, 1990.

65. Sobol WM, Bratton AR, Rivers MB, Weingeist TA: Morning glory disk syndrome associated with subretinal neovascular membrane formation. *Am J Ophthalmol* 110:93-94, 1990.

66. Steinkuller PG: The morning glory disk anomaly: case report and literature review. *J Pediatr Ophthalmol Strabismus* 17:81-87, 1980.

67. Sugar HS: Congenital pits in the optic disc and their equivalents (congenital colobomas and colobomalike excavations) associated with submacular fluid. *Am J Ophthalmol* 63:298-307, 1967.

68. Sugar HS: Congenital pits in the optic disc with acquired macular pathology. *Am J Ophthalmol* 53:307-311, 1962.

69. Theodossiadis G: Evolution of congenital pit of the optic disk with macular detachment in photocoagulated and nonphotocoagulated eyes. *Am J Ophthalmol* 84:620-631, 1977.

70. Theodossiadis G: Treatment of retinal detachment with congenital optic pit by krypton photocoagulation. *Graefes Arch Clin Exp Ophthalmol* 226:299, 1988.

71. Theodossiadis GP, Kollia AK, Theodossiadis PG: Cilioretinal arteries in conjunction with a pit of the optic disc. *Ophthalmologica* 204:115-121, 1992.

72. Theodossiadis GP, Koutsandrea C, Theodossiadis PG: Optic nerve pit with serous macular detachment resulting in rhegmatogenous retinal detachment. *Br J Ophthalmol* 77:385-386, 1993.

73. von Fricken MA, Dhungel R: Retinal detachment in the morning glory syndrome; pathogenesis and management. *Retina* 4:97-99, 1984.

74. Willis R, Zimmerman LE, O'Grady R, et al: Heterotopic adipose tissue and smooth muscle in the optic disc; association with isolated colobomas. *Arch Ophthalmol* 88:139-146, 1972.

75. Wise JB, MacLean AL, Gass DM: Contractile peripapillary staphyloma. *Arch Ophthalmol* 75:626-630, 1966.

76. Yedavally S, Frank RN: Peripapillary subretinal neovascularization associated with coloboma of the optic nerve. *Arch Ophthalmol* 111:552-553, 1993.

77. Zinn KM: Bilateral complete colobomas with a unilateral optic pit and recurrent retinal detachment; case report. *Mt Sinai J Med* 46:419-423, 1979.

Optic Disc Hypoplasia and Tilted Disc Syndrome

78. Barroso LHL, Ragge NK, Hoyt WF: Multiple cilioretinal arteries and dysplasia of the optic disc. *J Clin Neuro-Ophthalmol* 11:278-279, 1991.

79. Benner JD, Preslan MW, Gratz E, et al: Septo-optic dysplasia in two siblings. *Am J Ophthalmol* 109:632-637, 1990.

80. Beuchat L, Safran AB: Optic nerve hypoplasia: Papillary diameter and clinical correlation. *J Clin Neuro-Ophthalmol* 5:249-253, 1985.

81. Björk Å, Laurell C-G, Laurell U: Bilateral optic nerve hypoplasia with normal visual acuity. *Am J Ophthalmol* 86:524-529, 1978.

82. Brazitikos PD, Safran AB, Simona F, Zulauf M: Threshold perimetry in tilted disc syndrome. *Arch Ophthalmol* 108:1698-1700, 1990.

83. Brodsky MC, Glasier CM: Optic nerve hypoplasia; clinical significance of associated central nervous system abnormalities on magnetic resonance imaging. *Arch Ophthalmol* 111:66-74, 1993.

84. Brodsky MC, Glasier CM, Pollock SC, Angtuago EJC: Optic nerve hypoplasia; identification by magnetic resonance imaging. *Arch Ophthalmol* 108:1562-1567, 1990.

85. Buchanan TAS, Hoyt WF: Temporal visual field defects associated with nasal hypoplasia of the optic disc. *Br J Ophthalmol* 65:636-640, 1981.

86. Burke JP, O'Keefe M, Bowell R: Optic nerve hypoplasia, encephalopathy, and neurodevelopmental handicap. *Br J Ophthalmol* 75:236-239, 1991.

87. Edwards WC, Layden WE: Optic nerve hypoplasia. *Am J Ophthalmol* 70:950-959, 1970.

88. Frisén L, Holmegaard L: Spectrum of optic nerve hypoplasia. *Br J Ophthalmol* 62:7-15, 1978.

89. Kim RY, Hoyt WF, Lessell S, Narahara MH: Superior segmental optic hypoplasia; a sign of maternal diabetes. *Arch Ophthalmol* 107:1312-1315, 1989.

90. Layman PR, Anderson DR, Flynn JT: Frequent occurrence of hypoplastic optic disks in patients with aniridia. *Am J Ophthalmol* 77:513-516, 1974.

91. Margolis S, Aleksic S, Charles N, et al: Retinal and optic nerve findings in Goldenhar-Gorlin syndrome. *Ophthalmology* 91:1327-1333, 1984.

92. Mosier MA, Lieberman MF, Green WR, Knox DL: Hypoplasia of the optic nerve. *Arch Ophthalmol* 96:1437-1442, 1978.

93. Novakovic P, Taylor DSI, Hoyt WF: Localising patterns of optic nerve hypoplasia — retina to occipital lobe. *Br J Ophthalmol* 72:176-182, 1988.

94. Petersen RA, Holmes L: Optic nerve hypoplasia in infants of diabetic mothers. *Arch Ophthalmol* 104:1587, 1986.

95. Ragge NK, Hoyt WF, Lambert SR: Big discs with optic nerve hypoplasia. *J Clin Neuro-Ophthalmol* 11:137, 1991.

96. Romano PE: Simple photogrammetric diagnosis of optic nerve hypoplasia. *Arch Ophthalmol* 107:824-826, 1989.

97. Sherlock DA, McNicol LR: Anaesthesia and septo-optic dysplasia; implications of missed diagnosis in the perioperative period. *Anaesthesia* 42:1302-1305, 1987.

98. Stur M: Congenital tilted disk syndrome associated with parafoveal subretinal neovascularization. *Am J Ophthalmol* 105:98-99, 1988.

99. Walton DS, Robb RM: Optic nerve hypoplasia; a report of 20 cases. *Arch Ophthalmol* 84:572-578, 1970.

100. Young SE, Walsh FB, Knox DL: The tilted disk syndrome. *Am J Ophthalmol* 82:16-23, 1976.

101. Zeki SM: Optic nerve hypoplasia and astigmatism: a new association. *Br J Ophthalmol* 74:297-299, 1990.

102. Zeki SM: Optic nerve hypoplasia in children. *Br J Ophthalmol* 74:300-304, 1990.

103. Zeki SM, Dudgeon J, Dutton GN: Reappraisal of the ratio of disc to macula/disc diameter in optic nerve hypoplasia. *Br J Ophthalmol* 75:538-541, 1991.

104. Zeki SM, Hollman AS, Dutton GN: Neuroradiological features of patients with optic nerve hypoplasia. *J Pediatr Ophthalmol Strabismus* 29:107-112, 1992.

Drusen (Hyaline Bodies) of the Optic Nerve Head

105. Bec P, Adam P, Mathis A, et al: Optic nerve head drusen; high-resolution computed tomographic approach. *Arch Ophthalmol* 102:680-682, 1984.

106. Boldt HC, Bryne SF, DiBernardo C: Echographic evaluation of optic disc drusen. *J Clin Neuro-Ophthalmol* 11:85-91, 1991.

107. Boyce SW, Platia EV, Green WR: Drusen of the optic nerve head. *Ann Ophthalmol* 10:695-704, 1978.

108. Brodrick JD: Drusen of the disc and retinal haemorrhages. *Br J Ophthalmol* 57:299-306, 1973.

109. Carter JE, Merren MD, Byrne BM: Pseudodrusen of the optic disc; papilledema simulating buried drusen of the optic nerve head. *J Clin Neuro-Ophthalmol* 9:273-276, 1989.

110. Chern S, Magargal LE, Annesley WH: Central retinal vein occlusion associated with drusen of the optic disc. *Ann Ophthalmol* 23:66-69, 1991.

111. Friedman AH, Beckerman B, Gold DH, et al: Drusen of the optic disc. *Surv Ophthalmol* 21:375-390, 1977.

112. Friedman AH, Gartner S, Modi SS: Drusen of the optic disc; a retrospective study in cadaver eyes. *Br J Ophthalmol* 59:413-421, 1975.

113. Friedman AH, Henkind P, Gartner S: Drusen of the optic disc – a histopathological study. *Trans Ophthalmol Soc UK* 95:4-9, 1975.

114. Frisén L, Schöldström G, Svendsen P: Drusen in the optic nerve head; verification by computerized tomography. *Arch Ophthalmol* 96:1611-1614, 1978.

115. Gartner S: Drusen of the optic disk in retinitis pigmentosa. *Am J Ophthalmol* 103:845, 1987.

116. Gass JDM: Diseases of the optic nerve that may simulate macular disease. *Trans Am Acad Ophthalmol Otolaryngol* 83:OP763-OP770, 1977.

117. Gass JDM: *Stereoscopic atlas of macular diseases; diagnosis and treatment,* ed. 2, St. Louis, 1977, CV Mosby, p. 372.

118. Gittinger JW Jr, Lessell S, Bondar RL: Ischemic optic neuropathy associated with optic disc drusen. *J Clin Neuro-Ophthalmol* 4:79-84, 1984.

119. Harris MJ, Fine SL, Owens SL: Hemorrhagic complications of optic nerve drusen. *Am J Ophthalmol* 92:70-76, 1981.

120. Hitchings RA, Corbett JJ, Winkleman J, Schatz NJ: Hemorrhages with optic nerve drusen; a differentiation from early papilledema. *Arch Neurol* 33:675-677, 1976.

121. Hogan MJ, Zimmerman LE: *Ophthalmic pathology; an atlas and textbook,* ed. 2, Philadelphia, 1962, WB Saunders, p. 580.

122. Hoover DL, Robb RM, Petersen RA: Optic disc drusen and primary megalencephaly in children. *J Pediatr Ophthalmol Strabismus* 26:81-85, 1989.

123. Hoyt WF, Pont ME: Pseudopapilledema: anomalous elevation of the optic disk; pitfalls in diagnosis and management. *JAMA* 181:191-196, 1962.

124. Jonas JB, Gusek GC, Guggenmoos-Holzmann I, Naumann GOH: Optic nerve head drusen associated with abnormally small optic discs. *Int Ophthalmol* 11:79-82, 1987.

125. Kamin DF, Hepler RS, Foos RY: Optic nerve drusen. *Arch Ophthalmol* 89:359-362, 1973.

126. Karel I, Otradovec J, Peleška M: Fluorescence angiography in circulatory disturbances in drusen of the optic disk. *Ophthalmologica* 164:449-462, 1972.

127. Kelley JS: Autofluorescence of drusen of the optic nerve head. *Arch Ophthalmol* 92:263-264, 1974.

128. Kelley JS, Hoover RE, Robin A, Kincaid M: Laser scotometry in drusen and pits of the optic nerve head. *Ophthalmology* 86:442-447, 1979.

129. Knight CL, Hoyt WF: Monocular blindness from drusen of the optic disk. *Am J Ophthalmol* 73:890-892, 1972.

130. Lansche RK, Rucker CW: Progression of defects in visual fields produced by hyaline bodies in optic disks. *Arch Ophthalmol* 58:115-121, 1957.

131. Michaelson C, Behrens M, Odel J: Bilateral anterior ischaemic optic neuropathy associated with optic disc drusen and systemic hypotension. *Br J Ophthalmol* 73:762-764, 1989.

132. Moisseiev J, Cahane M, Treister G: Optic nerve head drusen and peripapillary central serous chorioretinopathy. *Am J Ophthalmol* 108:202-203, 1989.

133. Moody TA, Irvine AR, Cahn PH, et al: Sudden visual field constriction associated with optic disc drusen. *J Clin Neuro-Ophthalmol* 13:8-13, 1993.

134. Mooney D: Bilateral haemorrhages associated with disc drusen. *Trans Ophthalmol Soc UK* 93:739-743, 1973.

135. Mullie MA, Sanders MD: Scleral canal size and optic nerve head drusen. *Am J Ophthalmol* 99:356-359, 1985.

136. Newman NJ, Lessell S, Brandt EM: Bilateral central retinal artery occlusions, disk drusen, and migraine. *Am J Ophthalmol* 107:236-240, 1989.

137. Pietruschka G, Priess G: Zur klinischen Bedeutung und Prognose der Drusenpapille. *Klin Monatsbl Augenheilkd* 162:331-341, 1973.

138. Purcell JJ Jr, Goldberg RE: Hyaline bodies of the optic papilla and bilateral acute vascular occlusions. *Ann Ophthalmol* 6:1069-1076, 1974.

139. Reifler DM, Kaufman DI: Optic disk drusen and pseudotumor cerebri. *Am J Ophthalmol* 106:95-96, 1988.

140. Rosenberg MA, Savino PJ, Glaser JS: A clinical analysis of pseudopapilledema. I. Population, laterality, acuity, refractive error, ophthalmoscopic characteristics, and coincident disease. *Arch Ophthalmol* 97:65-70, 1979.

141. Rubinstein K, Ali M: Retinal complications of optic disc drusen. *Br J Ophthalmol* 66:83-95, 1982.

142. Rucker CW: Defects in visual fields produced by hyaline bodies in the optic disks. *Arch Ophthalmol* 32:56-59, 1944.

143. Sacks JG, O'Grady RB, Choromokos E, Leestma J: The pathogenesis of optic nerve drusen; a hypothesis. *Arch Ophthalmol* 95:425-428, 1977.

144. Sadun AA, Green RL, Nobe JR, Cano MR: Papillopathies associated with unusual calcifications in the retrolaminar optic nerve. *J Clin Neuro-Ophthalmol* 11:175-180, 1991.

145. Sanders MD, Ffytche TJ: Fluorescein angiography in the diagnosis of drusen of the disc. *Trans Ophthalmol Soc UK* 87:457-468, 1967.

146. Sanders TE, Gay AJ, Newman M: Hemorrhagic complications of drusen of the optic disk. *Am J Ophthalmol* 71:204-217, 1971.

147. Sarkies NJ, Sanders MD: Optic disc drusen and episodic visual loss. *Br J Ophthalmol* 71:537-539, 1987.

148. Scholl GB, Song H-S, Winkler DE, Wray SH: The pattern visual evoked potential and pattern electroretinogram in drusen-associated optic neuropathy. *Arch Ophthalmol* 110:75-81, 1992.

149. Spencer WH: Drusen of the optic disc and aberrant axoplasmic transport. *Am J Ophthalmol* 85:1-12, 1978.

150. Stevens RA, Newman NM: Abnormal visual-evoked potentials from eyes with optic nerve head drusen. *Am J Ophthalmol* 92:857-862, 1981.

151. Tso MOM: Pathology and pathogenesis of drusen of the optic nervehead. *Ophthalmology* 88:1066-1080, 1981.

152. Walsh FB, Hoyt WF: *Clinical neuro-ophthalmology,* ed. 3, Baltimore, 1974, Williams & Wilkins, p. 673.

153. Wilhelm JL, Gutman FA: Macular choroidal neovascular membrane with bilateral optic nerve drusen: case report. *Ann Ophthalmol* 15:48-51, 1983.

154. Wise GN, Henkind P, Alterman M: Optic disc drusen and subretinal hemorrhage. *Trans Am Acad Ophthalmol Otolaryngol* 78:OP212-OP219, 1974.

Hereditary Optic Neuropathies

155. Berninger TA, Jaeger W, Krastel H: Electrophysiology and colour perimetry in dominant infantile optic atrophy. *Br J Ophthalmol* 75:49-52, 1991.

156. Berninger TA, von Meyer L, Siess E, et al: Leber's hereditary optic atrophy: Further evidence for a defect of cyanide metabolism? *Br J Ophthalmol* 73:314-316, 1989.

157. Borruat F-X, Green WT, Graham EM, et al: Late onset Leber's optic neuropathy: a case confused with ischaemic optic neuropathy. *Br J Ophthalmol* 76:571-573, 1992.
158. Caldwell JBH, Howard RO, Riggs LA: Dominant juvenile optic atrophy; a study in two families and review of hereditary disease in childhood. *Arch Ophthalmol* 85:133-147, 1971.
159. de Gottrau P, Büchi ER, Daicker B: Distended optic nerve sheaths in Leber's hereditary optic neuropathy. *J Clin Neuro-Ophthalmol* 12:89-93, 1992.
160. Eliott D, Traboulsi EI, Maumenee IH: Visual prognosis in autosomal dominant optic atrophy (Kjer type). *Am J Ophthalmol* 115:360-367, 1993.
161. Glaser JS: Heredofamilial disorders of the optic nerve. *In:* Goldberg MF, editor: *Genetic and metabolic eye disease,* Boston, 1974, Little, Brown & Co, pp. 463-486.
162. Jacobson DM, Stone EM: Difficulty differentiating Leber's from dominant optic neuropathy in a patient with remote visual loss. *J Clin Neuro-Ophthalmol* 11:152-157, 1991.
163. Johns DR: The molecular genetics of Leber's hereditary optic neuropathy. *Arch Ophthalmol* 108:1405-1406, 1990.
164. Johns DR, Heher KL, Miller NR, Smith KH: Leber's hereditary optic neuropathy; clinical manifestations of the 14484 mutation. *Arch Ophthalmol* 111:495-498, 1993.
165. Johns DR, Smith KH, Miller NR: Leber's hereditary optic neuropathy; clinical manifestations of the 3460 mutation. *Arch Ophthalmol* 110:1577-1581, 1992.
166. Johns DR, Smith KH, Savino PJ, Miller NR: Leber's hereditary optic neuropathy; clinical manifestations of the 15257 mutation. *Ophthalmology* 100:981-986, 1993.
167. Kjer P: Infantile optic atrophy with dominant mode of inheritance; a clinical and genetic study of 19 Danish families. *Acta Ophthalmol Suppl* 54, 1959.
168. Kline LB, Glaser JS: Dominant optic atrophy; the clinical profile. *Arch Ophthalmol* 97:1680-1686, 1979.
169. Krill AE, Smith VC, Pokorny J: Further studies supporting the identity of congenital tritanopia and hereditary dominant optic atrophy. *Invest Ophthalmol* 10:457-465, 1971.
170. Leber T: Ueber hereditäre und congenital-angelegte Sehnervenleiden. *Albrecht von Graefes Arch Ophthalmol* 17(2):249-291, 1871.
171. Lopez PF, Smith JL: Leber's optic neuropathy; new observations. *J Clin Neuro-Ophthalmol* 6:144-152, 1986.
172. Lott MT, Voljavec AS, Wallace DC: Variable genotype of Leber's hereditary optic neuropathy patients. *Am J Ophthalmol* 109:625-631, 1990.
173. Manchester PT Jr, Calhoun FP Jr: Dominant hereditary optic atrophy with bitemporal field defects. *Arch Ophthalmol* 60:479-484, 1958.
174. McCluskey DAJ, O'Connor PS, Sheehy JT: Leber's optic neuropathy and Charcot-Marie-Tooth disease; report of a case. *J Clin Neuro-Ophthalmol* 6:76-81, 1986.
175. McLeod JG, Low PA, Morgan JA: Charcot-Marie-Tooth disease with Leber optic atrophy. *Neurology* 28:179-184, 1978.
176. Miller NR: *Walsh and Hoyt's clinical neuro-ophthalmology,* ed. 4, Baltimore, 1982, Williams and Wilkins, vol. 1, pp. 212-226.
177. Newman NJ, Lott MT, Wallace DC: The clinical characteristics of pedigrees of Leber's hereditary optic neuropathy with the 11778 mutation. *Am J Ophthalmol* 111:750-762, 1991.
178. Newman NJ, Wallace DC: Mitochondria and Leber's hereditary optic neuropathy. *Am J Ophthalmol* 109:726-730, 1990.
179. Nikoskelainen E, Hoyt WF, Nummelin K: Ophthalmoscopic findings in Leber's hereditary optic neuropathy. I. Fundus findings in asymptomatic family members. *Arch Ophthalmol* 100:1597-1602, 1982.
180. Nikoskelainen E, Hoyt WF, Nummelin K: Ophthalmoscopic findings in Leber's hereditary optic neuropathy. II. The fundus findings in the affected family members. *Arch Ophthalmol* 101:1059-1068, 1983.
181. Nikoskelainen E, Hoyt WF, Nummelin K, Schatz H: Fundus findings in Leber's hereditary optic neuroretinopathy. III. Fluorescein angiographic studies. *Arch Ophthalmol* 102:981-989, 1984.
182. Nikoskelainen E, Sogg RL, Rosenthal AR, et al: The early phase in Leber hereditary optic atrophy. *Arch Ophthalmol* 95:969-978, 1977.
183. Nikoskelainen EK, Savontaus M-L, Wanne OP, et al: Leber's hereditary optic neuroretinopathy, a maternally inherited disease; a genealogic study in four pedigrees. *Arch Ophthalmol* 105:665-671, 1987.
184. Ortiz RG, Newman NJ, Manoukian SV, et al: Optic disk cupping and electrocardiographic abnormalities in an American pedigree with Leber's hereditary optic neuropathy. *Am J Ophthalmol* 113:561-566, 1992.
185. Singh G, Lott MT, Wallace DC: A mitochondrial DNA mutation as a cause of Leber's hereditary optic neuropathy. *N Engl J Med* 320:1300-1305, 1989.
186. Smith JL, Hoyt WF, Susac JO: Ocular fundus in acute Leber optic neuropathy. *Arch Ophthalmol* 90:349-354, 1973.
187. Smith JL, Tse DT, Bryne SF, et al: Optic nerve sheath distention in Leber's optic neuropathy and the significance of the "Wallace mutation." *J Clin Neuro-Ophthalmol* 10:231-238, 1990.
188. Stehouwer A, Oosterhuis JA, Renger-van Dijk AH, Went LN: Leber's optic neuropathy. II. Fluorescein angiographic studies. *Doc Ophthalmol* 53:113-122, 1982.
189. Stone EM, Newman NJ, Miller NR, et al: Visual recovery in patients with Leber's hereditary optic neuropathy and the 11778 mutation. *J Clin Neuro-Ophthalmol* 12:10-14, 1992.
190. Uemura A, Osame M, Nakagawa M, et al: Leber's hereditary optic neuropathy: mitochondrial and biochemical studies on muscle biopsies. *Br J Ophthalmol* 71:531-536, 1987.
191. van Heuven GJ: Die Diagnose der hereditären Leberschen Sehnervenatrophie (abstract). *Klin Monatsbl Augenheilkd* 73:252-253, 1924.
192. Wallace DC, Singh G, Lott MT, et al: Mitochondrial DNA mutation associated with Leber's hereditary optic neuropathy. *Science* 242:1427-1430, 1988.
193. Weleber RG, Miyake Y: Familial optic atrophy with negative electroretinograms. *Arch Ophthalmol* 110:640-645, 1992.

Leber's Idiopathic Stellate Neuroretinitis and Multifocal Retinitus

194. Bar S, Segal M, Shapira R, Savir H: Neuroretinitis associated with cat scratch disease. *Am J Ophthalmol* 110:703-705, 1990.
195. Brazis PW, Stokes HR, Ervin FR: Optic neuritis in cat scratch disease. *J Clin Neuro-Ophthalmol* 6:172-174, 1986.
196. Carithers HA, Margileth AM: Cat-scratch disease; acute encephalopathy and other neurologic manifestations. *Am J Dis Child* 145:98-101, 1991.
197. Carroll DM, Franklin RM: Leber's idiopathic stellate retinopathy. *Am J Ophthalmol* 93:96-101, 1982.
198. Chrousos GA, Drack AV, Young M, et al: Neuroretinitis in cat scratch disease. *J Clin Neuro-Ophthalmol* 10:92-94, 1990.
199. Dreyer RF, Hopen G, Gass JDM, Smith JL: Leber's idiopathic stellate neuroretinitis. *Arch Ophthalmol* 102:1140-1145, 1984.
200. Fish RH, Hogan RN, Nightingale SD, Anand R: Peripapillary angiomatosis associated with cat-scratch neuroretinitis. *Arch Ophthalmol* 110:323, 1992.
201. Foster RE, Gutman FA, Meyers SM, Lowder CY: Acute multifocal inner retinitis. *Am J Ophthalmol* 111:673-681, 1991.

202. François J, Verriest G, De Laey JJ: Leber's idiopathic stellate retinopathy. *Am J Ophthalmol* 68:340-345, 1969.
203. Gass JDM: Fluorescein angiography in endogenous intraocular inflammation. *In:* Aronson SB, Gamble CN, Goodner EK, O'Connor GR, editors: *Clinical methods in uveitis: the Fourth Sloan Symposium on Uveitis.* St. Louis, 1968, CV Mosby, pp. 214-215.
204. Gass JDM: *Stereoscopic atlas of macular diseases; diagnosis and treatment,* ed. 2, St. Louis, 1977, CV Mosby, p. 376.
205. Gass JDM: *Stereoscopic atlas of macular diseases; diagnosis and treatment,* ed. 3, St. Louis, 1987, CV Mosby, pp. 748-749.
206. Glaser JS: Topical diagnosis: prechiasmal visual pathways. *In:* Glaser JS, editor: *Neuro-ophthalmology,* ed. 2, Philadelphia, 1990, JB Lippincott, p. 126.
207. Goldstein BG, Pavan PR: Retinal infiltrates in six patients with an associated viral syndrome. *Retina* 5:144-150, 1985.
208. Leber T: Die pseudonephritischen Netzhauterkrankungen, die Retinitis stellata; die Purtschersche Netzhautaffektion nach schwerer Schädelverletzung. *In:* Graefe AC, Saemisch T, editors: *Graefe-Saemisch Handbuch der Augenheilkunde,* ed. 2, Leipzig, 1916, Englemann, vol. 7, pt. 2, ch. 10, pp. 1349-1339.
209. Lesser RL, Kornmehl EW, Pachner AR, et al: Neuro-ophthalmologic manifestations of Lyme disease. *Ophthalmology* 97:699-706, 1990.
210. Maitland CG, Miller NR: Neuroretinitis. *Arch Ophthalmol* 102:1146-1150, 1984.
211. Miller NR: *Walsh and Hoyt's clinical neuro-ophthalmology,* ed. 4, Baltimore, 1982, Williams & Wilkins, vol. 1, p. 234.
212. Papastratigakis B, Stavrakas E, Phanouriakis C, Tsamparlakis J: Leber's idiopathic stellate maculopathy. *Ophthalmologica* 183:68-71, 1981.
213. Purvin VA, Chioran G: Recurrent neuroretinitis. *Arch Ophthalmol* 112:365-371, 1994.
214. Ulrich GG, Waecker NJ Jr, Meister SJ, et al: Cat scratch disease associated with neuroretinitis in a 6-year-old girl. *Ophthalmology* 99:246-249, 1992.
215. Weiss AH, Beck RW: Neuroretinitis in childhood. *J Pediatr Ophthalmol* 26:198-203, 1989.

Neuroretinopathy and Progressive Facial Hemiatrophy

216. Garcher C, Humbert P, Bron A, et al: Neuropathie optique et syndrome de Parry-Romberg. A propos d'un cas. *J Fr Ophtalmol* 13:557-561, 1990.
217. Gass JDM: *Differential diagnosis of intraocular tumors; a stereoscopic presentation,* St. Louis, 1974, CV Mosby, p. 256.
218. Gass JDM, Harbin TS Jr, Del Piero EJ: Exudative stellate neuroretinopathy and Coats' syndrome in patients with progressive hemifacial atrophy. *Eur J Ophthalmol* 1:2-10, 1991.
219. Josten K: Sclérodermie en coup de sabre und Auge. *Klin Monatsbl Augenheilkd* 133:567-570, 1958.
220. Meunier A, Toussaint D: Sclérodermie en "coup de sabre" avec lesion du fond d'oeil. *Bull Soc Belge Ophtalmol* 118(2): 369-377, 1958.
221. Parry CH: *Collections from the unpublished medical writings of the late Caleb Hillier Parry, M.D., F.R.S.,* vol. 1, London, 1825, Underwoods, p. 478.
222. Romberg MH: *Klinishe Ergebnisse,* Berlin, 1846, A. Forstner, p. 75.
223. Wartenberg R: Progressive facial hemiatrophy. *Arch Neurol Psychiatr* 54:75-96, 1945.

Anterior Ischemic Optic Neuropathy

224. Aiello AL, Sadun AA, Feldon SE: Spontaneous improvement of progressive anterior ischemic optic neuropathy: report of two cases. *Arch Ophthalmol* 110:1197-1199, 1992.

225. Aiello PD, Trautmann JC, McPhee TJ, et al: Visual prognosis in giant cell arteritis. *Ophthalmology* 100:550-555, 1993.
226. Albert DM, Searl SS, Craft JL: Histologic and ultrastructural characteristics of temporal arteritis; the value of the temporal artery biopsy. *Ophthalmology* 89:1111-1126, 1982.
227. Arnold AC, Hepler RS: Fluorescein angiography in acute nonarteritic anterior ischemic optic neuropathy. *Am J Ophthalmol* 117:220-230, 1994.
228. Barrett DA, Glaser JS, Schatz NJ, Winterkorn JMS: Spontaneous recovery of vision in progressive anterior ischemic optic neuropathy. *J Clin Neuro-Ophthalmol* 12:219-225, 1992.
229. Beck RW, Gamel JW, Willcourt RJ, Berman G: Acute ischemic optic neuropathy in severe preeclampsia. *Am J Ophthalmol* 90:342-346, 1980.
230. Beck RW, Savino PJ, Repka MX, et al: Optic disc structure in anterior ischemic optic neuropathy. *Ophthalmology* 91:1334-1337, 1984.
231. Beck RW, Servais GE, Hayreh SS: Anterior ischemic optic neuropathy. IX. Cup-to-disc ratio and its role in pathogenesis. *Ophthalmology* 94:1503-1508, 1987.
232. Beri M, Klugman MR, Kohler JA, Hayreh SS: Anterior ischemic optic neuropathy. VII. Incidence of bilaterality and various influencing factors. *Ophthalmology* 94:1020-1028, 1987.
233. Boghen DR, Glaser JS: Ischaemic optic neuropathy; the clinical profile and natural history. *Brain* 98:689-708, 1975.
234. Borchert M, Lessell S: Progressive and recurrent nonarteritic anterior ischemic optic neuropathy. *Am J Ophthalmol* 106: 443-449, 1988.
235. Brittain GPH, McIlwaine GG, Bell JA, Gibson JM: Plasma viscosity or erythrocyte sedimentation rate in the diagnosis of giant cell arteritis. *Br J Ophthalmol* 75:656-659, 1991.
236. Brown GC: Anterior ischemic optic neuropathy occurring in association with carotid artery obstruction. *J Clin Neuro-Ophthalmol* 6:39-42, 1986.
237. Burde RM: Optic disk risk factors for nonarteritic anterior ischemic optic neuropathy. *Am J Ophthalmol* 116:759-764, 1993.
238. Chung SM, Gay CA, McCrary JA III: Nonarteritic ischemic optic neuropathy; the impact of tobacco use. *Ophthalmology* 101:779-782, 1994.
239. Deutsch D, Eting E, Avisar R, et al: Familial anterior ischemic optic neuropathy and papillophlebitis. *Am J Ophthalmol* 110:306-308, 1990.
240. Eagling EM, Sanders MD, Miller SJH: Ischaemic papillopathy; clinical and fluorescein angiographic review of forty cases. *Br J Ophthalmol* 58:990-1008, 1974.
241. Ellenberger C Jr: Ischemic optic neuropathy as a possible early complication of vascular hypertension. *Am J Ophthalmol* 88:1045-1051, 1979.
242. Ellenberger C Jr, Keltner JL, Burde RM: Acute optic neuropathy in older patients. *Arch Neurol* 28:182-185, 1973.
243. Eshaghian J, Goeken JA: C-reactive protein in giant cell (cranial, temporal) arteritis. *Ophthalmology* 87:1160-1166, 1980.
244. Feit RH, Tomsak RL, Ellenberger C Jr: Structural factors in the pathogenesis of ischemic optic neuropathy. *Am J Ophthalmol* 98:105-108, 1984.
245. Flaharty PM, Sergott RC, Lieb W, et al: Optic nerve sheath decompression may improve blood flow in anterior ischemic optic neuropathy. *Ophthalmology* 100:297-305, 1993.
246. Fry CL, Carter JE, Kanter MC, et al: Anterior ischemic optic neuropathy is not associated with carotid artery atherosclerosis. *Stroke* 24:539-542, 1993.
247. Gartner S: Optic neuritis and macular edema following cataract extraction. *Eye Ear Nose Throat Month* 43(2):45-49, 1964.

248. Gass D: Ischemic optic neuropathy in aphakia (and phakia). *In:* Welsh RC, Welsh J, editors: *The new report on cataract surgery; proceedings of the first-biennial Cataract Surgical Congress, Miami Beach,* Miami, 1969, Miami Educational Press, pp. 84-86.

249. Giuffrè G, Brancato G: Subretinal neovascularization in anterior ischemic optic neuropathy. *Graefes Arch Clin Exp Ophthalmol* 229:19-23, 1991.

250. Glaser JS, Teimory M, Schatz NJ: Optic nerve sheath fenestration for progressive ischemic optic neuropathy; results in second series consisting of 21 eyes. *Arch Ophthalmol* 112:1047-1050, 1994.

251. Golnik KC, Newman SA: Anterior ischemic optic neuropathy associated with macrocytic anemia. *J Clin Neuro-Ophthalmol* 10:244-247, 1990.

252. Hamed LM, Purvin V, Rosenberg M: Recurrent anterior ischemic optic neuropathy in young adults. *J Clin Neuro-Ophthalmol* 8:239-246, 1988.

253. Hamed LM, Winward KE, Glaser JS, Schatz NJ: Optic neuropathy in uremia. *Am J Ophthalmol* 108:30-35, 1989.

254. Hayreh SS: Anterior ischemic optic neuropathy. IV. Occurrence after cataract extraction. *Arch Ophthalmol* 98:1410-1416, 1980.

255. Hayreh SS: Anterior ischemic optic neuropathy. V. Optic disc edema an early sign. *Arch Ophthalmol* 99:1030-1040, 1981.

256. Hayreh SS: Anterior ischemic optic neuropathy. VIII. Clinical features and pathogenesis of post-hemorrhagic amaurosis. *Ophthalmology* 94:1488-1502, 1987.

257. Hayreh SS: The role of optic nerve sheath fenestration in management of anterior ischemic optic neuropathy. *Arch Ophthalmol* 108:1063-1064, 1990.

258. Ischemic Optic Neuropathy Decompression Trial Research Group: Optic nerve decompression surgery for nonarteritic anterior ischemic optic neuropathy (NAION) is not effective and may be harmful. *JAMA* 273:625-632, 1995.

259. Jablons MM, Glaser JS, Schatz NJ, et al: Optic nerve sheath fenestration for treatment of progressive ischemic optic neuropathy; results in 26 patients. *Arch Ophthalmol* 111:84-87, 1993.

260. Jaffe G, Schatz H: Ocular manifestations of preeclampsia. *Am J Ophthalmol* 103:309-315, 1987.

261. Johnson LN, Arnold AC: Incidence of nonarteritic and arteritic ischemic optic neuropathy; population-based study in the state of Missouri and Los Angeles County, California. *J Neuro-Ophthalmol* 14:38-44, 1994.

262. Johnson LN, Kuo HC, Arnold AC: HLA-A29 as a potential risk factor for nonarteritic anterior ischemic optic neuropathy. *Am J Ophthalmol* 115:540-542, 1993.

263. Johnson MW, Kincaid MC, Trobe JD: Bilateral retrobulbar optic nerve infarctions after blood loss and hypotension; a clinicopathologic case study. *Ophthalmology* 94:1577-1584, 1987.

264. Josef JM, Burde RM: Editorial: Ischemic optic neuropathy of the young. *J Clin Neuro-Ophthalmol* 8:247-248, 1988.

265. Kalenak JW, Kosmorsky GS, Rockwood EJ: Nonarteritic anterior ischemic optic neuropathy and intraocular pressure. *Arch Ophthalmol* 109:660-661, 1991.

266. Katz B, Spencer WH: Hyperopia as a risk factor for nonarteritic anterior ischemic optic neuropathy. *Am J Ophthalmol* 116:754-758, 1993.

267. Katz B, Weinreb RN, Wheeler DT, Klauber MR: Anterior ischaemic optic neuropathy and intraocular pressure. *Br J Ophthalmol* 74:99-102, 1990.

268. Keltner JL: Giant-cell arteritis; signs and symptoms. *Ophthalmology* 89:1101-1110, 1982.

269. Kline LB: Progression of visual defects in ischemic optic neuropathy. *Am J Ophthalmol* 106:199-203, 1988.

270. Knox DL, Hanneken AM, Hollows FC, et al: Uremic optic neuropathy. *Arch Ophthalmol* 106:50-54, 1988.

271. Lavin PJM, Ellenberger C Jr: Recurrent ischemic optic neuropathy. *Neuro-Ophthalmol* 3:193-198, 1983.

272. Lieberman MF, Shahi A, Green WR: Embolic ischemic optic neuropathy. *Am J Ophthalmol* 86:206-210, 1978.

273. Mack HG, O'Day J, Currie JN: Delayed choroidal perfusion in giant cell arteritis. *J Clin Neuro-Ophthalmol* 11:221-227, 1991.

274. Mansour AM, Shoch D, Logani S: Optic disk size in ischemic optic neuropathy. *Am J Ophthalmol* 106:587-589, 1988.

275. McHenry JG, Spoor TC: The efficacy of optic nerve sheath decompression for anterior ischemic optic neuropathy and other optic neuropathies. *Am J Ophthalmol* 116:254-255, 1993.

276. Michaelson C, Behrens M, Odel J: Bilateral anterior ischaemic optic neuropathy associated with optic disc drusen and systemic hypotension. *Br J Ophthalmol* 73:762-764, 1989.

277. Naumann GOH, Jonas J: Optic disk size in ischemic optic neuropathy. *Am J Ophthalmol* 107:685, 1989.

278. Plotnik JL, Kosmorsky GS: Operative complications of optic nerve sheath decompression. *Ophthalmology* 100:683-690, 1993.

279. Portnoy SL, Beer PM, Packer AJ, Van Dyk HJL: Embolic anterior ischemic optic neuropathy. *J Clin Neuro-Ophthalmol* 9:21-25, 1989.

280. Quigley HA, Miller NR, Green WR: The pattern of optic nerve fiber loss in anterior ischemic optic neuropathy. *Am J Ophthalmol* 100:769-776, 1985.

281. Repka MX, Savino PJ, Schatz NJ, Sergott RC: Clinical profile and long-term implications of anterior ischemic optic neuropathy. *Am J Ophthalmol* 96:478-483, 1983.

282. Rizzo JF III, Lessell S: Optic neuritis and ischemic optic neuropathy; overlapping clinical profiles. *Arch Ophthalmol* 109:1668-1672, 1991.

283. Sadun AA: The efficacy of optic nerve sheath decompression for anterior ischemic optic neuropathy and other optic neuropathies. *Am J Ophthalmol* 115:384-389, 1993.

284. Schmidt D, Richter T, von Reutern G-M, Engelhardt R: Akute Durchblutungsstörungen des Auges; Klinische Befunde und Ergebnisse der Doppler-Sonographie der A. carotis Interna. *Fortsch Ophthalmol* 88:84-98, 1991.

285. Sergott RC, Cohen MS, Bosley TM, Savino PJ: Optic nerve decompression may improve the progressive form of nonarteritic ischemic optic neuropathy. *Arch Ophthalmol* 107:1743-1754, 1989.

286. Siatkowski RM, Gass JDM, Glaser JS, et al: Fluorescein angiography in the diagnosis of giant cell arteritis. *Am J Ophthalmol* 115:57-63, 1993.

287. Smith JL: Pseudohemangioma of the optic disc following ischemic optic neuropathy. *J Clin Neuro-Ophthalmol* 5:81-89, 1985.

288. Spedick MJ, Tomsak RL: Ischemic optic neuropathy following secondary intraocular lens implantation. *J Clin Neuro-Ophthalmol* 4:255-257, 1984.

289. Spoor TC, McHenry JG, Lau-Sickon L: Progressive and static nonarteritic ischemic optic neuropathy treated by optic nerve sheath decompression. *Ophthalmology* 100:306-311, 1993.

290. Spoor TC, Wilkinson MJ, Ramocki JM: Optic nerve sheath decompression for the treatment of progressive nonarteritic ischemic optic neuropathy. *Am J Ophthalmol* 111:724-728, 1991.

291. Tomsak RL: Ischemic optic neuropathy associated with retinal embolism. *Am J Ophthalmol* 99:590-592, 1985.

292. Tomsak RL, Remler BF: Anterior ischemic optic neuropathy and increased intraocular pressure. *J Clin Neuro-Ophthalmol* 9:116-118, 1989.

293. Traustason OI, Feldon SE, Leemaster JE, Weiner JM: Anterior ischemic optic neuropathy: classification of field defects by Octopus™ automated static perimetry. *Graefes Arch Clin Exp Ophthalmol* 226:206-212, 1988.

294. Wall M, Newman SA: Optic nerve sheath decompression for the treatment of progressive nonarteritic ischemic optic neuropathy. *Am J Ophthalmol* 112:741, 1991.

Idiopathic Optic Neuritis and Papillitis

295. Beck RW, Cleary PA, Trobe JD, et al: The effect of corticosteroids for acute optic neuritis on the subsequent development of multiple sclerosis; the Optic Neuritis Study Group. *N Engl J Med* 329:1764-1769, 1993.

296. Beck RW, Optic Neuritis Study Group: Editorial: The optic neuritis treatment trial; implications for clinical practice. *Arch Ophthalmol* 110:331-332, 1992.

297. Keltner JL, Johnson CA, Spurr JO, et al: Visual field profile of optic neuritis; one-year follow-up in the Optic Neuritis Treatment Trial. *Arch Ophthalmol* 112:946-953, 1994.

298. Optic Neuritis Study Group: The clinical profile of optic neuritis; experience of the Optic Neuritis Treatment Trial. *Arch Ophthalmol* 109:1673-1678, 1991.

299. Parmeley C, Schiffman JS, Maitland CG, et al: Does neuroretinitis rule out multiple sclerosis? *Arch Neurol* 44:1045-1048, 1987.

300. Trobe JD: High-dose corticosteroid regimen retards development of multiple sclerosis in optic neuritis treatment trial. *Arch Ophthalmol* 112:35-36, 1994.

Traumatic Optic Neuropathy

301. Kline LB, Morawetz RB, Swaid NS: Indirect injury of the optic nerve. *Neurosurgery* 14:756-764, 1984.

302. Lessell S: Indirect optic nerve trauma. *Arch Ophthalmol* 107:382-386, 1989.

303. Spoor TC, Hartel WC, Lensink DB, Wilkinson MJ: Treatment of traumatic optic neuropathy with corticosteroids. *Am J Ophthalmol* 110:665-669, 1990 (Correction 111:526, 1991).

304. Wolin MJ, Lavin PJM: Spontaneous visual recovery from traumatic optic neuropathy after blunt head injury. *Am J Ophthalmol* 109:430-435, 1990.

Optic Nerve Meningiomas

305. Alper MG: Management of primary optic nerve meningiomas; current status—therapy in controversy. *J Clin Neuro-Ophthalmol* 1:101-117, 1981.

306. Boschetti NV, Smith JL, Osher RH, et al: Fluorescein angiography of optociliary shunt vessels. *J Clin Neuro-Ophthalmol* 1:9-30, 1981.

307. Cibis GW, Whittaker CK, Wood WE: Intraocular extension of optic nerve meningioma in a case of neurofibromatosis. *Arch Ophthalmol* 103:404-406, 1985.

308. Cunliffe IA, Moffat DA, Hardy DG, Moore AT: Bilateral optic nerve sheath meningiomas in a patient with neurofibromatosis type 2. *Br J Ophthalmol* 76:310-312, 1992.

309. Dowhan TP, Muci-Mendoza R, Aitken PA: Disappearing optociliary shunt vessels and neonatal hydrocephalus. *J Clin Neuro-Ophthalmol* 8:1-8, 1988.

310. Dunn SN, Walsh FB: Meningioma (dural endothelioma) of the optic nerve; report of a case. *Arch Ophthalmol* 56:702-707, 1956.

311. Dutton JJ: Optic nerve sheath meningiomas. *Surv Ophthalmol* 37:167-183, 1992.

312. Dutton JJ, Anderson RL: Idiopathic inflammatory perioptic neuritis simulating optic nerve sheath meningioma. *Am J Ophthalmol* 100:424-430, 1985.

313. Frisén L, Hoyt WF, Tengroth BM: Optociliary veins, disc pallor and visual loss; a triad of signs indicating spheno-orbital meningioma. *Acta Ophthalmol* 51:241-249, 1973.

314. Hannesson OB: Primary meningioma of the orbit invading the choroid; report of a case. *Acta Ophthalmol* 49:627-632, 1971.

315. Hart WM Jr, Burde RM, Klingele TG, Perlmutter JC: Bilateral optic nerve sheath meningiomas. *Arch Ophthalmol* 98:149-151, 1980.

316. Hollenhorst RW Jr, Hollenhorst RW Sr, MacCarty CS: Visual prognosis of optic nerve sheath meningiomas producing shunt vessels on the optic disk; the Hoyt-Spencer syndrome. *Mayo Clin Proc* 53:8-92, 1978; also *Trans Am Ophthalmol Soc* 75:141-163, 1977.

317. Imes RK, Schatz H, Hoyt WF, et al: Evolution of optociliary veins in optic nerve sheath meningioma; evolution. *Arch Ophthalmol* 103:59-60, 1985.

318. Karp LA, Zimmerman LE, Borit A, Spencer W: Primary intraorbital meningiomas. *Arch Ophthalmol* 91:24-28, 1974.

319. Kennerdell JS, Maroon JC, Malton M, Warren FA: The management of optic nerve sheath meningiomas. *Am J Ophthalmol* 106:450-457, 1988.

320. Lindblom B, Truwit CL, Hoyt WF: Optic nerve sheath meningioma; Definition of intraorbital, intracanalicular, and intracranial components with magnetic resonance imaging. *Ophthalmology* 99:560-566, 1992.

321. Mark LE, Kennerdell JS, Maroon JC, et al: Microsurgical removal of a primary intraorbital meningioma. *Am J Ophthalmol* 86:704-709, 1978.

322. McNab AA, Wright JE: Cysts of the optic nerve three cases associated with meningioma. *Eye* 3:355-359, 1989.

323. Samples JR, Robertson DM, Taylor JZ, Waller RR: Optic nerve meningioma. *Ophthalmology* 90:1591-1594, 1983.

324. Schatz H, Green WR, Talamo JH, et al: Clinicopathologic correlation of retinal to choroidal venous collaterals of the optic nerve head. *Ophthalmology* 98:1287-1293, 1991.

325. Sibony PA, Kennerdell JS, Slamovits TL, et al: Intrapapillary refractile bodies in optic nerve sheath meningioma. *Arch Ophthalmol* 103:383-385, 1985.

326. Sibony PA, Krauss HR, Kennerdell JS, et al: Optic nerve sheath meningiomas; clinical manifestations. *Ophthalmology* 91:1313-1326, 1984.

327. Smith JL, Vuksanovic MM, Yates BM, Bienfang DC: Radiation therapy for primary optic nerve meningiomas. *J Clin Neuro-Ophthalmol* 1:85-99, 1981.

328. Spencer WH: Primary neoplasms of the optic nerve and its sheaths: clinical features and current concepts of pathogenetic mechanisms. *Trans Am Ophthalmol Soc* 70:490-528, 1972.

329. Strempel I: Rare choroidal tumour simulating a malignant melanoma. *Ophthalmologica* 202:110-114, 1991.

330. Walsh FB: Meningiomas, primary within the orbit and optic canal. *In:* Smith JL, editor: *Neuro-ophthalmology symposium of the University of Miami and the Bascom Palmer Eye Institute,* vol. 5, Hallendale, FL, 1970, Huffman Publishing, pp. 240-266.

331. Wright JE: Primary optic nerve meningiomas: clinical presentation and management. *Trans Am Acad Ophthalmol Otolaryngol* 83:OP617-OP625, 1977.

332. Wright JE, Call NB, Liaricos S: Primary optic nerve meningioma. *Br J Ophthalmol* 64:553-558, 1980.

333. Wright JE, McNab AA, McDonald WI: Primary optic nerve sheath meningioma. *Br J Ophthalmol* 73:960-966, 1989.

334. Zimmerman CF, Schatz NJ, Glaser JS: Magnetic resonance imaging of optic nerve meningiomas; enhancement with gadolinium-DTPA. *Ophthalmology* 97:585-591, 1990.

Optic Nerve Gliomas

335. Aoki S, Barkovich AJ, Nishimura K, et al: Neurofibromatosis types 1 and 2: cranial MR findings. *Radiology* 172:527-534, 1989.
336. Bouzas EA, Parry DM, Eldridge R, Kaiser-Kupfer MI: Visual impairment in patients with neurofibromatosis 2. *Neurology* 43:622-623, 1993.
337. de Keizer RJW, de Wolff-Rouendaal D, Bots GTAM, et al: Optic glioma with intraocular tumor and seeding in a child with neurofibromatosis. *Am J Ophthalmol* 108:717-725, 1989.
338. Hoyt WF, Baghdassarian SA: Optic glioma of childhood; natural history and rationale for conservative management. *Br J Ophthalmol* 53:793-798, 1969.
339. Mulvihill JJ, Parry DM, Sherman JL, et al: NIH Conference. Neurofibromatosis 1 (Recklinghausen disease) and neurofibromatosis 2 (bilateral acoustic neurofibromatosis); an update. *Ann Intern Med* 113:39-52, 1990.
340. Wright JE, McNab AA, McDonald WI: Optic nerve glioma and the management of optic nerve tumours in the young. *Br J Ophthalmol* 73:967-974, 1989.

Visual Loss Secondary to Papilledema Caused by Increased Intracranial Pressure

341. Brourman ND, Spoor TC, Ramocki JM: Optic nerve sheath decompression for pseudotumor cerebri. *Arch Ophthalmol* 106:1378-1383, 1988.
342. Coppeto JR, Monteiro MLR: Juxtapapillary subretinal hemorrhages in pseudotumor cerebri. *J Clin Neuro-Ophthalmol* 5:45-53, 1985.
343. Corbett JJ, Nerad JA, Tse DT, Anderson RL: Results of optic nerve sheath fenestration for pseudotumor cerebri; the lateral orbitotomy approach. *Arch Ophthalmol* 106:1391-1397, 1988.
344. Corbett JJ, Savino PJ, Thompson HS, et al: Visual loss in pseudotumor cerebri; follow-up of 57 patients from five to 41 years and a profile of 14 patients with permanent severe visual loss. *Arch Neurol* 39:461-474, 1982.
345. Gittinger JW Jr, Asdourian GK: Macular abnormalities in papilledema from pseudotumor cerebri. *Ophthalmology* 96:192-194, 1989.
346. Green GL, Lessell S, Loewenstein JI: Ischemic optic neuropathy in chronic papilledema. *Arch Ophthalmol* 98:502-504, 1980.
347. Gutgold-Glen H, Kattah JC, Chavis RM: Reversible visual loss in pseudotumor cerebri. *Arch Ophthalmol* 102:403-406, 1984.
348. Hayreh SS: Optic disc edema in raised intracranial pressure. V. Pathogenesis. *Arch Ophthalmol* 95:1553-1565, 1977.
349. Jamison RR: Subretinal neovascularization and papilledema associated with pseudotumor cerebri. *Am J Ophthalmol* 85:78-81, 1978.
350. Keane JR: Papilledema with unusual ocular hemorrhages. *Arch Ophthalmol* 99:262-263, 1981.
351. Keltner JL: Editorial: Optic nerve sheath decompression; how does it work? Has its time come? *Arch Ophthalmol* 106:1365-1369, 1988.
352. Liu GT, Glaser JS, Schatz NJ: High-dose methylprednisolone and acetazolamide for visual loss in pseudotumor cerebri. *Am J Ophthalmol* 118:88-96, 1994.
353. Mitchell DJ, Steahly LP: Pseudotumor cerebri and macular disease. *Retina* 9:115-117, 1989.
354. Mittra RA, Sergott RC, Flaharty PM, et al: Optic nerve decompression improves hemodynamic parameters in papilledema. *Ophthalmology* 100:987-997, 1993.
355. Morris AT, Sanders MD: Macular changes resulting from papilloedema. *Br J Ophthalmol* 64:211-216, 1980.
356. Morse PH, Leveille AS, Antel JP, Burch JV: Bilateral juxtapapillary subretinal neovascularization associated with pseudotumor cerebri. *Am J Ophthalmol* 91:312-317, 1981.
357. Orcutt JC, Page NGR, Sanders MD: Factors affecting visual loss in benign intracranial hypertension. *Ophthalmology* 91:1303-1312, 1984.
358. Paton L: Optic neuritis in cerebral tumours and its subsidence after operation. *Trans Ophthalmol Soc UK* 25:129-162, 1905.
359. Pollock SC: Acute papilledema and visual loss in a patient with pseudotumor cerebri. *Arch Ophthalmol* 105:752-753, 1987.
360. Rosenberg ML, O'Connor P, Carter J: Idiopathic unilateral disc edema; the big blind spot. *J Clin Neuro-Ophthalmol* 4:181-184, 1984.
361. Rush JA: Pseudotumor cerebri; clinical profile and visual outcome of 63 patients. *Mayo Clin Proc* 55:541-546, 1980.
362. Sergott RC, Savino PJ, Bosley TM: Modified optic nerve sheath decompression provides long-term visual improvement for pseudotumor cerebri. *Arch Ophthalmol* 106:1384-1390, 1988.
363. Spoor TC, McHenry JG: Long-term effectiveness of optic nerve sheath decompression for pseudotumor cerebri. *Arch Ophthalmol* 111:632-635, 1993.
364. Spoor TC, Ramocki JM, Madion MP, Wilkinson MJ: Treatment of pseudotumor cerebri by primary and secondary optic nerve sheath decompression. *Am J Ophthalmol* 112:117-185, 1991.
365. Tomsak RL, Niffenegger AS, Remler BF: Treatment of pseudotumor cerebri with diamox (acetazolamide). *J Clin Neuro-Ophthalmol* 8:93-98, 1988.
366. Troost BT, Sufit RL, Grand MG: Sudden monocular visual loss in pseudotumor cerebri. *Arch Neurol* 36:440-442, 1979.
367. Tse DT, Nerad JA, Anderson RL, Corbett JJ: Optic nerve sheath fenestration in pseudotumor cerebri; a lateral orbitotomy approach. *Arch Ophthalmol* 106:1458-1462, 1988.

Nutritional Amblyopia

368. Carroll FD: Jamaican optic neuropathy in immigrants to the United States. *Am J Ophthalmol* 71:261-265, 1971.
369. Carroll FD: Nutritional amblyopia. *Arch Ophthalmol* 76:406-411, 1966.
370. Cullom ME, Heher KL, Miller NR, et al: Leber's hereditary optic neuropathy masquerading as tobacco-alcohol amblyopia. *Arch Ophthalmol* 111:1482-1485, 1993.
371. Frisén L: Fundus changes in acute malnutritional optic neuropathy. *Arch Ophthalmol* 101:577-579, 1983.
372. Johns DR, Neufeld MJ, Hedges TR III: Mitochondrial DNA mutations in Cuban optic and peripheral neuropathy. *J Neuro-Ophthalmol* 14:135-140, 1994.
373. Johns DR, Sadun AA: Cuban epidemic optic neuropathy; mitochondrial DNA analysis. *J Neuro-Ophthalmol* 14:130-134, 1994.
374. Lessell S: Toxic and deficiency optic neuropathies. *In:* Smith JL, Glaser JS, editors: *Neuro-ophthalmology symposium of the University of Miami and the Bascom Palmer Eye Institute,* vol. 7, St. Louis, 1973, CV Mosby, pp. 21-37.
375. MacKenzie AD, Phillips CI: West Indian amblyopia. *Brain* 91:249-260, 1968.
376. Mackey D, Howell N: Tobacco amblyopia. *Am J Ophthalmol* 117:817-818, 1994.
377. Rizzo JF III, Lessell S: Tobacco amblyopia. *Am J Ophthalmol* 116:84-87, 1993.

14

Photocoagulation Treatment of Macular Diseases

With the introduction of photocoagulation techniques by Meyer-Swickerath[103] and fluorescein angiographic techniques by Novotny and Alvis,[111] the clinician was provided with tools for a new approach to early diagnosis and treatment of some of the choroidal and retinal exudative maculopathies. Controlled randomized clinical trials have demonstrated the effectiveness of argon and krypton laser treatment of choroidal neovascular membranes (CNVMs) in patients with age-related macular degeneration (see Chapter 3, p. 104), the presumed ocular histoplasmosis syndrome (see Chapter 3, p. 130), and idiopathic choroidal neovascularization (see Chapter 3, p. 248). The value of laser therapy in the treatment of CNVMs caused by other diseases is not known but, with the possible exception of high myopia and angioid streaks, probably would prove to be similar if sufficient cases were available for study.[84] Trials concerning diabetic retinopathy have found evidence that panretinal photocoagulation is useful in preventing severe loss of visual function in patients with proliferative retinopathy and that focal treatment is beneficial in treating patients with visual loss caused by background diabetic retinopathy (see Chapter 6, p. 523).[32-35,37-40] Other clinical trials have demonstrated the benefit of photocoagulation for some of the manifestations of branch retinal vein occlusion (see Chapter 6, p. 562),[11,12] central retinal vein occlusion (see Chapter 6, p. 555),[22,74] and sickle cell disease (see Chapter 6, p. 248).[27,67,68] Until further clinical trials are done in regard to the treatment of other diseases we have to rely on the published results of uncontrolled pilot studies. This chapter provides some general guidelines for photocoagulation based on these studies, my own clinical experience, and my interpretation of the results of treatment reported by others. While awaiting reliable guidelines for therapy, the clinician should be conservative in the use of photocoagulation, particularly in treating those disorders in which there is minimal evidence to support its value. In such cases we must be constantly aware that photocoagulation may not only fail to benefit the patient but may actually make the visual outcome worse.

▼ GENERAL PRINCIPLES OF PHOTOCOAGULATION

In the retina an intact vascular endothelium, the blood inner–retinal barrier, is vital in keeping serous fluid and blood from accumulating in the extracellular spaces of the retina. In the choroid, on the other hand, where large endothelial pores are normally present in the choriocapillaris, an intact retinal pigment epithelium (RPE), the blood–outer retinal barrier, is essential in preventing accumulation of serous fluid beneath the sensory retina (see Chapters 1 and 2). Any disease altering the permeability of the retinal vessels or the permeability of the RPE and its attachment to Bruch's membrane in the macular region may cause loss of central vision, in the former case because of intraretinal exudation and hemorrhage and in the latter instance because of serous and hemorrhagic detachment of the RPE or retina or both. Through use of a broad spectrum of wavelengths of light that are selectively absorbed by blood in the retinal and choroidal blood vessels or by melanin in the choroid and RPE, we are able to generate heat in sufficient quantities to coagulate tissue in the vicinity of the permeability alterations.*

The mechanisms by which photocoagulation prevents or inhibits exudation and hemorrhage are complex and incompletely understood. One of the primary effects of photocoagulation is to reduce blood flow through the abnormal vascular bed. In the case of abnormal retinal vessels this may be accomplished by any one or a combination of the following: (1) coagulation and thrombosis of the retinal vessels caused by absorption of light by hemoglobin within the retinal vessels, e.g., sharply focused argon or yellow dye laser[117]; (2) delayed closure of the retinal capillaries[145]; (3) coagulation and thrombosis caused by the inward spread of heat generated by absorption of light by melanin and hemoglobin in the RPE and choroid (Fig. 14-1); (4) retinal arterial narrowing induced by increased oxygen tension at the inner retinal level caused by photocoagulation destruction of the metabolically active RPE and outer retina[56,76,114,143]; and (5) damage to the outer blood–retinal barrier (RPE), allowing movement

*References 2, 3, 5, 6, 19, 28, 31, 42, 65, 66, 94, 96, 97, 102, 104, 105, 113, 124, 125, 128-130, 134, 136, 142, 148, 150.

FIG. 14-1   Diagram Showing Spread of Heat from the RPE, the Primary Site of Laser Light Absorption.

A, Short-duration, low-intensity argon laser application.

B, Longer duration, higher intensity application. The application in **A** may be effective in correcting choroidal vascular abnormalities but would be ineffective in coagulation of a retinal vascular lesion. The application in **B** may be effective in treating both choroidal and retinal vascular lesions but will cause a nerve fiber bundle visual field defect.

of antiangiogenic factors into the inner retina and vitreous.[95,126] In the choroidal exudative diseases, reduction of leakage may be accomplished primarily by (1) reestablishment of the blood–ocular barrier by debridement of the incompetent RPE cells and stimulation of the neighboring RPE cells to proliferate, and (2) reduction of blood flow by coagulation and thrombosis of the choroidal vessels or new vessels derived from the choroid. The use of either sharply focused small spot–size laser applications to occlude retinal neovascular arterial feeder vessels, or intense, long duration, large spot–size applications to occlude the entire retinal neovascular network is often unsuccessful and is fraught with potential complications. This direct approach to photocoagulation of retinal and optic disc new vessels has been replaced largely by the technique of panretinal photocoagulation in the case of diabetic retinopathy and by regional scatter coagulation of areas of capillary nonperfusion in other diseases, such as branch vein occlusion and sickle cell retinopathy. The mechanisms by which panphotocoagulation induces resolution of retinal neovascularization are unknown. Theories that have been postulated include the reduction in the amount of an as yet unidentified vasoproliferative substance produced by the ischemic retina, liberation of antiangiogenic substances by photocoagulation damage to the outer retina and RPE, and vasoconstriction that occurs because of greater diffusion of oxygen from the choroid to the inner retina after partial destruction of the metabolically active RPE and outer retina (see Chapter 6, diabetic retinopathy, p. 524).[56,76,112,114,143]

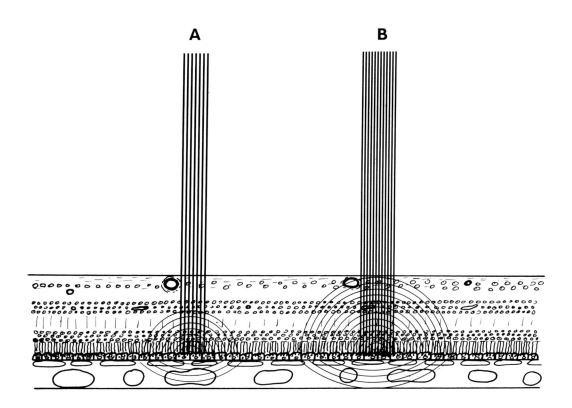

In the eye, photocoagulation is accomplished by irradiating the inner eye with a focused light beam of a single or multiple wavelengths. There is considerable information concerning the histopathology of laser irradiation of the animal and human retina and choroid.* The light is absorbed by the pigmented structures within the eye and is converted into thermal energy, which causes denaturation of tissue proteins and a coagulative necrosis in the tissue absorbing the light energy, as well as in surrounding tissue. The area of effective coagulation is directly related to the intensity and duration of the irradiation. The precise level of the photocoagulation is determined by the wavelength of the light used and the amount and distribution of the ocular and blood pigments in the area irradiated. In the eye three pigments that are primarily involved in photocoagulation are melanin in the RPE and choroid, hemoglobin in the retinal and choroidal blood vessels as well as in the extravascular tissues, and xanthophyll, which is concentrated in the central macular area. Figure 14-2 depicts the distribution of the pigments in the macula and demonstrates the relative effectiveness of the various light sources in causing photocoagulation at various levels in the choroid and retina. Outside the foveal avascular zone (FAZ), all the commercially available photocoagulators using continuous-wavelength visible or near-infrared light generate heat primarily by laser absorption by the melanin pigment in the RPE and choroid. The most widely used lasers for treatment of chorioretinal diseases include the argon blue-green (488 to 514 nm), argon green (514 to 527 nm), frequency doubling YAG (532 nm), krypton red (647 nm), diode (790 to 830 nm), and tunable dye laser (range from 577 nm to 630 nm). Inside the FAZ argon blue-green and to a lesser extent argon green are absorbed by the xanthophyll pigment, which is concentrated in the inner as well as the outer plexiform layers of the retina. This causes opacification and photocoagulation of the inner retina that inhibits transmission of the laser to the underlying RPE and choroid. Theoretically, the yellow dye laser should be ideal for treatment of juxtafoveal and subfoveal neovascular membranes because of its minimal absorption by the xanthophyll and maximal absorption by hemoglobin in the new vessels.[113,126,136,140] Argon green, although partly absorbed by xanthophyll, theoretically should be superior to krypton or the diode laser by

*References 3, 6, 19, 42, 94, 97, 102, 104, 105, 109, 114, 117, 128-130, 134, 140, 142.

FIG. 14-2 Diagrams Showing Differences in the Sites of Absorption (Indicated by Star Symbols) of Argon Blue-Green, Argon Green, and Krypton Red Laser in Eyes with Choroidal Neovascular Membranes *(CNVM)* that Extend into the Capillary-Free Zone *(CFZ)*. Black Dots in Retina Indicate Xanthophyll Pigment; *RPE,* Retinal Pigment Epithelium; *CH,* Choroid.

A, Argon blue-green laser outside CFZ absorbed primarily by outer retina, RPE, CNVM, and inner choroidal vessels and melanin.
B, Argon blue-green laser inside CFZ primarily absorbed by retinal xanthophyll.
C, Argon green laser inside CFZ absorbed primarily by RPE, CNVM, and inner choroidal vessels and melanin.
D, Krypton red laser inside CFZ absorbed primarily by RPE and choroidal melanocytes.

virtue of its absorption by hemoglobin. On the other hand, krypton red and yellow dye lasers are less likely to damage the inner retina and can be focused more precisely in the presence of any media haze. In practice, differences in the effectiveness of treatment of juxtafoveal neovascularization with these lasers has not been demonstrated.[13] The tunable dye laser has the advantage of the availability of a wide range of wavelengths, which in the occasional patient with peculiar structure of the neovascular membrane or the media may allow more intense photocoagulation. The major disadvantage of the dye laser is its predilection for breakdown. The author prefers use of the krypton red laser for treatment of juxtafoveal neovascularization and for large extrafoveal subretinal neovascular complexes in the papillomacular bundle because of the reduced risk of causing damage to the inner retina, the greater ease of focusing the laser in eyes with media changes, and, in the case of juxtafoveal membranes, better visibility of the edge of the membrane and better control of spread of the laser burn. I have had no experience with the diode laser, which produces comparable photocoagulation both clinically and experimentally.* The solid-state diode laser and the frequency-doubled YAG green laser have the advantage of greater portability and durability.[2,63,101] The diode laser has been adapted to the slit lamp, indirect ophthalmoscope, and endoscope.

*References 3, 59, 102, 127, 129, 135, 137, 138, 142.

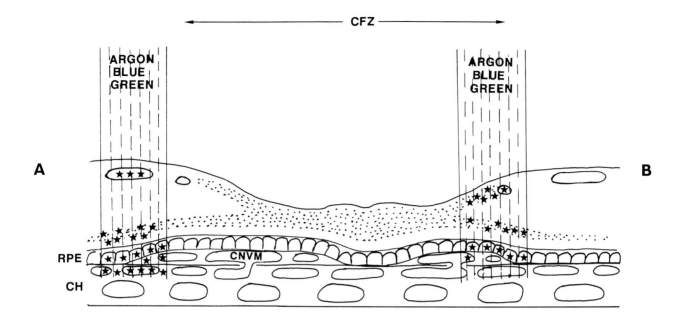

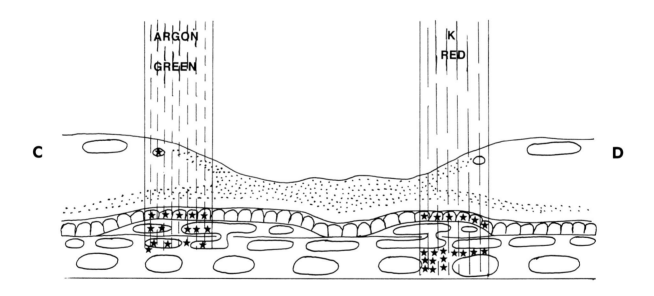

Although most of the early randomized trials for the treatment of extrafoveal neovascular membranes utilized argon blue-green laser, most physicians use argon green for treatment of extrafoveal lesions to reduce the chance of laser absorption by the small amount of xanthophyll outside the foveolar area. In the hypopigmented fundus, the argon green has the advantage over the krypton red laser, which is absorbed primarily by melanin. The neodymium-YAG laser has enjoyed limited use for photocoagulation of the retina and for vitreolysis.[31,65,100,132]

▼ VISUAL LOSS CAUSED BY PHOTOCOAGULATION

Photocoagulation burns involving only the outer retinal layers produce a scotoma that corresponds with the site of outer retinal destruction. In very mild, low-intensity, short-duration burns, the necrosis may involve only the RPE and outer segments of the visual cells and their regrowth may cause little or no functional loss in the area (Figs. 14-1 and 14-3, *A* to *C*).[116] More intense burns may cause a scotoma that corresponds with the area treated (Fig. 14-3, *D* to *F*). If the burn involves the inner retina (Fig. 14-1, *B*), the scotoma will also include the area supplied by the ganglion cells whose nerve fibers pass through the area of treatment. The distribution of nerve fibers in the papillomacular bundle is such that full-thickness retinal burns may be employed within an area not exceeding four clock hours of the nerve fiber layer temporal to the optic disc of the normal eye with minimal risk of impairment of the central visual acuity.[6] Burns involving the superior or inferior half of the central macular area interfere with the central visual function less than burns placed in the temporal or nasal margin of the center of the fovea. Parafoveal burns on the temporal side of the left eye and nasal side of the right eye are more likely to interfere with reading vision.

▼ TYPES OF PHOTOCOAGULATORS

The ideal instrument for photocoagulation of macular lesions should include the following features:

1. Patient and operator should be in a comfortable sitting position.
2. There should be easy stereoscopic viewing of the macula before, during, and after photocoagulation.
3. The instrument should have an accurate, easy to use aiming device.
4. The instrument should have a readily accessible control panel that includes a wide range of settings to accurately and easily control the power (up to at least 1 watt), spot size, and duration of photocoagulation, as well as an application counter.
5. The instrument should provide for the operative selection of a wide range of wavelengths of highly collimated light.
6. An illuminated stereoscopic viewer should be mounted conveniently for monitoring fluorescein angiograms during photocoagulation.
7. There should be a foot-controlled trigger.

FIG. 14-3 Histopathology of Photocoagulation Burns.

A to **D,** Ruby laser burns *(arrows)* in owl monkey after 15 minutes (**A** and **B**), and 20 hours (**C**), and 30 months (**D**). Note thrombus in choriocapillaris at 20 hours *(arrow,* **C**).
   E, Xenon lesion 1 day after treatment.
   F, Xenon lesion 5 weeks after treatment.

8. The procedure should produce no pain or photophobia and thus require no anesthesia.
9. There should be safety devices to prevent accidental photocoagulation of the patient and the operator.

My experience with photocoagulation has been limited to the West German Zeiss xenon photocoagulator, the American Optical ruby laser, Coherent Radiation argon and krypton lasers, and Coherent Radiation and Nidek dye lasers.

The argon and krypton laser instruments are equipped to produce highly collimated, bichromatic blue-green or monochromatic green light (in the case of the argon laser) or monochromatic red light (in the case of the krypton laser) of variable intensity, duration, and spot size. Recently developed dye lasers provide the clinician with a wide range of wavelengths. All the continuous-wave laser instruments have most of the ideal design features for photocoagulation. The physician and patient are comfortably seated, and the fundus is viewed stereoscopically through a slit lamp and contact lens. The instruments delivers a bichromatic or monochromatic light of variable intensity, duration, and spot size.

▼ PREOPERATIVE PHOTOGRAPHIC STUDIES

Before considering photocoagulation treatment in a patient with a macular lesion, the physician should ask the following questions:

1. Is the loss of central vision caused by exudation or bleeding into or beneath the retina?
2. Is the lesion responsible for the exudation or bleeding located primarily in the retina or choroid?
3. What is the lesion's position relative to the FAZ?
4. What are the chances of recovery or preservation of useful central vision if success in eliminating the source of blood and exudate is achieved?

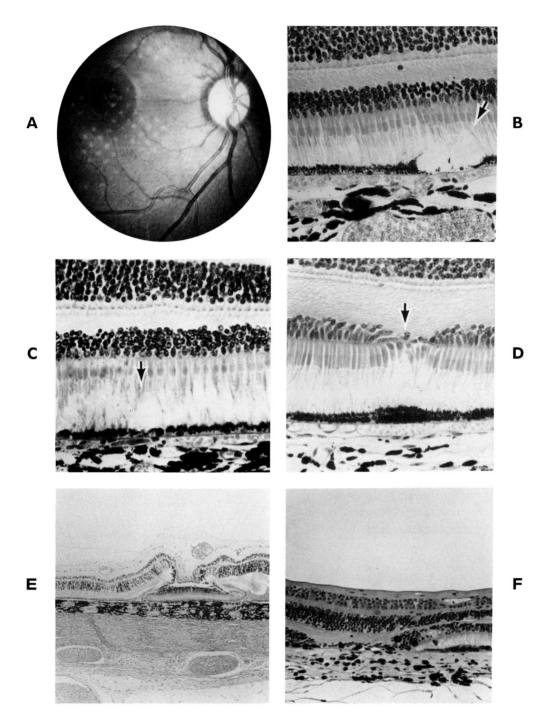

5. What are the chances of early spontaneous resolution of the exudation and blood and visual recovery?
6. What are the risks of photocoagulation?
7. What other methods of effective therapy are available?

With careful ophthalmoscopic and biomicroscopic examination using a fundus contact lens, the physician is usually able to determine the presence or absence of a macular lesion that may be amenable to photocoagulation. A large variety of fundus contact lenses and slit lamps are available for examination and treatment of macular lesions. The ideal contact lens–slit lamp combination is one that allows for a wide range of slit beam angles and magnification for stereoscopic viewing of the fundus through a non–hand held contact lens. This combination permits the examiner to use both hands to vary both the angle of the slit and the focus simultaneously. The author prefers the Haig-Streit fundus lens and Zeiss slit lamp for examination and treatment. A balanced salt solution rather than viscous preparations are used for contact lens examination for the following reasons: greater adherence of the lens to the cornea so that it is unnecessary to hold the lens during examination, rapid recovery of vision after lens removal without the need for irrigation and most importantly the possibility of obtaining excellent quality fundus photographs and angiographs soon after lens removal (Fig. 14-4).[17,48] Those patients with a lesion that either appears favorable or may be favorable for photocoagulation should have a thorough photographic and angiographic study to determine the precise origin of the exudate or blood in the macular area. This study should include color stereoscopic photographs and stereoscopic black and white fluorescein angiographic views of both maculae.

The following procedures are generally used at the Bascom Palmer Eye Institute. After clinical examination, color stereophotographs of the lesion in question as well as of the macular region of the opposite eye are made. Photographs with a fixation device in place are not reliable in determining the center of the foveola because the patient's fixation point in the presence of macular exudation or detachment is often eccentric. The fluorescein angiographic study includes rapid-sequence stereoangiography for a period of several minutes followed by stereophotographs at periodic intervals up to at least 10 minutes following injection. If the photographer sees no apparent leakage in the macula, he or she should include angiographic views of the fundus outside the disc–macular area. Biomicroscopy and ophthalmoscopy with blue filters in place may be necessary in such patients to identify peripheral areas of leakage. The black and white film is developed immediately and sent to the treating physician. The author infrequently uses digital fluorescein angiography because of the important disadvantage of lack of quality stereoscopic views.

Stereophotographs and angiograms are important in detecting minimal serous detachment of the macula, intraretinal extracellular edema, the location and size of the leaks, the differentiation of fluorescence caused by depigmentation or atrophy of the RPE from that caused by true leakage, the precise localization of the area of leakage and its relationship to the FAZ, and the presence and location of occult CNVMs, which often underlie

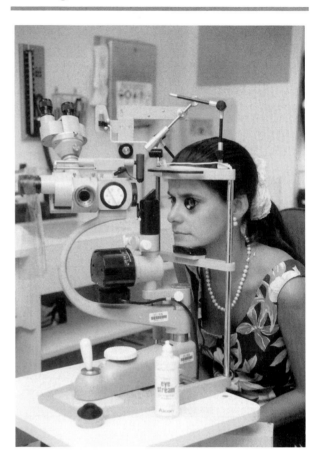

FIG. 14-4 Use of Balanced Salt Solution and Haig-Streit Contact Lens for Examination and Laser Photocoagulation of the Ocular Fundus.

areas of irregularly elevated RPE that fail to stain evenly and promptly. Review of the fluorescein angiographic negatives with either a stereoscopic viewer or +8.00 diopter stereo spectacles provides the physician with the optimum information needed for treatment (Fig. 14-5).

The photographic studies should be reviewed and compared simultaneously with biomicroscopic examination to determine the leakage sites and their relationship the center of the macula. This is particularly important in elderly patients, in whom angiography may fail to define this zone clearly.

Use of an illuminated projector is helpful in explaining to the patient and family the photographic findings, the cause for his or her visual problem, the proposed treatment, its advantages over alternative methods of management, the expected course if treatment is successful, the chances for success, and potential complications of the treatment (Fig. 14-6).

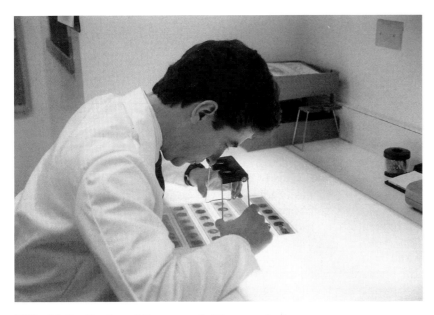

FIG. 14-5   Review of Stereoscopic Fluorescein Angiograms.

FIG. 14-6   Use of Illuminated View Box To Explain Findings and Proposed Treatment to Patients.

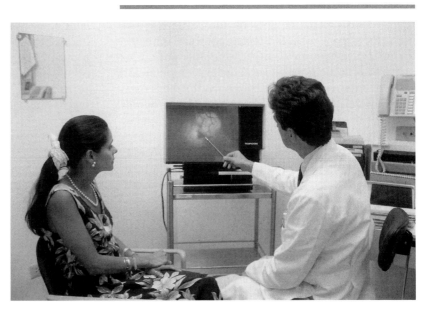

▼ TECHNIQUES OF PHOTOCOAGULATION

On the day of photocoagulation, the patient's best corrected visual acuity and Amsler grid findings are recorded. The pupil is maximally dilated. The stereophotographs are reviewed and compared with the biomicroscopic appearance of the patient's fundus. Angiography is usually repeated if there has been more than several days' delay in treatment or if there is any reason to suspect that a change has occurred in the fundus.

Laser photocoagulation

Before activating the instrument the operator should make certain that all instrument controls are properly set and that the foot switch is in a position where neither the patient nor the operator will accidentally activate it. The instrument is turned on and allowed to warm up for approximately 5 to 10 minutes. If the instrument is used before this warmup period, the operator may need to make frequent adjustments for the gradual increase in the wattage that occurs during this time. The 35-mm negative film strip of the angiogram is placed in the stereo viewer (Fig. 14-7) or, as some prefer, in a nonstereo projection device. The corneal epithelium should be clear and the pupil maximally dilated. Retrobulbar anesthesia is usually unnecessary but should be used whenever there is doubt as to the patient's ability to maintain steady fixation during treatment. This is most likely to occur in patients with poor vision in the fellow eye, in children, and in patients who are photophobic, particularly those with extensive retinal vascular leakage and secondary vitreous inflammatory cell infiltration, e.g., retinal angiomas and retinal telangiectasis. The heights of the patient's and operator's stools and the instrument are adjusted to ensure maximum comfort, and the patient is urged to breathe normally and to relax. A balanced saline solution rather than a viscous solution is used to apply the contact lens (Fig. 14-4). This provides greater lens adhesion to the cornea and makes possible clearer posttreatment fundus photographs. With the contact lens in place, the fundus is examined to check for any changes that may have occurred since the last examination and to compare important landmarks in the fundus with the stereoangiograms. Identification of the FAZ of the retina is the single most important landmark to determine the anatomic center of the macula. Less reliable landmarks include the determination of the patient's point of fixation and identification of the foveal reflex. The point of fixation is an

FIG. 14-7 **Electric Stereoscopic Viewer** *(arrow)* **Mounted Above the Slit-Lamp Binocular of the Argon Laser Instrument.**

unreliable landmark in patients with subnormal visual acuity. In patients, however, with minimal subfoveal fluid and nearly normal acuity fixation is relatively reliable. The foveal reflex, which ordinarily identifies the center of the macula in such patients, may be displaced eccentrically 100 μm or more away from the foveal center by an eccentric pigment epithelial or retinal elevation that is confined to the opposite side of the FAZ. The 50-μm-spot size aiming light can be used to check the locus of the patient's fixation and to check for visual function in areas of planned photocoagulation. If the patient appears to fixate eccentrically for no apparent reason, he or she may be the rare patient whose anatomic foveal center does not correspond with the center of the foveal avascular zone. The stereoangiogram that best depicts the lesion to be treated is selected. The intensity of the aiming light is reduced to the minimal level visible to the operator. Ideally, the aiming light should not be visible to the patient. If it is visible to the patient, he or she is advised to ignore it and to concentrate on the fixation light with the opposite eye. The spot size, power, and duration settings are rechecked, and the laser activator switch is turned to the "on" position. If the lesion to be treated is within one disc diameter of the center of the foveola, a test burn is placed somewhere in the vicinity of the major vascular arcades inferior to the macula. This is done not only to test the intensity and size of the burn but also to check for any spontaneous movement that the patient may make during the application. This is important even when using retrobulbar anesthesia since small ocular movements may still occur. It is essential that the patient show no or only minimal eye movement before proceeding with treatment near the FAZ.

The spot size, duration, and intensity selection depend primarily on the size, depth, and nature of the lesion to be treated. For a given spot size, duration, and power setting, the intensity of the burn obtained depends primarily on the clarity of the ocular media and the degree of pigmentation of the fundus of the particular eye. For any intensity setting, the same power is delivered over the total area of each of the possible spot size selections. To maintain comparable burn intensities when chang-

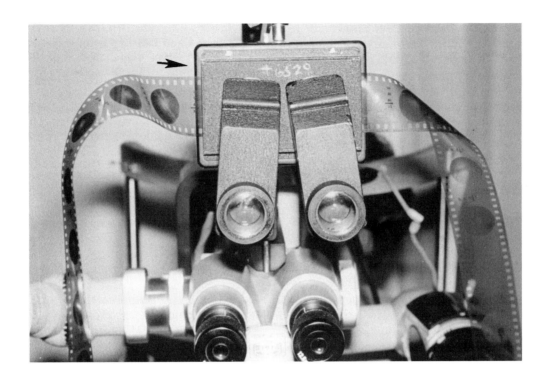

ing from one spot size to the next smaller spot size, the operator must reduce the power setting by at least 50%, and vice versa when increasing the spot size. In general, the spot size of 50 μm should be avoided because of the added risk of Bruch's membrane rupture and choroidal hemorrhage. The specifics in regard to spot size, intensity, and duration of photocoagulation applications depend primarily on the type of lesion being treated (see next section). During the course of photocoagulation, the operator should make frequent reference to the center of the foveola in the patient as well as the angiogram to make certain that it is not accidentally treated. After completion of treatment, the size, intensity, duration, number, and location of laser applications are recorded in the patient's chart as well as the laser log. Stereophotographs of the fundus are made immediately following treatment. If any doubt exists concerning adequate coverage of the subretinal CNVM with laser treatment, posttreatment photographs are compared with pretreatment angiogram using either an Aus Jena Dokumator DL-2 Microfilm Reader or the less time-consuming superimposition of instant Polaroid transparent posttreatment photographs and the angiogram.[18,23] If retrobulbar anesthesia is used, the eye is patched for approxi-

mately 3 hours. The patient is observed during this period until light perception returns. No topical or oral medications are routinely used. The patient is advised to avoid strenuous physical activity until at least the first postoperative visit.

Xenon photocoagulation

The technique of photocoagulation with the xenon light is the same as that with the argon laser with the following exceptions. The patient is in the reclining position. Retrobulbar anesthesia is required. Since small ocular movements are usually present even after the best retrobulbar anesthesia, the patient is asked to look in the direction corresponding to that of the center of the foveola from the area to be treated. Thus if a slight movement occurs during photocoagulation, the foveola will be carried away from rather than toward the light. For example, if the foveola of the right eye lies nasal to the area to be treated, the patient's gaze should be directed to the left. A test spot is made in the paramacular area. The desired size and intensity of the test spot depend on the size, location, and nature of the lesion to be treated. Before treating a small serous detachment of the RPE, a low-intensity setting to create a light gray outer retinal test burn is all that is required. To treat choroidal neovascularization, however, a higher intensity is needed to produce a definite white test burn. The intensity should be adjusted to achieve an exposure time of 1 second or less. Unlike the argon laser, the total power per unit time delivered to the fundus increases as the spot size increases. In the presence of a refractive error, xenon photocoagulation is done through either a contact lens, a hand-held lens, or the patient's spectacles. Because of the difficulty in judging the degree of photocoagulation through the direct ophthalmoscope, it is important to monitor the photocoagulation applications using the indirect ophthalmoscope and the +15.00 viewing lens. The use of a green filter is helpful in detecting minimal graying of the outer retinal layers. When making multiple applications of photocoagulation, it is important to identify the foveolar area between each application. With the direct ophthalmoscope and the xenon light, the concentrated xanthophyll pigment in the foveolar area is usually easy to identify and provides a valuable landmark. Following photocoagulation the eye is patched for approximately 3 hours to avoid corneal exposure. The activity of those patients with choroidal or retinal lesions that are normally prone to hemorrhage is curtailed until at least the first postoperative examination. Bilateral patches and pinholes are not used.

Ruby laser photocoagulation

My technique for use of the American Optical ruby laser to treat macular lesions has been described elsewhere.[50] Because the duration of the ruby laser pulse is fixed at 0.2 msec, the instrument is contraindicated in the treatment of retinal vascular or choroidal neovascular disease. Although the ruby laser is probably the ideal instrument for treating either large or small areas of serous detachment of the RPE in patients without evidence of choroidal neovascularization, such as in idiopathic central serous chorioretinopathy, I abandoned its use in favor of the argon laser instrument, which is effective and technically easier to use.

▼ TYPES OF MACULAR LESIONS AMENABLE TO PHOTOCOAGULATION

A large number of diseases produce a relatively small number of similar pathologic and physiologic alterations that are responsible for exudation and hemorrhage into the macular region. For the purposes of discussing general principles of pho-

FIG. 14-8   Diagrams Depicting the Probable Mode of Action of Low-Intensity Photocoagulation in the Treatment of Serous Detachment of the RPE in Causing Resolution of Serous Detachment of the Retina.

Small black and white arrows indicate direction of fluid movement caused by the RPE cell physiologic pump. *Large black arrows* indicate direction of movement of large proteins and fluid through the site of RPE detachment and defective physiologic pump. **A,** Photocoagulation of detached RPE. **B,** Necrosis of RPE after photocoagulation. **C,** Migration and proliferation of RPE covering the previous RPE defect, restoration of RPE pump, and resolution of subretinal fluid.

tocoagulation, these pathologic alterations can be subdivided into several groups. The reader may wish to review the concept of the RPE and retinal capillary endothelial cell physiologic pump, as well as the principles of interpretation of fluorescein angiography outlined in Chapters 1 and 2.

Subpigment epithelial and subretinal serous exudation derived from the choriocapillaris; Bruch's membrane intact

In patients with subpigment epithelial and subretinal serous exudation from the choriocapillaris, serous exudate gains entrance into the subretinal space either through a focal area of RPE detachment or through a focal defect in the RPE. The area of RPE detachment or defect is usually readily identifiable with fluorescein angiography. Small serous RPE detachments or defects that lie outside of the FAZ may be treated safely with photocoagulation (see Fig. 3-4, *H*). Only low-intensity, short-duration photocoagulation applications of any type are usually required in the area of the RPE detachment or leak (Fig. 14-8, *A* and *B*). Rapid proliferation of the surrounding, relatively normal RPE occurs and replaces the destroyed RPE. Usually within 1 to 3 weeks, the subretinal space is dry, presumably because of the restoration of the integrity of the RPE barrier to movement of large molecules and restoration of its physiologic pumping mechanisms (Fig. 14-8, *C*). Use of photocoagulation to renew the RPE is analogous to the use of mechanical debridement of the corneal epithelium in the treatment of recurrent corneal erosion. Presumably there is only minimal coagulation of the choriocapillaris by these low-intensity burns (see Chapter 3, idiopathic central serous chorioretinopathy).

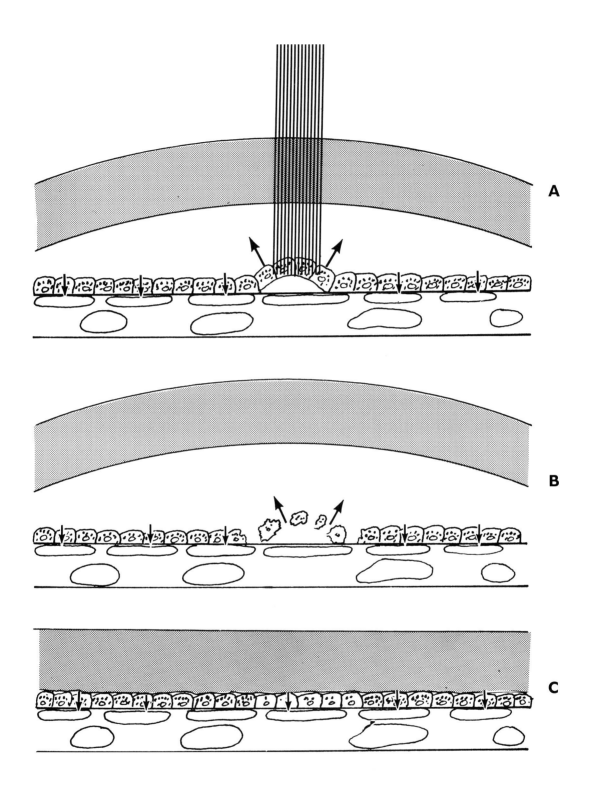

A

B

C

Large serous RPE detachment without evidence of neovascularization (avascular serous RPE detachment)

In patients with a large, oval or round serous RPE detachment that extends into the center of the macula, it is unnecessary to treat the entire area of the RPE detachment. In most cases, collapse of large areas of serous RPE detachment can be accomplished by placing moderate-intensity, noncontiguous, 100- to 200-μm spots of argon photocoagulation along and straddling the border of the RPE detachment (see Figs. 3-16, A to D; and 14-9).[46,50,121] This disrupts the RPE and allows serous exudate to leak into the surrounding subretinal space, where the neighboring RPE that is still anchored to Bruch's membrane can pump the exudate back into the choriocapillaris. In unusually large serous RPE detachments, a few photocoagulation applications scattered on the dome of the RPE detachment may be useful to promote RPE proliferation that may assist in anchoring the reattached RPE to Bruch's membrane. Photocoagulation should not be placed within the FAZ. Partial collapse of the RPE detachment and an increase in the surrounding subretinal fluid are often evident within 24 to 48 hours or sooner following treatment. It is probable that mechanical disruption of the RPE at the time of laser or xenon application is not necessary since even low-intensity burns probably devitalize the RPE sufficiently to allow passage of sub-RPE serous exudate into the subretinal space. Intense, small argon laser burns should not be directed to the attached RPE because of the possibility of disrupting the underlying Bruch's membrane and choriocapillaris. The prognosis for either spontaneous or postphotocoagulation reattachment of the RPE and return of visual function is best in the young or middle-aged patient who has recently developed a large, round or oval area of serous detachment of the RPE (see Chapter 3).

Older patients with macular drusen frequently develop serous detachments of the RPE either as a result of confluence of drusen or more frequently because of exudation from occult CNVMs. In the former case, nonvascularized RPE detachments are often round or oval with scalloped borders and may have a pigment figure on their surface. They are less likely to have underlying choroidal neovascularization, and angiography usually demonstrates prompt and even staining of the sub-RPE exudate. It is probably advisable to observe these

FIG. 14-9 Diagrams Depicting the Probable Mode of Action of Multiple Marginal Photocoagulation Applications in the Treatment of Large Areas of Serous Detachment of the RPE. Small Black and White Arrows Indicate the Direction of Fluid Movement Caused by the RPE Cell Physiologic Pump, Which Is Intact.

A, Multiple marginal photocoagulation applications.
B, Necrosis of RPE occurs after photocoagulation. Movement of proteinaceous fluid *(large black arrows)* from the sub-RPE space through the areas of damaged RPE into the subretinal space.
C, Reattachment of the RPE, migration, and proliferation of the RPE to replace the necrotic RPE; restoration of RPE pump; and resolution of subretinal fluid.

patients, who often maintain good acuity for many months or years. If the detachment shows evidence of progressive enlargement or if the vision deteriorates and there are no signs of underlying choroidal neovascularization, I would recommend photocoagulation as described above (see Figs. 3-14 and 14-9).

The clinical and angiographic features of serous RPE detachments caused by choroidal neovascularization are discussed later in this chapter.

Serous retinal detachment caused by multifocal areas of acute RPE damage

Multifocal areas of acute damage to the RPE may be caused by inflammatory cellular infiltration of the choroid (e.g., Harada's disease; see Fig. 3-60), neoplastic infiltration of the choroid (e.g., melanoma, metastatic carcinoma or leukemia; see Figs. 3-89 and 11-3, A and C), and multifocal areas of infarction of the RPE caused by fibrin–platelet occlusion of the choriocapillaris in systemic hypertension and collagen vascular disease (see Figs. 2-14, E to H, 3-66, and 3-67). Photocoagulation is infrequently indicated in treatment of these diseases. It may be used occasionally to cause resolution of prolonged exudative detachment of the macula associated with a choroidal tumor of uncertain nature (e.g., choroidal nevus; see Fig. 3-81, A to C). Multifocal pinpoint leaks in the RPE occasionally occur on the surface of organized RPE detachments, particularly when these detachments are adjacent to a larger area of serous RPE detachment.

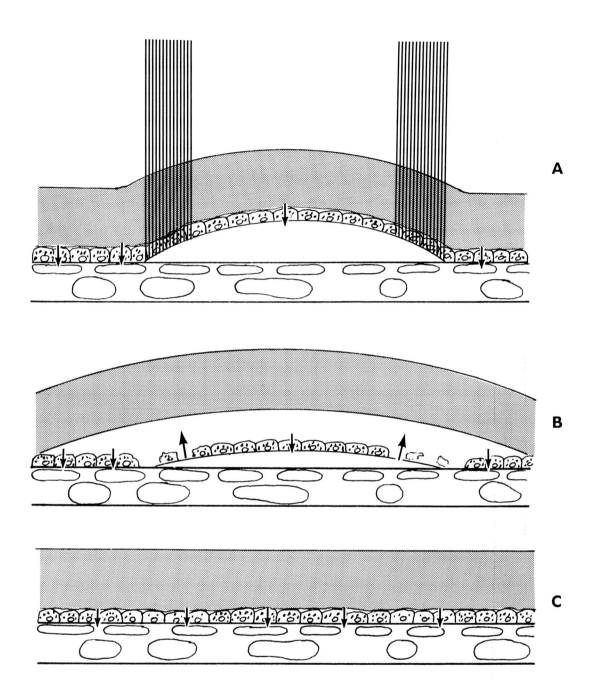

Large defects in the RPE with overlying cystic retina and serous retinal detachment

Certain choroidal lesions, particularly choroidal hemangiomas, may over a period of many years cause chronic and extensive degenerative changes in the overlying RPE and retina (see Fig. 3-74, *G* and *H*). Serous detachment of the overlying and surrounding retina, however, may not occur until middle or late adulthood. For reasons that are unknown, choroidal hemangiomas, unlike choroidal nevi, rarely cause breaks in Bruch's membrane and choroidal neovascularization. Intense, long-duration applications of xenon or argon photocoagulation to the surface of that portion of the hemangioma where angiography demonstrates leakage of dye is required in order to reattach the retina (see Fig. 3-73). Moderate- to high-intensity contiguous applications are necessary to partly coagulate the blood vessels on the inner surface of the tumor to reduce the influx of serous exudate into the subretinal space. In the author's experience, the long-duration xenon photocoagulation applications were more effective than argon laser in producing resolution of subretinal exudation caused by a choroidal hemangioma with one treatment. Moderately intense burns are required to cause collapse of the outer cystic layers of the retina and to stimulate glial proliferation, which provides adhesion of the surviving inner retina to the surface of Bruch's membrane (Fig. 14-10). This amount of photocoagulation does not reduce the size of the hemangioma. It is unnecessary to attempt to destroy the tumor.

FIG. 14-10   Diagram of Photocoagulation Treatment of Choroidal Hemangioma.

A, Cystoid retinal edema and degeneration and atrophy of the RPE are caused by chronic serous exudation derived from the hemangioma before the exudation extending into the surrounding subretinal space *(arrow)*.

B, Atrophic subretinal scar after moderately intense confluent photocoagulation. Retinal astrocytes attached to Bruch's membrane overlying the tumor probably replace the RPE cells as the barrier to the passage of choroidal exudate into the retina and subretinal space.

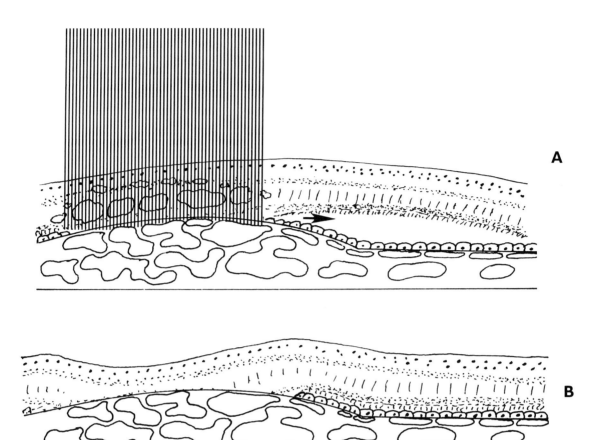

Subretinal and sub-RPE exudate and blood derived from choroidal neovascularization extending through breaks within or around the peripapillary end of Bruch's membrane into the sub-RPE or subretinal space

The reader should review the anatomy, physiology, and clinical and fluorescein angiographic features of choroidal neovascularization in Chapter 2. Choroidal neovascular membranes typically grow outward in a cartwheel fashion from the site of their ingrowth through Bruch's membrane, or in a tongue-shaped distribution from the optic disc margin into either the sub-RPE (type I neovascularization) or subretinal space (type II neovascularization). Initially this may be unassociated with exudation, visible changes in the RPE and retina, or loss of visual function. Exudation from these vessels, however, usually occurs and causes detachment of either the retina alone or the RPE and retina.

The rate of blood perfusion and the permeability alteration within these CNVMs are variable and are important in determining the ease with which the membrane may be detected angiographically. Early-phase angiograms are important in determining the precise location of these CNVMs and their proximity to the foveolar area. In some instances the capillary details of these membranes are readily visible angiographically. In others, because of poor perfusion of the new vessels or because of overlying blood or cloudy exudate, precise localization is not possible. If blood flow through a CNVM is minimal and there is no exudate surrounding the membrane, it may not be possible to detect its presence angiographically. Likewise, if the neovascular tuft is very small it may be clinically and angiographically invisible, or it may appear identical to a small drusen or a small RPE detachment identical to that seen in idiopathic central serous chorioretinopathy (Fig. 14-11). The biomicroscopic and fluorescein angiographic clues to the presence of choroidal neovascularization are discussed in detail in Chapter 2 and are summarized in Table 14-1. There is no problem requiring greater experience in the interpretation of fluorescein angiography than that of the detection and localization of poorly perfused or small occult CNVMs. Good-quality stereoscopic fundus photographs and angiograms are essential in such cases.

FIG. 14-11   Large Serous RPE Detachment Associated with Occult Choroidal Neovascular Membranes.

A and B, On initial examination the cause of the hyperfluorescent spot (A, *arrow*) within the area of RPE detachment was unrecognized. Several months later it is apparent that the hyperfluorescent spot in A was a small CNVM (B) that had enlarged.

C to F, Large serous RPE detachment in this elderly man with drusen in the opposite macula. *Arrows,* C and D, indicate location of new vessels. Following krypton red laser photocoagulation (E) the retinal RPE reattached (F) and 2 years later his visual acuity was 20/30.

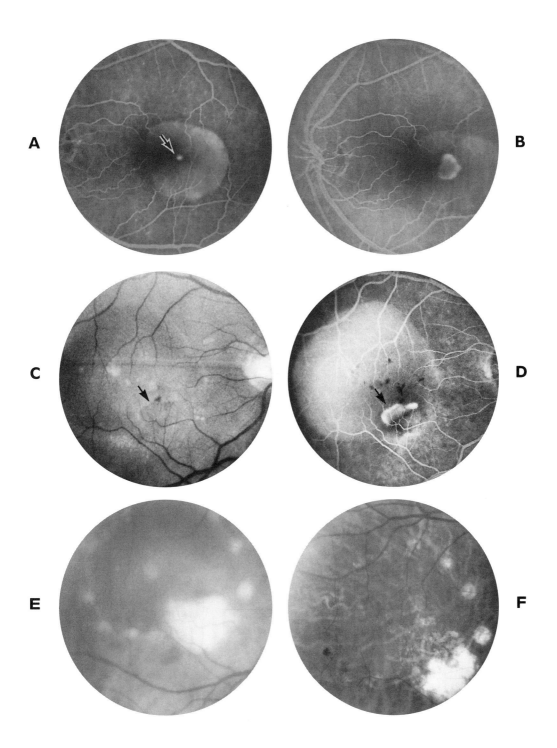

The visual prognosis in patients with choroidal neovascularization, with or without treatment, is directly related to the distance of the CNVM from the center of the fovea and to a lesser degree to the location of the CNVM in reference to the foveal center (Fig. 14-12). Paracentral burns applied in the horizontal median are more likely to be associated with visual disability. Randomized controlled clinical trials by the Macular Photocoagulation Study (MPS) and others have established the efficacy of laser photocoagulation treatment in symptomatic patients with well-defined CNVM located outside the FAZ (extrafoveal CNVM), for those extending into but not beneath the center of the FAZ (juxtafoveal CNVM), and for CNVM extending beneath the FAZ (subfoveal CNVM).[21,28,29,85-92,107] The MPS guidelines in reference to extrafoveal and juxtafoveal membranes apply to patients with age-related macular degeneration (AMD), presumed ocular histoplasmosis (POHS), and idiopathic CNVM. The MPS guidelines for subfoveal CNVM apply only to AMD in patients either with a primary CNVM or a recurrent CNVM after photocoagulation. Results of treatment of subfoveal CNVM in AMD should not be extrapolated to include subfoveal CNVM in other disorders, particularly in younger patients whose prognosis without treatment may be better. Likewise, the results of these trials do not apply to patients with ill-defined CNVM, with large areas of RPE detachment, or with inactive CNVM unassociated with exudate or blood irrespective of their location.

Photocoagulation of subfoveal CNVM appears to be of limited benefit for patients with CNVM greater than 2 optic disc areas in size.[90] The potential benefit is maximum in the patient with a small subfoveal CNVM (one disc area or less) and low visual acuity (20/200 or worse).[93] Although the MPS subfoveal study randomized patients with visual acuity as good as 20/30, most physicians are reluctant to recommend treatment until the patient has demonstrated a further decline in visual acuity.[149] Although the prognosis for patients with untreated subfoveal CNVM is poor,[14,15] some patients do retain or recover good central vision following spontaneous resolution of the subretinal fluid and exudate (see Figs. 3-21, *A* and *B*, and 3-45).

When the edge of the CNVM lies one disc diameter or more from the FAZ, the prognosis for spontaneous resolution of the macular detachment is relatively good and the patient may elect to be followed before considering treatment.

FIG. 14-12   Diagram Depicting the Relationship of Location of CNVMs and the Prognosis for the Recovery of Useful Central Vision Following Photocoagulation Treatment. Stippled Area *(CFZ)* Corresponds to the Capillary-Free Zone.

A, Small peripapillary CNVM: excellent prognosis.
B, Large peripapillary CNVM: good prognosis.
C, Extrafoveolar CNVM: fair to good prognosis.
D, Extrafoveolar CNVM: good prognosis.
E, Extrafoveal CNVM: very good prognosis.
F, Peripheral macular CNVM: excellent prognosis.
G, Juxtafoveolar CNVM: poor prognosis. **A** and **F** may be observed for evidence of growth before photocoagulation.

FIG. 14-13   Photocoagulation of Type 1 sub-RPE CNVM.

A, Diagram depicting moderately intense photocoagulation of CNVM.
B, Chorioretinal scar and partly obliterated CNVM after photocoagulation.

Before the availability of krypton red and yellow and argon green laser instruments, it was difficult to achieve effective photocoagulation burns at the level of the RPE in the area of the FAZ because absorption of the blue component of blue-green laser by the xanthophyll pigment produced superficial retinal burns. In spite of the theoretical advantages of krypton red and yellow over argon green in the treatment of juxtafoveal lesions, the treatment results are probably comparable.[13]

There is general agreement that coverage of the entire CNVM with moderately intense, overlapping, long-duration (0.2 second or longer) applications of laser is important in achieving a successful result (see Figs. 3-33, *G* to *L;* 3-37, *A* to *F;* 3-41, and 14-13). The spot size used depends on the proximity of the membrane to the center of the fovea as well as the size of the membrane. Smaller spot sizes (100 to 200 μm) may be used to delimit the membrane. Spot sizes of 200 or 500 μm are used to treat the central portion of the membrane. In general, the intensity of the photocoagulation application should be sufficiently intense to produce whitening that extends into the inner one-third of the retina. A test spot outside the area of the CNVM may be used to assure proper intensity of the applications

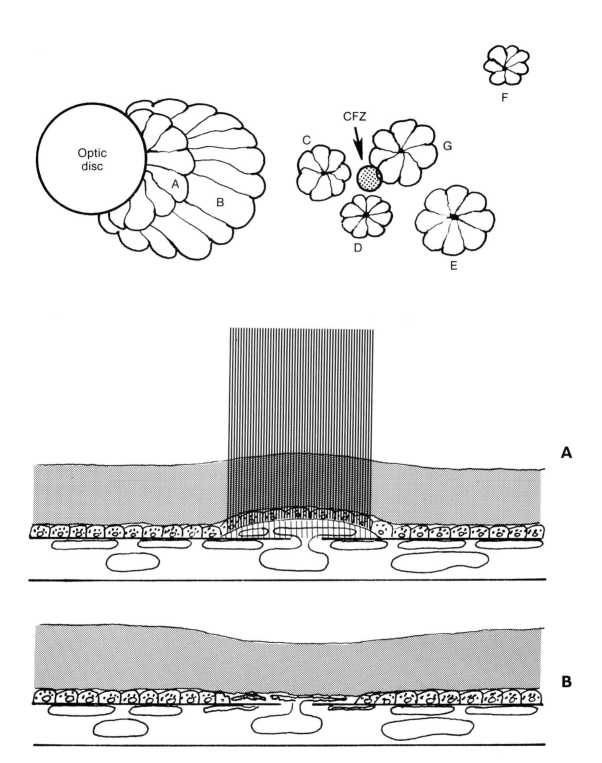

and to assess the patient's ability to maintain steady fixation. It is desirable to treat that portion of the CNVM near the center of the foveola first, since bleeding when it occurs during treatment frequently occurs from the periphery of the CNVM away from the site of photocoagulation. If bleeding occurs during photocoagulation, pressure should be applied to the contact lens and the area of bleeding should be treated rapidly to prevent blood from spreading beneath the foveolar area. To ensure complete treatment of the membrane it is advisable to include photocoagulation of a small margin of at least 75 μm in width of the retina surrounding the membrane. This margin may be reduced when treating some juxtafoveal CNVMs. If nuclear lens changes cause distortion of the burn during application of argon laser, it may be advisable to shift to krypton red laser. Since krypton red laser is primarily absorbed by choroidal melanocytes, the use of long-duration applications (0.2 second or longer), larger spot sizes (200 to 500 μm), and lower intensities, sufficient to produce a yellow-white burn that is confined to the outer one-half to two-thirds of the retina, will reduce the chances of choroidal hemorrhage and rupture of Bruch's membrane. If the edge of the CNVM closest to the foveola is covered by more than a thin film of blood, there is less chance that photocoagulation will be successful. Nevertheless if the extrafoveal area of neovascularization is reasonably well outlined, it may be advisable to apply Krypton red laser treatment rather than waiting for clearing of the blood, during which time the new vessels may extend beneath the foveal center (Fig. 14-14). The value of placing a delimiting line of photocoagulation as a barrier between an area of subretinal blood that obscures the underlying CNVM and the foveola as a means of preventing spread of the membrane and blood into the center of the fovea is unknown. There is little chance that such treatment provides an effective barrier for at least 6 to 8 weeks.

FIG. 14-14 Photocoagulation of Subretinal New Vessels Partly Obscured by Blood.

A, Sudden loss of vision occurred in the left eye of this woman with age-related macular degeneration and a disciform scar in the right eye. Fluorescein angiography (**B**) and indocyanine green angiography (**C**) indicated the approximate location of the subretinal neovascular membrane (*arrows,* **B** and **C**). Intense krypton red laser treatment (**D**) was successful in eradicating the membrane. Her visual acuity was 20/40 several months after treatment (**E**).

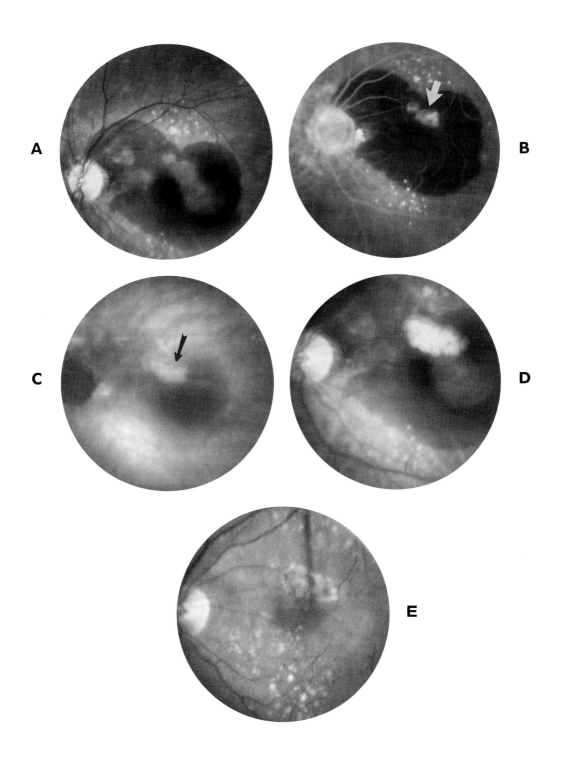

Large serous RPE detachments caused by type I choroidal neovascularization (vascularized serous RPE detachments)

The reader should review the discussion concerning the biomicroscopic and fluorescein angiographic signs of choroidal neovascularization accompanying serous RPE detachments on pp. 24-32. These are summarized in Table 14-1. If the locus of the CNVM can be determined with reasonable accuracy and if it lies outside the FAZ, intense argon laser or moderately intense krypton laser treatment to the membrane may be successful in causing resolution of the serous detachment of the RPE. Theoretically, krypton red should be superior to argon laser in treating that portion of the CNVM that extends beneath the serous RPE detachment. Supplemental use of noncontiguous burns along the border of the serous RPE detachment may or may not be required to produce flattening of the RPE (see Figs. 3-18, E and K; 3-19, D to I; and 14-11, E).[49,121] Patients with irregularly notched or elevated, partly organized serous RPE detachments are at risk of developing RPE tears either with or without photocoagulation treatment (see Figs. 3-19, 3-20, 3-91, and 14-18).[25,47,57] They also have a high incidence of continued or recurrent growth of sub-RPE fibrovascular tissue after treatment. The best technique of photocoagulation to avoid these complications is unclear. The author favors the technique illustrated in Figs. 3-18 E and K, and 14-11, E.

The value of photocoagulation in patients with large serous RPE detachments is uncertain. Although some studies have suggested a beneficial effect of photocoagulation,[5] the only controlled clinical trial to date found that use of a grid type of treatment to the surface of the serous RPE detachment in older patients with drusen was harmful.[106] In this latter study, I believe the authors' failure to recognize some of the signs of occult choroidal neovascularization and their protocol requirement for retreatment using a grid pattern at each visit when the detachment had not resolved were partly responsible for their adverse results.

TABLE 14-1
BIOMICROSCOPIC AND ANGIOGRAPHIC SIGNS OF CHOROIDAL NEOVASCULARIZATION

Biomicroscopic signs	Fluorescein angiogram signs	Comment
Elevation, often irregular, of RPE with preservation of fine details of RPE; evidence suggesting type 1 CNVM	May show no change or minimal irregular early fluorescence and late, often pinpoint areas of staining	Patient may be asymptomatic even when subfoveal CNVM is present; see Figs. 2-6 and 3-15
Cloudy subretinal exudate	Details of CNVM may be evident; late staining in area of CNVM	See Fig. 3-17
Subretinal pigmented ring, mound, or plaque; evidence suggesting type 2 CNVM	In presence of subretinal exudate, CNVM usually evident in area of or extending beyond RPE change; this sign most frequently seen in presumed ocular histoplasmosis syndrome and myopic degeneration	See Figs. 3-36; 3-37; 3-39; 3-45; 3-72, J to L; and 3-78, A to C
Yellow exudate in outer retina and subretinal space	Exudate obstructs background choroidal fluorescence and does not stain; staining occurs in area of CNVM that lies adjacent to yellow exudate	See Figs. 3-81, J to L; and 3-90, D
Blood in outer retina and subretinal space	Blood obstructs background fluorescence	See Figs. 2-8; 3-21; 3-33, A and B; 3-36, E and F; 3-39, G and H; and 3-54, A and B
Subretinal white or partly pigmented plaque or mound of fibrous tissue	Some details of hidden CNVM may be evident; lesion always stains	See Figs. 3-39, I and L; and 3-41, K and L
Subretinal and sub-RPE blood vessels	When associated with subretinal exudation, details of CNVM often evident; when unassociated with exudation, perfusion with dye may not be evident	See Figs. 3-17, A; 3-22, D to F; and 3-92, A to C
Cystoid macular edema associated with atrophic RPE changes	Evidence of CNVM extending close to or inside capillary-free zone usually present, as well as late staining of retinal cysts	See Fig. 2-15
Serous detachment of RPE with flattening or indentation of its margins ("notch" sign)	Uneven and delayed staining of sub-RPE exudate; irregular early hyperfluorescence and evidence of late staining may or may not occur in area of CNVM that lies primarily outside RPE detachment at site of notching	See Figs. 2-9, C to E; 2-10; 3-18; 3-19, A to C; 3-34, A to C; and 14-11
Round or oval serous detachment of RPE	Uneven and delayed staining of sub-RPE exudate	See Figs. 2-9, F; 2-10; and 3-19, D to F
Serous detachment of RPE with subretinal yellow exudate or blood near its margin	Blood and exudate obstruct background fluorescence; uneven and delayed staining of sub-RPE exudate	See Fig. 3-34, D and E
Serous and hemorrhagic detachment of RPE; blood usually dark gray or black and may show a fluid level	Uneven and delayed staining of sub-RPE exudate and obstruction of background fluorescence in area of blood	See Fig. 3-18, G to J
Organized RPE detachment: usually normal orange or brown color with preservation of fine details of RPE and drusen	Either no or minimal irregular or early hyperfluorescence either with or without late punctate or irregular staining	See Figs. 3-19, A to C; and 3-23, D to H
Combined serous and organized detachment of RPE; organized portion shows features above and is usually smaller and less elevated than area of RPE serous detachment	Organized portion of RPE detachment shows features above; serous RPE detachment shows slow and uneven staining	See Fig. 3-19
Radial chorioretinal folds surrounding partly organized serous RPE detachment	Stellate pattern of hyperfluorescent ridges around RPE detachment and irregular pattern of staining of RPE detachment	Folds are caused by contraction of Bruch's membrane–CNVM complex beneath RPE detachment; see Fig. 4-4, D to F

Localized paracentral retinal vascular alterations causing cystoid macular edema, exudation, and hemorrhage

Patients with loss of central vision caused by intraretinal and subretinal accumulation of exudate or blood caused by localized permeability alterations in the retinal vessels may regain vision following photocoagulation of the abnormal blood vessels if these are largely confined to the paracentral retina outside the papillomacular bundle area (see Figs. 6-31; 6-41, *D* to *G;* 6-43, *A* to *F;* and 6-59). Because of the unusual structure of the nerve fiber layer of Henle, exudate or blood derived from retinal blood vessels in the macular area tends to spread toward and to pool in the center of the macula, where it causes loss of visual acuity. Since photocoagulation adequate to correct retinal vascular permeability alteration also damages the nerve fiber layer of the retina, photocoagulation of retinal vascular abnormalities in the papillomacular bundle area must be limited in scope.

Favorable prognostic signs in regard to improvement of vision after photocoagulation of retinal vascular abnormalities include (1) preoperative visual acuity of 20/200 or better, (2) vascular abnormality confined to one-quarter of the macula, (3) typical pattern of polycystic edema without evidence of a large solitary cyst or inner lamellar hole formation, (4) a granular rather than globular pattern of yellowish intraretinal exudate in the foveolar area as part of a circinate ring surrounding a localized paramacular zone of abnormal capillaries outside the papillomacular bundle area, (5) angiographic evidence of perfusion of an intact perifoveolar capillary network, and (6) absence of evidence of significant disturbance of the RPE in the central macular area.

Before recommending photocoagulation the physician should recall the following:

1. The retina usually tolerates the presence of extracellular serous exudation, and to a lesser extent yellow circinate exudate, for a period of many months without sustaining significant permanent structural or functional damage (see Fig. 6-30).

2. Spontaneous improvement of intraretinal exudation and recovery of visual acuity may occur in some patients (see Fig. 6-30, *E* to *I*).

3. Complications of photocoagulation may occur (Figs. 14-16 to 14-19).

If photocoagulation of an area of retinal vascular leakage is undertaken, stereoangiograms provide a guide for placement of laser to those areas where maximum leakage of exudate is occurring. To effectively correct retinal vascular leakage of exudate with photocoagulation, it is desirable to observe some whitening of the inner retinal tissue and some narrowing and blanching of the abnormal blood vessels. Theoretically use of argon green or krypton yellow is preferable to krypton red or diode laser for the treatment of leaky retinal blood vessels. The favorable effect of laser, however, may be as much related to damage of the RPE as to the retinal vessels, since the longer wavelength lasers may also result in reduction of intraretinal exudation.[95] It is unnecessary to treat all areas of capillary dilation and mild leakage. To avoid causing a large paracentral scotoma, a noncontiguous pattern of photocoagulation burns may be used. It is advisable to avoid photocoagulation within one-third disc diameter from the center of the fovea during the first course of photocoagulation, even when the angiogram shows evidence of some dilation and dye leakage from the parafoveolar network. In such cases the central macular exudation may disappear and the patient may recover good visual acuity. Additional photocoagulation can be added later if the initial treatment fails to improve the degree of central macular exudation. The Branch Retinal Occlusion Study Group, on the basis of a randomized controlled clinical trial, has established guidelines for the treatment of macular edema and retinal neovascularization in patients with macular edema caused by branch retinal vein occlusion[11,12] (see Chapter 6, p. 562).

Generalized retinal vascular alterations causing cystoid macular edema, exudation, and hemorrhage

Patients with cystoid macular edema and exudation secondary to diffuse permeability alterations of the entire parafoveolar capillary network, e.g., aphakic cystoid macular edema, in general do not benefit by selective photocoagulation of portions of the capillary abnormality. The National Collaborative Diabetic Retinopathy Study and other clinical trials have demonstrated the value of peripheral panretinal photocoagulation in the treatment of proliferative diabetic retinopathy, and of focal and scatter photocoagulation in preserving central vision in patients with visual loss caused by background diabetic retinopathy.[16,24,32-35,37-40] (See Chapter 6, diabetic retinopathy, p. 523.) Diabetics with extensive cystoid macular edema and minimal ophthalmoscopic evidence of background retinopathy, however, usually fail to respond to photocoagulation treatment. The Central Retinal Vein Occlusion Study found that scatter treatment was ineffective in preserving or improving central visual acuity in patients with cystoid macular edema caused by central retinal vein occlusion (see Chapter 6).

Photocoagulation as a barrier to prevent retinal detachment and exudation or choroidal infiltration into the macular area

Photocoagulation to create a line of chorioretinal scarring and adhesion may be used as a barrier to the spread of rhegmatogenous retinal detachment, subretinal and intraretinal exudation, and choroidal infiltration into the central macular area in situations such as the following: (1) localized, long-standing, rhegmatogenous or tractional retinal detachment, usually in patients with demarcation lines and extensive retinal degeneration in the area of the detachment (see Fig. 12-27, *A*); (2) juxtapapillary retinal detachment associated with an optic pit; (3) retinal exudation and detachment caused by a juxtapapillary capillary angioma involving the temporal margin of the optic disc; and (4) juxtapapillary choroidal osteoma. Several rows of moderately intense, noncontiguous laser applications are usually adequate to prevent spread of long-standing rhegmatogenous or tractional retinal detachment. It may be necessary to use closely spaced or contiguous laser applications to prevent intraretinal and subretinal spread of exudation from a juxtapapillary angioma into the central macular area. It is not known whether or not creation of a chorioretinal scar at the edge of an expanding choroidal osteoma will prevent its growth.

Submacular exudation caused by peripheral retinal and choroidal vascular abnormalities

Yellow exudate may accumulate in the macula because of chronic exudative retinal detachment caused by peripheral retinal vascular abnormalities such as retinal telangiectasis (see Fig. 6-27, *A* to *F*) and angiomatosis retinae (see Fig. 10-22, *G* to *K*) or peripheral choroidal neovascularization (see Fig. 3-25, *A* to *C*). This macular deposit is caused by gravitation of the lipid- and protein-rich exudate from the peripheral lesion into the submacular region. These patients may recover some central vision following photocoagulation of the peripheral retinal vascular or choroidal neovascular abnormality (see Fig. 3-27, *J* to *L*). Recovery of useful central vision is unlikely, however, if there are large amounts of lipid exudation or evidence of organization of the exudate in the central macular area. Use of focal intense laser applications to the feeder artery leading to a large peripheral retinal capillary angioma to reduce blood flow to the angioma before direct treatment of the angioma may prevent massive exudative retinal detachment after treatment.[7,110]

▼ POSTPHOTOCOAGULATION EVALUATION

Providing the patient with a near-vision test card and several Amsler recording grids for use at home is worthwhile as a means of documenting the patient's course postoperatively (Fig. 14-15). The patient should be advised that visual function may decrease during the first few days following photocoagulation because of an increase in the amount of exudation. After this initial period, patients are advised to return promptly if they notice any further decrease in visual acuity or an increase in the size of the scotoma. The time of initial followup examination and the frequency of examinations depends on the patient's disease, the type of photocoagulation used, and the postoperative course.

After photocoagulation for idiopathic central serous chorioretinopathy, at least 6 weeks should be allowed for signs of resolution of the macular detachment. If no improvement in the degree of detachment occurs, angiography should be repeated and a careful search should be made for choroidal leaks outside the area of detachment, particularly in the area superior to the macula and disc. If resolution occurs following the initial treatment, it is unnecessary to repeat angiography, and the patient can be safely observed at yearly intervals as long as he or she has no recurrence of symptoms.

The patient should be reexamined within 1 to 3 weeks after photocoagulation of a CNVM. Biomicroscopic examination of the treated area is most important in determining the adequacy of treatment. The clinician should search for evidence of extension of the CNVM beyond the site of photocoagulation at each followup examination. Comparison of the biomicroscopic findings with stereophotographs made on each previous examination is important to detect the spread of the neovascular tissue, which usually appears as a grayish pseudopod of exudation extending from the zone of previous photocoagulation. If there is any evidence that suggests such an extension, angiography should be repeated. Three weeks after

FIG. 14-15 Amsler Grids and Near-Vision Chart.
Instructions for patients are written at bottom of chart.

treatment fluorescein angiography is usually repeated even if there is no evidence of either persistence or recurrence of the CNVM. If the CNVM has extended beyond the zone of treatment, it is usually readily apparent as a new area of fluorescein staining adjacent to the treatment zone. Interpretation of posttreatment angiograms done within the first 2 or 3 weeks after photocoagulation is difficult. The zone of previous photocoagulation treatment may or may not show evidence of fluorescein staining. As long as the staining is confined within the area of treatment, it is unnecessary to repeat the treatment. These patients should, however, be watched more carefully than those patients in whom repeat angiography shows no evidence of staining in the area of treatment. Even in a patient with the latter finding, however, subsequent growth of the CNVM from the edge of the prior treatment site may occur. It is important that the patient check his or her scotoma on the Amsler chart daily, particularly during the first several months after treatment. Resolution of all subretinal exudate and blood and return of visual function are the best and most reliable signs that treatment of a CNVM has been adequate.

A period of 8 to 12 weeks following photocoagulation of retinal vascular diseases may be required before the patient begins to show evidence of resolution of macular exudation and improvement of central function. If, after this time, biomicroscopic examination shows no evidence of resolution of edema or circinate exudate in the foveolar area, a repeat fluorescein angiogram should be obtained. If there is evidence of persistent dye leakage from the retinal capillaries that would explain the presence of the edema and exudation, then additional photocoagulation may be indicated.

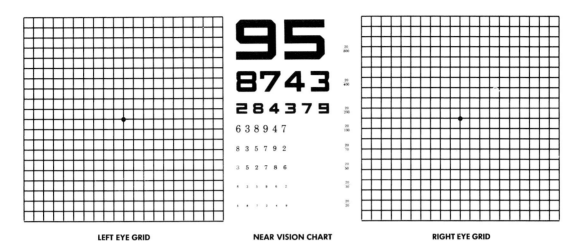

LEFT EYE GRID **NEAR VISION CHART** **RIGHT EYE GRID**

PROPER USE OF THESE GRIDS AND NEAR VISION CHART WILL ENABLE YOU TO DETECT CHANGES IN YOUR VISION.

1. PLACE IN SOME HANDY, WELL-LIGHTED PLACE, SUCH AS ON YOUR MIRROR, WHERE YOU CAN LOOK AT IT EACH MORNING, AT APPROXIMATELY 12 TO 14 INCHES FROM YOUR FACE.

2. WEAR THE GLASSES YOU NORMALLY WEAR FOR READING — IF YOU WEAR BIFOCALS, USE THE BOTTOM PORTION (THE READING PORTION) OF THE GLASS.

3. COVER ONE EYE AND WITH THE OTHER EYE LOOK AT THE CENTRAL BLACK DOT. ALL THE LINES SHOULD BE STRAIGHT AND NOT BROKEN. MARK WITH A PENCIL ANY AREAS OF DISTORTION, ANY GRAY OR BLURRED SPOTS WHERE THE LINES ARE MISSING. NOW CHECK YOUR OTHER EYE. IF ANY CHANGES ARE PRESENT AND YOUR DOCTOR IS NOT AWARE OF THEM, NOTIFY HIM PROMPTLY.

EACH MORNING, CHECK EACH EYE TO DETECT ANY CHANGES ON THE GRID AND THE NEAR VISION CHART. IF YOU NOTICE NEW AREAS OF DISTORTION (WAVY LINES INSTEAD OF STRAIGHT LINES, ENLARGEMENT OF THE BLANK SPOT — ESPECIALLY IN THE CENTRAL VISION AREA NEAR THE DOT), YOU SHOULD CONTACT YOUR DOCTOR IMMEDIATELY.

1-18-050   BPEI – 1983

▼ COMPLICATIONS OF PHOTOCOAGULATION THERAPY OF MACULAR LESIONS

Dyschromatopsia in the treating ophthalmologist

Arden et al. have demonstrated acute decrease in color contrast sensitivity (tritan axis) in all surgeons after operating blue-green laser instruments.[1] Sensitivity returned to baseline within 48 hours. There was a chronic sensitivity reduction proportional to duration of laser use. Bright reflections from the front surface of the contact lens appear to be the cause of loss of color contrast sensitivity. This effect was eliminated by using the lowest aiming beam intensity, blue absorbing filters, or green laser.

Corneal burns caused by indirect ophthalmoscopic delivery system

Severity of corneal damage varies from asymptomatic anterior stromal opacities to full-thickness coagulative necrosis and corneal edema requiring corneal transplantation.[64] Precautionary measures include avoidance of high power settings, optimization of aiming beam focus, and avoidance of treating through corneal edema.

Pupillary abnormalities

Iris burns may occur from use of any delivery system.[64,83,147] Partial sphincter palsies, cholinergic supersensitivity, and light-near dissociation (Adie's pupil) occurring after panretinal photocoagulation suggest that thermal damage to ciliary nerves in the suprachoroidal space may occur.

Lens burns

Focal lens opacifications occur most often in eyes with nuclear sclerosis treated with argon blue-green laser. Cataract pigments absorb blue and to a lesser degree green light, causing immediate but nonprogressive localized opacities. Longer wavelengths such as krypton red are minimally absorbed by lens pigments and are preferred in patients with nuclear cataracts. Krypton red laser may induce focal lens opacities in the presence of uveal pigment on the anterior lens capsule. Posterior capsulotomy may occur as a complication of indirect laser applications.[75]

Increased intraocular pressure

Most eyes after extensive panretinal photocoagulation experience a transient rise in intraocular pressure. In most cases the anterior chamber angle is open and the cause of the increased pressure is

FIG. 14-16 Complications of Photocoagulation Treatment.

A and **B**, Misplacement of photocoagulation. Early angiogram (**A**) showed fluorescein leakage from the perifoveal retinal capillaries in this patient who had bilateral aphakic cystoid macular edema. *Arrow* indicates center of fovea. A circular pattern of argon laser burns (**B**) was inadvertently placed too high. *Arrow* indicates center of fovea. One year later the cystoid macular edema had resolved in both eyes. Visual acuity in the right eye was 20/200 and in the untreated eye was 20/20.

C and **D**, Excessive xenon photocoagulation (**C**) used in treating a CNVM in the presumed ocular histoplasmosis syndrome. The retinal vessels are enveloped within the treated retina. Six months later the CNVM was destroyed. The visual acuity was 20/30, but there was metamorphopsia secondary to retinal traction lines radiating from the scar (**D**).

not known. In some cases ciliochoroidal effusion may cause closure of the anterior chamber angle and elevation of the intraocular pressure for several hours or days.[8] Medical treatment may be necessary in some cases. Dividing panretinal photocoagulation into two or more sessions reduces the chances of severe rise in intraocular pressure.

Accidental photocoagulation of the central macular area

Accidental photocoagulation of the foveolar area (Fig. 14-16, *A* and *B*) is most likely to occur in eyes with altered foveal anatomy, particularly in those with extensive remodeling of the retinal vasculature. Mistakes can be avoided by (1) adequate immobilization of the eye using retrobulbar anesthesia and sedation if necessary, (2) full pupillary dilation, (3) biomicroscopic study of the macula and comparison with good-quality stereoangiograms, (4) use of a stereo viewer or projector to monitor the angiogram during photocoagulation, (5) frequent reference to the foveolar area during photocoagulation, and (6) placement of the burns nearest to the center of the macula before doing treatment elsewhere.

Thermal papillitis from peripapillary treatment

Severe visual loss may occur after treatment in the peripapillary region.[9,132] The mechanism of this is not always clear. In some instances it may result from nerve fiber bundle damage to the juxtapapillary retina. In others injury to the optic nerve head itself occurs.

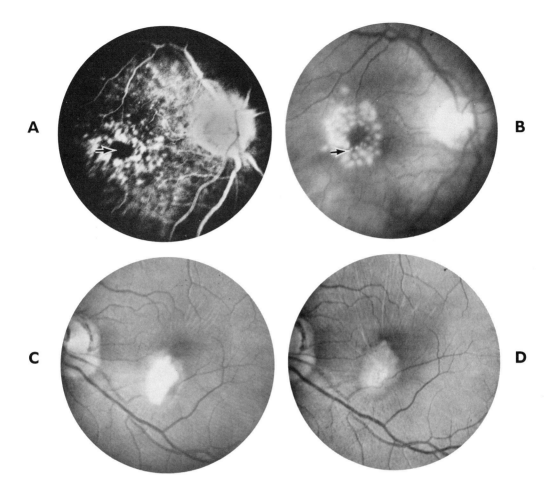

Hemorrhage

Hemorrhage may occur as an immediate or delayed complication of photocoagulation therapy.[50,53,55,57,82] Bleeding may occur from (1) the choriocapillaris, (2) a CNVM, (3) retinal blood vessels, or (4) retinal neovascular membranes. Subretinal bleeding caused by rupture of Bruch's membrane and the choriocapillaris is most likely to occur when using high-power, small-aperture (50 μm), long-wavelength photocoagulation laser applications. Bleeding from a CNVM during photocoagulation may occur either in the vicinity of or remote from the site of application of photocoagulation. Precautions include preliminary use of low power settings, reduction of power when reducing spot size (energy density varies inversely with the area of the laser spot), and avoidance of short-duration exposures (< 0.2 second) with long wavelengths. If bleeding occurs during treatment the operator should raise the intraocular pressure with pressure on the contact lens, readjust the treatment parameters, and make additional applications to the area until the bleeding stops. Bleeding from the retinal vessels into either the retina or the vitreous occurs infrequently during photocoagulation in the macular areas. It is most likely to occur with small-aperture, intense applications. It often stops spontaneously in a few seconds. Several applications of photocoagulation may be necessary to stop it. Delayed bleeding from an inadequately treated CNVM is one of the most common complications following photocoagulation. The use of intense, long-duration photocoagulation to cover the entire CNVM as well as a narrow zone of surrounding retina during the initial treatment is the best means of preventing this complication.

Choroidal neovascularization and subretinal fibrosis

The development of subretinal choroidal neovascularization and/or fibrous tissue proliferation may occur as a delayed complication following photocoagulation rupture of or damage to Bruch's membrane.* This complication often appears within several months after the treatment. Avoidance of small spot size (50 μm), intense burns, and repeated applications to the same area reduces the chance of subretinal neovascularization.

Choriovitreous neovascularization

Following intense photocoagulation burns, usually in the peripheral retina rather than the macula, proliferation of new vessels may occur from the choroid through the atrophic retina into the vitreous and cause vitreous hemorrhage.[4] Similar changes may rarely occur spontaneously.[123] Chorioretinal vascular anastomosis may become evident in photocoagulation scars.[44]

Retinal distortion

Distortion of the central retina after photocoagulation may be caused by (1) contraction of a chorioretinal scar with traction lines extending into the central foveolar area (Fig. 14-16, *C* and *D*) and (2) the formation and contraction of fibrocellular epiretinal membranes (Fig. 14-17).[45,60] Excessive photocoagulation in the paracentral area and, particularly, the retreating of a previously photocoagulated area are the most common causes of retinal, and in some cases chorioretinal, striae leading away from the site of a photocoagulation scar.[57] Contraction of an epiretinal membrane is most likely to occur following photocoagulation treatment of retinal vascular diseases, particularly when they are associated with inner retinal hemorrhages (Fig. 14-17).[51,62] This probably results from damage to the internal limiting membrane.

---

*References 4, 41, 43, 58, 61, 79, 118, 120, 133, 139, 141, 144.

FIG. 14-17   Complication of Photocoagulation Treatment.

A to **C**, Macular pucker (**C**) developing 2 months following photocoagulation of an area of retinal capillary leakage caused by a branch retinal vein occlusion (**A** and **B**).

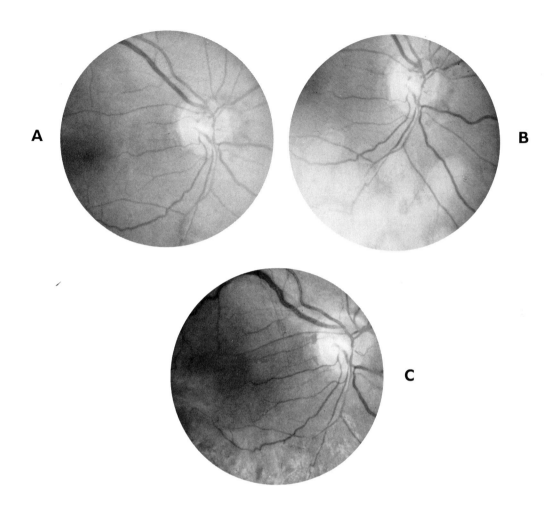

Acute RPE tear

During or after photocoagulation of a partly organized serous detachment of the RPE, a tear may occur along the edge of the RPE detachment and cause precipitous loss of central vision as well as a characteristic funduscopic appearance (see Figs. 3-19, *J* to *K,* and 3-91). During the course of krypton laser treatment to a relatively thick, often hypopigmented CNVM, abrupt contraction of the membrane may cause an acute dehiscence in the relatively normal RPE near the edge of the membrane (Fig. 14-18).[47,57,73,80]

Cystoid macular edema

Cystoid macular edema may occur following excessive photocoagulation in the paracentral retina or panretinal photocoagulation, particularly when the photocoagulation has partly obstructed the retinal venous outflow of the macula.[98] The development of or worsening of cystoid macular edema is a frequent complication of panretinal photocoagulation (PRP) for diabetic retinopathy.[99] Possible causes for this phenomenon include increased macular blood flow and inflammation induced by the laser treatment. Chances for this latter complication may be reduced by use of scatter photocoagulation to the macular area for background retinopathy before PRP, or the use of a more peripherally placed pattern of PRP. Cystoid macular edema, macular holes, peripheral retinal holes, and retinal detachment may occasionally occur soon after YAG laser opening of the posterior lens capsule.[146]

Paracentral scotoma

Despite preservation of excellent visual acuity, some patients experience great difficulty in reading because of large paracentral scotomata following photocoagulation. This complication is best avoided by using only the minimal photocoagulation required to treat the original lesion successfully. Some paracentral scotomas, including those induced with grid therapy, often become less apparent to the patient with passage of time.

Nerve fiber bundle defect causing loss of central vision

Excessive photocoagulation in the papillomacular bundle region may cause loss of central vision. No more than four clock hours of the fundus adjacent to the optic nerve on the temporal side should be treated with intense photocoagulation. Use of longer wavelength, moderately intense burns is helpful in reducing the changes of this complica-

FIG. 14-18 Complication of Photocoagulation Treatment.

A to D, Intraoperative RPE tear occurring during krypton laser photocoagulation. An angiogram made several weeks before treatment showed a CNVM (*arrow,* **A**) and neighboring serous RPE detachment. A repeat angiogram on the day of treatment showed a small spontaneous tear in the RPE (*arrow,* **B**). Postoperative photographs showed RPE tear (*arrows,* **C** and **D**) that occurred during treatment.

(From Gass, J.D.M.: Am. J. Ophthalmol. 98:700, 1984; published with permission from The American Journal of Ophthalmology; copyright by The Ophthalmic Publishing Co.[47])

tion. Particular care is required in treating lesions in the papillomacular bundle in patients with previous arcuate visual field caused by glaucoma or other optic nerve disease.

Vascular occlusion

Transient closure of large choroidal vessels, particularly during krypton laser photocoagulation, may cause large zones of delayed perfusion of the choroidal circulation angiographically (see Fig. 2-1, *E*).[26,57,69] Closure of choroidal vessels is usually unassociated with either biomicroscopic or functional changes. Biomicroscopic and angiographic evidence of wedge-shaped zones of choroidal vascular occlusion and functional damage have been observed after heavy argon and xenon photocoagulation of peripheral retinal vascular lesions.[52] Excessive laser treatment to the major retinal vessels, particularly with green or yellow wavelengths, may occasionally cause prolonged occlusion of the blood vessel. Severe loss of vision after panretinal photocoagulation may also be caused by choroidal ischemia in some cases.[72] Patients with collagen vascular disease may be particularly susceptible to ischemic damage.[70]

Macular hole formation

Macular hole formation may be the direct result of a central foveal burn.[54,81] I have observed the development of a full-thickness macular hole soon after ruby laser treatment of an extrafoveolar leak in a patient with idiopathic central serous chorioretinopathy. There was evidence that vitreous traction played a role in the hole formation. This traction may also have been partly responsible for the serous detachment. The photocoagulation may have played no role in causing the hole. I have been told of one other similar occurrence in a patient following photocoagulation for idiopathic central serous chorioretinopathy.

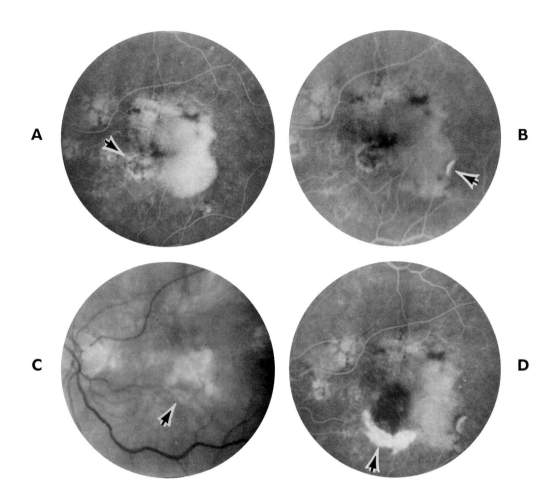

Progressive enlargement of photocoagulation scar

Many months following an apparently successful photocoagulation of a paracentral CNVM, the patient may notice the slowly progressive loss of central vision associated with concentric enlargement of the area of RPE and retinal atrophy surrounding the area of initial photocoagulation (Fig. 14-19).* This appears to be independent of the wavelength of laser used, the patient's age, or the size of the neovascular membrane treated. This apparently may occur in the absence of further exudation or hemorrhage from the site of the original CNVM. It is more likely to occur in highly myopic eyes. Progressive enlargement of the RPE atrophy into the center of the fovea is not always accompanied by a decrease in the visual acuity.

Lacquer crack formation or expansion

In eyes with myopic degeneration lacquer cracks may appear or preexisting cracks may elongate or widen after laser treatment.

Central binocular diplopia

Binocular vertical diplopia may occur either spontaneously or following treatment of patients with parafoveal CNVMs.[20] It is caused by displacement of the photoreceptors toward the CNVM. The patient may be unable to superimpose paracentral and more peripheral images simultaneously. This is usually not relieved by prism therapy. Monocular diplopia may also occur transiently in patients who develop a parafoveolar CNVM. They may see a faint, distorted image that is displaced slightly from the more normal image.

Visual loss caused by retrobulbar anesthesia

Although not a direct complication of photocoagulation, visual loss caused by complications of the preoperative administration of retrobulbar anesthesia represents one of the important risks to the patient undergoing photocoagulation. The complications of anesthesia include retrobulbar hemorrhage, optic nerve sheath hemorrhage, central retinal artery occlusion, ocular penetration or

*References 10, 30, 108, 115, 118, 119, 122.

FIG. 14-19   Progressive Enlargement of Photocoagulation Scar.

A to **D,** This middle-aged woman with a type 2 subretinal neovascular membrane (**A**) had argon-green laser photocoagulation (**B**). Postoperatively her visual acuity was 20/60 (**C**). It declined slowly to 20/200 associated with progressive enlargement of the scar over the subsequent 4 years (**D**).

E to **G,** Argon laser treatment in March of 1981 (**E**), seventeen months after treatment (**F**), and three years after treatment (**G**). The visual acuity declined from 20/30 to 20/60.

perforation, and brainstem anesthesia (see discussion, p. 758).[71]

Loss of peripheral visual field and development of nyctalopia

After panretinal photocoagulation approximately 5% of patients have constriction of the peripheral visual field to large isopters, and many patients are aware of nyctalopia.

Other complications

Transient myopia,[77] uveal effusion, and light-induced seizures[36] are other complications that usually occur only in patients receiving extensive panretinal photocoagulation. Severe unexplained transient visual loss may occur in patients after panretinal photocoagulation for diabetic retinopathy.[72]

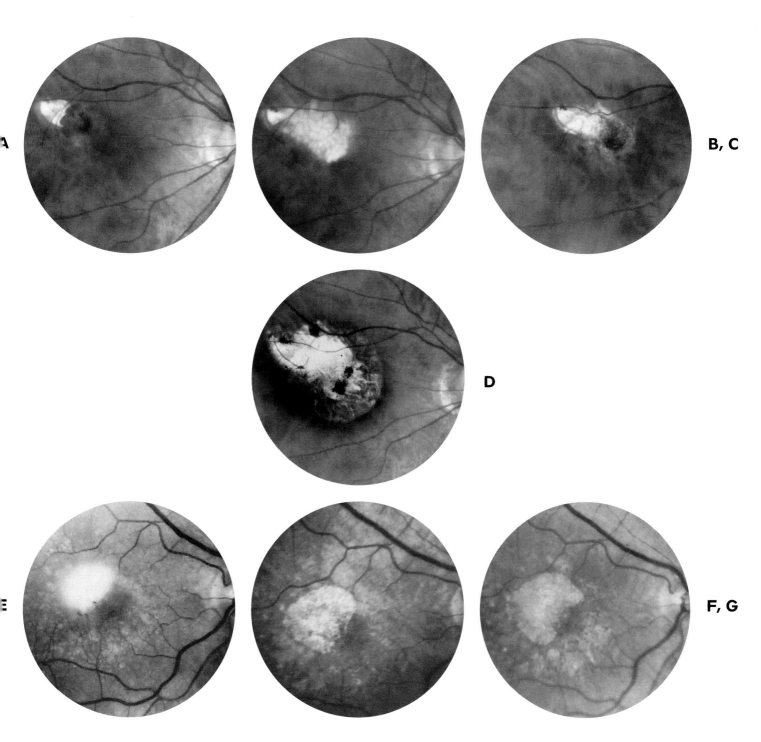

A

B, C

D

E

F, G

1057

REFERENCES

1. Arden GB, Berninger T, Hogg CR, Perry S: A survey of color discrimination in German ophthalmologists; changes associated with the use of lasers and operating microscopes. *Ophthalmology* 98:567-575, 1991.

2. Balles MW, Puliafito CA, D'Amico DJ, et al: Semiconductor diode laser photocoagulation in retinal vascular disease. *Ophthalmology* 97:1553-1561, 1990.

3. Benner JD, Huang M, Morse LS, et al: Comparison of photocoagulation with the argon, krypton, and diode laser indirect ophthalmoscopes in rabbit eyes. *Ophthalmology* 99:1554-1563, 1992.

4. Benson WE, Townsend RE, Pheasant TR: Choriovitreal and subretinal proliferations: Complications of photocoagulation. *Ophthalmology* 86:283-289, 1979.

5. Bird AC, Grey RHB: Photocoagulation of disciform macular lesions with krypton laser. *Br J Ophthalmol* 63:669-673, 1979.

6. Blair CJ, Gass JDM: Photocoagulation of the macula and papillomacular bundle in the human. *Arch Ophthalmol* 88:167-171, 1972.

7. Blodi CF, Russell SR, Pulido JS, Folk JC: Direct and feeder vessel photocoagulation of retinal angiomas with dye yellow laser. *Ophthalmology* 97:791-797, 1990.

8. Blondeau P, Pavan PR, Phelps CD: Acute pressure elevation following panretinal photocoagulation. *Arch Ophthalmol* 99: 1239-1241, 1981.

9. Bloom SM: Thermal papillitis after dye red photocoagulation of a peripapillary choroidal neovascular membrane. *Retina* 10:261-264, 1990.

10. Brancato R, Pece A, Avanza P, Radrizzani E: Photocoagulation scar expansion after laser therapy for choroidal neovascularization in degenerative myopia. *Retina* 10:239-243, 1990.

11. Branch Vein Occlusion Study Group: Argon laser photocoagulation for macular edema in branch vein occlusion. *Am J Ophthalmol* 98:271-282, 1984.

12. Branch Vein Occlusion Study Group: Argon laser scatter photocoagulation for prevention of neovascularization and vitreous hemorrhage in branch vein occlusion; a randomized clinical trial. *Arch Ophthalmol* 104:34-41, 1986.

13. Bressler SB: Editorial: Does wavelength matter when photocoagulating eyes with macular degeneration or diabetic retinopathy? *Arch Ophthalmol* 111:177-180, 1993.

14. Bressler SB, Bressler NM, Fine SL, et al: Natural course of choroidal neovascular membranes within the foveal avascular zone in senile macular degeneration. *Am J Ophthalmol* 93:157-163, 1982.

15. Bressler SB, Bressler NM, Fine SL, et al: Subfoveal neovascular membranes in senile macular degeneration; relationship between membrane size and visual prognosis. *Retina* 3:7-11, 1983.

16. British Multicentre Study Group: Photocoagulation for diabetic maculopathy; a randomized controlled clinical trial using xenon arc. *Diabetes* 32:1010-1016, 1983.

17. Brod RD, Lightman DA: Effect of contact lens biomicroscopy on the clarity of fluorescein angiography. *Ophthalmology* 98:532-534, 1991.

18. Brod RD, Lightman DA: A simple method for assessing laser photocoagulation coverage of choroidal neovascular membranes. *Am J Ophthalmol* 110:313, 1990.

19. Brooks HL Jr, Eagle RC Jr, Schroeder RP, et al: Clinicopathologic study of organic dye laser in the human fundus. *Ophthalmology* 96:822-834, 1989.

20. Burgess D, Roper-Hall G, Burde RM: Binocular diplopia associated with subretinal neovascular membranes. *Arch Ophthalmol* 98:311-317, 1980.

21. Canadian Ophthalmology Study Group: Argon green vs krypton red laser photocoagulation of extrafoveal choroidal neovascular lesions; one-year results in age-related macular degeneration. *Arch Ophthalmol* 111:181-185, 1993.

22. Central Vein Occlusion Study Group: Baseline and early natural history report; the central Vein Occlusion Study. *Arch Ophthalmol* 111:1087-1095, 1993.

23. Chamberlin JA, Bressler NM, Bressler SB, et al: The use of fundus photographs and fluorescein angiograms in the identification and treatment of choroidal neovascularization in the Macular Photocoagulation Study. *Ophthalmology* 96: 1526-1534, 1989.

24. Cheng H: Response of proliferative diabetic retinopathy to xenon-arc photocoagulation; a multicentre randomized controlled trial; second interim report. *Trans Ophthalmol Soc UK* 96:224-227, 1976.

25. Chuang EL, Bird AC: Bilaterality of tears of the retinal pigment epithelium. *Br J Ophthalmol* 72:918-920, 1988.

26. Cohen SMZ, Fine SL, Murphy RP, et al: Transient delay in choroidal filling after krypton red laser photocoagulation for choroidal neovascular membranes. *Retina* 3:284-290, 1983.

27. Condon P, Jampol LM, Farber MD, et al: A randomized clinical trial of feeder vessel photocoagulation of proliferative sickle cell retinopathy. II. Update and analysis of risk factors. *Ophthalmology* 91:1496-1498, 1984.

28. Coscas G, Soubrane G: Photocoagulation des néovaisseaux sous-rétiniens dans la dégénérescence maculaire sénile par laser à argon; résultats de l'étude randomisée de 60 cas. *Bull Mem Soc Fr Ophthalmol* 94:149-154, 1982, publ. 1983.

29. Coscas G, Soubrane G, Ramahefasolo C, Fardeau C: Perifoveal laser treatment for subfoveal choroidal new vessels in age-related macular degeneration; results of a randomized clinical trial. *Arch Ophthalmol* 109:1258-1265, 1991.

30. Dastgheib K, Bressler SB, Green WR: Clinicopathologic correlation of laser lesion expansion after treatment of choroidal neovascularization. *Retina* 13:345-352, 1993.

31. De Jong PTVM, Vrensen GFJM, Willekens BLJC, Mooy CM: Free running neodymium-YAG laser coagulation of the human fovea; a light and electron microscopic study. *Retina* 9:312-318, 1989.

32. Diabetic Retinopathy Study Research Group: Four risk factors for severe visual loss in diabetic retinopathy; the third report from the Diabetic Retinopathy Study. *Arch Ophthalmol* 97:654-655, 1979.

33. Diabetic Retinopathy Study Research Group: Photocoagulation treatment of proliferative diabetic retinopathy; clinical application of Diabetic Retinopathy Study (DRS) findings, DRS report number 8. *Ophthalmology* 88:583-600, 1981.

34. Diabetic Retinopathy Study Research Group: Photocoagulation treatment of proliferative diabetic retinopathy: the second report of Diabetic Retinopathy Study findings. *Ophthalmology* 85:82-106, 1978.

35. Diabetic Retinopathy Study Research Group: Preliminary report on effects of photocoagulation therapy. *Am J Ophthalmol* 81:383-396, 1976.

36. Duffey RJ: Grand mal seizure during argon laser panretinal photocoagulation. *Am J Ophthalmol* 103:116-117, 1987.

37. Early Treatment Diabetic Retinopathy Study Research Group: Early photocoagulation for diabetic retinopathy; ETDRS report number 9. *Ophthalmology* 98:766-785, 1991.

38. Early Treatment Diabetic Retinopathy Study Research Group: Fluorescein angiographic risk factors for progression of diabetic retinopathy; ETDRS report number 13. *Ophthalmology* 98:834-840, 1991.

39. Early Treatment Diabetic Retinopathy Study Research Group: Photocoagulation for diabetic macular edema; Early Treatment Diabetic Retinopathy Study report number 1. *Arch Ophthalmol* 103:1796-1806, 1985.

40. Early Treatment Diabetic Retinopathy Study Research Group: Treatment techniques and clinical guidelines for photocoagulation of diabetic macular edema; Early Treatment Diabetic Retinopathy Study report number 2. *Ophthalmology* 94:761-774, 1987.

41. Fine SL, Patz A, Orth DH, et al: Subretinal neovascularization developing after prophylactic argon laser photocoagulation of atrophic macular scars. *Am J Ophthalmol* 82:352-357, 1976.

42. Folk JC, Sneed SR, Folberg R, et al: Early retinal adhesion from laser photocoagulation. *Ophthalmology* 96:1523-1525, 1989.

43. François J, De Laey JJ, Cambie E, et al: Neovascularization after argon laser photocoagulation of macular lesions. *Am J Ophthalmol* 79:206-210, 1975.

44. Galinos SO, McMeel JW, Trempe CL, Schepens CL: Chorioretinal anastomoses after argon laser photocoagulation. *Am J Ophthalmol* 82:241-245, 1976.

45. Gass JDM: Options in the treatment of macular diseases. *Trans Ophthalmol Soc UK* 92:449-468, 1972.

46. Gass JDM: Photocoagulation of macular lesions. *Trans Am Acad Ophthalmol Otolaryngol* 75:580-608, 1971.

47. Gass JDM: Retinal pigment epithelial rip during krypton red laser photocoagulation. *Am J Ophthalmol* 98:700-706, 1984.

48. Gass JDM: Saline for contact lens ophthalmoscopy and photocoagulation. *Am J Ophthalmol* 108:742, 1989.

49. Gass JDM: Serous retinal pigment epithelial detachment with a notch; a sign of occult choroidal neovascularization. *Retina* 4:205-220, 1984.

50. Gass JDM: *Stereoscopic atlas of macular diseases; diagnosis and treatment*, ed. 2, St. Louis, 1977, CV Mosby, pp. 382-401.

51. Gloor B, Werner H: Postkoagulative und spontan auftretende internoretinale Fibroplasie mit Maculadegeneration. *Klin Monatsbl Augenheilkd* 151:822-845, 1967.

52. Goldbaum MH, Galinos SO, Apple D, et al: Acute choroidal ischemia as a complication of photocoagulation. *Arch Ophthalmol* 94:1025-1035, 1976.

53. Goldberg MF, Herbst RW: Acute complications of argon laser photocoagulation; epipapillary and peripapillary neovascularization. *Arch Ophthalmol* 89:311-318, 1973.

54. Goldberg MF, Young RSL, Read J, Cunha-Vaz JG: Macular hole caused by a 589-nanometer dye laser operating for 10 nanoseconds. *Retina* 3:40-44, 1983.

55. Gole GA: Massive choroidal haemorrhage as a complication of krypton red laser photocoagulation for disciform degeneration. *Aust NZ J Ophthalmol* 13:37-38, 1985.

56. Gottfredsdóttir MS, Stefánsson E, Jónasson F, Gislason I: Retinal vasoconstriction after laser treatment for diabetic macular edema. *Am J Ophthalmol* 115:64-67, 1993.

57. Grabowski WM, Decker WL, Annesley WH Jr: Complications of krypton red laser photocoagulation to subretinal neovascular membranes. *Ophthalmology* 91:1587-1591, 1984.

58. Guyer DR, D'Amico DJ, Smith CW: Subretinal fibrosis after laser photocoagulation for diabetic macular edema. *Am J Ophthalmol* 113:652-656, 1992.

59. Haller JA, Lim JI, Goldberg MF: Pilot trial of transscleral diode laser retinopexy in retinal detachment surgery. *Arch Ophthalmol* 111:952-956, 1993.

60. Han DP, Folk JC: Internal limiting membrane wrinkling after argon and krypton laser photocoagulation of choroidal neovascularization. *Retina* 6:215-219, 1986.

61. Han DP, Mieler WF, Burton TC: Submacular fibrosis after photocoagulation for diabetic macular edema. *Am J Ophthalmol* 113:513-521, 1992.

62. Hövener G: Koagulationsbehandlung bei der Periphlebitis retinae (mit Auftreten einer internoretinalen Fibroplasie). *Klin Monatsbl Augenheilkd* 165:271-274, 1974.

63. Hunter DG, Repka MX: Diode laser photocoagulation for threshold retinopathy of prematurity; a randomized study. *Ophthalmology* 100:238-244, 1993.

64. Irvine WD, Smiddy WE, Nicholson DH: Corneal and iris burns with the laser indirect ophthalmoscope. *Am J Ophthalmol* 110:311-313, 1990.

65. Jagger JD, Hamilton AMP, Polkinghorne P: Q-switched neodymium YAG laser vitreolysis in the therapy of posterior segment disease. *Graefes Arch Clin Exp Ophthalmol* 228:222-225, 1990.

66. Jalkh AE, Pflibsen K, Pomerantzeff O, et al: A new solid-state, frequency-doubled neodymium-YAG photocoagulation system. *Arch Ophthalmol* 106:847-849, 1988.

67. Jampol LM, Condon P, Farber M, et al: A randomized clinical trial of feeder vessel photocoagulation of proliferative sickle cell retinopathy. I. Preliminary results. *Ophthalmology* 90:540-545, 1983.

68. Jampol LM, Farber M, Rabb MF, Serjeant G: An update on techniques of photocoagulation treatment of proliferative sickle cell retinopathy. *Eye* 5:260-263, 1991.

69. Johnson R, Schatz H: Delayed choroidal vascular filling after krypton laser photocoagulation. *Am J Ophthalmol* 99:154-158, 1985.

70. Jost BF, Olk RJ, Patz A, et al: Anterior segment ischaemia following laser photocoagulation in a patient with systemic lupus erythematosus. *Br J Ophthalmol* 72:11-16, 1988.

71. Klein ML, Jampol LM, Condon PI, et al: Complications of retrobulbar anesthesia given prior to photocoagulation. In: Fine SL, Owens SL, editors: *Management of retinal vascular and macular disorders,* Baltimore, 1983, Williams & Wilkins, pp. 208-212.

72. Kleiner RC, Elman MJ, Murphy RP, Ferris FL III: Transient severe visual loss after panretinal photocoagulation. *Am J Ophthalmol* 106:298-306, 1988.

73. Koenig F, Soubrane G, Coscas G: Déchirures de l'épithélium pigmentaire après photocoagulation au cours de la dégénérescence maculaire liée à l'âge. *J Fr Ophtalmol* 12:775-780, 1989.

74. Laatikainen L, Kohner EM, Khoury D, Blach RK: Panretinal photocoagulation in central retinal vein occlusion: a randomised controlled clinical study. *Br J Ophthalmol* 61:741-753, 1977.

75. Lakhanpal V, Husain D, Schocket SS: Posterior capsulotomy as a complication of indirect laser photocoagulation. *Am J Ophthalmol* 114:600-602, 1992.

76. Landers MB III, Stefansson E, Wolbarsht ML: Panretinal photocoagulation and retinal oxygenation. *Retina* 2:167-175, 1982.

77. Lerner BC, Lakhanpal V, Schocket SS: Transient myopia and accommodative paresis following retinal cryotherapy and panretinal photocoagulation. *Am J Ophthalmol* 97:704-708, 1984.

78. Lewis H, Resnick SC, Flannery JG, Straatsma BR: Tissue plasminogen activator treatment of experimental subretinal hemorrhage. *Am J Ophthalmol* 111:197-204, 1991.

79. Lewis H, Schachat AP, Haimann MH, et al: Choroidal neovascularization after laser photocoagulation for diabetic macular edema. *Ophthalmology* 97:503-511, 1990.

80. Lim JI, Blair NP, Liu SJ: Retinal pigment epithelium tear in a diabetic patient with exudative retinal detachment following

panretinal photocoagulation and filtration surgery. *Arch Ophthalmol* 108:173-174, 1990.

81. Lim JI, Schachat AP, Conway B: Macular hole formation following laser photocoagulation of choroidal neovascular membranes in a patient with presumed ocular histoplasmosis. *Arch Ophthalmol* 109:1500-1501, 1991.

82. Little HL, Zweng HC: Complications of argon laser retinal photocoagulation. *Trans Pac Coast Oto-Ophthalmol Soc* 52: 115-129, 1971.

83. Lobes LA Jr, Bourgon P: Pupillary abnormalities induced by argon laser photocoagulation. *Ophthalmology* 92:234-236, 1985.

84. Macular Photocoagulation Study Group: Argon laser photocoagulation for idiopathic neovascularization; results of a randomized clinical trial. *Arch Ophthalmol* 101:1358-1361, 1983.

85. Macular Photocoagulation Study Group: Argon laser photocoagulation for neovascular maculopathy; three-year results from randomized clinical trials. *Arch Ophthalmol* 104:694-701, 1986.

86. Macular Photocoagulation Study Group: Argon laser photocoagulation for ocular histoplasmosis; results of a randomized clinical trial. *Arch Ophthalmol* 101:1347-1357, 1983.

87. Macular Photocoagulation Study Group: Krypton laser photocoagulation for idiopathic neovascular lesions; results of a randomized clinical trial. *Arch Ophthalmol* 108:832-837, 1990.

88. Macular Photocoagulation Study Group: Krypton laser photocoagulation for neovascular lesions of ocular histoplasmosis; results of a randomized clinical trial. *Arch Ophthalmol* 105:1499-1507, 1987.

89. Macular Photocoagulation Study Group: Laser photocoagulation of subfoveal neovascular lesions in age-related macular degeneration; results of a randomized clinical trial. *Arch Ophthalmol* 109:1220-1231, 1991.

90. Macular Photocoagulation Study Group: Laser photocoagulation of subfoveal neovascular lesions in age-related macular degeneration; updated findings from two clinical trials. *Arch Ophthalmol* 111:1200-1209, 1993.

91. Macular Photocoagulation Study Group: Laser photocoagulation of subfoveal recurrent neovascular lesions in age-related macular degeneration; results of a randomized clinical trial. *Arch Ophthalmol* 109:1232-1241, 1991.

92. Macular Photocoagulation Study Group: Subfoveal neovascular lesions in age-related macular degeneration; guidelines for evaluation and treatment in the Macular Photocoagulation Study. *Arch Ophthalmol* 109:1242-1257, 1991.

93. Macular Photocoagulation Study Group: Visual outcome after laser photocoagulation for subfoveal choroidal neovascularization secondary to age-related macular degeneration; the influence of initial lesion size and initial visual acuity. *Arch Ophthalmol* 112:480-488, 1994.

94. Marshall J, Bird AC: A comparative histopathological study of argon and krypton laser irradiations of the human retina. *Br J Ophthalmol* 63:657-668, 1979.

95. Marshall J, Clover G, Rothery S: Some new findings on retinal irradiation by krypton and argon lasers. *Doc Ophthalmol Proc Ser* 36:21-37, 1984.

96. Marshall J, Hamilton AM, Bird AC: Histopathology of ruby and argon laser lesions in monkey and human retina; a comparative study. *Br J Ophthalmol* 59:610-630, 1975.

97. Marshall J, Hamilton AM, Bird AC: Intra-retinal absorption of argon laser irradiation in human and monkey retinae. *Experientia* 30:1335-1337, 1974.

98. McDonald HR, Schatz H: Macular edema following panretinal photocoagulation Study Group: Visual outcome after laser. *Retina* 5:5-10, 1985.

99. McDonald HR, Schatz H: Visual loss following panretinal photocoagulation. for proliferative diabetic retinopathy. *Ophthalmology* 92:388-393, 1985.

100. McMullen WW, Garcia CA: Comparison of retinal photocoagulation using pulsed frequency-doubled neodymium-YAG and argon green laser. *Retina* 12:265-269, 1992.

101. McNamara JA, Tasman W, Vander JF, Brown GC: Diode laser photocoagulation for retinopathy of prematurity; preliminary results. *Arch Ophthalmol* 110:1714-1716, 1992.

102. Menchini U, Trabucchi G, Brancato R, Cappellini A: Can the diode laser (810 nm) effectively produce chorioretinal adhesion? *Retina* 12(Suppl):S80-S86, 1992.

103. Meyer-Schwickerath G: *Light coagulation* (translated by S.M. Drance), St. Louis, 1960, CV Mosby.

104. Michels M, Flannery JG, Lewis H: Noncontact transscleral neodymium-YAG laser photocoagulation of the pigmented rabbit retina. *Arch Ophthalmol* 110:395-398, 1992.

105. Miller H, Miller B: Photodynamic therapy of subretinal neovascularization in the monkey eye. *Arch Ophthalmol* 111:855-860, 1993.

106. Moorfields Macular Study Group: Retinal pigment epithelial detachments in the elderly: a controlled trial of argon laser photocoagulation. *Br J Ophthalmol* 66:1-16, 1982.

107. Moorfields Macular Study Group: Treatment of senile disciform macular degeneration: a single-blind randomised trial by argon laser photocoagulation. *Br J Ophthalmol* 66:745-753, 1982.

108. Morgan CM, Schatz H: Atrophic creep of the retinal pigment epithelium after focal macular photocoagulation. *Ophthalmology* 96:96-102, 1989.

109. Naveh N, Bartov E, Weissman C: Subthreshold argon-laser irradiation elicits a pronounced vitreal prostaglandin E_2 response. *Graefes Arch Clin Exp Ophthalmol* 229:178-181, 1991.

110. Nicholson DH: Induced ocular hypertension during photocoagulation of afferent artery in angiomatosis retinae. *Retina* 3:59-61, 1983.

111. Novotny HR, Alvis DL: A method of photographing fluorescence in circulating blood in the human retina. *Circulation* 24:82-86, 1961.

112. Patz A: Clinical and experimental studies on retinal neovascularization. *Am J Ophthalmol* 94:715-743, 1982.

113. Peyman GA, Raichand M, Zeimer RC: Ocular effects of various laser wavelengths. *Surv Ophthalmol* 28:391-404, 1984.

114. Pournaras CJ, Tsacopoulos M, Strommer K, et al: Scatter photocoagulation restores tissue hypoxia in experimental vasoproliferative microangiopathy in miniature pigs. *Ophthalmology* 97:1329-1333, 1990.

115. Rice TA, Murphy RP, Fine, SL, Patz A: Stability of size of argon laser photocoagulation scars in ocular histoplasmosis. *In:* Fine SL, Owens SL, editors: *Management of retinal vascular and macular disorders,* Baltimore, 1983, Williams & Wilkins, pp. 187-190.

116. Roider J, Michaud NA, Flotte TJ, Birngruber R: Response of the retinal pigment epithelium to selective photocoagulation. *Arch Ophthalmol* 110:1786-1792, 1992.

117. Royster AJ, Nanda SK, Hatchell DL, et al: Photochemical initiation of thrombosis; fluorescein angiographic, histologic, and ultrastructural alterations in the choroid, retinal pigment epithelium, and retina. *Arch Ophthalmol* 106:1608-1614, 1988.

118. Rutledge BK, Wallow IHL, Poulsen GL: Sub-pigment epithelial membranes after photocoagulation for diabetic macular edema. *Arch Ophthalmol* 111:608-613, 1993.

119. Schatz H, Madeira D, McDonald HR, Johnson RN: Progressive enlargement of laser scars following grid laser photocoagulation for diffuse diabetic macular edema. *Arch Ophthalmol* 109:1549-1551, 1991.

120. Schatz H, Yannuzzi LA, Gitter KA: Subretinal neovascularization following argon laser photocoagulation treatment for central serous chorioretinopathy: complication or misdiagnosis? *Trans Am Acad Ophthalmol Otolaryngol* 83:OP893-OP906, 1977.

121. Schmidbauer JM, Daus W, Krastel H, Völker HE: Krypton-Lasertherapie; Anwendung bei sekundärer seröser Abhebung des retinalen Pigmentepithels (RPE) und bei multiplen idiopathischen serösen Abhebungen des RPE. *Ophthalmologe* 89:437-440, 1992.

122. Shah SS, Schachat AP, Murphy RP, Fine SL: The evolution of argon laser photocoagulation scars in patients with the ocular histoplasmosis syndrome. *Arch Ophthalmol* 106:1533-1536, 1988.

123. Sinclair SH, Salmenson BD: Idiopathic choriovitreal membrane – a case report. *Br J Ophthalmol* 76:567-568, 1992.

124. Singerman LJ: Red krypton laser therapy of macular and retinal vascular diseases. *Retina* 2:15-28, 1982.

125. Singerman LJ, Kalski RS: Tunable dye laser photocoagulation for choroidal neovascularization complicating age-related macular degeneration. *Retina* 9:247-257, 1989.

126. Singh A, Boulton M, Lane C, et al: Inhibition of microvascular endothelial cell proliferation by vitreous following retinal scatter photocoagulation. *Br J Ophthalmol* 74:328-332, 1990.

127. Smiddy WE: Diode endolaser photocoagulation. *Arch Ophthalmol* 110:1172-1174, 1992.

128. Smiddy WE, Fine SL, Green WR, Glaser BM: Clinicopathologic correlation of krypton red, argon blue-green, and argon green laser photocoagulation in the human fundus. *Retina* 4:15-21, 1984.

129. Smiddy WE, Hernandez E: Histopathologic results of retinal diode laser photocoagulation in rabbit eyes. *Arch Ophthalmol* 110:693-698, 1992.

130. Smiddy WE, Patz A, Quigley HA, Dunkelberger GR: Histopathology of the effects of tunable dye laser on monkey retina. *Ophthalmology* 95:956-963, 1988.

131. Stempels N, Tassignon MJ, Worst J: Les hémorrhagies dans la bourse prémaculaire traitées par le Q-switched Nd-YAG laser. *Ophtalmolgie* 4:314-316, 1990.

132. Swartz M, Apple DJ, Creel D: Sudden severe visual loss associated with peripapillary burns during panretinal photocoagulation. *Br J Ophthalmol* 67:517-519, 1983.

133. Takeda M: Clinical investigation of choroidal neovascularization. Part 1. Choroidal neovascularization after xenon arc photocoagulation. *Folia Ophthalmol Jpn* 33:24-34, 1982.

134. Thomas EL, Apple DJ, Swartz M, Kavka-Van Norman D: Histopathology and ultrastructure of krypton and argon laser lesions in a human retina-choroid. *Retina* 4:22-39, 1984.

135. Thomas MA, Ibanez HE: Subretinal endophotocoagulation in the treatment of choroidal neovascularization. *Am J Ophthalmol* 116:279-285, 1993.

136. Trempe CL, Mainster MA, Pomerantzeff O, et al: Macular photocoagulation; optimal wavelength selection. *Ophthalmology* 89:721-728, 1982.

137. Ulbig MW, McHugh DA, Hamilton AMP: Photocoagulation of choroidal neovascular membranes with a diode laser. *Br J Ophthalmol* 77:218-221, 1993.

138. Uram M: Ophthalmic laser microendoscope endophotocoagulation. *Ophthalmology* 99:1829-1832, 1992.

139. Varley MP, Frank E, Purnell EW: Subretinal neovascularization after focal argon laser for diabetic macular edema. *Ophthalmology* 95:567-573, 1988.

140. Vogel M, Schäfer FP, Stuke M, et al: Animal experiments for the determination of an optimal wavelength for retinal coagulations. *Graefes Arch Clin Exp Ophthalmol* 227:277-280, 1989.

141. Wallow IHL, Myers FL, Kim YM, Bindley C: Subretinal new vessels after krypton laser photocoagulation. *Arch Ophthalmol* 103:1844-1848, 1985.

142. Wallow IHL, Sponsel WE, Stevens TS: Clinicopathologic correlation of diode laser burns in monkeys. *Arch Ophthalmol* 109:648-653, 1991.

143. Weiter JJ, Zuckerman R: The influence of the photoreceptor-RPE complex on the inner retina; an explanation for the beneficial effects of photocoagulation. *Ophthalmology* 87:1133-1139, 1980.

144. Wilkinson CP: Stimulation of subretinal neovascularization. *Am J Ophthalmol* 81:104-106, 1976.

145. Wilson DJ, Finkelstein D, Quigley HA, Green WR: Macular grid photocoagulation; an experimental study on the primate retina. *Arch Ophthalmol* 106:100-105, 1988.

146. Winslow RL, Taylor BC: Retinal complications following YAG laser capsulotomy. *Ophthalmology* 92:785-789, 1985.

147. Woon WH, ffytche TJ, Hamilton AMP, Marshall J: Iris clipping of a diode laser beam when performing retinal photocoagulation. *Br J Ophthalmol* 75:386-390, 1991.

148. Yannuzzi LA: Krypton red laser photocoagulation for subretinal neovascularization. *Retina* 2:29-46, 1982.

149. Yannuzzi LA: A new standard of care for laser photocoagulation of subfoveal choroidal neovascularization secondary to age-related macular degeneration. *Arch Ophthalmol* 112:462-464, 1994.

150. Yannuzzi LA, Shakin JL: Krypton red laser photocoagulation of the ocular fundus. *Retina* 2:1-14, 1982.

Index

I-9

I-11

I-15

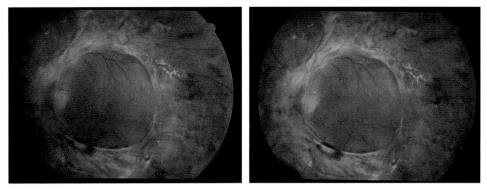

PLATE 65 Cicatricial diabetic proliferative retinopathy.

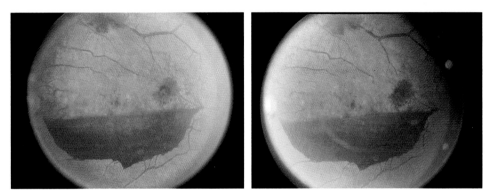

PLATE 66 X-ray irradiation retinopathy. Subhyaloid hematoma.

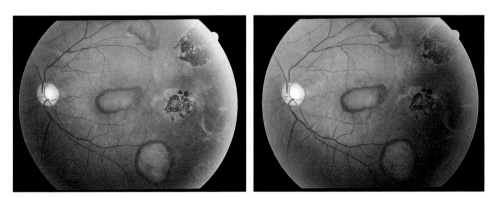

PLATE 67 Sickle cell C retinopathy.

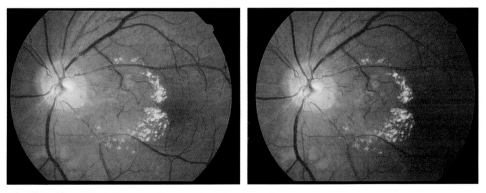

PLATE 68 Eales' disease with macular telangiectasis.

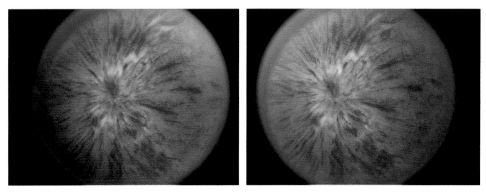

PLATE 69   Central retinal vein obstruction.

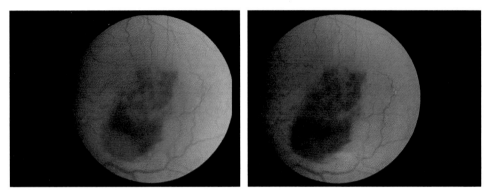

PLATE 70   Acute branch retinal vein obstruction.

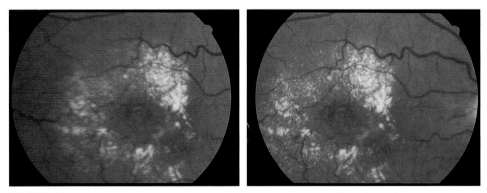

PLATE 71   Old branch retinal vein obstruction, leaking venous collateral vessels.

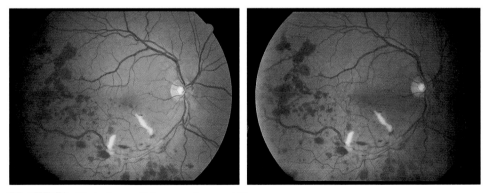

PLATE 72   Retinal vasculitis, secondary syphilis.

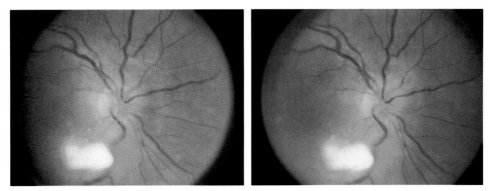

PLATE 73 Monilia retinitis.

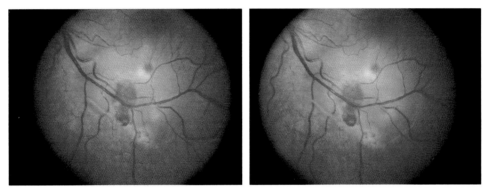

PLATE 74 Toxoplasmosis retinitis and macular detachment.

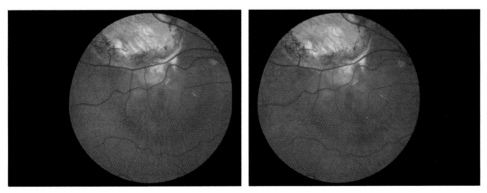

PLATE 75 Toxoplasmosis chorioretinal scar, type 2 SRN.

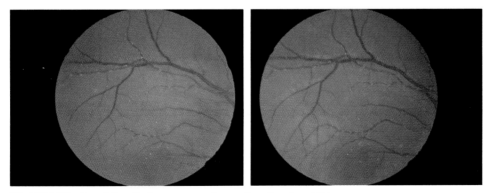

PLATE 76 Arterial wall plaques, toxoplasmosis retinochoroiditis.

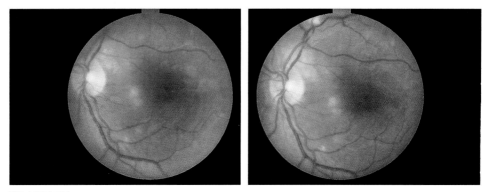

PLATE 77 Subfoveal nematode, small type, DUSN.

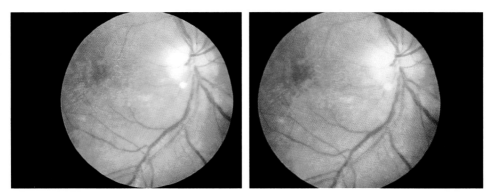

PLATE 78 Subfoveal nematode, large type, DUSN.

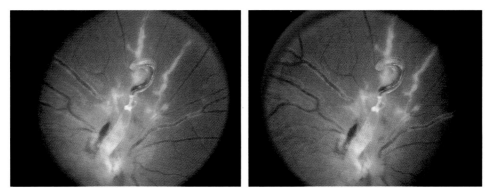

PLATE 79 *Gnathostoma spinigerum.*

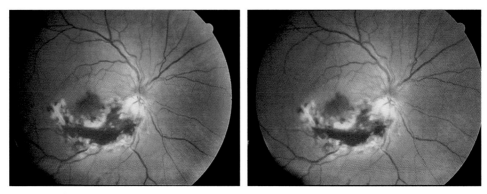

PLATE 80 Cytomegalovirus neuroretinitis.

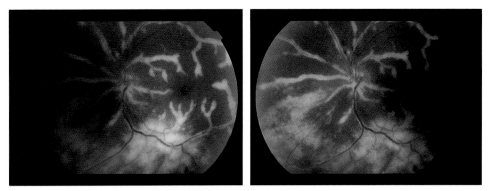

PLATE 81 Cytomegalovirus retinitis, frosted retinal angiitis.

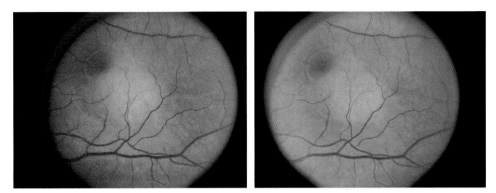

PLATE 82 Chicken pox, focal choroiditis.

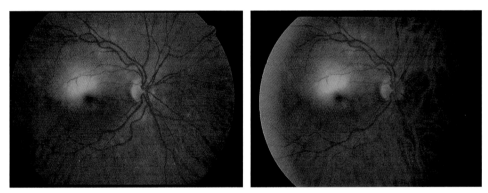

PLATE 83 Herpes zoster acute retinitis in AIDS. Posterior outer retinal necrosis (PORN).

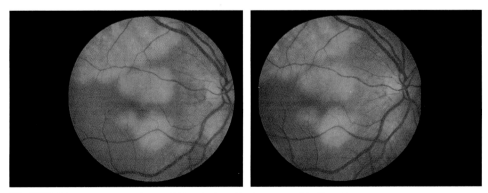

PLATE 84 Acute posterior multifocal placoid pigment epitheliopathy.

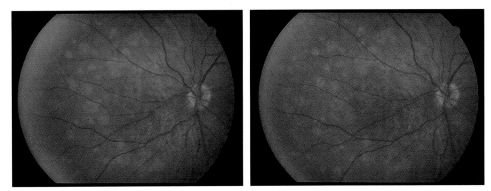

PLATE 85   Multiple evanescent white dot syndrome.

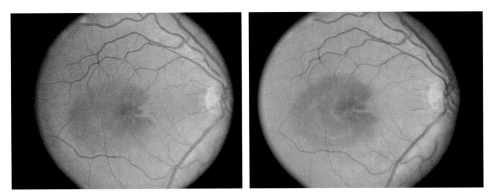

PLATE 86   Acute macular neuroretinopathy.

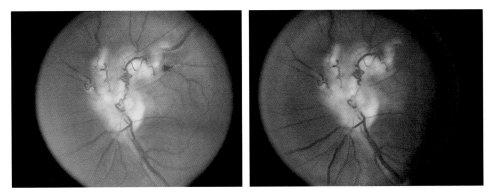

PLATE 87   Sarcoid neuroretinitis.

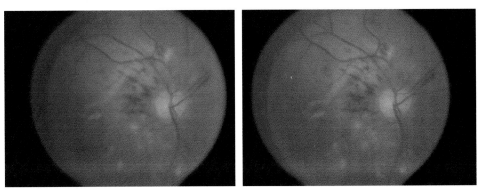

PLATE 88   Behçet's disease.

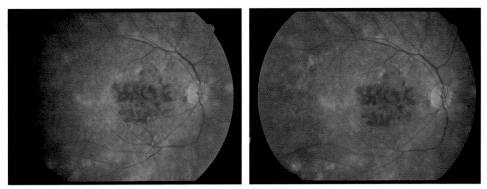

PLATE 89   Vitiliginous chorioretinitis.

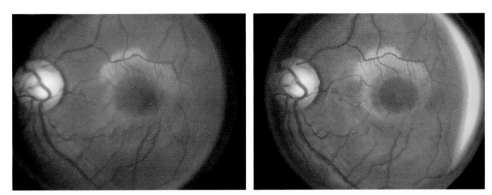

PLATE 90   Berlin's edema.

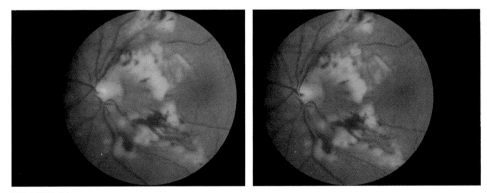

PLATE 91   Purtscher's retinopathy.

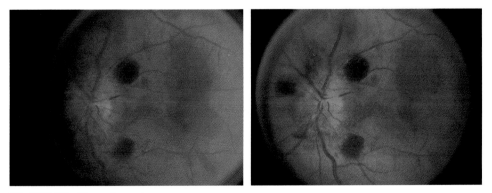

PLATE 92   Terson's syndrome.

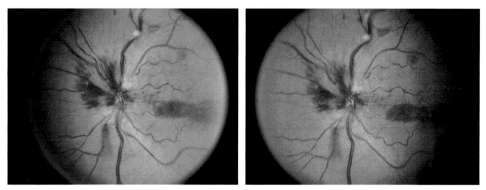

PLATE 93 Postcontusion hemorrhagic neuroretinopathy.

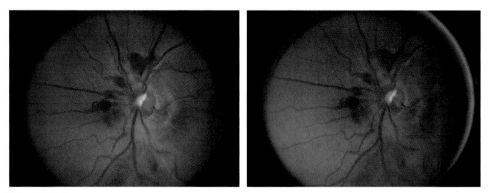

PLATE 94 Valsalva retinopathy

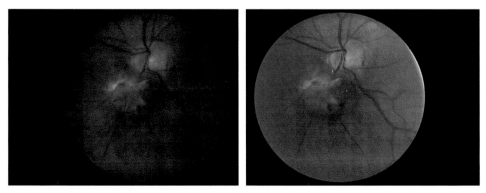

PLATE 95 Evulsion of optic nerve head.

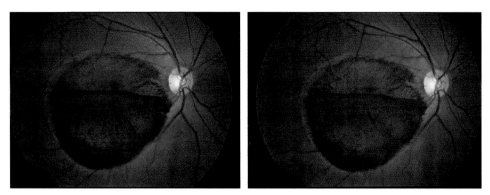

PLATE 96 Intraocular iron foreign body, pseudomelanoma.

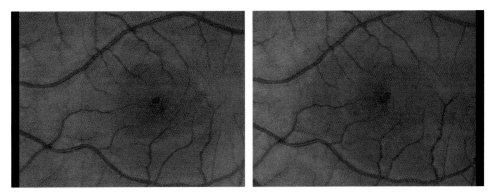

PLATE 97   Sun gazing maculopathy, outer lamellar foveolar facet.

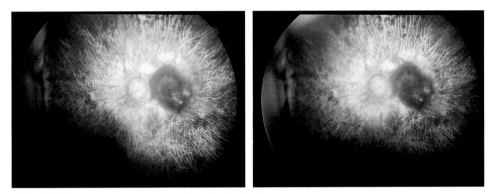

PLATE 98   Siderosis, intraocular iron foreign body.

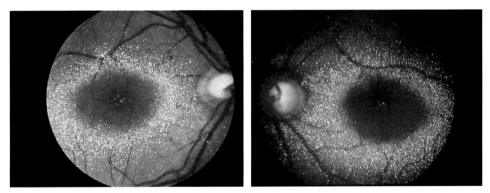

PLATE 99   Canthaxanthin retinopathy (right and left eye) (**nonstereo**).

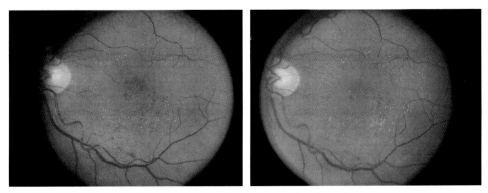

PLATE 100   Canthaxanthin retinopathy, old branch retinal vein occlusion.

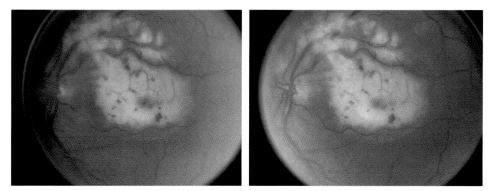

PLATE 101   Gentamicin retinal toxicity.

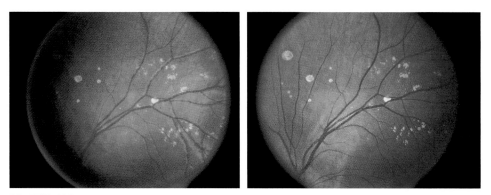

PLATE 102   Congenital grouped albinotic RPE nevi.

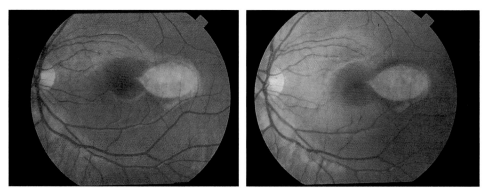

PLATE 103   Amelanotic RPE nevus.

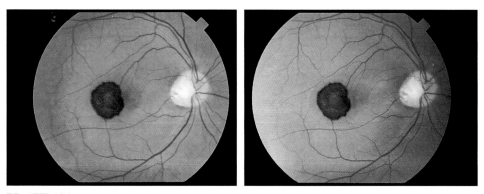

PLATE 104   Congenital RPE hyperplasia.

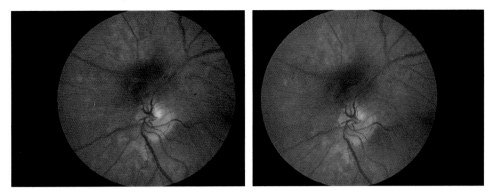

PLATE 105   Combined RPE and retinal hamartoma, papillary type.

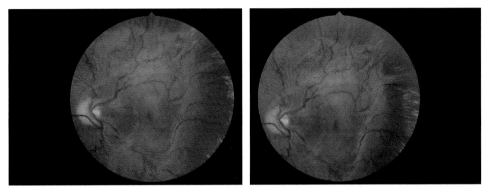

PLATE 106   Combined RPE and retinal hamartoma, macular type.

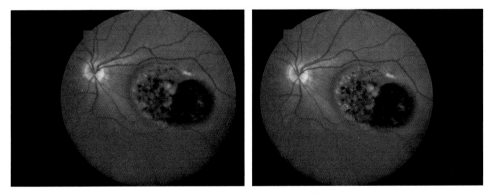

PLATE 107   Reactive RPE hyperplasia, familial macular staphyloma.

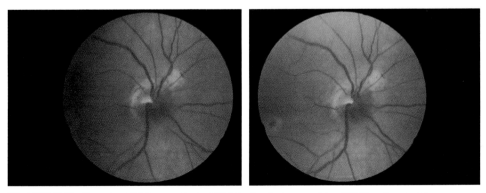

PLATE 108   Reactive RPE hyperplasia, POHS, simulating combined RPE and retinal hamartoma.

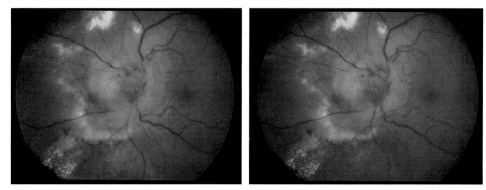

PLATE 109   Reactive RPE hyperplasia, POHS, pseudomelanoma.

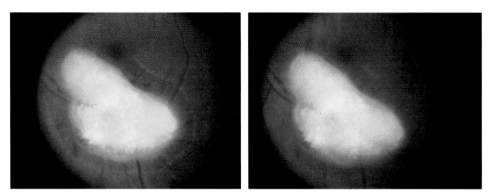

PLATE 110   Astrocytic hamartoma, retina.

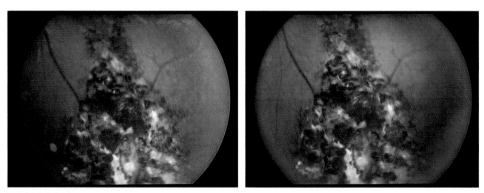

PLATE 111   Cavernous hemangioma, retina.

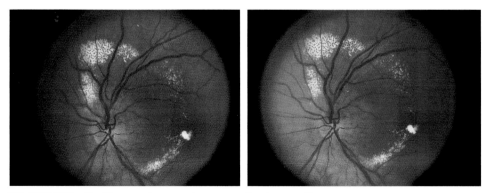

PLATE 112   Capillary angioma, optic nerve and retina, sessile type.

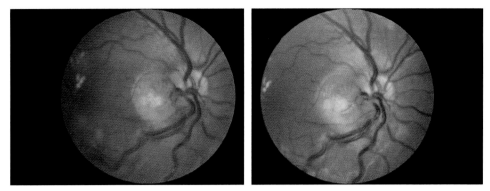

PLATE 113 Capillary angioma, optic nerve, endophytic type.

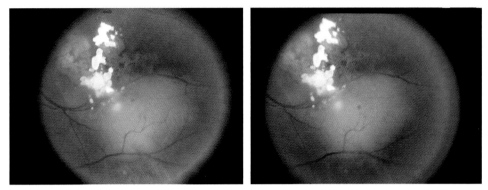

PLATE 114 Retinoma ("regressed retinoblastoma").

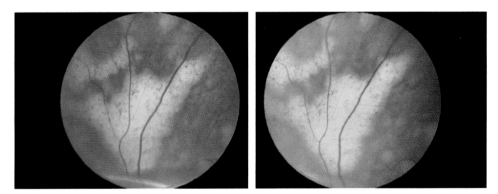

PLATE 115 Non-Hodgkin's lymphoma (reticulum cell sarcoma).

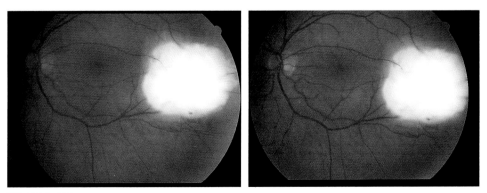

PLATE 116 Metastatic carcinoma to retina.

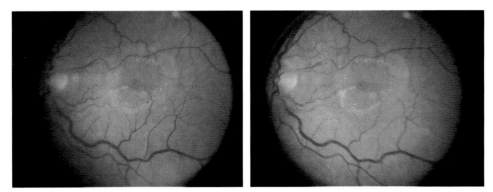

PLATE 117 Vitreous traction maculopathy.

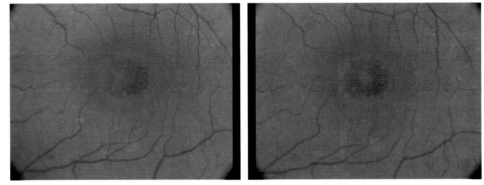

PLATE 118 Stage 1-B lesion (impending or occult macular hole).

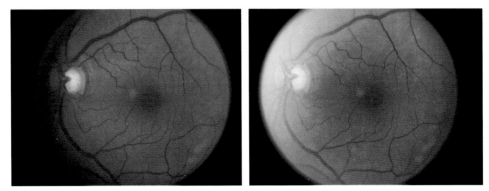

PLATE 119 Stage 2 macular hole, "can-opener" type.

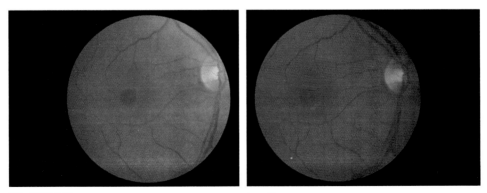

PLATE 120 Stage 3 macular hole with "operculum."

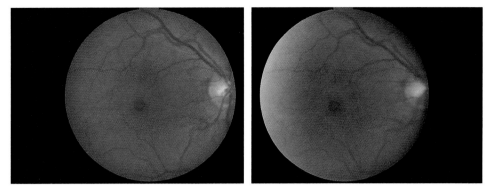

PLATE 121 Pseudomacular hole (hole in epiretinal membrane).

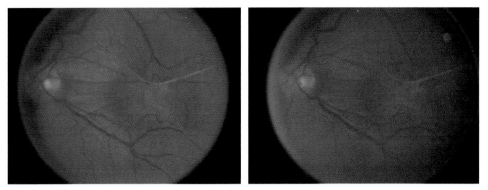

PLATE 122 Macular pucker, partly separated epiretinal membrane.

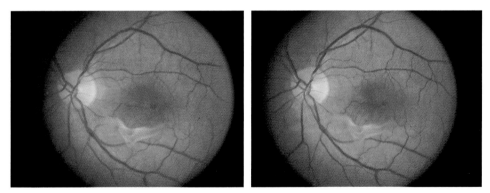

PLATE 123 Spontaneous separation of epiretinal membrane.

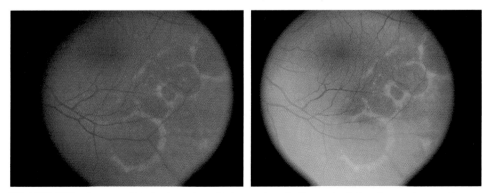

PLATE 124 Outer wall holes in retinoschisis causing shallow retinal detachment in macula.

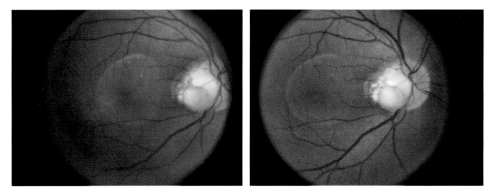

PLATE 125 Congenital optic disc pit with macular detachment.

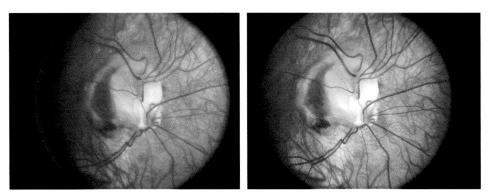

PLATE 126 Bifid optic disc anomaly.

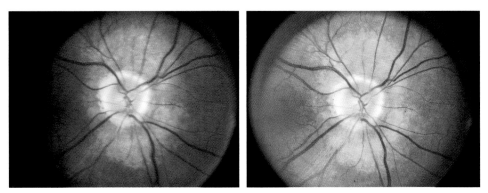

PLATE 127 Peripapillary staphyloma causing transient obscurations.

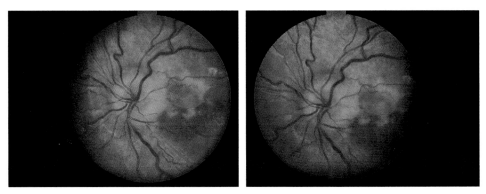

PLATE 128 Optic disc drusen, type 2 SRN.